DIABETES

DIABETES

PROCEEDINGS OF THE EIGHTH CONGRESS
OF THE INTERNATIONAL DIABETES FEDERATION

Brussels, July 15–20, 1973

EDITORS

W. J. MALAISSE
Brussels

J. PIRART
Brussels

CO-EDITOR

J. VALLANCE-OWEN
Belfast

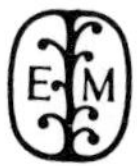

1974

EXCERPTA MEDICA, AMSTERDAM
AMERICAN ELSEVIER PUBLISHING COMPANY, INC., NEW YORK

INTERNATIONAL CONGRESS SERIES No. 312

ISBN EXCERPTA MEDICA 90 219 0235 4
ISBN AMERICAN ELSEVIER 0 444 15074 9
LIBRARY OF CONGRESS CATALOG CARD NUMBER 74–77386

Publisher:

EXCERPTA MEDICA
335 Jan van Galenstraat
Amsterdam
P.O. Box 1126

Sole Distributors for the USA and Canada:

AMERICAN ELSEVIER PUBLISHING COMPANY, INC.
52 Vanderbilt Avenue
New York, N.Y. 10017

Printed in The Netherlands by Casparie Alkmaar B.V.

TABLE OF CONTENTS

PLENARY LECTURES

PANELS

BETA CELL 1973

THE ROLE OF GLUCAGON IN HEALTH AND DIABETES

REGULATION OF METABOLIC FUELS SUPPLY

TABLE OF CONTENTS

PLENARY LECTURES

IMMUNITY, AUTOIMMUNITY, AND DIABETES*

P. A. BASTENIE

Laboratoire de Médecine Expérimentale, Université de Bruxelles, Belgique

It is easily thought, said and even written that diabetes mellitus, like other conditions of ill-defined etiology, may be (some say is) an autoimmune disease. Such a definite statement might correspond to some sort of fashionable thinking, rather than to a critical evaluation of proved facts. As professor Heremans (1973) recently said: 'Immunology is like a fungus the mycelium of which pervades the whole dignified building of medicine, suddenly producing crops of mushroom in areas where its presence was least expected, for instance endocrinology'. As far as diabetes is concerned, one may still wonder about the quality of this mushroom. To ascertain this, it seemed necessary to bring together not only diabetologists and pathologists interested in the subject but also, and foremost, basic immunologists. Thanks to the generous support of the Francqui Foundation, such a meeting was organized a few months ago by doctor Willy Gepts and myself. For the greater part of this talk I shall only be the spokesman of the distinguished participants of this Colloquium. However, I shall have to accept the responsibility for most of the conclusions and final considerations.

This review will be divided into 3 parts:

1. The initial, already 10 years old, concept of autoimmunity, on which the assumption is based that diabetes mellitus in itself is an autoimmune disease.
2. The present concepts of autoimmunity.
3. The discussion, on the basis of these concepts, of the data which argue in favour of autoimmune processes playing a part in the pathology of diabetes mellitus.

THE INITIAL CONCEPTS OF AUTOIMMUNITY

Autoimmune diseases entered medical thinking only 17 years ago when Roitt et al. (1956) discovered the presence of thyroid antibodies in the serum of patients affected with Hashimoto's goiter while Rose and Witebsky (1956) produced lymphocytic thyroiditis in the experimental animal by injecting homologous thyroglobulin. Some time afterwards autoimmunity was defined as a condition in which 'structural or functional damage is produced by the action of immunologically competent cells or antibodies against normal components of the body' (Mackay and Burnet, 1963).

It was then proposed to separate such conditions into 2 distinct groups: the acquired

* Presidential Adress.

TABLE 1
Secondary, acquired or transient autoimmune diseases

Syndrome	Tissue affected	Induced by
Dressler	Pericardium Myocardium	Necrosis Virus Trauma
Endophthalmia	Lens	Infection Trauma
Hemolytic anemia	Red cells	Ovarian tumor Lymphoma Mononucleosis infection
Male sterility	Testicles	Stasis in vas deferens

or transient and the idiopathic diseases. In the first group (Table 1) the pathological process was recognized as the result of a primary anomaly arising in the tissues. Despite the normal working of the immune system, assuring tolerance of all the body components, the abnormal antigen admittedly induced an autoimmune reaction, i.e., an immune reaction against a tissue component of the body itself. Peri- and myocarditis, arising after myocardial damage by viral attack, surgery or infarct, is the best example of such a condition.

The second group, that of idiopathic diseases (Table 2), includes several conditions which are often associated. Here organ-specific autoimmunity and tissue damage are supposed to be related to the spontaneous loss of the normal tolerance of these tissue components. This loss of tolerance was thought to be due to a sudden abnormality arising within the immune system, i.e., proliferations of immunologically competent cells active against certain constituents of the body. Normally such forbidden clones should have been eliminated once and for all during fetal life (Burnet, 1959a, b; Mackay and Burnet, 1963).

According to criteria set forth by Witebsky, Feltkamp (1966) and others, idiopathic autoimmune diseases have a series of common characteristics (Table 3): the serum contains specific antibodies and thus increased levels of IgG. In the tissues one finds destructive cell lesions and characteristic lymphocytes and plasma cells infiltrations. Moreover, similar lesions can be reproduced by injecting in the experimental animal extracts of its own tissues. On the clinical side, one finds that these autoimmune diseases are more frequent in women than in men and that their incidence increases with age.

Another important trait is the occurrence in the patients thus affected of other so-called autoimmune diseases or at least of antibodies pertaining to these diseases. Among

TABLE 2
Idiopathic autoimmune diseases

Tissue or organ affected	Disease
Blood	Idiopathic hemolytic anemia Idiopathic thrombocytopenia
Collagen	Rheumatoid arthritis Lupus erythematosus diffusus etc.
Thymus	Myasthenia gravis
Gastric mucosa	*Pernicious anemia*
Adrenal cortex	*Addison's disease*
Thyroid	*Thyroiditis and hypothyroidism*

the close relatives of such patients one finds a high incidence of: (1) the same disease; (2) antibodies characteristic of that disease; and (3) other autoimmune diseases. The best example of this pathology is autoimmune thyroiditis, leading to spontaneous myxedema. All stages have now been studied from normality to asymptomatic thyroiditis and to clinical hypothyroidism (Bastenie et al., 1972a). Not only the morphological changes in the thyroid and in the pituitary induced by the progressive thyroiditis and parenchyme destruction, but all criteria set forth for idiopathic autoimmune diseases are fulfilled (Feltkamp, 1966).

How far does diabetes mellitus conform to these criteria? Admittedly the overall incidence of diabetes is highest in women and increases with age (Table 4). Insulitis has been described, albeit almost exclusively in juvenile diabetics. Insulitis has been reproduced experimentally and in a few animals has led to the development of diabetes. Moreover, the association of diabetes with other autoimmune diseases has repeatedly been shown, mostly with thyroiditis. Diabetes itself runs in families.

It is easy to understand that many are inclined to include diabetes among the idiopathic autoimmune diseases.

THE PRESENT CONCEPTS OF IMMUNITY AND AUTOIMMUNITY

The new knowledge which has upset this assumption results from the shifting of the study of antibodies to that of the cellular reactions to the antigens. Only recently was delayed hypersensitivity (i.e. specific cell-mediated immunity) considered in the pathogenesis of human autoimmune disorders. The mobilization of cellular defenses was first studied in experimental autoimmunity in the rejection of homografts. These studies have led to the already classical knowledge concerning the cellular basis of immune responses as reviewed by Roitt et al. (1969).

TABLE 3
Characteristics of idiopathic autoimmune diseases (AID)

Serum
- Antibodies: IgG ↗
- Complement ↘

Tissues
- Parenchyme destruction
- Lymphoblasmatocytes infiltrations

Experimental reproduction
- Tissue lesions
- Antibodies

Clinic
- F > M
- ↗ with age

Associations
- *In patient:* other AID antibodies
- *In close relatives:* same AID
  other AID antibodies

TABLE 4
Diabetes mellitus as an idiopathic AID

Criteria of AID	Diabetes
F > M	+
Incidence ↗ with age	+
Lymphocytic infiltrates	+ (Only juvenile diabetes)
Experimental production	+
Association-other AID	+
Association in close relatives Diabetes; other AID	+
Antibodies in serum IgG ↗	0?

The small lymphocytes belong to 2 distinct populations: one dependent on the presence of the thymus and therefore called T lymphocytes and the other independent of the thymus and originating from the bone marrow, called B lymphocytes. The T lymphocytes constitute the greater part of the small lymphocytes circulating in the blood. B lymphocytes appear to be more restricted to lymphoid tissue.

The T lymphocytes can be non-specifically stimulated in cultures by phytohemagglutinin, a non-specific mitogen which acts on other receptor sites besides those which are antigen-sensitive. This response to non-specific mitogens provides some measure of the overall activity of T lymphocytes in the blood but need not necessarily reflect their ability to react to specific antigens (Fudenberg et al., 1971).

The small T lymphocytes can also be stimulated into blast cells by the action of an antigen, which has been processed by the action of macrophages and thereby transformed into an immunogen. The clones of cells which stem from the immunogen-stimulated T lymphocytes will differentiate into 'killer cells'. The effects of these cells have been well studied in graft rejections, in human thyroiditis and in tissue cultures of Hashimoto goitre.

The immunogen-stimulated T lymphocytes further secrete soluble factors which have several properties: distention and increased permeability of the capillaries, and stimulation or inhibition of macrophages. There is further evidence that the immunogen-stimulated T cells can cooperate with the B cells and control their activity (Allison et al., 1971).

The B cells, stimulated by an immunogen (transformed antigen) can also differentiate into blast cells which will produce cell clones resulting in the formation of plasmatocytes. These specialized cells are the seat of synthesis and secretion of specific antibodies. It is now clear that the production of antibodies, important as it may be in certain cases (as for instance in hemolytic anemia), is in many cases of little direct pathogenic significance. The antibodies may, however, stimulate inactive tolerant T lymphocytes into immune reactions (cf. Heremans, 1973).

Research has now turned to the study of the action of antigens in calling forth the reactions of immunocytes and to the study of these reactions in order to explain the disappearance of the normal state of tolerance, which the immunocytes normally display

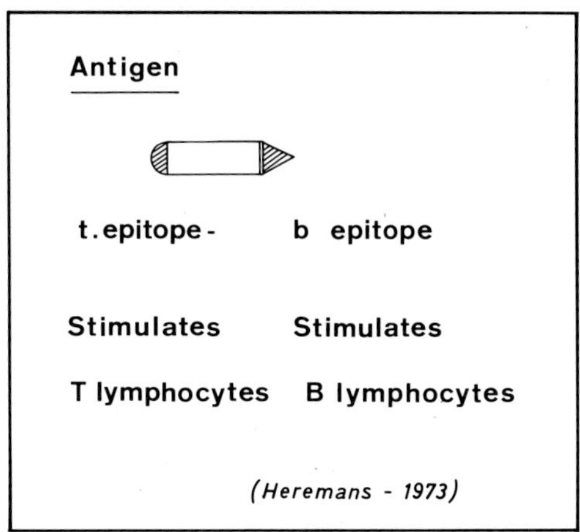

FIG. 1. Epitopes of antigens (after Heremans, 1973).

towards the various components of 'self'. Antigens are considered as possessing epitopes (Fig. 1), which are the immunogenic sites directed against T or B lymphocytes and are therefore called t or b epitopes. These epitopes are composed of proteins, polysaccharides or nucleic acids. Many epitopes are normally hidden and are brought to light only after partial enzymatic breakdown or denaturation (i.e. uncoiling) of the macromolecule.

Even resting immunocytes exhibit a low level of immunoglobulin synthesis. A fraction of this immunoglobulin is incorporated into their cell membrane, where it stays for a period of hours before being lost (Fig. 2). The combination on these receptor sites of the

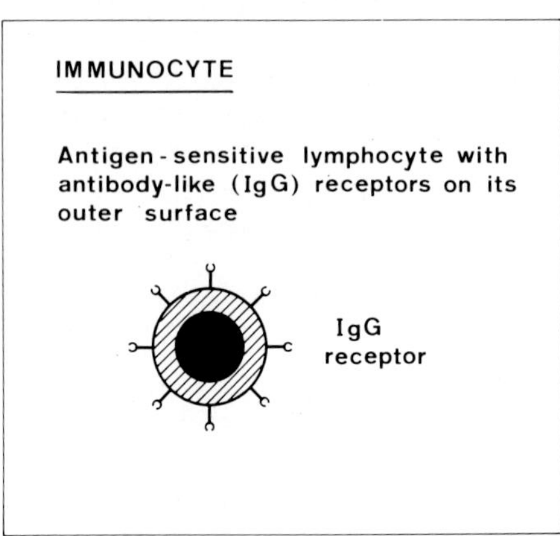

FIG. 2. Schematic representation of an immunocyte.

immunoglobulin with the antigen can be observed in autoradiographic preparations seen in electron microscopy: when the antigen is marked with radioiodine, it impresses a silver reagent. The black dots which then appear on the cellular membrane are the results of the combination with the Ag on the receptor sites. Such a combination may result in: (1) induction of immune reactions; and (2) inhibition of immune reactions.

The first possibility has already been discussed. In the second possibility the immunocyte fails to undergo induction and becomes refractory to subsequent stimulation: the antigen has behaved as a tolerogen. In other words: immunocytes may become tolerant to antigens which in other circumstances might induce immune reactions. They do so when submitted to excess stimulation; cells so impressed will die or become inactive. However, tolerance is maintained only in so far as the supply of antigen is kept up.

T and B cells do not react in the same way nor to the same antigens. T tolerance is faster in onset, more protracted and obtained with lower concentrations. Therefore T lymphocytes are tolerant to normal self-antigens which are present in low concentrations in the circulating blood. Moreover, according to many observations in vivo (see Heremans. 1973), T cells are necessary both for induction of immune responses and for immune tolerance. They effect these actions by the secretion of associative antibodies. This is shown experimentally since transfers of thymus cells from young to old mice reduce the incidence of autoimmune manifestations.

Tolerance to self-antigens thus appears as an intricate process, which must continuously be acquired, renewed and maintained (Fig. 3). In the concept of balanced self-tolerance, proposed by Heremans, self-antigens present in small quantities in the serum

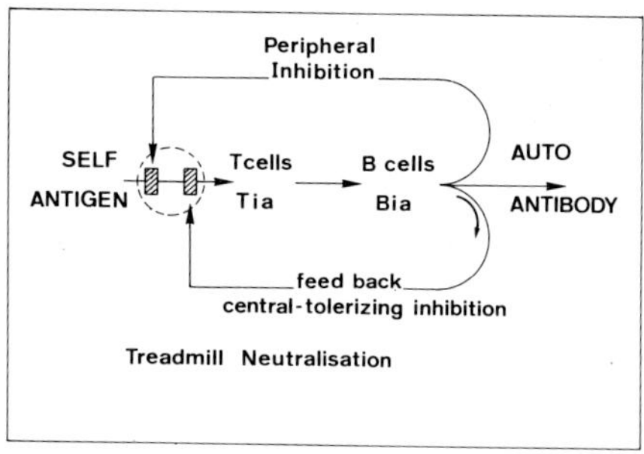

FIG. 3. The concept of balanced self-tolerance in the normal state (Heremans, 1973).

would partly activate the inactive T cells (Ti) and B cells (Bi) so that some slight degree of antibody formation would be produced. However, this autoimmune reaction eliminates part of antigen, and on the other hand the auto-antibodies exert a negative feed-back on the production of antibodies. Thus in the normal state self-antigens and autoimmune reactions at every moment neutralize each other as in a kind of treadmill. Autoimmunity results from the break-down of this balance, which can be due to changes in the quality or the quantity of the self-antigens – or to an alteration in the immune system – often an immune deficiency, cellular or humoral (Table 5).

TABLE 5
Breakdown of tolerance of self-antigens

Factors affecting	– antibody forming cells – cell mediated immune reactions
Defect of *control mechanism*	– genetic – acquired
Altered *antigens*	– chemical drugs – infections (viral) – metabolic processes – cell death

An important byproduct of the experimental work just reviewed consists of a series of tests of cell-mediated immunity that can now be applied to clinical studies. The rosettes formation test only detects the presence of sensitized cells. These cells have immunoglobulins at their surface. When brought into contact with red cells coated with the antigen, the red cells will form a ringlet or rosette around the sensitized lymphocytes.

A more specific test of cellular immunity is the leukocyte migration test (LMT) based on the principle that sensitized T lymphocytes, when in contact with the sensitizing factor, secrete a polypeptide that inhibits the migration of guinea pig macrophages and also of human leukocytes.

Normal migration of leukocytes in a migration chamber is markedly reduced when

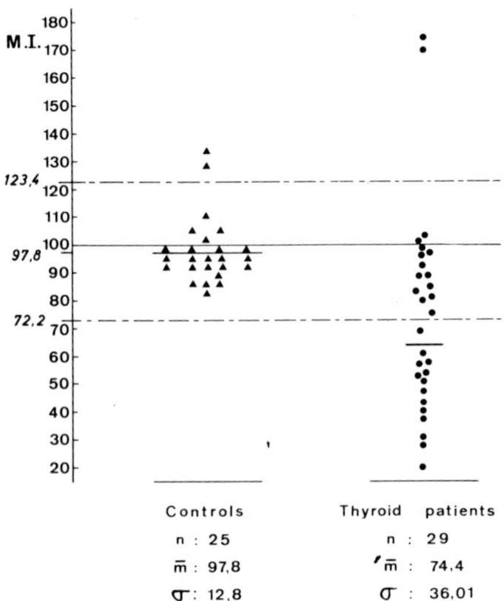

FIG. 4. Migration index (surface with antigen/surface without antigen) in normal and thyroid patients; the antigen used is thyroglobulin (From Delespesse et al., 1973, by courtesy).

antigen to which the cells are sensitized is added to the medium. Results of the test are easily expressed as a migration index, as seen in Figure 4 comparing results of normal controls and patients affected with various thyroid diseases: a group of the latter display definite reactions against thyroglobulin.

The third test, admitted as specific of cell-mediated immunity, is the lymphoblast transformation test (LTT). When lymphocytes of a subject sensitized to a given antigen are cultured in the presence of this antigen, lymphoblastic transformation is induced. This can be studied by the morphological changes, for instance the number of mitoses, or by the measurement of the tritiated thymidine incorporated into the lymphocytes culture.

With these new concepts in mind and techniques at hand we can turn back to our problem, the study of autoimmunity in diabetes.

THE STUDY OF AUTOIMMUNITY IN DIABETES

As recalled earlier, clear-cut autoimmune diseases like lymphocytic thyroiditis have definite clinical, biological, serological and epidemiological characteristics. At first sight diabetes mellitus responds to these criteria. However, on a closer look, discrepancies become apparent (Table 6).

The clinical characteristics of autoimmune diseases (age and sex incidence) are found only in the adult-onset type: no other signs of immune abnormality can be detected in this form of diabetes except for the possibility of an immune complex disease and the association with other so-called idiopathic autoimmune conditions. It is clear that the immune complexes formed in insulin-treated patients are related to exogenous insulin and that deposition of this material in the capillary walls is by no means a true autoimmune process. As to the association of diabetes with other autoimmune conditions, we shall

TABLE 6
Signs of autoimmunity in diabetes mellitus

	Diabetes		
	Juvenile-onset		Adult-onset
Criteria of autoimmune diseases	No insulin	Insulin	
1. F > M	–	–	+
age ↗	–	–	+
2. Insulitis pathology	+	–	–
Experimental production	+		
3. Antibodies			
IgG ↗	–	?	
Ab to insulin	–	+	(+)
Im to non-insulin Ag	+	+ Transient	–
4. Associations with other AID	+	+	+
? Immune complex diseases	0	+	(+)

shortly see that this is a consequence of diabetes and certainly not a proof of the autoimmune nature of the disease.

In the juvenile-onset form we shall have to discuss 3 points:

1. Insulitis, detected at the autopsy of a number of these patients;
2. The presence of antibodies or cell-mediated reactions against pancreas antigens;
3. The frequent association of immunological and clinical signs of other autoimmune conditions.

Insulitis

Insulitis, i.e. round cell infiltrates in the islets of Langerhans had been described from time to time, when its interest was revived by the now classical paper of Gepts (1965) suggesting that the condition is more frequent than hitherto believed and underlining its striking resemblance with the lesions observed in immunological experiments. Here are 2 examples of insulitis, taken from Gepts' material. In the first one*, the lesions comprise inflammatory reactions characterized by infiltrates of mononuclear cells, mostly lymphocytes, around and within the Langerhans islets, and changes of increased cell activity in the beta cells already reduced in number. In the second example*, the cell infiltrates are less dense and the beta cells have almost disappeared; fibrous tissue is dense. This is clearly a later stage of the process, leading from subacute inflammation to atrophy and scarring of the islets.

Insulitis was found by Gepts in 15 out of 22 (68%) cases of juvenile diabetes, who had died within 6 months of the acute onset of their disease. This high incidence came as a surprise, most authors considering the condition as rare. Doniach (1973), reviewing the autopsy material of the London Hospital dating back to the pre-insulin era, found no example of insulitis but did see the same atrophy and fibrous retraction. All authors agree that in juvenile diabetics dying later in the course of the disease only atrophy is seen and no insulitis has ever been encountered.

The discrepancies may be due to the lack of systematic studies or, more likely, to the transient nature of the inflammatory process, rapidly ending into cell destruction and atrophy of the islet tissue. It may be of interest to note that similar lesions are almost never found in adult-onset diabetes, where moreover no scarring or atrophy of the islets is observed (Doniach, 1973).

TABLE 7
Experimental autoimmune insulitis

1963–1968 Ag = insulin-homo-heterologous antigen

Authors	Species	Lesions	Antibodies	Metabolic changes
Renold et al., 1963, 1964, 1966	Cattle	++	+	0
Grodsky et al., 1966	Rabbit	+++	+	++ D.M.
Renold, 1967; Federlin et al., 1968	Sheep	++	+	0

D.M. = diabetes mellitus.

To what extent do experimental autoimmune processes induce a similar condition? Renold et al. (1963) (Table 7) were the first to observe lymphocytic insulitis in cattle injected with heterologous or even homologous insulin over periods of 4 months to 2

* The micrographs have kindly been provided for this lecture by Professor W. Gepts. They can be fond in his own publication (Gepts, 1973).

years. The infiltration was typically composed of small lymphocytes (cf. Gepts, 1973). In some islets there was pronounced fibrosis and scarring, while intermediate stages with associated infiltrations and beginning scarring were seen. However marked the lesions were, no alterations in carbohydrate tolerance were observed. Contrariwise, in experiments by Grodsky et al. (1966) the immunization of rabbits with heterologous insulin resulted in insulitis and abnormalities of glucose tolerance, including frank diabetes in 2 of the animals treated. The formation of antibodies was thereby induced, which not only reacted with the exogenous heterologous insulin, but also with the animal's own insulin (Federlin et al., 1968; Renold et al., 1969).

Further experimental work (Klöppel et al., 1972; Jansen et al., 1973; Nerup et al., 1973) is summarized in Table 8. Once-crystallized insulin and highly purified insulin have been compared in their effects of inducing insulitis, antibody production and glucose metabolism alterations. Much of this work is to be presented at this Congress by the group of Jansen and Freytag. I shall only give a very brief preview here so as to whet your appetite but leave you with your hunger.

Clearly, insulin-contaminating agents must be responsible. Probably more than one factor is at work since in certain conditions a dissociation can be produced between the development of antibodies and that of islets lesions. It is interesting to see that in the first case carbohydrate intolerance has been produced, apparently by cross-reaction of insulin antibodies with endogenous insulin. However, true diabetes mellitus has only been found in animals with severe insulitis.

A most interesting finding is that of Nerup et al. (1973) of insulitis produced in mice and rats by an endocrine-pancreas extract, different from biologically active insulin. Lymphocytic insulinitis has also been produced by viral infections. This was done for the

TABLE 8
Experimental autoimmune insulitis

1969–1973					
Authors	Species	Antigen	Insulitis	Antibody	Metabolic changes
Klöppel et al., 1972	Rabbit	Bovine insulin	++	++	+ (10%)
Jansen et al., 1973	Mice	1 X crist. insulin M.C. insulin	++ –	No correlation	+ D.M.
Nerup et al., 1973	Mice Rat	Islet tissue extract	++		0

D.M. = diabetes mellitus; M.C. = monocomponent.

first time by Craighead and McLane in 1968. An outbreak of new findings wil be reviewed in this Volume bv Craighead, Müntefering. Taylor and Freytag.

The possible relationship in human pathology between viral infections and diabetes mellitus has been at the origin of several studies (Table 9). Gamble and Taylor (1969)

TABLE 9
Viral infections → human diabetes mellitus (D.M.)

Older observations	: Mumps → D.M.
Gamble and Taylor, 1969	: Viral antibodies in D.M. serum
Craighead et al., 1973	: D.M. ↔ Coxsackie virus

showed the presence of high titers of virus antibodies in young diabetics. Craighead et al. (1973) called attention to the association of the juvenile type of diabetes with past infections by Coxsackie viruses.

In the experimental animal, the chain of events is almost complete (Fig. 5). It has now been proved that certain viruses have the capacity to invade specifically islets of Langerhans and to damage their structures. As a result, a disease develops that morphologically and clinically is 'strikingly similar to juvenile diabetes with sudden onset' (Craighead, 1973).

The role of genetic and metabolic factors has been demonstrated: all strains of mice are not susceptible and Craighead showed that experimental hypothalamic obesity (with hyperfunctioning beta cells) enhances the development of insulitis.

How viruses may serve as mediators of immunological reactions is a difficult problem, which I think will be the subject of further exciting discussions.

In the human, only parts of the puzzle fall into place, although impressive evidence has been forwarded, including the demonstration of viral particles in beta cells, viral antibodies in the serum and finally the finding in non-insulin-treated juvenile diabetics of a transient cell-mediated immune reaction to an islet tissue extract.

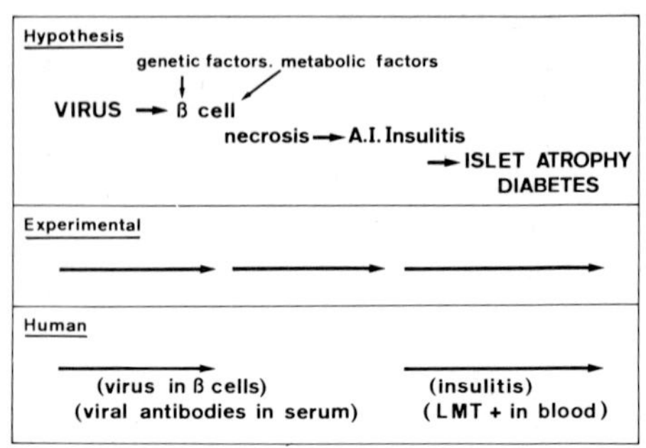

FIG. 5. Viral origin of autoimmune insulitis?

The presence of antibodies or cell-mediated reactions against pancreas antigens

This brings us to the next point of our discussion. Indeed, no insulin antibodies have been detected in the serum of diabetics, except when treated with insulin. Reports to the contrary are admittedly due to non-specific techniques (Deckert, 1967). However, in contrast with these negative findings, Nerup et al. (1973) report on a specific immunological reactivity observed in 1/3 of diabetic subjects, predominantly patients with juvenile diabetes of short duration.

The precise nature of the antigen is not yet known but the antigenic reactivity, demonstrated by the leukocyte migration test, was associated with organ-specific, species non-specific tissue components of the endocrine pancreas, differing from insulin. As indicated in Figure 6, the analogy of the pathological and immunological findings is impressive and suggests that the observations of Nerup and his colleagues may be relative to patients surviving the islets lesions described by Gepts (Gepts, 1965, 1973)!

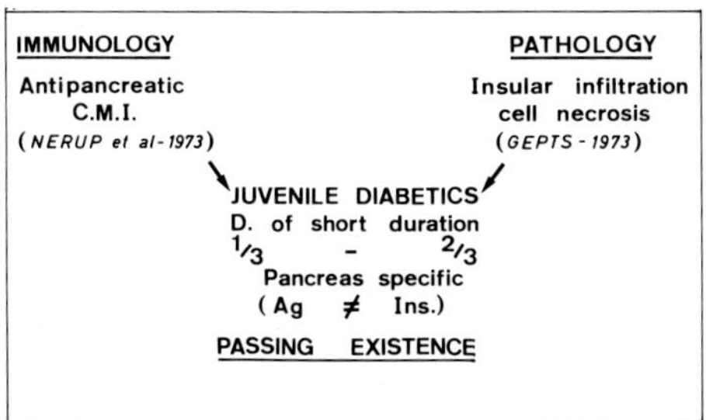

FIG. 6. Antipancreatic cell-mediated immunity (C.M.I.) and insulitis in juvenile diabetics.

The frequent association of immunological and clinical signs of other autoimmune conditions

We now come to the last part of this presentation: the association of diabetes mellitus with other autoimmune processes. As already pointed out by Feltkamp (1963), the so-called idiopathic autoimmune diseases are frequently found in association (Fig. 7). Diabetes was not mentioned at that time. However, it has now been found that there is a significant association between diabetes mellitus and several of these diseases, particularly thyroiditis, gastritis (i.e. pernicious anemia), and adrenalitis. Pernicious anemia has been studied by Whittingham et al. (1971), Mathews et al. (1973), and Irvine et al. (1969). Both groups found biological signs of latent pernicious anemia in about 4% of diabetic women over the age of 40. For Addison's disease also (in most cases a lymphocytic adrenalitis, accompanied by signs of humoral and cellular autoimmunity) the relationship with diabetes is significantly above chance coincidence as demonstrated by Irvine et al. (1970) and by Nerup et al. (1973). It is not exceptional to find diabetes, Addison's disease and hypothyroidism described in one patient (Schmidt's syndrome; Carpenter et al., 1972). Indeed the most frequent and most studied association is that of diabetes and lymphocytic thyroiditis (Bastenie et al., 1972b).

Among diabetics, hypothyroidism was encountered by Pirart (1965) in 0.3–0.4% contrasting with the less than 0.1% incidence in a general control population (Table 10).

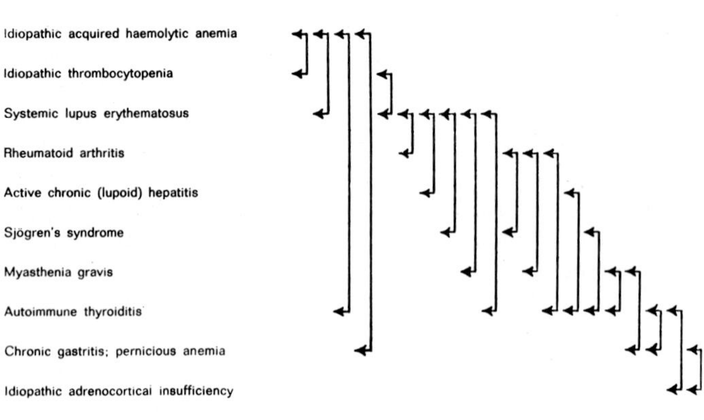

FIG. 7. Associations between the so-called idiopathic autoimmune diseases, according to Feltkamp (1963).

TABLE 10
Association of diabetes and hypothyroidism. Pirart – Bastenie

Population	N	*Cases of hypothyroidism*	*Frequency °/oo*
General	420,000	32	0.7
Diabetic clinic	2,819	11	4
Population	N	*Cases of diabetes*	*Frequency °/oo*
General	2,000	60	30
Hypothyroid	80	11	140

Correspondingly, in a group of hypothyroid patients, associated diabetes was observed in 14% of the cases, the incidence of this disease being 3% in a general population of 2,000 patients examined (Bastenie, 1971). The same incidence was found by Andreani (1973). If myxedema is indeed the end result of a process of thyroid destruction by latent autoimmune thyroiditis, one should find diabetes also associated with the latent process.

Many authors have found thyroid antibodies with higher frequency in diabetic subjects than in non-diabetic, as indicated by a review of the literature (Bastenie et al., 1972c).

Results similar to ours have been reported by Whittingham et al. (1971) who found the frequency of thyroid and gastric mucosa antibodies in the general population, rising with age. Contrariwise, in the diabetic population a high incidence was already found in the younger age groups, this incidence dropping slightly in the older age group. This, according to the authors and recently emphasized by Mathews (Mathews et al., 1973;

1973; Mathews, 1974) might be due to the higher mortality induced by the associated autoimmune disorders.

These autoimmune processes are not inborn; in the younger age group their incidence increases with the duration of diabetes. The 5% incidence in the non-diabetic controls increases to 10% in subjects with diabetes of less than 10 years, it goes up to 50% in the juvenile-onset diabetes of more than 20 years duration. The same phenomenon was observed when diabetic patients, normal subjects and patients affected with thyroid disease were submitted to one or more of the tests of cellular immune recognition (rosettes) or immune reaction (leukocyte migration and lymphoblast transformation tests). As shown in Figure 8, the diabetic patients have a markedly increased incidence of positive reactions (Bastenie et al., 1972c).

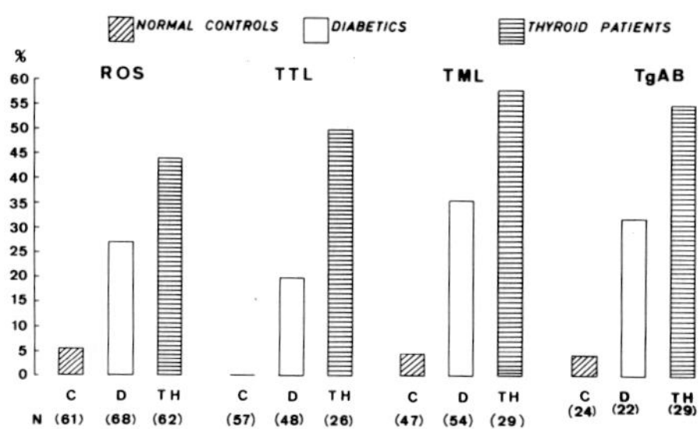

FIG. 8. Prevalence of positive cellular immunity reactions: rosette formation test (ROS), lymphoblast transformation test (TTL), and leukocytes migration test (TML) against thyroglobulin in normal controls (C), diabetic patients (D) and patients with various thyroid diseases (TH) compared with the incidence of cases with circulating thyroglobulin antibodies (TgAB).

When the diabetics thus studied are grouped into age classes, there is no increase with age in the frequency of the cell-mediated reactions. (Admittedly the number of patients under the age of 40 is too small to allow for statistical calculations.) The reason for the occurrence of the thyroid autoimmune reactions in diabetes has been further investigated by Delespesse et al. (1973). In the first place the capacity of T lymphocyte to respond to phytohemagglutinin (PHA) has been studied in 21 diabetic patients, compared with 25 normal female and 20 male control subjects. The PHA test has been measured by the uptake of tritiated thyroidine in the lymphocytic cultures. No statistical analysis was necessary to bring out the gradual fall of the PHA test in the normal population, in relation with age. This fall was more marked in the female than in the male subjects. The response of the diabetics, whatever their age or sex, was at the low level observed in old non-diabetic subjects. It was found at its lowest level in patients with severe insulin-dependent diabetes.

And this brings me to propose a hypothesis. In Figure 9, for this purpose, 3 series of data are superimposed. The data were obtained by the workers of our group in 3 different studies. The first series is related to the frequency of thyroglobulin antibodies, studied in 1277 females and 421 male patients hospitalized for various non-thyroid diseases. The frequency in % is indicated in white columns in the different age groups. The second series of data is related to the normal subjects submitted to cell-mediated immune reac-

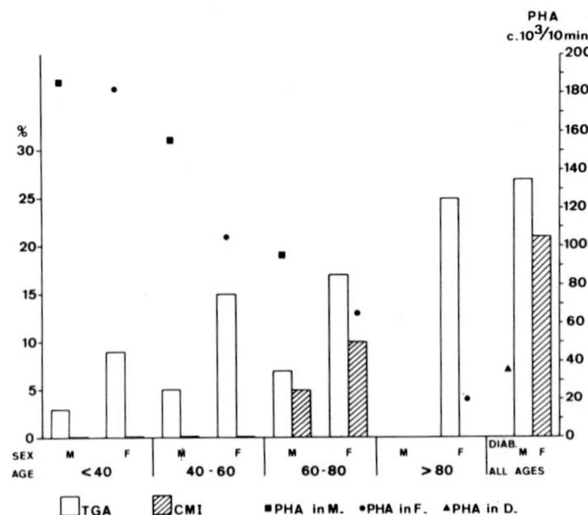

FIG. 9. Composite Figure resulting from 3 different studies performed by the same workers on 3 different but comparable populations. The Figure is only presented to suggest a hypothesis. The white columns indicate the occurrence of circulating thyroglobulin antibodies (TGA) in 1277 female and 421 male patients affected with various non-endocrine diseases. The striped columns indicate the incidence of cell-mediated immune reactions (CMI) found in 57 normal subjects, divided into age groups. The black dots (squares for males, circles for females) indicate the mean value of tritiated thymidine uptake in PHA lymphocytes cultures in normal male and female subjects. In the right part of the Figure the overall incidence (in %) of thyroglobulin antibodies in 200 diabetic patients, the frequency of cell-mediated immune reactions to thyroglobulin in 60 diabetics, and the mean value of PHA response observed in 21 diabetics, are indicated.

tions to thyroid extract, as just demonstrated: the frequency in percentage is indicated in the striped columns: it is only observed in the old age group. The third series corresponds to the results of the PHA tests shown above in the normal population, also classed in age groups. The dots (round for females, triangular for males) represent the counts (X 1000) per 10 minutes.

In the right part of the Figure the results obtained in diabetic patients are indicated: thyroid antibodies in 200 patients, cellular immune reactions in 60, PHA test in 21, marked as black triangles.

There appears to be an inverse relationship between the frequency of thyroid autoimmunity (humoral and cellular) on the one hand and the capacity of the lymphocytes to react with PHA on the other hand. In normal populations signs of autoimmunity increase with age and are parallelled by the reduction of the PHA test. In diabetic populations, regardless of sex and age, autoimmunity is at the highest frequency and PHA response at its lowest level.

According to recent concepts, immune deficiency (humoral or cellular) is a predisposing cause of autoimmunity. As T lymphocytes play a major role in the control of immune and autoimmune reactions, the thyroid autoimmune processes observed in diabetics might be due to the overall lowered activity of the diabetic's T lymphocytes. Preliminary work of members of our group (Duchâteau, Kennes and Hubert) suggest that this is not due to a reduction in the number but to a depression of the function of the diabetic lymphocytes. Thus autoimmune thyroiditis in diabetes – and the same might apply to gastritis and adrenalitis – appears as a secondary phenomenon, partly due to an acquired anomaly of the T lymphocytes.

In summing up, I would like to stress 3 points. The first point is that diabetes mellitus is certainly not an idiopathic autoimmune disease. However, in the juvenile-onset type an autoimmune process seems to be an important step in the process of beta cell destruction. This is probably (but as yet not certainly) initiated by a common viral infection.

The second point is that recent data point to the concept that other autoimmune diseases associated with diabetes are to a large extent consequences of the diabetic state, since these disorders increase in frequency and intensity with the duration and severity of the diabetes.

Finally and in conclusion, I would like to stress that autoimmunity, thanks to the advances of basic immunology, has lost its character of idiopathic, mysterious, genetically-inborn doom!

Undoubtedly genetic factors play an important part in the development of diabetes. However, exogenous agents may be equally important and they may prove amenable to therapy, or even to prevention.

In ending this address I feel that I have oversimplified certain aspects of this intriguing problem and perhaps have been rash in drawing conclusions. My excuse may be that its challenge is so exciting and the grounds for hope so great.

REFERENCES

ALLISON, A. C., DENMAN, A. M. and BARNES, R. D. (1971): Cooperating and controlling functions of thymus derived lymphocytes in relation to autoimmunity. *Lancet, II,* 135.

ANDREANI, D. (1973): Discussion on the association of hypothyroidism and diabetes. In: *Francqui Foundation Colloquium on Immunity, Autoimmunity and Diabetes,* 1973. Editors: P. A. Bastenie and W. Gepts. Excerpta Medica, Amsterdam, in press.

BASTENIE, P. A. (1971): Endocrine disorders and diabetes. In: *Handbook of Diabetes,* p. 871. Editor: E. F. Pfeiffer. Lehmann's Verlag, Munich.

BASTENIE, P. A., BONNYNS, M. and VANHAELST, L. (1972a): Thyroiditis and acquired hypothyroidism in adults. In: *Thyroiditis and Thyroid Function,* p. 211. Editors: P. A. Bastenie and A. M. Ermans. Pergamon Press, Oxford.

BASTENIE, P.A., BONNYNS, M., VANHAELST, L. and NEVE, P. (1972b): Diseases associated with autoimmune thyroiditis. In: *Thyroiditis and Thyroid Function,* p. 261. Editors: P. A. Bastenie and A. M. Ermans. Pergamon Press, Oxford.

BASTENIE, P. A., DELESPESSE, G., DUCHATEAU, J. and KENNES, B. (1972c): Autoimmunité cellulaire antihyroïdienne dans le diabète. *Bull. Acad. Roy. Méd. Belg., 12/7,* 687.

BASTENIE, P. A. and GEPTS, W. (1973): Editors of: *Francqui Foundation Colloquium on Immunity, Autoimmunity and Diabetes.* Excerpta Medica, Amsterdam, in press.

BURNET, F. M. (1959a): Autoimmune disease. *Brit. med. J., II,* 645.

BURNET, F. M. (1959b): *The Clonal Selection Theory of Acquired Immunity.* Cambridge University Press, London.

CARPENTER, C. C. J., SOLOMON, N., SILVERBERG, S. G., BLEDSOE, T., NORTHCUTT, R. C., KLINENBERG, J. R., BENNETT I. L. and HARVEY, A. M. (1964): Schmidt's syndrome: a review of the literature and a report of fifteen new cases including ten instances of coexisting diabetes mellitus. *Medicine, 43,* 153.

CRAIGHEAD, J. E. (1973): Insulitis associated with viral injection. In: *Francqui Foundation Colloquium on Immunity, Autoimmunity and Diabetes, 1973.* Editors: P. A. Bastenie and W. Gepts. Excerpta Medica, Amsterdam, in press.

CRAIGHEAD, J. E. and McLANE, M. F. (1968): Diabetes mellitus: induction in mice by encephalo-myocarditis. *Science, 62,* 913.

CRAIGHEAD, J. E., STEINKE, J. and GAMBLE, D. R. (1973): Association of juvenile type diabetes mellitus with past injection by Coxsackie virus group B. Submitted for publication.

DECKERT, T. (1967): Autoimmunological aspects of diabetes mellitus. *Acta med. scand., Suppl. 476,* 30.

DELESPESSE, G., DUCHATEAU, J., KENNES, B., GOVAERTS, A. and BASTENIE, P. A. (1973): The leucocyte migration test in human thyroid autoimmunity. *Hormone metabol. Res., 5,* 176.

DELESPESSE, G., DUCHATEAU, J., BASTENIE, P. A., LAUVAUX, J. P., GOVAERTS, A. and COLLET, H. (1974): Cell mediated immunity in diabetes mellitus. In: *Francqui Foundation Colloquium on Immunity, Autoimmunity* and *Diabetes, 1973.* Editors: P. A. Bastenie and W. Gepts. Excerpta Medica, Amsterdam, in press.

DONIACH, I. (1973): Pathology of the islets of Langerhans in diabetes mellitus. In: *Francqui Foundation Colloquium on Immunity, Autoimmunity and Diabetes, 1973.* Editors: P. A. Bastenie and W. Gepts. Excerpta Medica, Amsterdam, in press.

FEDERLIN, K., RENOLD, A. E. and PFEIFFER, E. F. (1968): Antigen binding leucocytes in patients and in insulin sensitized animals with delayed insulin allergy. In: *Proceedings of the 5th International Symposium on Immunopathology,* p. 107. Editors: Grabar and Miescher. Grune and Sratton, New York, N.Y.

FELTKAMP, T. E. W. (1966): *Idiopathic Autoimmune Diseases.* Drukkerij Aemstelstad, Amsterdam.

FREYTAG, G. (1973): Do viruses serve as mediators of immunologic reactions? In: *Francqui Foundation Colloquium on Immunity, Autoimmunity and Diabetes, 1973.* Editors: P. A. Bastenie and W. Gepts. Excerpta Medica, Amsterdam, in press.

FUDENBERG, H. H., GOOD, R. A. GOODMAN, H. C., HITZIG, W., KUNKEL, H. G., ROITT, I. M., ROSEN, F. S., ROWE, D. S., SELIGMANN, M. and SOOTHILL, J. R. (1971): Primary immunodeficiencies. Report of a W.H.O. Committee. *Pediatrics, 47,* 927.

GAMBLE, D. R. and TAYLOR, K. W. (1969): Seasonal incidence of diabetes mellitus. *Brit. med. J., III,* 631.

GEPTS, W. (1965): Pathology of the pancreas in juveniles. *Diabetes, 14,* 619.

GEPTS, W. (1973): Insulitis. Introduction. In: *Francqui Foundation Colloquium on Immunity, Autoimmunity and Diabetes, 1973.* Editors: P. A. Bastenie and W. Gepts. Excerpta Medica, Amsterdam, in press.

GRODSKY, G. M., FELDMAN, R., TORESON, W. E. and LEE, J. C. (1966): Diabetes mellitus in rabbits immunized with insulin. *Diabetes, 15,* 579.

HEREMANS, J. F. (1973): Antigens, immunogens and autoimmunity. In: *Francqui Foundation Colloquium on Immunity, Autoimmunity and Diabetes, 1973.* Editors: P. A. Bastenie and W. Gepts. Excerpta Medica, Amsterdam, in press.

IRVINE, W. J., CLARKE, B. F., SCARTH, L., CULLEN, D. R. and DUNCAN L. J. P. (1970): Thyroid and gastric autoimmunity in patients with diabetes mellitus. *Lancet, 11,* 163.

IRVINE, W. J., STEWART, A. G. and SCARTH, L. (1969): A clinical and immunological study of adrenocortical insufficiency. *Clin. exp. Immunol., 2,* 31.

JANSEN, F. K., FREYTAG, G., KLOPPEL, G. and HERBERG, L. (1973): A specific insulitis-producing antigen, different from the true Sanger insulin. In: *Francqui Foundation Colloquium on Immunity, Autoimmunity and Diabetes, 1973.* Editors: P. A. Bastenie and W. Gepts. Excerpta Medica, Amsterdam, in press.

KLÖPPEL, G., ALTENAHR, E. and FREYTAG, G. (1972): Studies on the insulitis in rabbits sensitized with insulin. *Virchow's Arch. path. Anat. Abt. A, 356,* 1.

MACKAY, I. R. and BURNET, F. M. (1963): *Autoimmune Diseases.* C. C. Thomas. Springfield, Ill.

MATHEWS, J. D. (1974): *Autoimmunity and The Pathogenesis of Cardiovascular Diseases.* Hypothesis. Unpublished.

MATHEWS, J. D., WHITTINGHAM, S., HOOPER, B., MACKAY, I. R. and CULLEN, K. J. (1973): Diabetes, autoantibodies and vascular disease in Australia. In: *Abstracts, 8th Congress of the International Diabetes Federation, Brussels, 1973,* p. 134. Editors: J. J. Hoet and P. Lefebvre. International Congress Series No. 280, Excerpta Medica, Amsterdam.

MÜNTEFERING, H. (1973): Experimental virus-induced diabetes mellitus accompanied by insulitis. In: *Francqui Foundation Colloquium on Immunity, Autoimmunity and Diabetes, 1973.* Editors: P. A. Bastenie and W. Gepts. Excerpta Medica, Amsterdam, in press.

NERUP, J. (1973): On the clinical and immunological association of diabetes mellitus and Addison's disease. In: *Francqui Foundation Colloquium on Immunity, Autoimmunity and Diabetes, 1973.* Editors: P. A. Bastenie and W. Gepts. Excerpta Medica, Amsterdam, in press.

NERUP, J., ANDERSEN, O. D., BENDIXEN, G., EGEBERG, J., KROMANN, H. and POULSEN, J. E. (1973): Spontaneous and experimental antipancreatic cellular hypersensitivity in man and rodents. In: *Abstracts, 8th Congress of the International Diabetes Federation, Brussels, 1973,* p. 134. Editors: J. J. Hoet and P. Lefebvre. International Congress Series No. 280, Excerpta Medica, Amsterdam.

PIRART, J. (1965): Action diabétogène de la thyroïde. *Ann. Endocr. (Paris), 62,* 27.

RENOLD, A. E., GONET, A. G. and VECCHIO, D. (1969): Immunopathology of the endocrine pancreas. In: *Textbook of Immunopathology, Vol. II,* p. 595. Editors: P. A. Mescher and H. I. Müller Eberhard. Grune and Stratton, New York.

RENOLD, A. E., STEINKE, J., SOELDNER, J. S., SMITH, R. and ANTONIADES, H. N. (1963): Immunologic responses of heifers to the administration of porcine and bovine (homologous) insulin (abstract). *J. clin. Invest., 42,* 969.

ROITT, I. M., DONIACH, D., CAMPBELL, P. N. and HUDSON, R. V. (1956): Autoantibodies in Hashimoto's disease (lymphadenoid goitre). *Lancet, II,* 820.

ROITT, I. M., GREAVES, M. F., TORRIGIANI, G., BROSTOFF, J. and PLAYFAIR, J. H. L. (1969): The cellular bases of immune serological responses. *Lancet, II,* 367.

ROSE, N. R. and WITEBSKY, E. (1956): Changes in the thyroid gland of rabbits following active immunization with rabbit thyroid extracts. *J. Immunol., 76,* 417.

WHITTINGHAM, S., MATHEWS, J. D., MACKAY, I. R., STOCKS, A. E., UNGAR, B. and MARTIN, F. I. R. (1970): Diabetes mellitus, autoimmunity and ageing. *Lancet, 1,* 764.

SPONTANEOUS AND EXPERIMENTAL DIABETIC SYNDROMES IN ANIMALS. A RE-EVALUATION OF THEIR USEFULNESS FOR APPROACHING THE PHYSIOPATHOLOGY OF DIABETES*

ALBERT E. RENOLD, ALEXANDER RABINOVITCH**, CLAES B. WOLLHEIM, MASATOSHI KIKUCHI, ARNDT H. GUTZEIT, MYLENE AMHERDT, FRANCINE MALAISSE-LAGAE and LELIO ORCI

Institut de Biochimie Clinique, Department of Medicine, and Institut d'Histologie et d'Embryologie, Department of Morphology, University of Geneva Medical School, Geneva, Switzerland

I feel greatly honored to have been asked by the Council of the European Association for the Study of Diabetes to deliver the Claude Bernard Lecture for 1973. That I should also feel terriby awed by association with so formidable a name as that of Claude Bernard is only natural. Also, I am of course aware of the fact that my collaborators and I have already quite often reviewed *spontaneous* diabetes in animals (Cameron et al., 1972; Renold and Dulin, 1967; Renold, 1968; Renold et al., 1970a, b, 1972; Stauffacher et al., 1971) as well as some aspects of *experimental* diabetes mellitus (Junod et al., 1969; Stauffacher et al., 1970, 1972; Veleminsky et al., 1970). And yet, in any occasion that has to be considered a great occasion in one's life, it does seem best to follow Shakespeare and 'to thine own self be true'; and that, as all my friends know, makes it impossible for me to leave out fat, diabetic or spiny mice whether from Bar Harbor, New Zealand, the Negev desert or the Nile delta, or even hamsters from China.

The bibliographical references to previous and extensive reviews from our laboratory having just been listed, interested readers are referred to these for detailed documentation of the extensive literature. Only new or recent findings will be specifically listed at the end of this text.

SPONTANEOUS INAPPROPRIATE HYPERGLYCEMIA

Although most physicians are familiar with the occasional diabetic or, more properly, inappropriately hyperglycemic dog, cat or monkey, it usually comes as a surprise to realize just how widespread syndromes resembling human diabetes are in the animal kingdom. To be sure, the species concerned and shown in Table 1 are all closely associated with man and thus share some of man's habits, at least those acquired in the so-called developed areas of the world, in particular inadequate physical activity and

* The Claude Bernard Lecture is sponsored by the Foundation Paul Neumann, Paris. The studies which are the basis of this report have been supported in part by grants from the Fonds National Suisse de la Recherche Scientifique (No. 3.384.70, 3.541.71, 3.0310.73 and 3.8030.72) Berne, Switzerland, the Fondation Education et Recherche, Basel, Switzerland, grants-in-aid from Hoffmann-La-Roche, Basel, Switzerland, and Hoechst Pharmaceuticals, Frankfurt-Hoechst, Federal Republic of Germany.

** Centennial Fellow of the Canadian Medical Research Council.

relatively excessive intake of food. It should be realized, however, that the 'wisdom' just expressed is only apparent, since few animals *not* closely associated with man have ever been examined in large, or even modest numbers for the presence of diabetes. Of special interest is the recent recognition by Yokote, in Japan, that Sekoke disease in carps exhibits many of the characteristics of diabetes (Yokote, 1970a, b) and that this is true for at least one other fish as well (Yokote, personal communication). Both syndromes in fish occur in colonies undergoing accelerated forced growth induced by qualitatively appropriate and abundant food.

Of special importance to research workers, of course, are smaller rodents suitable for breeding in the laboratory, and thus for study under conditions of controlled genetic as well as environmental conditions (Table 2). The best known of these rodents are the several mutants or inbred strains available in mice, many having originated at the Jackson Laboratories in Bar Harbor, Maine; others in New Zealand, Denmark or Japan; the Chinese hamsters studied in such exemplary fashion by Dulin and Gerritsen in Kalamazoo; the sand rats first described by Hackel and Schmidt-Nielsen, and, with your permission, our Geneva pet, Acomys cahirinus, the spiny mouse. Although we are now conditioned to think of animals which have been inbred or transplanted from a desert environment into the very different one of a laboratory, it is of interest that simple Swiss field mice

TABLE 1
Spontaneous inappropriate hyperglycemia in animals, excluding small rodents

Dogs, cats
Cattle, sheep, horses, pigs
Monkeys, shrews
Hippopotamus, fox
Dolphins
Fish: sekoke carp, ayu-fish

TABLE 2
Spontaneous inappropriate hyperglycemia, often associated with obesity, in small rodents

Mice – at least 8 or more mutants or strains
Rats – 2 or more mutants or strains
Chinese hamsters (cricetulus)
Sand rats (Psammomys)
Spiny mice (Acomys)
Tuco-tuco, gerbils
Guinea pigs
South-African hamsters (Mystromys)
Swiss field mice

(mulots) caught in the fields surrounding Lausanne and studied in a quite large terrarium reproducing their normal environments, in Professor Dolivo's Department of Physiology, similarly may develop quite severe diabetes, usually with obesity, and only when caught at specific periods of the year (Schenk and Dolivo, unpublished observations).

Genetic aspects

Genetically at least 3 groups – one might say 3 degrees of complexity – should be distinguished: Firstly, animals, mostly mice, carrying a double dose of an abnormal mutant gene such as db or ob. All hereditary aspects of these and similar syndromes appear to be explicable on the basis of transmission as a simple recessive somatic gene. There are also dominant variants of this, the simplest genetic profile.

Secondly, diabetes and obesity frequently appear in certain inbred strains, probably not as a result of mutation but as genetic information previously available is unmasked by inbreeding. For example, the inbred Japanese strain usually designated by the initials KK has been shown to transmit the characteristics of modest obesity with inappropriate hyperglycemia as a major dominant somatic gene, which is in turn greatly influenced by several recessive modifiers; the latter usually (in the absence of inbreeding) inhibit the expression of the major gene.

Thirdly, the most complex situation and that of which the complete definition represents, in my opinion, one of the most important genetic analyses carried out with relation to diabetes, whether in animals or in man, concerns the Chinese hamster, *Cricetulus griseus.* In collaboration with Dulin and Gerritsen, Butler, of Toronto, has established beyond reasonable doubt that the tendency to hyperglycemia, which becomes apparent during inbreeding of sublines of this species requires, if all observed facts are to be explained, that at least 4 pairs of recessive alleles be involved. If any 2 of these are homozygous abnormal, hyperglycemia is seen, while the most severe syndrome associated with ketosis is more frequent when 3 of the 4 alleles are homozygous abnormal. 'Clinical' variants exist between different inbred sublines and are likely to be related to just whichever 2 or 3 of the 4 alleles are involved in each instance.

Before leaving the contribution of hereditary mechanisms to spontaneous hyperglycemia in rodents, an important additional and recently reported observation (Coleman and Hummel, 1973) deserves mention, since it may well provide an explanation for the great individuality of the expression of diabetes in animals, and also in different men, women, or children. Coleman, from the Jackson Laboratories at Bar Harbor, established that a double dose of the *very same mutant gene* introduced into different inbred strains may lead to greatly different syndromes. In other words, given a particular potentially diabetogenic gene, whether or not, and just how and when it will find phenotypic expression, will be the result of multiple and quite inconspicuous differences within the individual genome. This largely resembles the much used but little understood clinical concept of incomplete and variable penetrance.

Some possible pathogenetic mechanisms

Even leaving genetics aside, the models represented by the spontaneous and predictable occurrence of hyperglycemia in animals haunts my collaborators and myself, because of the permissible hope that they – any one of them – might yield useful leads and indications as to possible pathogenetic mechanisms operative in human diabetes. Some of the pathogenetic mechanisms for which some evidence has been produced in one or more animal syndromes are summarized in Table 3. However, let me introduce the consideration of several of these possible mechanisms by recalling, that in any study of this nature it is difficult to distinguish a primary from a modifying mechanism. Also, while purely genetic and purely environmental syndromes may occasionally be recognized, the presence of *both* types of components is probably the rule, and in any case difficult to exclude.

TABLE 3
Some possible pathogenetic mechanisms (primary or modulating; all may have genetic and environmental components)

	Hyperinsulinism
1. Infections (viral)	?
2. Food intake: calories	+
3. Food intake: qualitative, e.g. sucrose	+
4. Obesity	+
5. Insensitivity of some tissues (primary or secondary) to insulin (e.g. adipose, muscle, liver)	+
6. Primary hyperinsulinism	+
7. Abnormal insulin	(+)

The first pathogenetic mechanism listed seems clearly environmental at first sight: *viral infection.* Infection has been considered quite often in human diabetes, especially for juvenile-type diabetes, which has from time to time been reported to occur with greater frequency after epidemics of, for example, mumps. More recently, experimental viral infections exhibiting considerable specificity for the islets of Langerhans were reported in mice (Craighead, 1972; Barboni and Manocchio, 1962) and suggested in guinea pigs. Similarly, there now exists a growing body of information, greatly stimulated by Taylor and his collaborators in the United Kingdom (Gamble et al., 1969, 1973) lending clinical support to such a concept and implicating viruses of the Coxsackie type; these have just been reported to be insulinotropic in mice as well (Coleman et al., 1973).

Of course, viruses may also produce apparently 'spontaneous' hyperglycemic syndromes in animals. Thus, Like observed and reported viral particles in his colony of db mice, but refrained from implicating them in the pathogenesis of the db syndrome more generally. It is of course understood that unequivocal evidence for the hereditary transmission of a mutant gene does not exclude infection, since what the mutation may have altered may be precisely the susceptibility of islet cells to a given virus.

Figure 1 presents a chance observation made by Orci in one of a few spiny mice relatively recently transferred from the slopes of the Dead Sea to a laboratory environment in Jerusalem and bred there for a few generations. The A2 cell shown here contains a cluster of viral particles. Again, however, it is unlikely that the observation is of pathogenetic importance even though a specific viral infection should be considered in each syndrome.

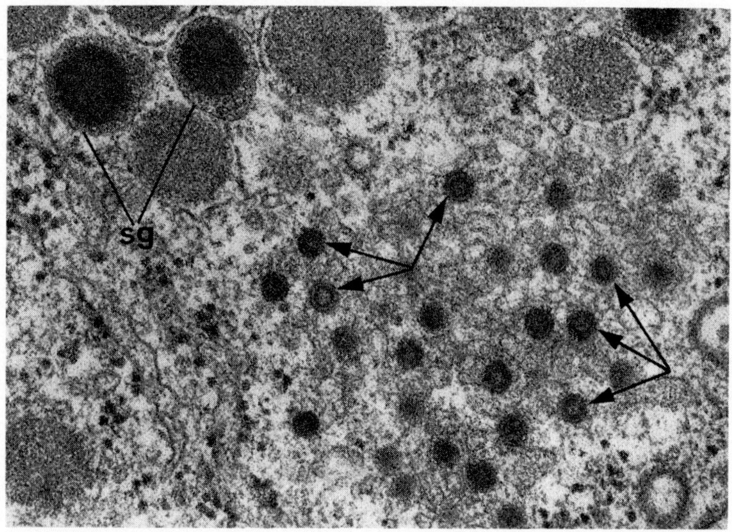

FIG. 1. Pancreatic islet from Acomys recently arrived from Israel. Field from an A2 cell showing a cluster of viral particles (arrows) associated with smooth membranous profiles. sg = secretory granules (X 52,000).

The next 2 pathogenetic factors listed are both environmental ones and concern *alteration of either quantitative or qualitative food intake.* There is much evidence in favor of the frequent contribution of these factors to many syndromes in several species, yet perhaps the most instructive example is that of the unexpectedly significant role of what seems a surprisingly small and rather short-lived increase in food intake in the Chinese hamster; Gerritsen and Dulin (1972) have shown that prediabetic and non-prediabetic Chinese hamsters have the same weight at birth but that, at 15 and 25 days of age, the prediabetic animals weigh about 2 g (20%) more than their non-prediabetic partners. The prediabetic animals also exhibit a greater food intake but the difference in both food intake and weight gradually disappears after 1 month and does not recur. Except for this brief period, hyperglycemic Chinese hamsters are never fat! Gerritsen and Dulin also observed that the simple expedient of slightly curtailing the food available to the prediabetic group, so as to return their early body weight curve to that of the non-prediabetic group, results in a considerable decrease in the severity and incidence of later glucosuria. When food intake is increased after 150 days, there may be a sudden increase in the incidence of glucosuria even though the syndrome remains less severe than in prediabetic animals not having been subjected to modest but early food restrictions.

Obesity is often associated with glucose intolerance and especially with hyperinsulinemia. The best known example, apart from obesity in man, remains the obob mutant in the mouse. When given the same dose of glucose intravenously as the controls, plasma IRI of the obob animals responds rather as in principally obese than in principally hyperglycemic animals. In particular, there is a prompt and sharp early rise of plasma IRI, within one minute of glucose administration, as well as prolonged late hyperinsulinemia (Cameron et al., 1972). This type of circulating IRI response to glucose is likely to be related to the frequent presence in most of these animals, either permanently or transiently, of *insensitivity to insulin* of some or all of their tissues, as predominantly studied for adipose tissue, muscle, and liver. For adipose tissue, a strong claim has been made for insensitivity to insulin being the consequence of dilution of insulin receptors on the plasma membrane (Kahn et al., 1973). Similar decreases in the density of receptor sites have been reported for other cells, including circulating ones such as lymphocytes, and have also been observed in man. Appealing as the concept is, it is still necessary, for the time being, to treat it with the same caution as all other concepts which have been put forward so far.

Primary hyperinsulinism as well as *secretion or accumulation of an abnormal insulin,* or of other abnormal pancreatic factors, has also been suggested and in 2 reported instances the transplantation of normal mouse islets into obob or NZO mice has led to at least partial normalization (Strautz, 1968; Gates et al., 1972). Similarly, Mahler and his collaborators reported extensively on the effects of betacytoxic agents upon insulin resistance in obob and other hyperinsulinemic mice (Mahler and Szabo, 1971)

It may be worth while to suggest one generalization at this stage: excepting infection, all other mechanisms considered have been or may be associated with *long-lasting or transient hyperinsulinemia, without hypoglycemia,* and thus with relative resistance to insulin action. It is quite uncertain, however, whether this generalization concerns a primary event, since subsequent manipulations have often revealed hyperinsulinism and resistance to insulin action to be secondary, reversible events, for example as a result of diminished food intake.

The mechanisms described so far were not characterized by an absolute, or an early decrease of insulin secretion. Now, however, I shall emphasize 3 syndromes which are associated with a *relatively early* – again not necessarily primary – *decrease of insulin release* (Table 4). The first of these is the syndrome in Chinese hamsters, even though we have already described the still earlier and clearly transient phase of overeating and overweight, associated with an equally transient increase in circulating insulin levels. A few weeks after weaning, however, and in animals genetically predestined to become diabetic, insulin secretion is clearly decreased, when compared with hamsters from control lines, free of glucosuria or hyperglycemia for 10 generations or more. It is of con-

TABLE 4
Syndromes associated with relatively early (not necessarily primary) decrease of insulin release

1. *Chinese hamsters*: (a) The very early hyperphagic phase, associated with elevated circulating insulin is brief; (b) later insulin secretion is markedly decreased; (c) glucagon secretion is increased.
2. *NZO mice*: insulin secretion decreased in response to glucose and tolbutamide, not in response to arginine.
3. *Spiny mice* (Acomys cahirinus).

siderable interest that this may also be demonstrated in vitro and that Grodsky (this Volume, pp. 304-315) will report on the convincing results obtained with perfused pancreas. He also noted another pathogenetic possibility: *relative increase of glucagon secretion.* .The very same suggestion had already been made on exclusively ultrastructural grounds and as early as 1969 by Orci et al. (1970, 1971). Orci then showed that in Chinese hamsters with early hyperglycemia the A2 cells were well granulated and, indeed, showed evidence of autophagy of alpha granules. In more severely diabetic animals, especially ketotic ones, A2 cells were extensively degranulated, while exhibiting striking evidence of continued synthesis and packaging of alpha granules, presumably containing glucagon, as suggested by the frequent occurrence of rapidly maturing alpha granules within the Golgi cisterns.

Secondly, Larkins and Martin reported early in 1972 that, when compared with non-obese mice, the insulin response of *New Zealand obese mice* to intraperitoneally administered glucose and tolbutamide was grossly diminished, whereas the plasma insulin response to arginine was entirely normal or, rather, exaggerated.

Finally, the third syndrome presently considered as clearly exhibiting decreased insulin release is our Geneva mascot, *the spiny mouse.* The Geneva colony derives from a few individuals trapped probably in the Negev desert and subsequently exposed to typical laboratory mouse existence, first in Basel, then in Geneva. The total duration of their separation from the desert is at least 15 years, or some 50 generations or so. All spiny mice from our colony exhibit grossly hyperplastic islets with considerable increase in the number, volume and insulin content of islets. By contrast, their in vivo insulin response to the administration of glucose is both delayed and decreased when compared not only to normal mice but also to several types of obese and inappropriately hyperglycemic mice. This lack of responsiveness extends also, when tested in vivo, to isoproterenol, where the response is *slow,* even more than it is *low,* and to aminophylline and cAMP. Accordingly, it was of considerable interest to observe (Fig. 2) that isolated Acomys islets perifused in vitro, when compared with the same number of islets from normal mice, responded very differently to glucose, arginine and tolbutamide. The difference is not the result of a simple, general depression of insulin release, but rather a clear-cut delay or suppression of the primary, early phase, with much less impairment of the secondary, late phase of insulin secretion in the dynamic system used (Rabinovitch and Gutzeit, unpublished observations).

At present, the data obtained in spiny mice suggest at least 2 possible specific mechanisms for the difficulty in release of stored hormone, possibilities which I should like to document briefly, as summarized in Table 5. The first line of evidence suggests that there might be, in spiny mouse B cells, an alteration, or a quantitative decrease in microtubular protein needed for translocation and secretion. This suggestion derives from the observation of Malaisse-Lagae, Amherdt and Orci, which is shown in Figure 3: morphometric analysis of islets from several strains and species, all exposed in vitro to vincristine, 10^{-5} M, for 180 minutes, reveals that, when compared with rats, Swiss albino mice, or C57 black and DBM mice, the B cells of spiny mice exhibit a gross decrease in the number of tubulin crystals formed (Malaisse-Lagae et al., in preparation).

The second pathogenetic possibility and presently that which we perhaps tend to favour, because of the uniqueness of the finding underlying it, concerns the hitherto complete lack of evidence of autonomic type nerve endings in close proximity of endocrine pancreatic cells *in this and only this species.* This has already been emphasized in the past and Orci and Amherdt have by now examined a very large number of Acomys

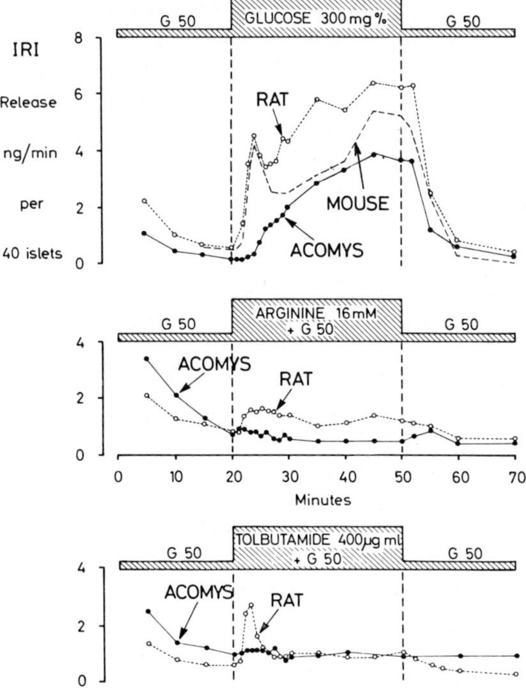

FIG. 2. IRI secretory responses to glucose, arginine and tolbutamide by perifused islets. Comparison of islets from Acomys and from rats or mice. (From Rabinovitch and Gutzeit, unpublished observations.)

TABLE 5
Spiny mice (Acomys)

Insulin release defect more pronounced during 'early' or first phase; there is some evidence for the following mechanisms:

1. Functional alteration or decrease of microtubular protein.
2. Decreased or absent B cell-associated autonomic nerve endings.

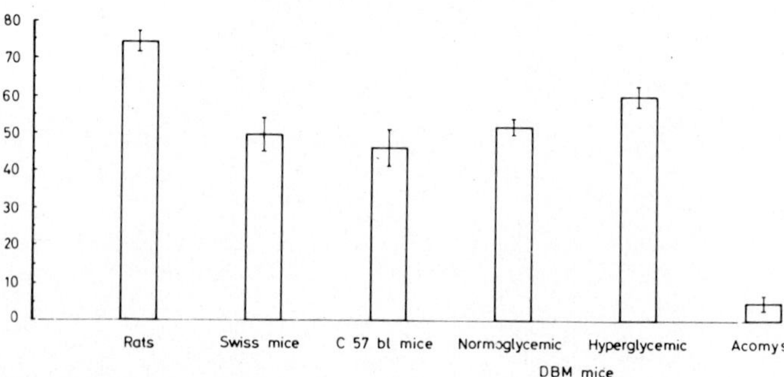

FIG. 3. Mean incidence (± S.E.M.) of crystal-containing B cells in various species, expressed in per cent of the total number of B cells examined in each islet (n = 5). (From Malaisse-Lagae et al., in preparation.)

islets in order to look for nerve endings. They have found none!

Although I can only qualify as a morphologist by avocation, not by professional competence, it nevertheless seems clear to me that the implications of this last finding greatly exceed the problems of the spiny mouse, with islet cells so far entirely devoid of such nerve endings. The observation tends to contribute to the growing body of evidence suggesting that we have yet to unravel the full story of the autonomic nervous system control of activity and state of responsiveness of groups of cells such as islets, where in all species so far examined, with the only exception of the spiny mouse, at least one cholinergic or adrenergic nerve ending has usually been found in each islet.

Before closing the subject of spontaneous diabetes in animals, I should like to mention one more ultrastructural observation: in mice homozygous for the db gene, Orci et al. have seen that despite ultrastructural evidence of active packaging and storage in granule form, the B cells of these animals often exhibit marked dilatation of the rough endoplasmic reticulum, without any sign of disorganization, swelling or membrane damage. Amherdt et al. (1973) reviewed their confirmation and extension of observations from other laboratories that the prolonged oral administration of the drug cyproheptadine in rats produces very similar (Fig. 4) changes to those in dbdb mice, together with autoradiographic evidence for possible interference at the level of transfer from RER to the Golgi complex. It may be very tentatively suggested that the anomaly in dbdb could be at that level also.

Summarizing, I might now state that, although diabetogenic events elsewhere than in the B cells of the islets of Langerhans may well be of importance, perhaps even of primary importance in several of the spontaneously hyperglycemic animals, in many the center of the stage is still occupied by the function of their B cells. Ultrastructurally, and soon we hope biochemically as well, we may distinguish possible candidates for interference with the insulin secretion process at different levels: for example, it would seem that the alterations seen in spiny mice best fit a relatively late interference with release,

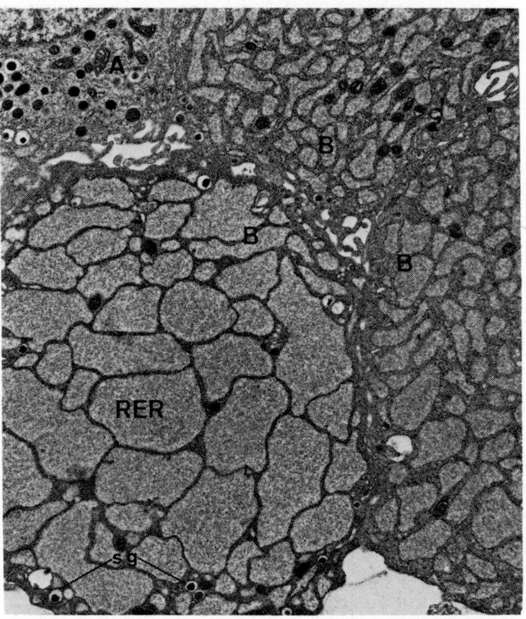

FIG. 4. Part of a pancreatic islet from a cyproheptadine-treated rat (8 days, 45 mg/kg/day, per os). The B cells (B) contain only a few secretory granules (sg). The rough endoplasmic reticulum cisternae (RER) are variably distended and filled with a flocculent material. In the upper lefthand corner, part of a normal appearing A2 cell. (X 5,840). (From Amherdt et al., 1973, by courtesy.)

rather than with synthesis or packaging, either at the level of microtubular function or at that of autonomous nervous system-induced modifications of the plasma membrane. On the other hand, in the dbdb mouse the rate limiting step is more likely to be in the region of, or just before the packaging process in the Golgi, with damming up of precursors in the rough endoplasmic reticulum.

EXPERIMENTAL DIABETES

Although the main emphasis of this paper is on spontaneous animal syndromes, I should not like to leave unmentioned the continued usefulness of experimental diabetic models, not spontaneous but induced, lest you think that they are of lesser value, a judgement which I do not personally share. Since I consider it my responsibility in this Lecture to present overall opinions and evaluations, hopefully balanced ones, I should now like to add a few relatively new examples of the usefulness of a diabetogenic chemical agent which has proved of great interest to us and to others during the past 10 years or so. Streptozotocin, the N-nitroso derivative of glucosamine, shares many but quite pointedly not all of the properties which characterize the diabetogenic activity of the classic agent of this field, alloxan (Junod et al., 1969; Stauffacher et al., 1970, 1972; Veleminsky et al., 1970).

Overall, alloxan and streptozotocin have similar diabetogenic activities and the depletion in pancreatic insulin, measured 48 hours after the administration of either drug, is approximately the same. The principal practical difference is that most streptozotocin-treated animals survive even 2 or 3 times the full diabetogenic dose, provided that they are treated with insulin as needed, whereas many of the alloxan-injected animals are likely to die from renal or other extrapancreatic causes within the first week after injection, even when the dose was no greater than a really diabetogenic one. Despite a number of potentially helpful leads – mostly concerned with the maintenance of the levels of the essential cofactors NAD and NADP, or with preservation of the plasma membrane integrity – it remains true that the precise mechanism of the diabetogenic action of streptozotocin on insulin-producing B cells is not fully understood. However, it is also likely, in my opinion, that considerable progress has already been and is about to be made, and that understanding of the precise reasons for the high degree of specificity for the type of damage done to B cells by this agent, as well as adequate understanding of just why a number of quite surprisingly heterogeneous substances inhibit its diabetogenic activity, that this knowledge will yield information of true significance about the metabolic machinery of the ever elusive, because so well hidden, insulin-secreting cells.

When a diabetogenic dose of streptozotocin is administered i.v. and food is withheld for the next 10 hours, the early blood glucose and plasma insulin profiles are rather surprising: there is an early increase in blood glucose during 2 hours, without either the usual parallel increase in plasma insulin, or a significant decrease of the latter. The lack of insulin response at this stage has led to the suggestion that streptozotocin almost immediately paralyzes insulin release, and indications for this early paralysis have indeed been reported by Lazarow's group (Dixit, 1972). The precise reason for the hyperglycemia has been left unexplained, I believe, although adrenal activation has been both claimed and refuted. If insulin release stops immediately, the absence of an initial plasma insulin decrease remains to be explained.

Rabinovitch and Kikuchi (unpublished observations) have carefully analyzed the sequence of events in vivo during the first 60 minutes and have come up with what would seem an entirely reasonable explanation, illustrated by Figure 5. When measured sufficiently accurately, it may be shown that plasma insulin levels do, in fact, decrease significantly by the end of one hour, despite a significant increase in plasma glucose. The latter may be related to decreased plasma insulin but also, and perhaps more so, to the simultaneously increased plasma glucagon levels and thus to a clearly increased plasma glucagon to insulin ratio. In vitro, Rabinovitch and Kikuchi have been able to demonstrate with the perifusion system adapted to rat islets that isolated islets prepared from the pancreas of animals having received streptozotocin as little as 10 minutes before being killed, are already almost completely paralyzed with regard to their insulin response to glucose (Fig. 6). This is even more pronounced after 60 minutes and, in exact concordance with the in vivo observations just described, there is a paradoxical glucose-induced pancreatic glucagon release from the islets removed 60 minutes after streptozotocin injection.

The likelihood of a specially useful role for streptozotocin in the analysis of B cell biology is greatly enhanced by the ability to use it in vitro. Our laboratory now uses a monolayer culture of newborn rat pancreas which yields, after one to several days of culture, reaggregated clusters of endocrine cells (Orci et al., 1973; Marliss et al., 1973; Hilwich and Schuster, 1971). Figure 7 shows the insulin secretory response of such cells to glucose with or without streptozotocin treatment (Marliss and Wollheim, unpublished observations). As with other preparations (Golden et al., 1971), a clear-cut direct effect

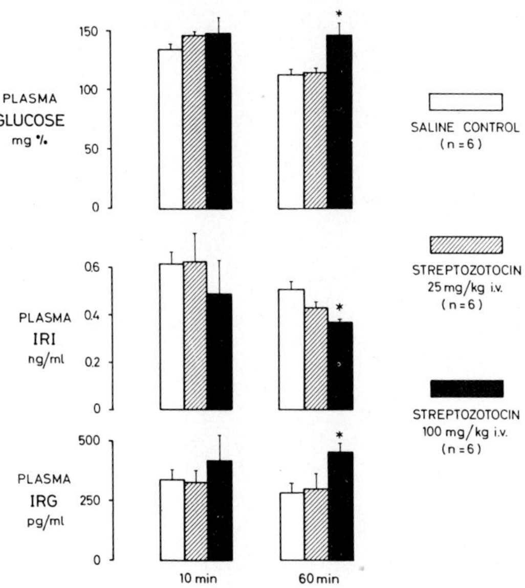

FIG. 5. Acute effects of streptozotocin in the rat (fasted 16 hours) in vivo.

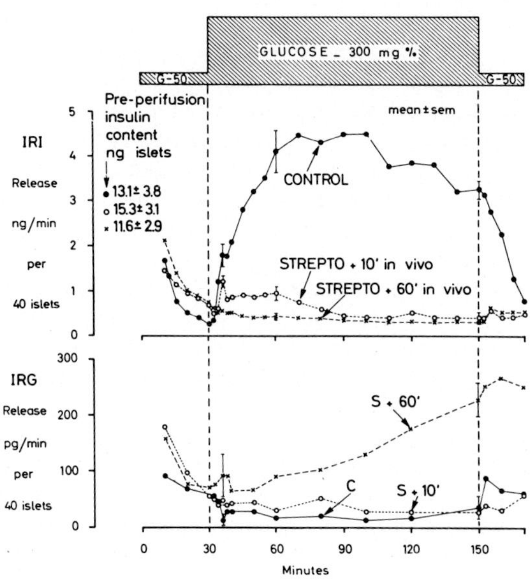

FIG. 6. Effect of streptozotocin (100 mg/kg i.v.) in vivo on subsequent IRI and IRG release from perifused rat islets.

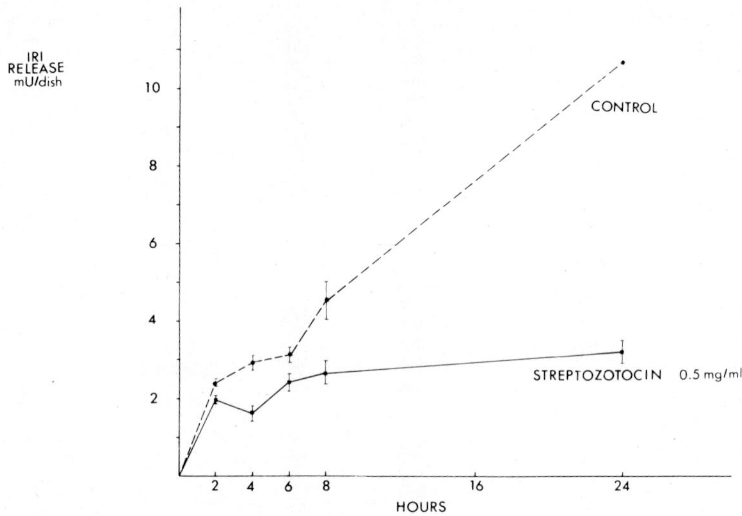

FIG. 7. Streptozotocin in pancreas monolayer cultures: Effect on IRI release into medium.

upon isolated endocrine cells may thus be considered as established for streptozotocin, and also for alloxan, although no data to support the latter is shown here. An interesting new finding concerns the likely importance of streptozotocin and alloxan effects on membrane-associated particles within the plasma membranes of endocrine cells (Fig. 8; Orci et al., unpublished observations). The exciting aspect of this contribution of the ultrastructural approach, using the freeze-etching technique, is the likelihood that membrane-associated particles represent proteins, such as multienzymes or other biologically active substances within membranes such as transporters, for example.

Finally, streptozotocin may also be used to obtain preparations of endocrine pancreatic cells enriched in A2 cells. This has been reported for isolated islets by Petersson (1970) whereas Wollheim (unpublished observations) first obtained a striking and selective effect on B cells in newborn rats; there was almost complete destruction of insulin-containing elements, while pancreatic glucagon, by contrast, increased – presumably as a result of glucose-induced inhibition of release. When Wollheim used such pancreases as starting material for monolayer cultures, they obtained a preparation containing only a few insulin-storing and insulin-releasing cells, yet a nearly normal number of glucagon-producing cells (Fig. 9), resulting in a major shift in the molar ratio of insulin to glucagon, either within the cultured cells or as released into the medium.

In closing this 5th Claude Bernard Lecture, I should like to be permitted to make 2 further points: firstly, it should be evident to you that a Lecture of this type, touching on a number of related but different observations, is of necessity the product of a team of research workers for whom I have simply acted as spokesman. This collaborative aspect of biological research is one that is most dear to me, and I am truly grateful to all of my collaborators, past and present, first for their contributions and also for allowing me to speak for them. This applies quite particularly, of course, to my colleagues from the Department of Morphology: I consider it one of the lucky events of my career that I

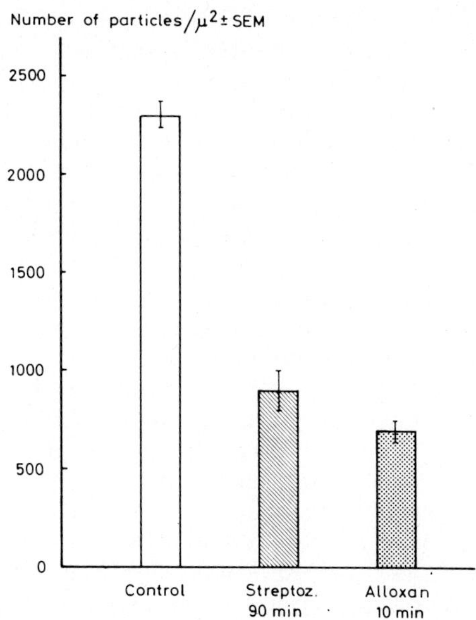

FIG. 8. Results of counting the membrane-associated particles on fracture face A of islet cells of Acomys Cahirinus treated with diabetogenic doses of streptozotocin (150 mg/kg i.p.) and alloxan (200 mg/kg i.p.). These preliminary results suggest that alloxan and streptozotocin induce a structural disarray and possibly an impairment of islet cell plasma membrane, early in the course of events which lead to B cell necrosis. (From Orci, unpublished observations.)

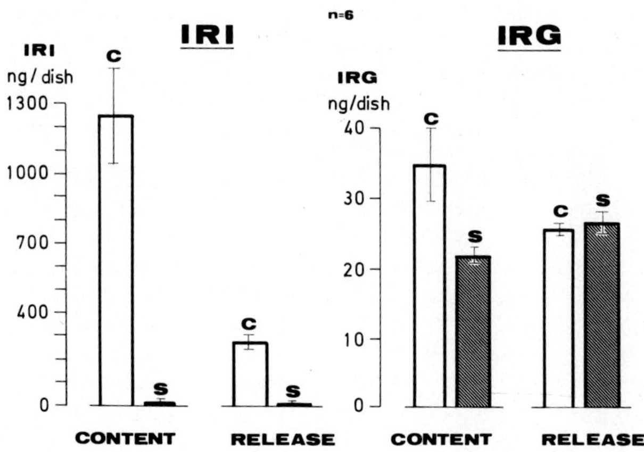

FIG. 9. Monolayer culture of pancreas from newborn streptozotocin-treated rats (150 mg/kg i.p.) 5.6 mM glucose.

should have been able to establish promptly upon my return to Geneva such close ties of mutual respect, friendship, and common investigative interest with Charles Rouiller, Lelio Orci and their stimulating and understanding group.

Secondly, I should like to generalize that the complexity which seems increasingly to characterize the search for complete understanding of diabetes mellitus may well prove to be typical of the major *chronic* syndromes and diseases which will most likely dominate biomedical research efforts during the next several, I suspect many, decades. Just how complex most of these chronic syndromes are, associating several hereditary and many environmental components – and not always the same ones – is only now beginning to be truly understood. Under these circumstances, it is my firm conviction that relevant research cannot afford to ignore any promising lead, some of which may be lying around, waiting to be noticed by the often conformist research community. The spontaneous animal syndromes are such a lead, a gift of Nature of which the importance is only slowly becoming appreciated. They may well provide us with *possible* (no more) models of, in the instance discussed here, the chronic disease diabetes mellitus and some of its complications in the areas of blood vessels, aging, and obesity. We simply must prove perceptive, inventive and persistent enough to take advantage of such leads!

Similarly, the availability of chemicals which affect insulin-secreting B cells with a high degree of specificity presents us with the evident challenge to arrive at full understanding of their mechanism(s) of action and, when that day dawns, at least better understanding of just what the evident specificity of such highly specialized cells is based on.

REFERENCES

AMHERDT, M., HUMBERT, F. RABINOVITCH, A., ORCI, L. and RENOLD, A. E. (1973): Alteration of the insulin-secretory process by cyproheptadine: a correlative ultrastructural and biochemical study. In: *Abstracts, VIII Congress of the International Diabetes Federation,* p. 1. Editors: J. J. Hoet and P. Lefebvre. International Congress Series No. 280, Excerpta Medica, Amsterdam.

BARBONI, E. and MANOCCHIO, I. (1962): Pancreatic lesions in cattle with diabetes mellitus following hoof and mouth disease. *Arch. vet. ital., 13,* 447.

CAMERON, D. P., STAUFFACHER, W. and RENOLD, A. E. (1972): Spontaneous hyperglycemia and obesity in laboratory rodents. In: *Handbook of Physiology, Section 7, Endocrinology, Vol. 1.,* Chapter 39, p. 611. Editors: D. Steiner, N. Freinkel, R. Greep and E. Astwood. Williams and Wilkins Co., Baltimore, Md.

CAMERON, D. P., STAUFFACHER, W., ORCI, L., AMHERDT, M. and RENOLD, A. E. (1972): Defective immunoreactive insulin secretion in the Acomys Cahirinus. *Diabetes, 21/11,* 1060.

COLEMAN, D. L. and HUMMEL, K. P. (1973): The influence of genetic background on the expression of the obese (ob) gene in the mouse. *Diabetologia, 9/4,* 287.

COLEMAN, T. J., GAMBLE, D. R. and TAYLOR, K. W. (1973): Diabetes in mice after Coxsackie B4 virus infection. *Brit. med. J.,* 3, 25.

CRAIGHEAD, J. E. (1972): Inflammatory lesions of the islets of Langerhans. In: *Handbook of Physiology, Section 7, Endorinology, Vol. 1,* Chapter 19, p. 315. Editors: D. Steiner, N. Freinkel, R. Greep and E. Astwood. Williams and Wilkins Co., Baltimore, Md.

DIXIT, P., TAM, B. B. and HERNANDEZ, R. E. (1972): Comparison of the effect of diabetogenic agents on the microdissected pancreatic islet tissue of the rat. *Proc. Soc. exp. Biol. (N.Y.), 140/4,* 1418.

GAMBLE, D. R., KINSLEY, M. L., FITZGERALD, M. G., BOLTON, R. and TAYLOR, K. W. (1969): Viral antibodies in diabetes mellitus. *Brit. med. J., 3,* 627.

GAMBLE, D. R., TAYLOR, K. W. and CUMMING, H. (1973): Coxsackie viruses and diabetes mellitus. *Brit. med. J., 4,* 250.

GATES, R. J., HUNT, M. I., SMITH, R. and LAZARUS, N. R. (1972): Return to normal of blood-glucose, plasma-insulin, and weight gain in New Zealand obese mice after implantation of islets of Langerhans. *Lancet, 2,* 567.

GERRITSEN, G. A. and DULIN, W. E. (1972): Effect of diet restriction on onset of development of diabetes in prediabetic Chinese hamsters. *Acta diabet. lat., 9, Suppl. 1,* 597.

GOLDEN, P., BAIRD, L., MALAISSE, W. J., MALAISSE-LAGAE, F. and WALKER, M. M. (1971): Effect of streptozotocin on glucose-induced insulin secretion by isolated islets of Langerhans. *Diabetes, 20,* 513.

HILWIG, I. and SCHUSTER, S. (1971): In: *Handbuch der experimentellen Pharmakologie, Neue Serie, Vol. XXXII/1,* p. 109. Editors: O. Eichler, A. Farah, H. Herken and A. D. Welch. Springer-Verlag, Heidelberg.

JUNOD, A., LAMBERT, A. E., STAUFFACHER, W. and RENOLD, A. E. (1969): Diabetogenic action of streptozotocin: relationship of dose to metabolic response. *J. clin. Invest., 48,* 2129.

KAHN, C. R., NEVILLE Jr, D. H. and ROTH, J. (1973): Insulin-receptor interaction in the obese-hyperglycemic mouse. *J. biol. Chem., 248/1,* 244.

MAHLER, R. J. and SZABO, O. (1971): Amelioration of insulin resistance in obese mice. *Amer. J. Physiol., 221/4,* 980.

MARLISS, E. B., WOLLHEIM, C. B., BLONDEL, B., ORCI, L., LAMBERT, A. E., STAUFFACHER, W., LIKE, A. A. and RENOLD, A. E. (19173): Insulin and glucagon release from monolayer cell cultures of pancreas from newborn rats. *Europ. J. clin. Invest., 3/1,* 16.

ORCI, L., LIKE, A. A., AMHERDT, M., BLONDEL, B., KANAZAWA, Y., MARLISS, E. B., LAMBERT, A. E., WOLLHEIM, C. B. and RENOLD, A. E. (1973): Monolayer cell culture of neonatal rat pancreas: an ultrastructural and biochemical study of functioning endocrine cells. *J. Ultrastruct. Res., 43,* 270.

ORCI, L., STAUFFACHER, W., DULIN, W. E. and RENOLD, A. E. and ROUILLER, C. (1970): Ultrastructural changes in A-cells exposed to diabetic hyperglycaemia. Observations made on pancreas of Chinese hamsters. *Diabetologia, 6/3,* 199.

ORCI, L., STAUFFACHER, W., RENOLD, A. E. and ROUILLER, C. (1971): Ultrastructural aspect of A-cells of non-ketotic and ketotic animals: indication for stimulation and inhibition of glucagon production. In: *Current Topics on Glucagon,* p. 15. Editors: M. Austoni, G. Scandellari, G. Federspil and A. Trisotto. Cedam, Padua.

PETERSSON, B. (1970): Intracellular 'X-granulolysis' in X-cells of diabetic animals. In: *The Structure and Metabolism of the Pancreatic Islets,* p. 123. Editors: S. Falkmer, B. Helleman and I.-B. Täljedal. Wenner-Gren Center International Symposium Series Vol. 16, Pergamon Press, London – Oxford – New York – Toronto.

RENOLD, A. E. (1968): Spontaneous diabetes and/or obesity in laboratory rodents. In: *Advances in Metabolic Disorders, Vol. 3,* p. 49. Editors: R. Levine and R. Luft. Academic Press, New York, N. Y.

RENOLD, A. E., BURR, I. M. and STAUFFACHER, W. (1970*a*): On the pathogenesis of diabetes mellitus: possible usefulness of spontaneous hyperglycemic syndromes in animals. In: *Pathogenesis of Diabetes Mellitus. Proceedings, XIII Nobel Symposium,* p. 215. Editors: E. Cerasi and R. Luft. Almqvist and Wiksell, Stockholm.

RENOLD, A. E., CAHILL Jr, G. F. and GERRITSEN, G. C. (1970*b*): Second Brook Lodge Workshop on spontaneous diabetes. In: *Diabetologia, 6/3,* 153.

RENOLD, A. E., CAMERON, D. P., AMHERDT, M., STAUFFACHER, W., MARLISS, E., ORCI, L. and ROUILLER, C. (1972): Endocrine-metabolic anomalies in rodents with hyperglycemic syndromes of hereditary and/or environmental origin. *Israel J. med. Sci., 8/3*, 189.

RENOLD, A. E. and DULIN, W. E. (1967): Spontaneous diabetes in laboratory animals. Introduction by Workshop Editors. *Diabetologia, 3/2,* 63.

STAUFFACHER, W., BALANT, L., AMHERDT, M., CAMERON, D. P. and ORCI, L. (1972): Mode of action of streptozotocin: indication for accelerated NAD-destruction. (Abstract). *Diabetologia, 8/1,* 68.

STAUFFACHER, W., BURR, I. M., GUTZEIT, A., BEAVEN, D., VELEMINSKY, J. and RENOLD, A. E. (1970): Streptozotocin diabetes: time course of irreversible B-cell damage; further observations on prevention by nicotinamide. *Proc. Soc. exp. Biol. (N.Y.), 133,* 194.

STAUFFACHER, W., ORCI, L., CAMERON, D. P., BURR, I. M. and RENOLD, A. E. (1971): Spontaneous hyperglycemia and/or obesity in laboratory rodents: an example of the possible usefulness of animal disease models with both genetic and environmental components. *Recent Progr. Hormone Res., 27,* 41.

STRAUTZ, R. L. (1968): Islet implants: reduction of glucose levels in the hereditary obese mouse. *Endocrinology, 83,* 975.

VELEMINSKY, J., BURR, I. M. and STAUFFACHER, W. (1970): Comparative study on early metabolic events resulting from the administration of the two diabetogenic agents alloxan and streptozotocin. *Europ. J. clin. Invest., 1/2,* 104.

YOKOTE, M. (1970a): Sekoke disease, spontaneous diabetes in carp, Cyprinus carpio, found in fish farms. I. Histological study. *Bull. Freshwater Fisheries Res. Lab., 20,* 39.

YOKOTE, M. (1970b): Sekoke disease, spontaneous diabetes in carp found in fish farms. II. Some metabolic aspects. *Bull. Jap. Soc. scient. Fisheries, 36,* 1214.

CLINICAL RESEARCH ON THE MOLECULAR LEVEL*

ROLF LUFT

Department of Endocrinology and Metabolism, Karolinska Hospital,
Stockholm, Sweden

The investigation and elucidation of clinical problems in the field of internal medicine today often requires advanced and refined techniques. Sometimes, especially when dealing with obscure or ambiguous and perhaps previously undescribed clinical entities, we may have to use methods of investigation that belong to preclinical research, which is often called 'basic research'. What then distinguishes the clinical scientist from the preclinical one is not the investigative technique but the objective. The clinical scientist tackles *clinical* problems, problems that emanate from the diseased person, with methods that make it possible for him to carry out his intentions. The technique by itself is not of great importance to him – it only becomes of great value when it helps him to shed some light on his particular problem.

I shall exemplify this idea by describing how my co-workers and I have investigated two clinical problems. When stating in the title of this lecture that this has been performed on the 'molecular level', my intention has been to emphasize that clinical research in these instances has been dealing with problems that belong partly to clinical medicine and partly to molecular biology. It is concerned firstly with the combined effects of biological processes and their dependence on cell structures, and secondly with events in cells related to such hypothetical concepts as cell receptors.

LOOSE-COUPLING OF OXIDATIVE PHOSPHORYLATION AS A CLINICAL ENTITY (LUFT'S DISEASE)

The first example considered will be a clinical entity originally described by us, and which we designated 'severe hypermetabolism of unknown origin' (Luft et al., 1962). The following is a brief outline of the approach we used in elucidating the nature of this new disease.

In 1960 a 30-year-old woman entered the Department of Endocrinology of the Karolinska Hospital. She had been examined numerous times in different hospitals since the age of 7 for a strange clinical picture, the most characteristic features of which were: (1) intense and profuse *perspiration* which made it necessary for her to change her clothes several times a day; (2) *polydipsia* but with small urinary volumes; (3) *polyphagia* with an intake of 3500–4000 calories a day in spite of the sedentary life; and (4) *thinness* and

* The Solomon A. Berson Memorial Lecture presented on the occasion of the 8th Congress of the International Diabetes Federation.

progressing asthenia despite the polyphagia: body weight 35 kg at a body height of 165 cm.

The main laboratory finding was a basal metabolic rate (BMR) of about +200%. Had the basal oxygen consumption been calculated in relation to cell mass – which was markedly reduced – instead of body surface area, the BMR would have been found to be about +300 to +400%.

The patient was studied with respect to all conditions which could possibly be connected with hypermetabolism. All results were negative. All other laboratory tests of thyroid function were normal, and measures that normally depress thyroid hormone production had no or only moderate effect on the BMR. The net result of this extended and laborious study was unequivocal: the patient presented with hypermetabolism of a degree hitherto never encountered, that was independent of thyroid function, and the origin of which was completely unclear.

It soon became clear to us that the defect in this patient might lie in the regulation of oxygen consumption. It was obvious that she was unable to adjust the energy metabolism to the circumstances and demands of the moment. Oxygen consumption occurs in subcellular elements, the mitochondria, which thereby provide the cells with the energy they need. These mitochondria had not been studied biochemically in man. Our first task was therefore to elaborate methods for the isolation of mitochondria from human muscle biopsies, and for the measurement of their functions. Basic studies on muscle and liver mitochondria from rat had led to a picture of the energy metabolism as it occurs normally in mitochondria and thereby in the cell, as shown in Figure 1. We found, of course, that the same principles were valid for human muscle mitochondria.

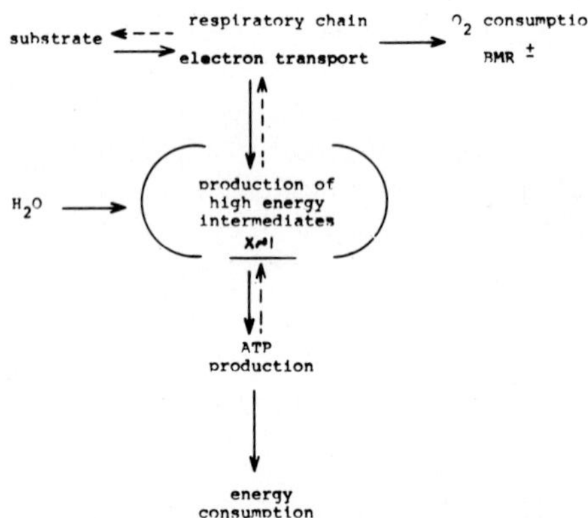

FIG. 1. Schematic illustration of the principles for oxidative phosphorylation and respiratory control.

Cellular metabolism leads to the formation of substrates that are taken up by the mitochondria, and are oxidated there by way of enzymes of the so-called *respiratory chain.* This process involves consumption of oxygen. This oxygen consumption – *respiration* – constitutes the basis of the BMR. According to a widely held hypothesis, energy liberated during respiration is conserved in the inner membranes of mitochondria in the form of labile high-energy compounds (denoted in Fig. 1 as X~I), which are there protected from access to water and thereby from spontaneous hydrolysis. From these compounds energy is liberated, whenever necessary, for the formation of ATP from ADP and inorganic phosphate (P_i). In this way, the oxidation of the respiratory chain is coupled to the phosphorylation of ADP by a process called *oxidative phosphorylation.* When energy is required by the organism, ATP is split with the liberation of energy. The more energy needed, the more ATP split, and the more respiration activated. This feed-back of oxygen consumption, which is effected by the energy demand, is called *respiratory control.*

Figure 2 shows an experiment performed with the purpose of examining the respiratory control of mitochondria isolated from skeletal muscle of a healthy person and of our patient. The normal mitochondria utilized only little oxygen, unless phosphate and ADP were added to make possible the utilization of respiratory energy for ATP synthesis.

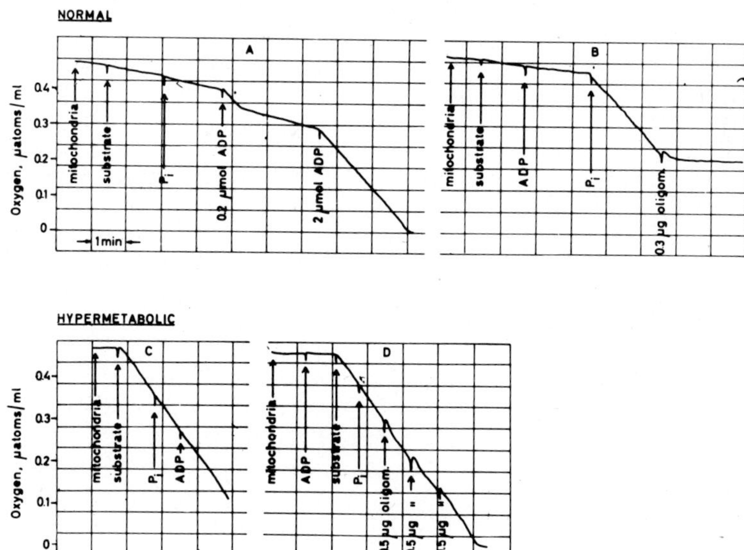

FIG. 2. Polarographic demonstration of lack of respiratory control in skeletal muscle mitochondria from a patient with severe hypermetabolism.

Thus, in the normal subject, oxidative phosphorylation and respiratory control are dependent on adequate amounts of ADP and P_i. However, the patient's mitochondria behaved in an entirely different way: they began to use O_2 at a high rate as soon as substrate was added, without the presence of ADP and P_i. Oxidation was thus loose-coupled from phosphorylation; there was no normal respiratory control.

We postulated that the function of the mitochondria of our patient was defective in the way illustrated in Figure 3 (Ernster and Luft, 1963).

The primary defect was probably a leakage in the waterproof structures surrounding the loci of the labile high-energy compound X~I. This leakage would permit water to enter these loci and cause spontaneous hydrolysis of X~I. The energy thereby liberated would be utilized only to a small extent for ATP synthesis. The major fraction would be given off as heat. Thus, the energy demand of the body would no longer regulate the

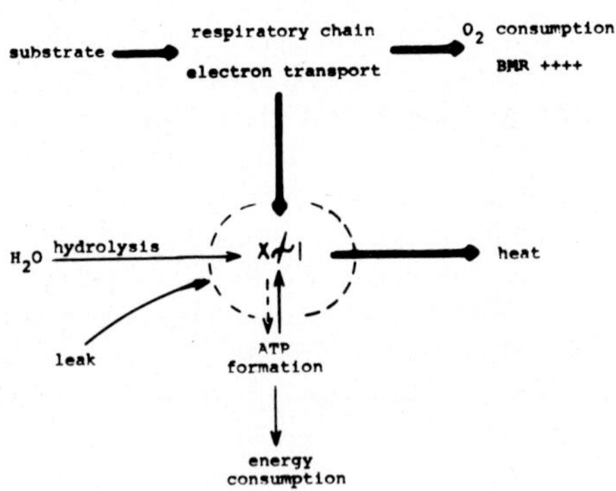

FIG. 3. Schematic illustration of the postulated defect in the function of the mitochondria of a patient with severe hypermetabolism.

respiratory chain, and the oxygen consumption would then proceed at a high level in an uncontrolled fashion.

This finding of a loose-coupling of respiration from phosphorylation gave a plausible explanation of the patient's syndrome: (1) *perspiration* – in order to eliminate the excess of heat produced; (2) *thirst* – to compensate for the loss of fluid through perspiration; (3) *polyphagia* – to compensate for the enormous loss of energy.

Continued studies of this syndrome led us over into the field of molecular biology. A series of observations constituted the basis for these new approaches. Figure 4 shows the structure of normal muscle mitochondria as revealed by the electron microscope, and Figures 5a and b demonstrate similar studies of the patient's muscle. The most conspicuous differences are as follows: (1) an enormous increase of the number of mitochondria in the patient's muscle; (2) an enormous variation and increase in the size of mitochondria, indicating increased production and turnover of mitochondria; (3) an aggregation of mitochondria which was particularly striking in the perinuclear area; (4) an increase in size of the nucleoli, indicating a high RNA content; (5) an increased content of RNA as also found by chemical determination in the muscle homogenate; and (6) an increased content of respiratory enzymes (e.g., cytochrome oxidase) in the mitochondria.

Since RNA presumably regulates the synthesis of mitochondria and of respiratory enzymes, we postulated the following mechanism for this regulation (Fig. 6) (Ernster and Luft, 1964): There should exist a feed-back mechanism between energy demand (corresponding to O_2 consumption) and the induction of the synthesis of m-RNA, mitochondria and respiratory enzymes in the mitochondria. This process would be modified in the patient as shown in Figure 7. The primary defect would be a loose-coupling of oxidation from phosphorylation, with a strong release of a 'metabolite' that acts as an inducer for the synthesis of m-RNA. This, in turn, would lead to increased synthesis of mitochondria and respiratory enzymes, resulting in a great increase in oxygen consumption. The latter would not be controlled by the energy demand, because of the loose-coupling of respiration from phosphorylation.

Provided this explanation is correct, treatment of the patient might be effected by diminishing protein synthesis. However, administration of a specific inhibitor of m-RNA formation, actinomycin D, proved unsuccessful. Recently, a second patient with this

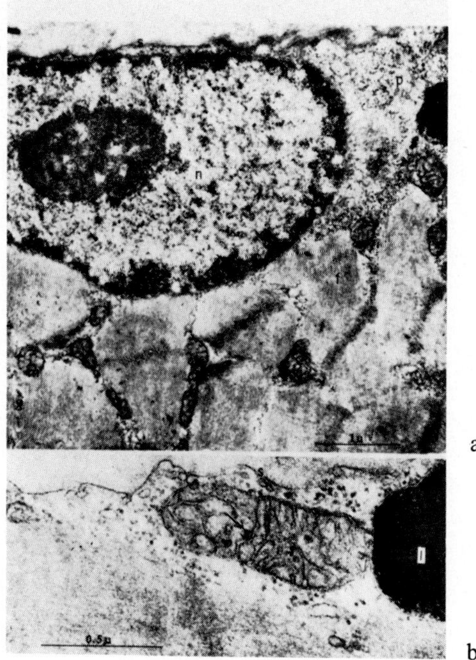

FIG. 4*a*. Electron micrograph of a thin section through the peripheral portion of a muscle fiber from a healthy subject. The myofibrils (f) are tightly packed and there are only a few mitochondria (m) between the myofibrils or between the sarcolemma (s) and the myofibrils. The nucleus (n) with its dense nucleolus is seen close to the sarcolemma. Magnification X 7,000.

FIG. 4*b*. A portion of the same muscle as in *a,* reproduced at higher magnification (X 28,500) so as to show the details of the morphology of the mitochondria. The outer membrane and the many inner membranes (cristae) can be seen.

syndrome was described (Haydar et al., 1971). In this patient, a young girl, it was possible, at least temporarily, to lower the BMR by the administration of very large doses of chloramphenicol, which is a specific inhibitor of mitochondrial protein synthesis. Attempts to reproduce this therapeutic effect in our patient, using lower doses of the drug, were unfortunately unsuccessful.

Clearly, more basic research in this field is required to further our understanding of this syndrome and to develop improved therapy.

This study demonstrates in a striking manner the necessary interrelationship between clinical problems and basic research, in this particular case bioenergetics and molecular biology.

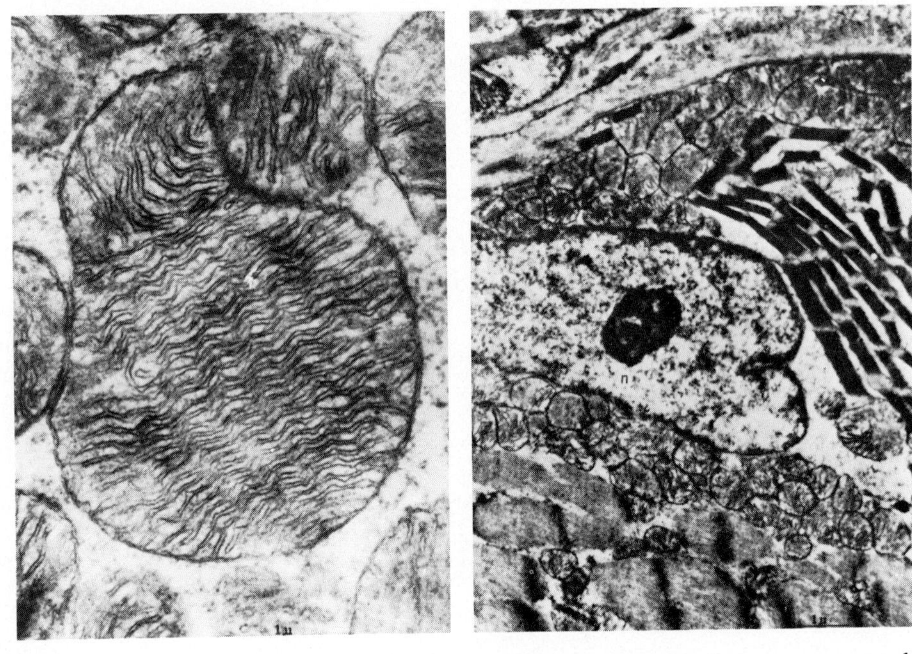

FIG. 5*a*. Low magnification electron micrograph (X 4,440) from a muscle fiber of the hypermetabolic patient. The Figure shows the cell nucleus (n) in the center and a multitude of mitochondria (m) surrounding it. Below this mitochondrial zone there are the myofibrils with some mitochondria intermingled. In the right part of the Figure there is a bundle of dense cell inclusions of unknown character.

FIG. 5*b*. Mitochondria from the mitochondrial zones of the hypermetabolic patient. The zig-zag arrangement of the densely packed cristae is evident. Magnification X 26,000.

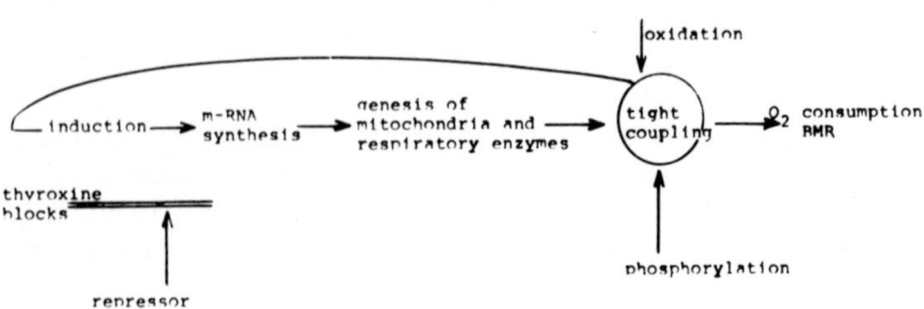

FIG. 6. Scheme for the normal course of the synthesis of mitochondria and respiratory enzymes.

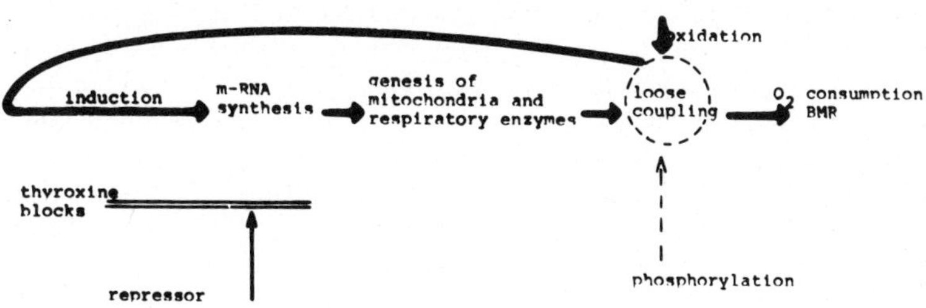

FIG. 7. Scheme for the deranged course of the synthesis of mitochondria and respiratory enzymes.

THE MOLECULAR BASIS OF THE PATHOGENESIS OF DIABETES MELLITUS

The first example illustrated clinical research directed towards an extremely rare disease. However, the elucidation of the pathophysiology of this syndrome opened the road to a new approach to our understanding of problems in bioenergetics. My second example, on the other hand, refers to a very common disease, diabetes mellitus. Diabetes in most instances is an inherited disease, but the genetic basis for the disease and the biological significance of the diabetic predisposition remain by and large unsolved problems. In 1967 we presented the hypothesis that genetic diabetes mellitus in all its stages of development is characterized by an absolute or relative insulin deficiency (Cerasi and Luft, 1967a). This hypothesis was based on the following observations: (1) the insulin response to glucose infusion, measured under dynamic conditions and in relation to the degree of stimulation, is subnormal in all patients with juvenile or maturity-onset diabetes (Cerasi and Luft, 1967b); (2) a similar deficiency in insulin response is found in subjects with minimal derangement of carbohydrate metabolism (latent or chemical diabetes) (Cerasi and Luft, 1967b); (3) the majority of healthy monozygotic twin sibs of diabetic patients (i.e., genetic prediabetics) show the same diabetic type of insulin response to glucose as the above groups (Cerasi and Luft, 1967c).

We suggested that this diminution of the insulin secretory capacity might be a basic and probably genetic mechanism in the pathogenesis of diabetes. A similar deficiency in insulin response was also found in about 20% of normal adults and children with normal i.v. glucose tolerance (Cerasi and Luft, 1967b, 1970d). Thus, a low response is not restricted to subjects with genetic prediabetes but is also present in a considerable number of people in the normal population. We suggested that these latter subjects represent the prediabetics in the normal population. However, since the majority of these will never develop diabetes, the term *low insulin responder* seems more adequate.

An important question is whether the secretion of insulin from the pancreatic beta cells is indeed reduced in diabetes, or if the observed hypoinsulinemia reflects an increased retention and destruction of insulin in the liver. This latter alternative is less probable, however, since we and others have shown that insulin response, as measured in portal vein blood, is also subnormal in those instances where it is subnormal in the peripheral circulation. It was also suggested that the deficient insulin response might be due to anatomical changes in the capillaries of the islets of Langerhans (thickening of the basal membranes). Such alterations would lead to difficulties in the exchange of glucose and insulin across the capillary wall. Such an explanation seems rather unlikely since, as will be discussed below, acute administration of pharmacological and physiological agents may normalize the decreased insulin response. Similar reasons also exclude the possibility that the reduced insulin secretion in diabetes is due to a gross defect in insulin synthesis.

The above discussion made it plausible that the foundation for the disturbed insulin secretion was to be found among those mechanisms which participate in the release of insulin secretion on stimulation with glucose. This makes a discussion of the processes that govern the liberation of insulin in normal subjects imperative.

The generally accepted view until recently was that one or several of the products of glycolysis in the beta cell is the signal that elicits the release of insulin. However, several observations in our laboratory and elsewhere were difficult to explain on the basis of the above view: (1) kinetic studies show that the insulin response to glucose infusion is a very rapid phenomenon, the maximal secretion rate being reached within 1–2 minutes after the start of glucose administration (Fig. 8). (2) The normal insulin response can be inhibited by administering agents which do not influence the glucose metabolism of the beta cells. Thus, the infusion of as little as 1–3 ng of epinephrine per kg body weight reduced the ability of glucose to release insulin by 50% (Cerasi et al., 1971). Similar

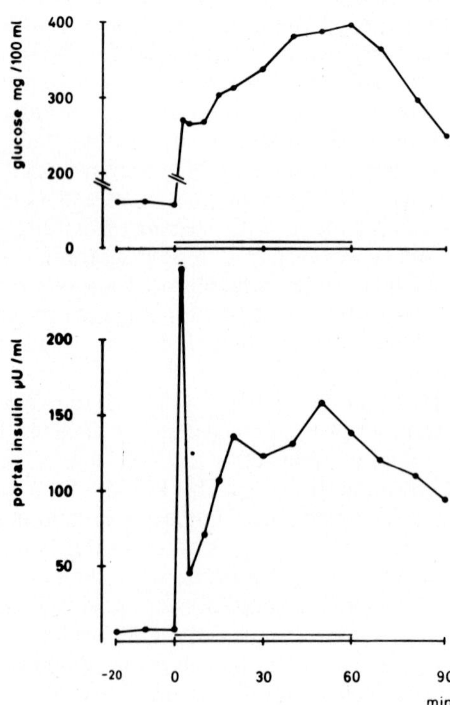

FIG. 8. Changes in portal vein insulin concentration during glucose infusion in a healthy subject. Glucose was injected intravenously and was constantly infused from 0 to 60 min. (horizontal line). The first sample was taken at 2 min. after the beginning of the glucose injection.

inhibition of the insulin response could be obtained with small doses of the beta-adrenergic antagonist propranolol (Cerasi et al., 1969, 1972a). This inhibition could be reversed if the subjects were pretreated with theophylline (Cerasi and Luft, 1969). (3) More direct evidence against the role of glycolysis in insulin secretion is the finding that glycolytic intermediates accumulate in the beta cells only after long-term stimulation with glucose; furthermore, some non-metabolizable analogues of glucose and amino acids may induce insulin release.

On the basis of our observations we suggested that the secretion of insulin may be controlled by two partially independent processes (Cerasi and Luft, 1970a, b, c, 1973): (1) a *bioenergetic* system including the several steps of glycolysis, and (2) a system of *cybernetic* nature. The latter would comprise a signal system initiated by glucose itself and leading to the release of insulin. According to this hypothesis glucose would, on the one hand, act as a substrate and be metabolized in the beta cell as in all other cells. On the other hand, perhaps by an allosteric action, glucose would act on a cell membrane receptor, inducing an insulinogenic signal (Fig. 9). The mode of transmission of this signal in the beta cell is not clear. It is known that the cyclic AMP (cAMP) system is of importance for the secretion of insulin and, consequently, we suggested that the cAMP system could be one of the links of the signal chain. Recently, studies from our laboratory have shown a direct glucose effect on intracellular cAMP in isolated rat islets (Grill and Cerasi, 1973) (Fig. 10).

Thus, our original hypothesis that *glucose has a direct insulin-releasing action while*

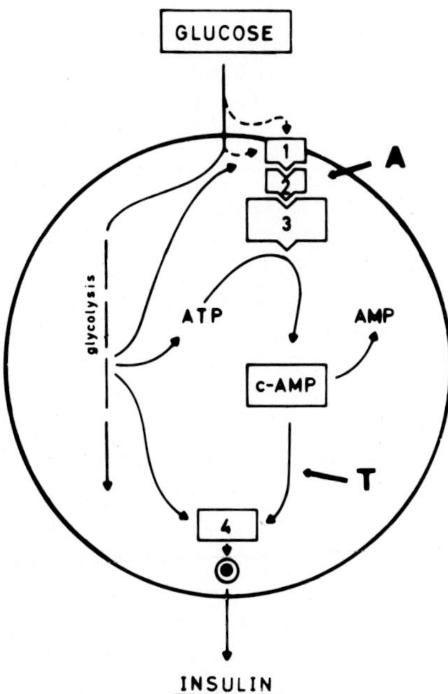

FIG. 9. Suggested mode of action of glucose on insulin release. The signal chain to the right, the metabolic chain to the left. 1 = glucose receptor; 2 = transmitter unit; 3 = adenyl cyclase; 4 = insulin releasing unit; A = arginine; T = tolbutamide.

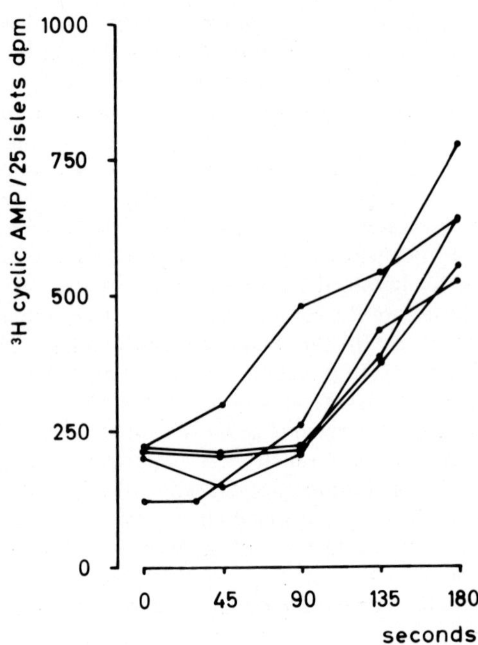

FIG. 10. Accumulation of tritiated cyclic AMP in isolated islets from rat pancreas. Glucose, 5 mg/ml together with 0.1 mmol 3-isobutyl-1-methyl xanthine was added to the medium at time zero.

glycolysis in the beta cell plays a secondary role, probably as an amplifier of the glucose signal, continues to gain experimental support.

The deficient insulin secretion in prediabetes and diabetes, against the background of the above discussion, may be explained by one of the following alternatives: (1) reduction of the number of beta cells in the pancreas; (2) reduction of the amount of insulin in the beta cells; (3) derangement of glycolysis in the beta cell, hence inability to amplify the glucose signal; and (4) deficiency in the initiation and/or transmission of the glucose signal.

We and other authors have shown that both diabetics and prediabetics may respond with almost normal insulin secretion following glucagon (Goldfine et al., 1972) or tolbutamide administration (Cerasi et al., 1969; Widström and Cerasi, 1973) or when glucose infusion is preceded by the administration of theophylline (Cerasi and Luft, 1969) or growth hormone (Luft et al., 1969). These findings exclude the first two alternative explanations given above.

The third alternative, i.e., incapacity to amplify the glucose signal, could also be excluded on the basis of some recent findings. Thus, we have demonstrated that arginine, which increases insulin release by a multiplicative potentiation of the glucose signal, exerts the same degree of potentiation in healthy as well as in diabetic and prediabetic individuals (Efendic et al., 1971, 1972). The well-known potentiation of insulin release by intestinal humoral factors was found to be equally effective in these three groups of subjects (Cerasi et al., 1972b). Finally, preliminary experiments indicate that pretreatment with glucose potentiates the insulin response to a second glucose pulse to the same degree in prediabetics as in healthy individuals. All these data favor the idea that the cellular mechanisms, which on activation by amino acids, intestinal hormones or glycolysis in the beta cell enhance the insulinogenic signal of glucose, are intact in diabetes and prediabetes.

These results enable us to delimit the defect in the beta cell in prediabetes and diabetes to the transmission of the insulinogenic signal of glucose, i.e., the fourth of the above alternatives. This assumption is supported by the finding that, in prediabetics and diabetics, a normal insulin response to glucose can be obtained without the above pretreatments, provided that blood glucose will be raised to very high levels (Cerasi et al., 1973). The dose-response relationship between blood glucose and plasma insulin shows a parallel displacement to the right in the prediabetics and diabetics (Fig. 11). This indicates that the sensitivity – or affinity – of the beta cell receptor for glucose is decreased in diabetes.

From the above discussion, it can be derived that *the beta cell defect in diabetes is a very selective one and limited to the transmission of information from the extracellular space. However, by being so strategically located, it impairs grossly the regulation of the secretion of insulin.*

We have presented a dynamic picture of the pathogenesis of genetic diabetes mellitus, and defined a defect in the beta cell leading to a reduction of insulin secretion, the common denominator of the preclinical and clinical stages of diabetes. It is probable that further characterization of the cellular mechanisms involved may facilitate the development of pharmacological agents capable of favorably influencing the release of insulin. A future implication of this might be the prevention not only of manifest diabetes but also, and more important, of the metabolic consequences of insulin deficiency.

ON THE THRESHOLD OF A NEW ERA

This presentation is a brief and simplified description of some aspects of clinical research emanating from my laboratory during the past 13 years. Two examples have been chosen to indicate the depth and breadth of clinical investigation. Clinical research has been concerned with attempts to understand the physiology of normal and pathologic states on an organ or tissue basis. In addition, it has long been clear that the interrelationships between organs through hormonal interactions and other mechanisms require study of the organism as a whole.

Recently, a new era has been opened in clinical research with an appreciation that the complete elucidation of disease processes is coming to depend more and more on an intimate knowledge of the molecular biology of the cell. This revolutionary new approach requires an understanding of physiologic and pathophysiologic processes at the molecular level and in terms of macromolecular structure. Nonetheless, the opening of a new approach to clinical research on the molecular level does not imply neglect of studies involving the total organism or its individual components. Modern clinical investigation requires an integrated approach ranging from study at the molecular level to the study of the entire organism, and perhaps even study of the interrelationship among organisms.

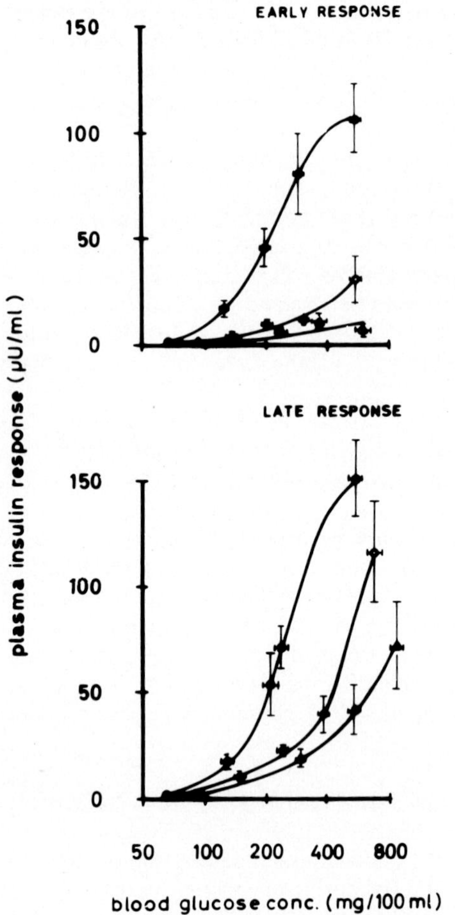

FIG. 11. Glucose-insulin dose-response curves for the early (10 min.) and late (60 min.) phases of insulin release on glucose administration. Solid circles represent the curves of the control group, open circles those of the prediabetics, and solid triangles the curves obtained in the group of diabetics. Insulin response is given as values above the fasting level, the glycemic stimulus as the logarithm of absolute blood glucose concentrations. Vertical bars denote ± S.E.M. insulin response, horizontal bars ± S.E.M. blood glucose concentration reached at each dose level.

REFERENCES

CERASI, E., CHOWERS, I., LUFT, R. and WIDSTRÖM, A. (1969): The significance of the blood glucose level for plasma insulin response to intravenously administered tolbutamide in healthy subjects. *Diabetologia, 5,* 343.

CERASI, E., EFENDIĆ, S. and LUFT, R. (1969): Role of adrenergic receptors in glucose-induced insulin secretion in man. *Lancet, ii,* 301.

CERASI, E., EFENDIC, S. and LUFT, R. (1973): Dose-response relation between plasma-insulin and blood-glucose levels during oral glucose loads in prediabetic and diabetic subjects. *Lancet, i,* 794.

CERASI, E. and LUFT, R. (1967a): 'What is inherited – what is added' hypothesis for the pathogenesis of diabetes mellitus. *Diabetes, 16,* 615.

CERASI, E. and LUFT, R. (1967b): Plasma insulin response to glucose infusion in healthy subjects and in diabetes mellitus. *Acta endocr. (Kbh.), 55,* 278.

CERASI, E. and LUFT, R. (1967c): Insulin response to glucose infusion in diabetic and non-diabetic monozygotic twin pairs. Genetic control of insulin response? *Acta endocr. (Kbh.), 55,* 330.

CERASI, E. and LUFT, R. (1967d): Further studies on healthy subjects with low and high insulin response to glucose infusion. *Acta endocr. (Kbh.), 55,* 305.

CERASI, E. and LUFT, R. (1969): The effect of an adenosine 3′,5′,-monophosphate diesterase inhibitor (aminophylline) on the insulin response to glucose infusion in prediabetic and diabetic subjects. *Hormone metabol. Res., 1,* 162.

CERASI, E. and LUFT, R. (1970a): Diabetes mellitus, a disorder of cellular information transmission. In: *Pathogenesis of Diabetes Mellitus. Nobel Symposium 13,* pp. 17-43, 349-354. Editors: E. Cerasi and R. Luft. Almqvist and Wiksell, Stockholm.

CERASI, E. and LUFT, R. (1970b): Is diabetes mellitus a disorder of cellular information transmission? *Acta diabet. lat., 7,* 278.

CERASI, E. and LUFT, R. (1970c): Diabetes mellitus – a disorder of cellular information transmission? *Hormone metabol. Res., 2,* 246.

CERASI, E. and LUFT, R. (1970d): The occurrence of low insulin response to glucose infusion in children. *Diabetologia, 6,* 85.

CERASI, E. and LUFT, R. (1973): Pathogenesis of genetic diabetes mellitus. Further development of a hypothesis. *Mt Sinai J. Med., 40,* 334.

CERASI, E., LUFT, R. and EFENDIC, S. (1971): Antagonism between glucose and epinephrine regarding insulin secretion. *Acta med. scand., 190,* 411.

CERASI, E., LUFT, R. and EFENDIC, S. (1972a): Effect of adrenergic blocking agents on insulin response to glucose infusion in man. *Acta endocr. (Kbh.), 69,* 335.

CERASI, E., LUFT, R. and EFENDIC, S. (1972b): Decreased sensitivity of the pancreatic beta cells to glucose in prediabetic and diabetic subjects. A glucose dose-response study. *Diabetes, 21,* 224.

EFENDIC, S., CERASI, E. and LUFT, R. (1971): Role of glucose in arginine-induced insulin release in man. *Metabolism, 20,* 568.

EFENDIC, S., CERASI, E. and LUFT, R. (1972): Arginine-induced insulin release in relation to the cyclic AMP system in man. *J. clin. Endocr., 34,* 67.

ERNSTER, L. and LUFT, R. (1963): Further studies on a population of human skeletal mitochondria lacking respiratory control. *Exp. Cell Res., 32,* 26.

ERNSTER, L. and LUFT, R. (1964): Mitochondrial respiratory control: biochemical, physiological and pathological aspects. In: *Advances in Metabolic Disorders, 1,* pp. 95-123. Editors: R. Levine and R. Luft. Academic Press, New York, N.Y.

GOLDFINE, I. D., CERASI, E. and LUFT, R. (1972): Glucagon stimulation of insulin release in man: Inhibition during hypoglycemia. *J. clin. Endocr., 35,* 312.

GRILL, W. and CERASI, E. (1973): Activation by glucose of adenyl cyclase in pancreatic islets of the rat. *FEBS Letters (Amst.), 33,* 311.

HAYDAR, N. A., CONN Jr., H. L., AFIFI, A., WAKID, N., BALLAS, S. and FAWAZ, K. (1971): Severe hypermetabolism with primary abnormality of skeletal muscle mitochondria. *Ann. int. Med., 74,* 548.

LUFT, R., CERASI, E. and WERNER, S. (1969): The effect of moderate and high doses of human growth hormone on the insulin response to glucose infusion in prediabetic subjects. *Hormone metabol. Res., 1,* 111.

LUFT, R., IKKOS, D., PALMIERI, G., ERNSTER, L. and AFZELIUS, B. (1962): A case of severe hypermetabolism of nonthyroid origin with a defect in the maintenance of mitochondrial respiratory control: a correlated clinical, biochemical and morphological study. *J. clin. Invest., 41,* 1776.

WIDSTRÖM, A. and CERASI, E. (1973): On the action of tolbutamide in normal man. I, II, III. *Acta endocr. (Kbh.), 72,* 506, 519, 532.

DIABETES, INSULIN AND FUTURE DEVELOPMENTS*

GEORGE F. CAHILL Jr.

Joslin Research Laboratories, Harvard Medical School and the Peter Bent Brigham Hospital, Boston, Mass., U.S.A.

Your Majesty, members of the Committee of Honor, members and guests of the Congress, and particularly Mrs. Hoet and members of the Hoet family, I had the great pleasure of knowing Dr. J. P. Hoet and it is a major distinction for me to present the first lecture named in his honor before this assembly. Professor Hoet had innumerable honors bestowed during his lifetime, and a select few I have listed below. I refer the reader to a brief article written by Sir Frank Young (1968) in honor of Professor Hoet for a more detailed biographical summary. I would like to emphasize, however, his unique and rapid academic progress: professor at the age of 29! This progress was particularly noteworthy in the face of the then traditional European medical establishment. What is not mentioned below are his many other humanitarian efforts in addition to those in medical science, particularly during the time of the Second World War. All this speaks of the power and enthusiasm of the man; indeed, we in Boston cherished each of his frequent visits and were left on every occasion infected by his enthusiasm and intellect.

Turning back the clock approximately half a century, two classical articles appeared in the Proceedings of the Royal Society (Best et al., 1926a, b) ascribing the peripheral effects of insulin not only to augmentation of glucose uptake and conversion to glycogen, but also to accelerated combustion. Figure 1 is taken from one of these, and illustrates the increased rate of glucose assimilation provoked by insulin. Of more interest to me, however, is the physiologic use of the 'steady state' as well as the principle of 'clearance' in the steady state, two concepts which required another 2–4 decades for appropriate development and acceptance as prerequisites for sophisticated physiologic studies. Professor Hoet and colleagues, particularly Dr. Charles Best, were not only chronologically young, but conceptually well ahead of their time. Parenthetically, Dr. Best has written a lovely letter concerning his unavoidable absence on this occasion, particularly in view of his extreme respect and affection for his former colleague in the laboratory of Sir Henry Dale and subsequently long-time personal friend, Dr. Joseph Hoet.

Now, turning to my task of presenting an overview on diabetes and diabetes research, I would like to say a few simple words about insulin, the beta cells and fuel homeostasis. In Figure 2 I have sketched a hypothetical day's activity in a normal man, demonstrating how the beta cells, as evidenced by insulin levels, closely monitor and respond to changes in fuel intake and circulating fuel concentrations, although only glucose concentration is

* The J. P. Hoet Memorial Lecture, sponsored by the International Diabetes Federation, and attended by Her Majesty the Queen of the Belgians.

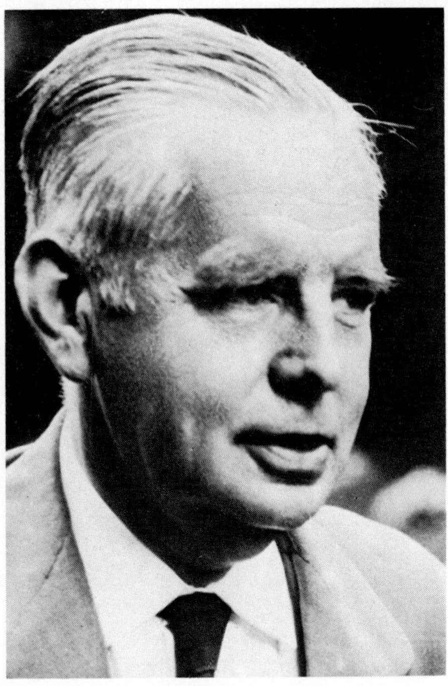

Joseph Pierre Hoet, 1899–1968

M.D. - Louvain	1923
Traveling Fellow of the Rockefeller Foundation - Henry Dale, Charles Best	
Ph.D. Cambridge	1926
Prof. Therapeutics, Louvain	1928
Prof. Internal Medicine	1934
Chief of Medicine, Hôpital St. Pierre	1948
President - IDF	1958
Honorary President, IDF	1961
Honorary Doctorate, Toronto	1964
First President, European Diabetes Association etc.	1965

illustrated. Thus, like a thermostat in a room, the beta cells are always 'at work', measuring and responding to the richness of the circulating fuel. Injection of a bolus of glucose into normal man results in an almost immediate increase in insulin levels, showing a very rapid time response of the beta cells, and this is followed by a rapid decrease in insulin levels, thanks to the short half-life of the hormone of some 8–10 minutes. Infusion of small amounts of glucose to normal man at rates sufficient to increase glucose levels with 3–5% provokes measurable increases in insulin levels, demonstrating the beta cells to be as capable of detecting minimally altered glucose levels as the scientist with his glucose analytic techniques (Cahill, 1972a). Many studies, which I shall not recount, have shown the diabetic to release too little insulin too late relative to a comparable but

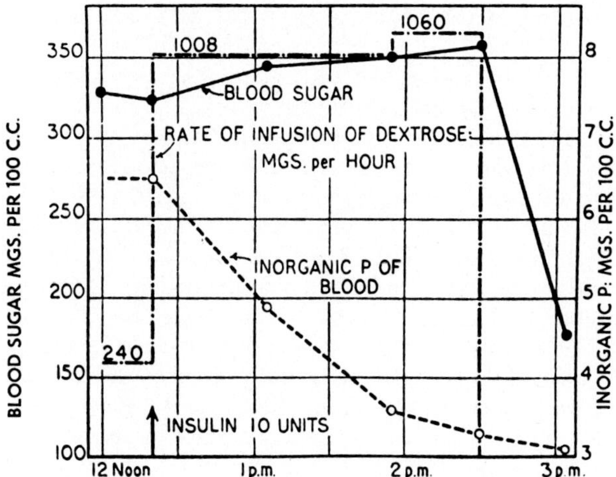

FIG. 1. Experiment of Best, Hoet and Marks (1926) showing the accelerated rate of glucose clearance from the blood after administration of insulin.

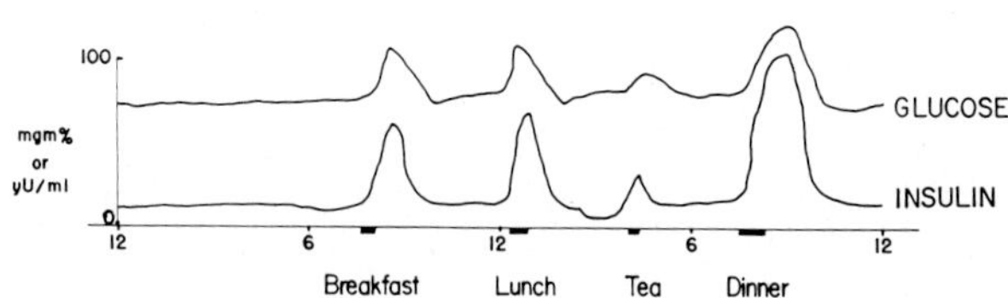

FIG. 2. Hypothetical correlation between levels of glucose and insulin in normal man.

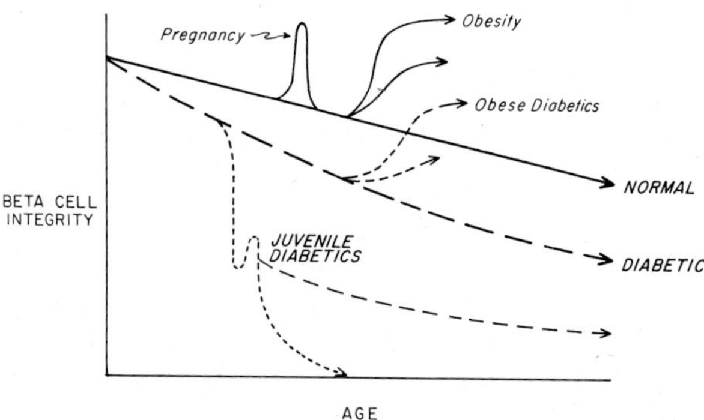

FIG. 3. Beta cell integrity in normal man, and in subjects with diabetes, showing the increased need during pregnancy or obesity and the deficiency in meeting this need in the diabetic. Also shown is the rapid demise in the juvenile diabetic, a transient improvement or perhaps even remission, and the eventual total demise or prolonged deficiency.

non-diabetic individual. Thus an abnormality in the beta cell appears central to the disease.

We know little of the beta cell except that morphologically it appears damaged or, at least, reduced in number in diabetics. In Figure 3, I have sketched a theoretical natural history of the beta cells in normal man, showing the transient increase in times of extra insulin need, such as pregnancy, or for a more prolonged period of time, in obesity. Also shown is the decrease in integrity in the diabetic, particularly the relatively rapid downhill course in the juvenile diabetic. There is much recent evidence to suggest a viral etiology of juvenile diabetes (Gamble and Taylor, 1969; Craighead and Steinke, 1971; Craighead, 1972), and an engrossing hypothesis would be that the underlying hereditary defect is an increased susceptibility to damage or possibly an earlier senescence of the beta cells themselves. A virus would cause an early rapid and irreversible demise in this hereditary milieu. Otherwise, advancing age, and particularly an increase in insulin need, as in obesity, would unmask the beta cell deficiency. Although this is conjecture, this 'beta cell fragility' hypothesis would explain the higher concurrence of juvenile and maturity-onset diabetes in a given kindred than either type of diabetes in the general population. If a virus does not destroy the cells in youth, this earlier demise would result in maturity-onset type of diabetes later in life.

There are many theories as to why the beta cell is so susceptible (Fig. 4) and diabetes therefore so relatively common. We know very little of the natural history of the beta

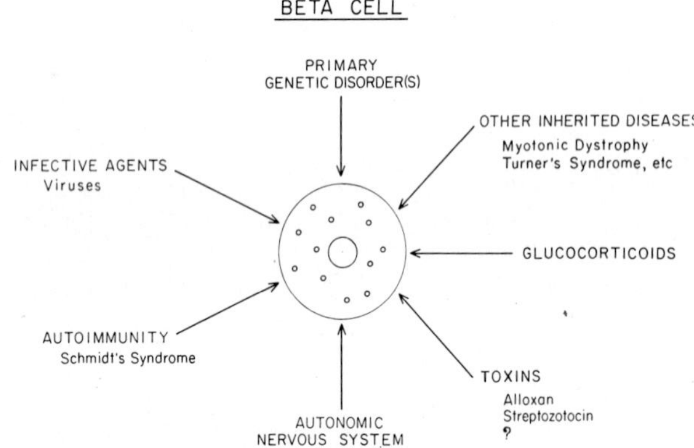

FIG. 4. Various factors altering beta cell integrity.

cell, except for several studies by Logothetopoulos (1972) and my colleagues Like and Chick (1969). Apparently beta cells regenerate by mitosis of former beta cells and not ductular or other cells. If one measures islet cell mitosis in the db mutant mouse, restriction of food markedly reduces mitosis, followed by mitotic resumption after reinitiation of ad lib feeding. Chick and Like (1970) have shown dietary protein to be more important than carbohydrate in inducing mitosis. What tells the beta cell to undergo mitosis or even how long a beta cell survives is unknown. There is no doubt, however, that there must be a feedback mechanism of some sort, analogous to the control of liver cellularity. After subtotal hepatectomy, regeneration occurs rapidly until the original liver mass is matched. It may even be possible that lack of this signal may, for the beta cell, be the primary inherited deficiency in diabetes.

The capacity to maintain beta cells in tissue culture, as developed by the Geneva group under Professor Renold and the late Professor Rouiller (Marliss et al., 1973) has now provided an excellent tool to dissect the various factors which initiate beta cell mitosis (Chick et al., 1973). If the beta cell is the primary site of the abnormalities in diabetes, one must accept that the complications result directly from the abnormal metabolism secondary to the beta cell deficiency. I think the general consensus is that this is the case, and the recent studies by investigators such as my colleague Dr. Robert Spiro (1973) on the enzymes involved in formation of the accumulating material in the basement membrane concur with this hypothesis.

Returning to Figure 1, any depot form of insulin lacks the feed-back regulation of the normal, and therefore any attempt at mimicking the normal requires a system capable of feed-back control. Two routes are available (Table 1), mechanical (or inorganic) and biologic (Felts, 1973). The latter, to be discussed first, involves either transplantation of

TABLE 1
Approaches to insulin administration

Inorganic	Mechanical pancreas	enzymatic detector catalytic detector
Organic	Pancreatic transplantation Islet transplantation Beta cell transplantation Beta cell rejuvenation	

the entire pancreas, or, more recently, of isolated islets and, better yet, of isolated beta cells themselves. Many laboratories are currently involved in these procedures (Table 2).

Concerning total organ transplantation in man, 32 have been registered with the Transplant Registry in Chicago as of July, 1973. Three patients are currently alive, 2 for a year and one for several weeks. The original largest series by Lillehei and Goetz and associates in Minnesota (1972) involved total pancreas transplantation plus segments of intestine in order to provide egress to the exocrine fluid. The 3 transplant patients now living, 2 in New York and one in Chicago, received a cadaver transplant according to an ingenious technique recently devised by Gliedman and associates at the Montefiore Hospital in New York (Gliedman et al., 1973a, b), whereby only a portion of the pancreas was transplanted and the exocrine fluid diverted via a small catheter into the ureter. The lower urinary system appears to be undisturbed by the presence of the pancreatic juice, and, even better, measurement of urinary pancreatic enzyme provides daily appraisal of the integrity of the transplant. One of the patients receiving this one year ago has done remarkably well and has normal glucose homeostasis. Of course, immunosuppression continues to be mandatory to prevent rejection. Again, one should be reminded of the experimental autotransplants made by Foglia and Houssay decades ago and the resulting normal glucose homeostasis, showing the beta cell to be both detector and responder, independent of innervation.

Even more exciting are the recent experimental approaches whereby isolated islets are injected intraperitoneally or even intraportally. Dr. Chick (personal communication) has even injected beta cells grown in monolayer culture into the portal vein of a diabetic animal. The diabetes was corrected by the numerous 'metastatic' beta cells located in the

TABLE 2
Some methods of beta cell transplantation

1965	Fetal pancreas	Gonet and Renold, Geneva
1966	Neonatal pancreas	Sak et al., Boston
1972/1973	Intraperitoneal islets	Reckard et al., Philadelphia Ballinger and Lacy, St. Louis
1973	Intraperitoneal neonatal minced pancreas	Leonard et al., Minneapolis
1973	Intraportal islets	Lacy et al., St. Louis
1973	Intraportal beta cells from tissue culture	Chick, Boston

portal radicals releasing insulin in a feed-back fashion. Dr. Paul Lacy had previously injected isolated islets with similar results. But again, these techniques, to be adapted to homotransplantation (heterogeneic), require immunosuppression.

An almost unbelievable observation has recently been reported in abstract form by Summerlin and colleagues (1973) whereby skin maintained in organ culture for several weeks can be transplanted even in other species and maintained without immunosuppression. Transplants across even classes can be made such as chicken skin into a mammal! Years ago, Jacobs and Huseby (1967) showed that tumors maintained in tissue culture could be allogeneically transplanted. We now await whether beta cells or islets maintained for prolonged periods of time in vitro can be heterogeneically transplanted, such as from monkey or rat to man.

Another recent development is the capacity to measure endogenous insulin production in the presence of exogenously administered insulin, by following the circulating levels of C-peptide. Thus Black et al. (1973) can monitor beta cell integrity in juvenile diabetics receiving insulin treatment. This can provide the researcher with a measure of not only the functional state of a transplant, but also the capacity to see if endogenous beta cells are still viable prior to transplantation. If so, the development of maneuvers to increase their mitotic potential is obviously a challenge for study. Perhaps more practical will be excision, growth in tissue culture and rejuvenation by hybridization with other cells, techniques now in use by the cellular biologists, and then re-implantation into the patient. Immunosuppression would obviously not be necessary in such a procedure.

In parallel with the race toward the development of an insulin system with feed-back control is the effort being made toward construction of a mechanical pancreas. The major hurdle has been the design of a stable, riliable glucose detector. Several techniques have been attempted. One is a glucose electrode which catalyzes the oxidation of glucose to gluconic acid and in so doing produces an electric current, a so-called glucose fuel cell (Wolfson and Strohl, 1967; Bessman and Schultz, 1972). Another is to enzymatically oxidize the glucose by glucose oxidase derived from bacteria or yeast (Gough and Andrade, 1973), and to measure the alteration in oxygen tension. My colleague, Dr. J. Stuart Soeldner has headed a team of bio-engineers and physiologists and in collaboration with Dr. Richard Egdahl's Department of Surgery at Boston University has developed a glucose detector (Soeldner et al., 1973; Chang et al., 1972, 1973; Cahill et al., 1972b). Studies over the past year have shown its long-term stability in experimental animals

(Fig. 5). Its use, however, has until recently necessitated egress of wires from the animal; so the next development has been the addition of a small FM radiotransmitter, the entire implantable package being slightly smaller than a pack of cigarettes. This apparatus has so far been in experimental animals for over 6 months, continuously emitting an intermittent radio signal, or 'beep', the rate of which is linearly proportional to the concentration of glucose in the animal. The power for the radio is derived from a mercury battery, similar to that used for cardiac pacemakers, and has an expected life of approximately two years (Fig. 6). The next step, of course, is to connect the glucose

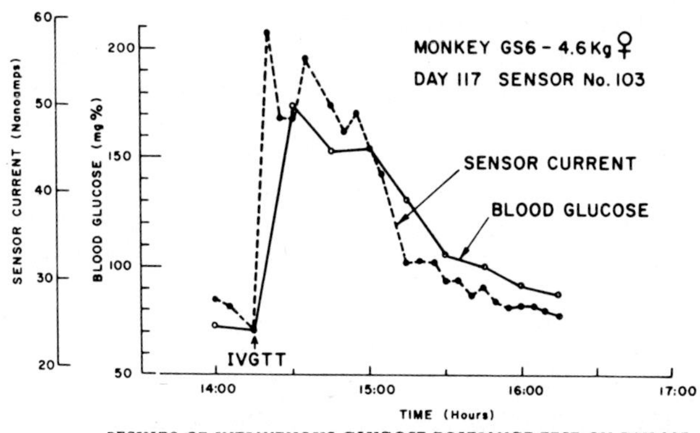

RESULTS OF INTRAVENOUS GLUCOSE TOLERANCE TEST ON DAY 117

FIG. 5. Comparison of blood glucose determined chemically and tissue fluid glucose determined by the glucose electrode 117 days after implantation into a monkey. The monkey received an intravenous glucose tolerance test. (From Soeldner et al., 1973, by courtesy.)

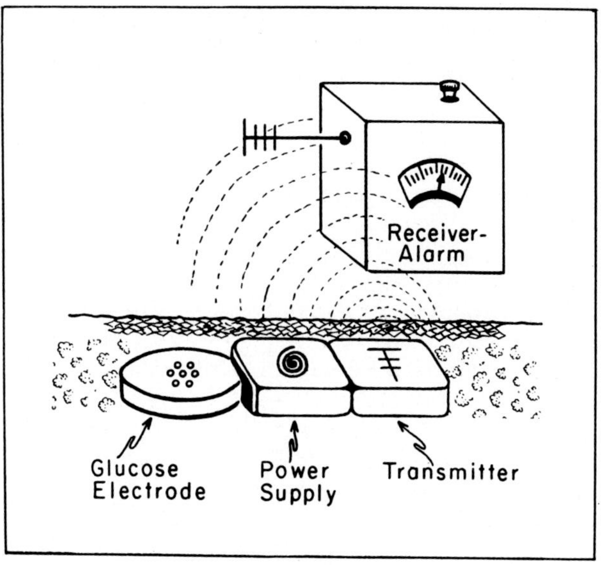

FIG. 6. Schematic drawing of the glucose monitor. (From Soeldner et al., 1973, by courtesy.)

detector, not to a radio, but to a small implantable computer and an insulin depot, and one has a mechanical insulin mechanism with feed-back control.

These developments, all now shown to be feasible, were considered too impractical, perhaps even illogical, several years ago, but science has made tremendous strides. I so far have emphasized only the palliative approaches to replacing insulin deficits with feed-back control; I have not discussed the more fascinating approaches toward clarification of the noxious stimulus to the beta cell itself which initiates its rapid demise in the juvenile diabetic. As stated earlier many data point to a viral insult as discussed by Craighead (this Volume, pp. 287-291). This therefore offers the opportunity of immunization in susceptible kindreds, if, of course the susceptible kindred and virus can be identified. The fascinating work of Goldstein and colleagues (1969) showing a decreased viability of fibroblasts in tissue culture, the fibroblasts having been derived from otherwise normal offspring of diabetic parents, must be mentioned as one of several routes to detect the susceptible population. These studies also corroborate the possibility that the initial diabetic lesion is a more susceptible beta cell, or one with a decreased mitotic potential. Other approaches include the interesting finding of DeMoor and Van Mieghem (1973) of abnormal levels of transcortin in diabetes-prone communities.

Perhaps the next J. P. Hoet Memorial Lecturer at the Ninth Congress of the International Diabetes Federation will describe one of the aforementioned routes as being successful in its direct application to the diabetic patient. At the rate science is moving, this is a reasonable possibility.

Your Majesty, and members and guests of the Congress, this has been a fascinating week, and we have heard many new advances in our knowledge of diabetes and its related problems. I must point out, however, the tremendous strides made by your own people, many of whom, such as the late Dr. Hoet, I cherish as personal friends. Such productivity by your country can only be derived from two factors: one is a people driven by intellect and personal industry, exemplified by Dr. Hoet, and the other, of course, is a climate created by a government and society aware of the talents of its people and willing, therefore, to provide the support for these great advances, not only for the benefit of the Belgians but for the well-being of the entire world. This Congress certainly attests to my comment. Thank you.

REFERENCES

BALLINGER, W. G. and LACY, P. E. (1972): Transplantation of intact pancreatic islets in rats. *Surgery, 72,* 175.

BESSMAN, S. P. and SCHULTZ, R. D. (1972): Sugar electrode sensor for the 'artificial pancreas'. *Hormone metabol. Res., 4,* 413.

BEST, C. H., HOET, J. P. and MARKS, H. P. (1926a): The fate of sugar disappearing under the action of insulin. *Proc. roy. Soc. (Lond.), 100B,* 32.

BEST, C. H., DALE, H. H., HOET, J. P. and MARKS, H. P. (1926b): Oxidation and storage of glucose under the action of insulin. *Proc. roy. Soc. (Lond.), 100B,* 55.

BLOCK, M. B., ROSENFIELD, R. L., MAKO, M. E., STEINER, D. F. and RUBENSTEIN, A. H. (1973): Sequential changes in beta-cell function in insulin-treated diabetic patients assessed by C-peptide immunoreactivity. *New Engl. J. Med., 288,* 1144.

CAHILL Jr., G. F. (1972a): The physiology of insulin in man. *Diabetes, 20,* 785.

CAHILL Jr., G. F., SOELDNER, J. S., HARRIS, G. W. and FOSTER, R. O. (1972b): Practical developments in diabetes research. *Diabetes, 21/Suppl. 2,* 703.

CHANG, K. W., AISENBERG, S. and SOELDNER, J. S. (1972): In vitro tests of implantable glucose sensor. In: *Proceedings of the 25th Annual Conference on Engineering in Medicine and Biology,* p. 58. Alliance for Engineering in Medicine and Biology, Arlington, Va.

CHANG, K. W., AISENBERG, S., SOELDNER, J. S. and HIEBERT, J. M. (1973): Validation and bio-engineering aspects of an implantable glucose sensor. *Trans. Amer. Soc. Artif. Int. Organs, 19,* 352.

CHICK, W. L. and LIKE, A. A. (1970): Studies in the diabetic mutant mouse. III. Physiological factors associated with alterations in beta cell proliferation. *Diabetologia, 6,* 243.

CHICK, W. L., LAURIS, V., FLEWELLING, J. H., ANDRES, K. A. and WOODRUFF, J. M. (1973): Effects of glucose on beta cells in pancreatic monolayer cultures. *Endocrinology, 92,* 212.

CRAIGHEAD, J. E. and STEINKE, J. (1971): Diabetes mellitus-like syndrome in mice infected with encephalomyocarditis virus. *Amer. J. Pathol., 63,* 119.

CRAIGHEAD, J. E. (1972): Workshop on viral infection and diabetes mellitus in man. *J. infect. Dis., 125,* 568.

DeMOOR, P. and VAN MIEGHEM, W. (1973): The apparent affinity of plasma transcortin (CBA) in inbred Tamilian Hindus belonging either to a diabetes-prone community or to a group without family history of diabetes. *J. clin. Endocr., 36,* 1100.

FELTS, P. W. (1973): Pancreas transplantation and the artificial pancreas. *South. med. J., 66,* 66.

GAMBLE, D. R. and TAYLOR, K. W. (1969): Seasonal incidence of diabetes mellitus. *Brit. med. J., 3,* 631.

GLIEDMAN, M. L., GOLD, M., WHITTAKER, J., RIFKIN, H., SOBERMAN, R., FREED, S., TELLIS, V. and VEITH, F. J. (1973a): Pancreatic duct to ureter anastomosis for exocrine drainage in pancreatic transplantation. *Amer. J. Surg., 125,* 245.

GLIEDMAN, M. L., RIFKIN, H., ROSS, H., SOBERMAN, R., ZARDAY, A., TELLIS, V., FREED, S. and VEITHER, F. J. (1973b): Clinical segmental pancreatic transplantation with ureter to pancreatic duct anastomosis for exocrine drainage (Abstract #26). *Diabetes, 22/Suppl. 1,* 295.

GOLDSTEIN, S., LITTLEFIELD, J. W. and SOELDNER, J. S. (1969): Diabetes mellitus and aging: diminished plating efficiency of cultured human fibroblasts. *Proc. nat. Acad. Sci. U.S.A., 64,* 155.

GONET, A. E. and RENOLD, A. E. (1965): Homografting of fetal rat pancreas. *Diabetologia, 1,* 91.

GOUGH, D. A. and ANDRADE, J. D. (1973): Enzyme electrodes. *Science, 180,* 380.

JACOBS, B. B. and HUSEBY, R. A. (1967): Growth of tumors in allogeneic hosts following organ culture explantation. *Transplantation, 5/3,* 410.

LEONARD, R. J., LAZAROW, A. and HEGRE, O. D. (1973): Pancreatic islet transplantation in the rat. *Diabetes, 22,* 413.

LIKE, A. A. and CHICK, W. L. (1969): Mitotic division in pancreatic beta cells. *Science, 163,* 941.

LILLEHEI, R. C. and GOETZ, F. C. (1972): Communicated at the symposium on Pancreas Transplantation and the Artificial Pancreas, Birmingham, Alabama.

LOGOTHETOPOULOS, J. (1972): Islet cell regeneration and neogenesis. In: *Handbook of Physiology, Section 7, Endocrinology, Vol. 1, Endocrine Pancreas,* pp. 67–76. Editors: R. O. Greep and E. B. Astwood. American Physiological Society, Washington, D. C.

MARLISS, E. B., WOLLHEIM, C. B., BLONDEL, B., ORCI, L., LAMBERT, A. E., STAUFFACHER, W., LIKE, A. A. and RENOLD, A. E. (1973): Insulin and glucagon release from monolayer cell cultures of pancreas from newborn rats. *Europ. J. clin. Invest., 3,* 16.

RECKARD, C. R., ZIEGLER, M. M. and BARKER, C. F. (1973): Islet transplantation in streptozotocin-induced diabetes in rats (Abstract #25). *Diabetes, 22/Suppl. 1,* 295.

SAK, M. F., MACCHI, I. A. and BEASER, S. B. (1966): Structural and functional characteristics of neonatal pancreas homografts in alloxan diabetic golden hamsters. *Diabetes, 15,* 51.

SOELDNER, J. S., CHANG, K. W., AISENBERG, S. and HEIBERT, J. M. (1973): Progress toward an implantable glucose sensor and an artificial beta cell. Temporal aspects of therapeutics. In: *Proceedings of the Second Alza Research Conference,* pp. 181-204. Editors: J. Urquhart and F. E. Yates. Plenum Press, New York, N.Y.

SPIRO, R. G. (1973): Biochemistry of the renal glomerular basement membrane and its alterations in diabetes mellitus. *New Engl. J. Med., 288,* 1337.

SUMMERLIN, W. T., MILLER, G. E. and GOOD, R. A. (1973): Successful tissue and organ allotransplantation without immunosuppression. *J. clin. Invest., 52/6,* 83a.

WOLFSON Jr., S. K. and STROHL Jr., C. K. (1967): Bioautofuel cell as a possible power source for cardiac pacemakers. *Circulation, 36/Suppl. 2,* 273.

YOUNG, F. G. (1968): Professor J. P. Hoet 1899–1968. *Diabetologia, 4,* 109.

BETA CELL 1973

MEMBRANE SULPHYDRYL GROUPS AND THE PANCREATIC BETA CELL RECOGNITION OF INSULIN SECRETAGOGUES*

BO HELLMAN, LARS-ÅKE IDAHL, ÅKE LERNMARK, JANOVE SEHLIN and INGE-BERT TÄLJEDAL

Department of Histology, University of Umeå, Umeå, Sweden

It is not clear how the pancreatic beta cells recognize and quantify the various stimuli for insulin release. Attention has been given to the hypothesis that glucose is recognized as an insulin secretagogue by virtue of its metabolism (Grodsky et al., 1963; Hellman, 1970; Ashcroft et al., 1972). Alternatively the insulin-releasing capacity of this and other compounds could be due to their interaction with specific receptors, perhaps in the cell membrane (Christensen and Cullen, 1969; Cerasi and Luft, 1970; Hellman et al., 1971, 1972b, c; Ashcroft et al., 1972; Matschinsky et al., 1972). However, there is no direct evidence that the beta cell plasma membrane is equipped with specific receptors for the recognition of insulin secretagogues other than glucagon (Goldfine et al., 1972).

Our recent approach to the problem of stimulus recognition included the testing of organic mercurials as possible inhibitors of glucose-stimulated insulin release. The finding that these compounds did not inhibit but markedly stimulated insulin release led us to investigate other classes of sulphydryl reagents as well. The results of these studies are summarized here and discussed with a view to the possible involvement of membrane sulphydryl groups in the beta cell recognition of glucose and sulfonylureas.

SULPHYDRYL REAGENTS WITH LIMITED ABILITY TO PENETRATE THE BETA CELLS

Binding of glucose to cell membranes may depend on the integrity of sulphydryl groups (Thomas et al., 1972). Sulphydryl reagents with a limited ability to penetrate the beta cells could therefore be useful in studying membrane binding sites that are involved in the recognition of glucose as an insulin secretagogue. Four electronegative membrane probes (Fig. 1) were selected for these studies. While chloromercuribenzene-p-sulphonic acid (CMBS) readily forms mercaptides, the 2 disulphides tested, 5,5′-dithiobis-(2-nitrobenzoic acid) (DTNB) and 6,6′-dithiodinicotinic acid (CPDS), are assumed to form disulphide bridges between membrane and reagent or between neighbouring membrane sulphydryl groups (Grasetti, 1969; Grasetti and Murray, 1970). The fourth compound under study, 4-acetamido-4′-isothiocyanostilbene-2,2′-disulphonic acid (SITS), is a rather non-specific sulphydryl reagent (Marinetti and Gray, 1967) that may react preferentially with super-

* This study has been supported by the Swedish Medical Research Council (12x-562).

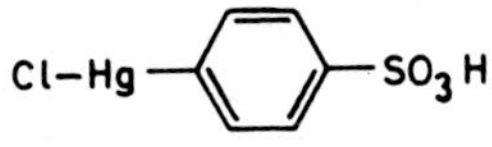

CMBS
chloromercuribenzene-p-sulphonic acid

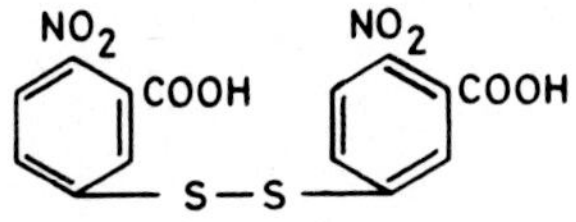

DTNB
5,5′-dithiobis-(2-nitrobenzoic acid)

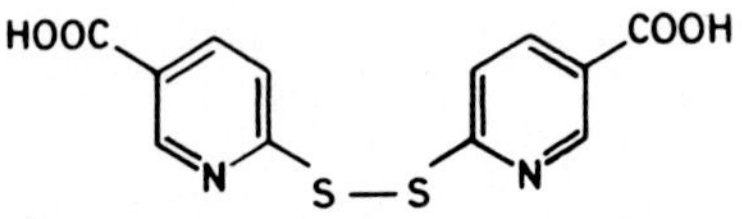

CPDS
6,6′-dithiodinicotinic acid

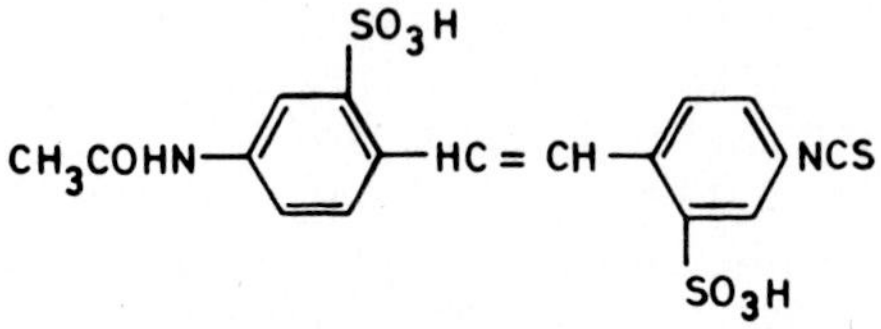

SITS
4-acetamido-4′-isothicyanostilbene-2,2′-disulphonic acid

FIG. 1. Structural formulae of the membrane probes tested.

ficial amino groups (Maddy, 1964; Knauf and Rothstein, 1971a; Cabantchik and Rothstein, 1972). SITS was tested mainly because it has been found to modify the permeation paths for CMBS in erythrocytes (Knauf and Rothstein, 1971b).

It was felt that a rapid inhibition of glucose-stimulated insulin release by slowly permeating sulphydryl reagents would provide suggestive evidence for the presence of a superficial glucose recognition site in the beta cells. Much to our surprise, however, all reagents proved to be potent stimulators of insulin release. The most striking effects were noted with CMBS (Bloom et al., 1972). Studies on erythrocytes have indicated that this compound binds rapidly to the cell membrane and then permates slowly through anion channels in the plasma membrane (Rothstein, 1970; Knauf and Rothstein, 1971b). This might also be the case in pancreatic beta cells as suggested by the biphasic uptake of (^{203}Hg)CMBS in microdissected islets (Fig. 2). As would be expected, if CMBS reacts with sulphydryl groups in the beta cell membrane, the islet content of (^{203}Hg)CMBS was drastically reduced after addition of L-cysteine. Figure 3 shows that 0.1 mM CMBS caused an almost instantaneous liberation of insulin, resulting in a very high initial peak followed by sustained release at a suprabasal rate. Stimulation by CMBS was additive to that exerted by glucose and could be demonstrated with a concentration as low as 0.01 mM. There is much to indicate that the increased discharge of insulin induced by CMBS is not due to passive diffusion of the hormone through a leaky beta cell membrane. Stimulation occurred within 60 seconds and with much lower concentrations than those which made the beta cells permeable to extracellular space markers such as sucrose and mannitol. Insulin release in response to CMBS was not only reversible (Fig. 4) but was also

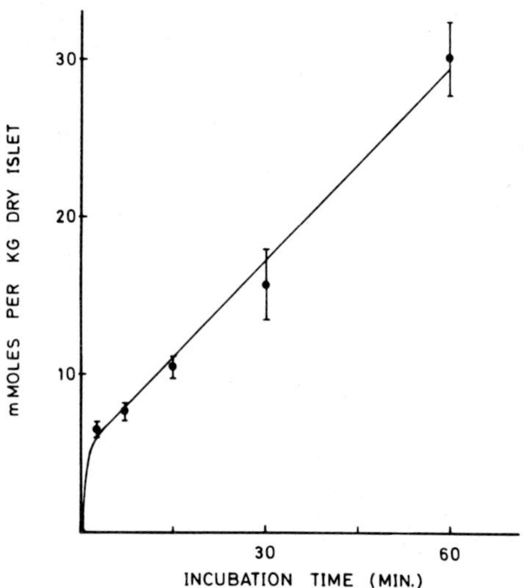

FIG. 2. Islet uptake of CMBS with time. The islets were incubated for different periods of time in Krebs-Ringer bicarbonate buffer supplemented with 0.2 mM (^{203}Hg)CMBS and 0.1 mM (6,6′-^{3}H)sucrose. The points represent the islet uptake of CMBS after correction for ^{203}Hg in the sucrose space. Mean values ± S.E.M.(Reproduced form Hellman et al., 1973e, by courtesy.)

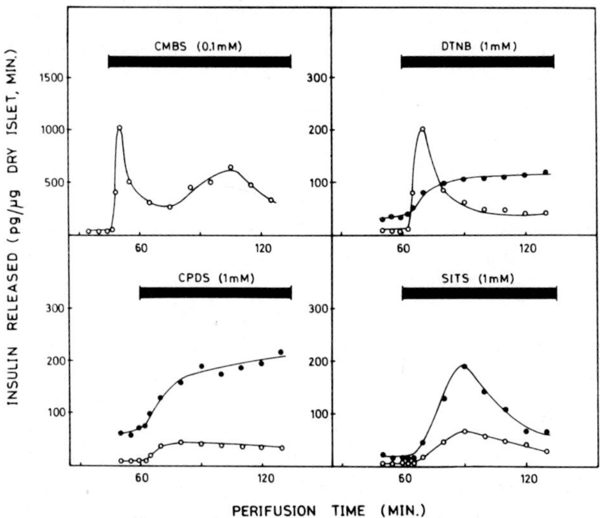

FIG. 3. Dynamics of insulin release induced by membrane probes. Islets were first perifused with albumin-containing bicarbonate buffer containing 3 (○) or 17 (●) mM glucose. The perifusion medium was then switched to the same kind of medium supplemented with 0.1 mM CMBS (upper left), 1 mM CPDS (lower left), 1 mM DTNB (upper right) or 1 mM SITS (lower right). The time of exposure to each reagent is indicated by the bar. The points represent the average rate of insulin release during sampling periods of 1–10 minutes.

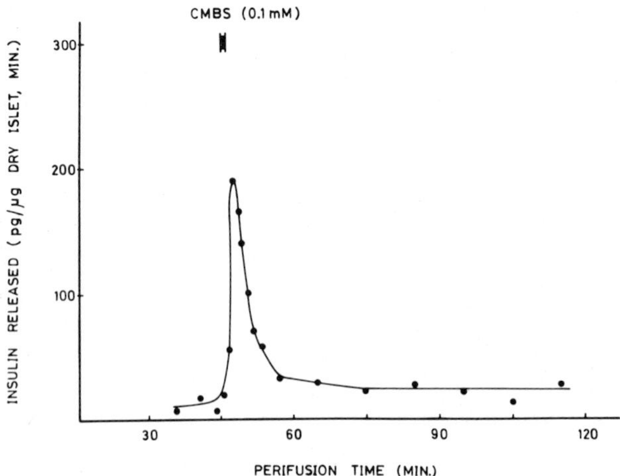

FIG. 4. Reversibility of CMBS-induced insulin release. Islets were perifused with albumin-containing bicarbonate buffer containing 3 mM glucose. After 45 minutes the perifusion medium was switched to the same type of medium supplemented with 0.1 mM CMBS. Perifusion with CMBS (bar) lasted for only 1 minute after which the experiment was continued with the CMBS-free medium. (Reproduced from Bloom et al., 1972, by courtesy.)

markedly reduced by the omission of Ca^{++} or the addition of epinephrine, diazoxide or dinitrophenol; all these conditions inhibit glucose-stimulated insulin release. Moreover, after exposure for 60 minutes to 0.1 mM CMBS the islet production of $^{14}CO_2$ from D-(U-^{14}C)glucose was unaffected and most beta cells were morphologically intact as revealed by electron microscopy.

The observations made with CMBS suggested that insulin release may be regulated by superficial sulphydryl groups in the beta cell membrane. The results obtained with the other sulphydryl-reactive membrane probes corroborate this idea (Hellman et al., 1973b, c). As shown in Figure 3, 1 mM CPDS rapidly stimulated insulin release at both high and low glucose concentrations. Stimulation with CPDS was evident during the whole perifusion period; there were no signs of a multiphasic release pattern similar to that seen with CMBS. In the case of DTNB the stimulatory pattern was markedly affected by glucose. Figure 3 shows that 1 mM DTNB generated a distinct initial peak in the presence of 3 mM glucose, whereas its secretagogic effect was manifested as a gradual increase to a plateau level when the incubation was performed in presence of 17 mM glucose. When microperifused islets were exposed to 1 mM SITS they responded within 6 minutes with a marked enhancement of insulin release (Fig. 3). The statistical treatment of a series of experiments indicated a synergism between SITS and glucose as insulin secretagogues. A significant stimulation was noted with as little as 0.01 mM SITS in the presence of 10 mM glucose. In contrast to glucose, CPDS and DTNB generated a distinct initial peak also when the islets were perifused with a medium deficient in Ca^{++}. However, with all membrane probes tested the rate of insulin release was significantly inhibited by Ca^{++} deficiency. Stimulation of insulin release by CPDS, DTNB or SITS did not appear to be caused by enhanced beta cell metabolism of glucose. At a concentration of 1 mM these 3 sulphydryl reagents did not affect or slightly inhibited the formation of $^{14}CO_2$ from D-(U-^{14}C)glucose.

SITS has been reported to block one of the anion channels by which CMBS permeates into the plasma membrane of erythrocytes (Rothstein, 1970; Knauf and Rothstein, 1971b). Similarly, SITS inhibited the membrane permeation of CMBS in beta cells (Hellman et al., 1973e). In addition, SITS markedly inhibited CMBS-induced insulin release (Table 1). The islet uptake of CMBS was also inhibited by glucose (Table 1), whereas glucose had no effect on the insulin-releasing action of CMBS (Blood et al., 1972). Since the effect of glucose on CMBS uptake was as great as that of glucose in combination with SITS, the 2 compounds may inhibit the same path of CMBS permeation. It is likely that the sulphydryl groups responsible for CMBS-induced insulin release are reached through this channel and the question therefore arises how glucose could inhibit the permeation but not the secretagogue action of CMBS. A tentative explanation might be that the target sulphydryl groups are located somewhere between the diffusion barriers caused by SITS and glucose.

TABLE 1

Effects of SITS on the uptake and insulin-releasing action of CMBS

Compounds tested	CMBS uptake (mmol/kg dry islet)		P value
	Test value	Difference from control	
Glucose, 20 mM	17.1 ± 1.8 (13)	−7.9 ± 1.4 (13)	<0.001
SITS, 1 mM	16.4 ± 1.2 (12)	−8.6 ± 2.3 (12)	<0.01
Glucose, 20 mM, plus SITS, 1 mM	13.5 ± 0.8 (6)	−6.7 ± 1.6 (6)	<0.01
	Insulin release (ng/μg dry islet per hr)		
CMBS, 0.05 mM	5.9 ± 0.9		
CMBS, 0.05 mM, plus SITS, 1 mM	2.9 ± 0.6		<0.001

In uptake experiments the islets were preincubated in bicarbonate buffer containing 3 mM glucose (control), 3 mM glucose plus 1 mM SITS, 20 mM glucose, or 20 mM glucose plus 1 mM SITS. Incubation was then performed for 45 minutes in the same type of media to which had been added 0.2 mM (^{203}Hg)CMBS and 0.1 mM (6,6′-^{3}H)sucrose. The values denote islet uptake of CMBS in excess of the sucrose space and represent the mean values ± S.E.M. for the numbers of experiments stated in parentheses. In addition to the value recorded with test compounds, the differences between parallel test and control incubations are presented. In studies of insulin release, the islets were preincubated for 40 minutes in bicarbonate buffer containing 1 mg/ml serum albumin as well as 0 or 1 mM SITS. They were then incubated for 60 minutes in the same types of media also supplemented with 0.05 mM CMBS. Amounts of insulin released during the 60-minutes period are given as mean values ± S.E.M. for 13 separate experiments.

SULFONYLUREA COMPOUNDS

Recent studies suggest that the beta cell plasma membrane may also play an important role in the recognition of insulin-releasing sulfonylurea derivatives. Studies with perfused pancreas preparations revealed that the sulfonylureas cause a prompt insulin secretory response, which starts even earlier than that induced by glucose (Curry, 1971; Gabbay and Tze, 1972). Available data on the uptake of sulfonylurea by islets suggest that these drugs do not readily enter the beta cells (Hellman et al., 1971, 1973i). This is particularly obvious in the case of tolbutamide. The time course of (^{35}S)tolbutamide uptake from an albumin-containing bicarbonate buffer is shown in Figure 5. Evidently the tolbutamide space approaches the extracellular sucrose space but is considerably smaller than the total water space as estimated with 3-O-methylglucose.

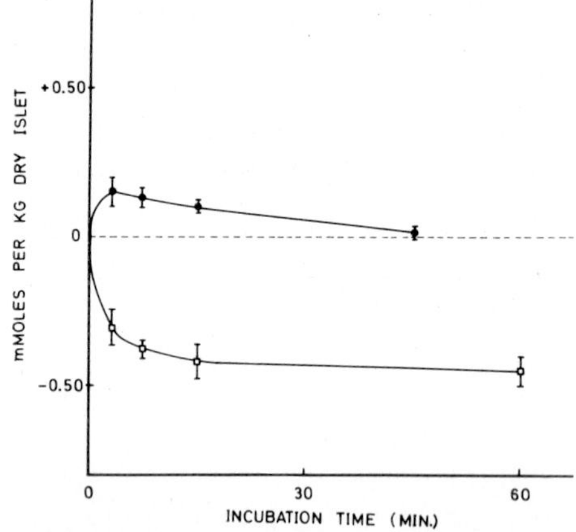

FIG. 5. Islet uptake of tolbutamide with time. The islets were incubated for different periods of time in bicarbonate medium containing 0.3% serum albumin and supplemented with 0.3 mM (^{35}S)tolbutamide and 0.1 mM of either (6,6′-^{3}H)sucrose or 3-*O*-methyl-D-(1-^{3}H)glucose. Islet uptake of tolbutamide is presented after correction for ^{35}S in the sucrose (upper curve) and 3-*O*-methyl-D-glucose (lower curve) spaces. Mean values ± S.E.M.

Further insight into the mechanism by which the beta cells recognize the sulfonylureas was obtained by studying how these compounds interact with SITS (Hellman et al., 1973f). As pointed out above, this membrane probe is an insulin secretagogue in itself but also inhibits both the permeation and the insulin-releasing action of CMBS. As can be seen in Figure 6, SITS also inhibits the islet uptake of glibenclamide. Furthermore the combination of SITS and glibenclamide resulted in a secretory rate no greater than the rate induced by SITS alone. These observations reinforce the hypothesis that sulfonylureas act on the beta cell membrane. In addition they focus attention on the possible involvement of membrane amino and sulphydryl groups in the secretagogue recognition of sulfonylureas and on the possibility that the site of recognition is associated with an anion diffusion channel. It is noteworthy that the islet uptake of glibenclamide, like that of CMBS, is significantly reduced when the islets are exposed to L-cysteine (Hellman, 1974).

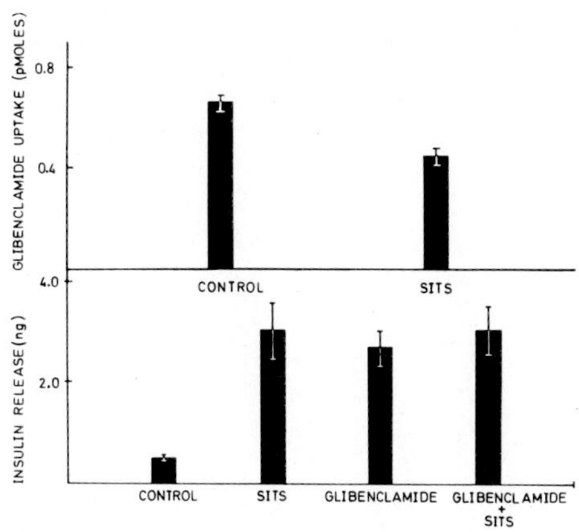

FIG. 6. Effects of SITS on the islet uptake (upper panel) and the insulin-releasing activity (lower panel) of glibenclamide. In the uptake experiments the islets were preincubated for 30 minutes with or without 1 mM SITS and then incubated for 60 minutes in the same type of medium supplemented with 0.02 mM (^{3}H)glibenclamide. Results are expressed as pmoles of glibenclamide taken up per μg islet dry weight. In the release experiments preincubation with or without SITS was followed by incubation for 60 minutes with the indicated combinations of 0.1 mM glibenclamide and 1 mM SITS. The amounts of insulin released are given as ng per μg islet dry weight. The observed release rates are well below the maximum secretory responses induced by glucose or glucose plus SITS indicating a negative interaction between glibenclamide and SITS.

ALKYLATING SULPHYDRYL REAGENTS

The reagents discussed above are believed to react essentially with sulphydryl groups located in the plasma membrane. If insulin release can be triggered by the blocking of such groups, more readily penetrating sulphydryl reagents might also stimulate insulin release during their passage through the cell membrane. Studies in our laboratory indicate that this is indeed the case (Hellman et al., 1973a). Dynamic recordings of how iodoacetamide influences glucose-stimulated insulin release are presented in Figure 7. At a concentration of 0.1 mM, iodoacetamide clearly stimulated insulin release, in contrast to the non-halogenated acetamide. When the islets were perifused with 0.3 or 1.0 mM iodoacetamide, stimulation was followed by a significant inhibition. The inhibitory action was found to be concentration-dependent in a way that agreed well with the effects of different concentrations of iodoacetamide on the islet content of fructose-1,6-diphosphate as well as on glucose oxidation. Thus, the biphasic release pattern observed with high concentrations of iodoacetamide suggests that stimulation, presumably brought about by the alkylation of superficial sulphydryl groups, is overcome when iodoacetamide had penetrated so deeply into the beta cells as to inhibit glycolysis.

The effects of different glucose concentrations on the stimulatory action of 0.1 mM iodoacetamide during 60 minutes of incubation are shown in Figure 8. It is evident that stimulation by iodoacetamide requires a certain concentration of glucose to be present and that the iodoacetamide-induced response increases with rising glucose concentration.

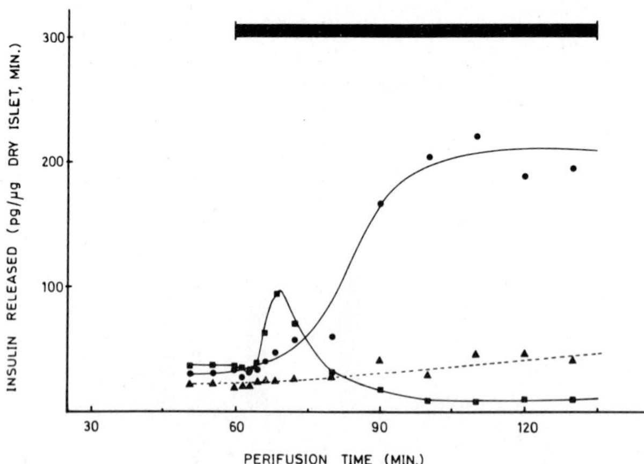

FIG. 7. Dynamics of insulin release induced by iodoacetamide. Islets were first perifused for 60 minutes with albumin-containing bicarbonate buffer supplemented with 17 mM glucose. The perifusion medium was then switched to the same kind of medium also supplemented with 0.1 mM iodoacetamide (●), 1.0 mM iodoacetamide (■) or 0.1 mM acetamide (▲). Exposure to iodoacetamide or acetamide is indicated by the bar.

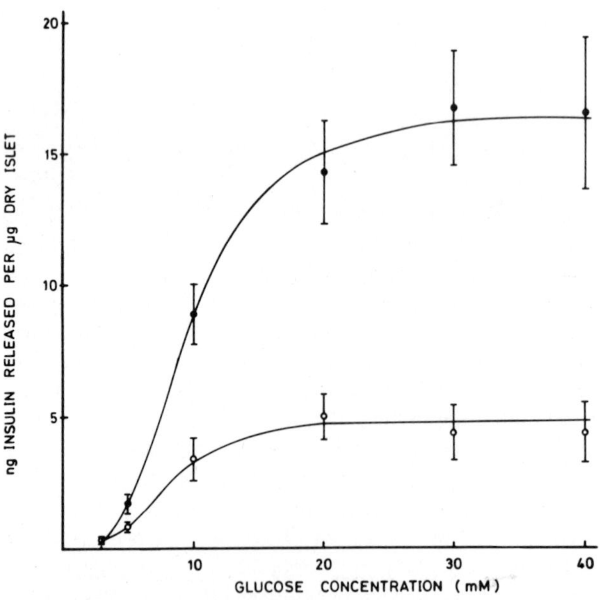

FIG. 8. Effects of different concentrations of glucose on iodoacetamide-induced insulin release. Incubation was performed for 60 minutes in media containing glucose as indicated. Parallel incubations were performed in media containing no further additives (○) and in media also contaning 0.1 mM iodoacetamide (●). Mean values ± S.E.M. (Reproduced from Hellman et al., 1973a, by courtesy.)

The general appearance of the curves suggests that iodoacetamide increases the V_{max} of glucose-stimulated insulin release with little or no effect on the apparent K_m. The permissive action of glucose on iodoacetamide-induced insulin release resembles the insulin-releasing action of glucose alone in being inhibited by mannoheptulose and in being rapidly reversible on withdrawal of glucose. It seems unlikely that iodoacetamide stimulates insulin release by increasing the beta cell content of cyclic 3,5-AMP. The stimulatory effect of theophylline, which is usually attributed to inhibition of cyclic nucleotide phosphodiesterase, was not enhanced but significantly inhibited by iodoacetamide.

It should be emphasized that at sufficiently low concentrations iodoacetamide and related halogenated compounds only amplify a physiological glucose stimulus, the beta cell function being unaffected at non-stimulatory glucose concentrations. Although iodoacetamide is quite toxic, its nature as a pure potentiator of glucose-stimulated release may be of interest in the development of new antidiabetic drugs; the currently employed sulfonylurea derivatives have a certain stimulatory effect in the absence of glucose. The principle of sensitizing the beta cells by alkylating their membrane sulfhydryl groups has up to now been tested as a means of improving the deficient beta cell response to glucose seen in normal, fetal and newborn mice and in adult diabetic mice carrying the mutated gene *db*. Figure 9 illustrates the secretory response observed after exposing islets microdissected from the diabetic mice to iodoacetamide (Boquist et al., 1974). Evidently the secretory machinery is sensitized to glucose only in those animals whose beta cells exhibit some capacity to respond to glucose alone. Principally the same conclusion emerged from the experiments with fetal and newborn mice.

GLUCOSE

Grodsky et al. (1963) suggested that only those sugars which are metabolized in the beta cells can elicit a secretory response. Subsequent studies have demonstrated close correlations between the rates of insulin release and glucose utilization (Ashcroft et al., 1972). Mannoheptulose (Coore and Randle, 1964; Hellman et al., 1972a) and 5-thio-D-glucose (Hellman et al., 1973g) inhibit both glucose oxidation and insulin release. It was suggested that a secretory signal may arise from glycolysis below fructose-1,6-diphosphate, and that the enzyme sequence phosphoglyceraldehyde dehydrogenase/phosphoglycerate kinase may represent a control site of direct significance for the regulation of insulin release (Hellman, 1970). These ideas are supported by the observations that D-glyceraldehyde mimics the electrophysiological effects of glucose on the beta cells (Dean and Matthews, 1972) and stimulates insulin release (Ashcroft et al., 1973; Hellman et al., 1973d), presumably by giving rise to 3-phosphoglyceraldehyde.

Matschinsky et al. (1972) reported that galactose and other poorly metabolized sugars stimulate insulin release from the rat pancreas, and that in this species glucose stimulates insulin release without raising the islet content of glucose-6-phosphate. The results were interpreted as showing that the essential feature of glucose recognition is the interaction of glucose molecules with direct receptors, as opposed to metabolic degradation. With the beta cell-rich islets of *ob/ob* mice we observed no effects of galactose on insulin release; a rise of glucose-6-phosphate was recorded even prior to the glucose-induced secretory response (Idahl, 1973). However, 2 other phenomena were encountered that draw attention to the possible existence of a direct receptor mechanism also in these islets. First, phlorizin and phloretin stimulate insulin release in the absence of glucose, effects that are

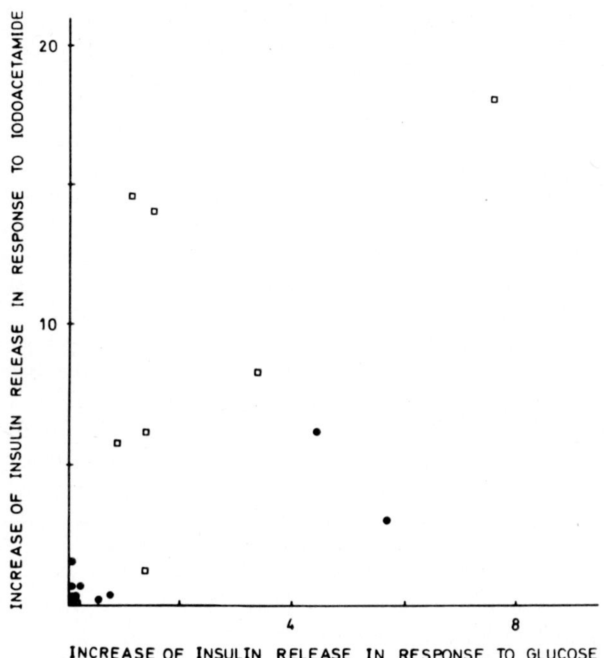

FIG. 9. Effect of iodoacetamide on insulin release from islets with different capacities for responding to glucose. The islets were microdissected from 19 diabetic mutant mice with the genotype C57Bl/KsJ-*db/db* (●) or C57Bl/6J-*db/db* (□). After preliminary incubation for 30 minutes in 3 mM glucose the islets were exposed for 60 minutes to one of the following combinations: (a) 3 mM glucose, (b) 20 mM glucose, (c) 20 mM glucose and 0.1 mM iodoacetamide. The amounts of insulin released in each of these media were calculated as ng per μg dry islet. Response to glucose was defined as the difference between the amounts of insulin released in 20 and 3 mM glucose and plotted on the abscissa. Response to iodoacetamide is plotted on the ordinate and represents the difference between insulin release with and without iodoacetamide at 20 mM glucose.

inhibited by mannoheptulose (Hellman et al., 1972b, c). Second, mannoheptulose apparently exerts a prompt inhibitory action on glucose-stimulated insulin release (Hellman et al., 1972a), whereas a significant inhibition of glucose oxidation was not observed until more than 15 minutes after the exposure to mannoheptulose (Sehlin, 1973). However, although mannoheptulose may be a fairly specific inhibitor of glucose recognition, it also inhibits endogenous metabolism in the islets (Hellerström, 1967). Since, in addition, phlorizin and phloretin may have several effects on cell membranes, the results observed with these compounds should be interpreted with caution. Although there is strong evidence that the beta cells are equipped with a transport system for D-glucose, there is also much to suggest that these glucose-binding sites are not identical with the recognition system for glucose as insulin secretagogue. For example, 3-*O*-methyl-D-glucose is readily transported by the same system as D-glucose in the islets of *ob/ob* mice but has no effect on insulin release from these islets (Hellman et al., 1973h). Thus several observations

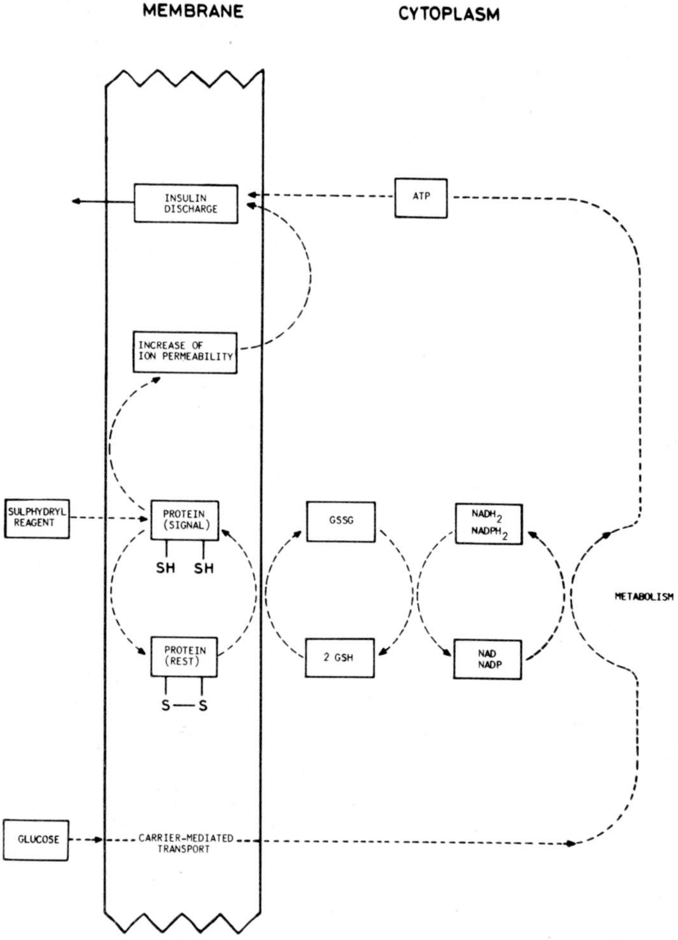

FIG. 10. Schematic illustration of a sulphydryl-disulphide bridge model for regulation of insulin release. It is speculated that the beta cell membrane contains disulphide bridges which prevent the occurrence of secretagogic ionic fluxes. These bridges can be reversibly split to sulphydryl groups, but under resting conditions the equilibrium is in favour of the disulphide bridge. Insulin release is envisaged as resulting from a shift of equilibrium away from the disulphide bridge state. Such a shift might result from the blockade of sulphydryl groups by sulphydryl reagents or from the production of reduced pyridine nucleotides in glucose metabolism. The effect of pyridine nucleotides may be mediated by glutathione, since it is recognized that sulphydryl compounds are the most specific reagents for the reduction of protein disulphide groups.

support the idea that glucose stimulates insulin release by virtue of its metabolism in the beta cells, while at least in the *ob/ob* mice there is so far less evidence for secretagogue receptors for the glucose molecule as such.

A COMPREHENSIVE MODEL FOR THE RECOGNITION OF SULPHYDRYL REAGENTS AND OF GLUCOSE

Electrophysiological studies suggest that insulin secretagogues directly or indirectly change the conformation of the beta cell membrane, resulting in altered ionic fluxes that in turn activate the mechanism for insulin discharge (Matthews and Dean, 1970). It is conceivable that sulphydryl groups play a role in the regulation of ionic fluxes and that the secretagogic effect of sulphydryl reagents is due to an interaction with these groups. Schwartz et al. (1960) discussed in general terms how the flux of Na^+ may depend on sulphydryl-disulphide interchanges in biological membranes. As a guide to our further work, we have considered the as yet highly speculative possibility of ion permeability in beta cells being dependent on the redox equilibrium between sulphydryl groups and disulphide bridges. In such a model, sulphydryl reagents may enhance insulin release by shifting the equilibrium away from the disulphide bridge conformation, which is assumed to be associated with a resting state of the beta cells (Fig. 10).

There is no experimental evidence for the existence in the beta cells of such a regulatory protein as depicted in Figure 10. Therefore the model may appear unnecessarily complex in comparison with the alternative possibility of the secretory signal depending only on the reaction of sulphydryl reagent with specific sulphydryl groups. However, because insulin release can be stimulated by sulphydryl reagents with different modes of reaction, the secretagogic effect may not be caused by a specific type of reaction but more probably results from the mere blockade of certain groups. Moreover, we feel that our scheme can well incorporate the idea that glucose is recognized as an insulin secretagogue by virtue of its metabolism. One result of glucose metabolism in the beta cells is the rapid and striking increase of reduced pyridine nucleotides (Panten et al., 1971). This might provide the reductive potential necessary for the sulphydryl-disulphide bridge model to work as a physiological mechanism. Ammon and Steinke (1972) suggested that NADPH plays an important role in insulin release by keeping glutathione in a reduced state. Because reduced glutathione is a potent reductant of protein disulphides, we have included it in Figure 10, although the possibility of more specific and enzyme-catalyzed reactions is not excluded.

REFERENCES

AMMON, H. P. T. and STEINKE, J. (1972): 6-Aminonicotinamide (6-AN) as a diabetogenic agent. In vitro and in vivo studies in the rat. *Diabetes, 21,* 143.

ASHCROFT, S. J. H., BASSETT, J. M. and RANDLE, P. J. (1972): Insulin secretion mechanisms and glucose metabolism in isolated islets. *Diabetes, 21,* 538.

ASHCROFT, S. J. H., WEERASINGHE, L. C. C. and RANDLE, P. J. (1973): Interrelationship of islet metabolism, adenosine triphosphate content and insulin release. *Biochem. J., 132,* 223.

BLOOM, G. D., HELLMAN, B., IDAHL, L.-Å LERNMARK, Å., SEHLIN, J. and TÄLJEDAL, I.-B. (1972): Effects of organic mercurials on mammalian pancreatic β-cells. *Biochem. J., 129,* 241.

BOQUIST, L., HELLMAN, B., LERNMARK, Å. and TÄLJEDAL, I.-B. (1974): Influence of the mutation 'diabetes' on insulin release and islet morphology in mice of different genetic backgrounds. Submitted for publication.

CABANTCHIK, Z. I. and ROTHSTEIN, A. (1972): The nature of the membrane sites controlling anion permeability of human red blood cells as determined by studies with disulfonic stilbene derivatives. *J. Membrane Biol., 10,* 311.

CERASI, E. and LUFT, R. (1970): Diabetes mellitus – a disorder of cellular information transmission. *Hormone metabol. Res., 2,* 246.

CHRISTENSEN, H. N. and CULLEN, A. M. (1969): Behaviour in the rat of a transport-specific bicyclic amino acid. *J. biol. Chem., 244,* 1521.

COORE, H. G. and RANDLE, P. J. (1964): Regulation of insulin secretion studied with pieces of rabbit pancreas incubated in vitro. *Biochem. J., 93,* 66.

CURRY, D. L. (1971): Is there a common beta cell insulin compartment stimulated by glucose and tolbutamide? *Amer. J. Physiol., 220,* 319.

DEAN, P. M. and MATTHEWS, E. K. (1972): The bioelectric properties of pancreatic islet cells. Effect of diabetogenic agents. *Diabetologia, 8,* 173.

GABBAY, K. H. and TZE, W. J. (1972): Inhibition of glucose-induced insulin release by aldose reductase inhibitors. *Proc. nat. Acad. Sci. U.S.A., 69,* 1435.

GOLDFINE, I. D., ROTH, J. and BIRNBAUMER, L. (1972): Glucagon receptors in β-cells. Binding of ^{125}I-glucagon and activation of adenylate cyclase. *J. biol. Chem., 247,* 1211.

GRODSKY, G. M., BATTS, A. A., BENNETT, L. L., VCELLA, C., McWILLIAMS, N. B. and SMITH, D. F. (1963): Effects of carbohydrates on secretion of insulin from isolated rat pancreas. *Amer. J. Physiol., 205,* 638.

GRASETTI, D. R. (1969): Some biochemical effects of thione-forming disulfides and their use in the study of cell thiols. *Ann. Ist. Sup. Sanità, 5,* 645.

GRASETTI, D. R. and MURRAY Jr., J. F. (1970): Modification of external sulfhydryl groups of Ehrlich ascites tumor cells with 6,6′-dithiodinicotinic acid. *Biochem. Pharmacol., 19,* 1836.

HELLERSTRÖM, C. (1967): Effects of carbohydrates on the oxygen consumption of isolated pancreatic islets of mice. *Endocrinology, 81,* 105.

HELLMAN, B. (1970): Methodological approaches to studies on the pancreatic islets. *Diabetologia, 6,* 110.

HELLMAN, B. (1974): Factors affecting the uptake of glibenclamide in microdissected pancreatic islets rich in β-cells. *Pharmacology,* in press.

HELLMAN, B., IDAHL, L.-Å., LERNMARK, Å., SEHLIN, J., SIMON, E. and TÄLJEDAL, I.-B. (1972a): The pancreatic β-cell recognition of insulin secretagogues. I. Transport of mannoheptulose and the dynamics of insulin release. *Molec. Pharmacol., 8,* 1.

HELLMAN, B., IDAHL, L.-Å., LERNMARK, Å., SEHLIN. J. and TÄLJEDAL, I.-B. (1973a): Iodoacetamide-induced sensitization of the pancreatic β-cells to glucose stimulation. *Biochem. J., 132,* 775.

HELLMAN, B., IDAHL, L.-Å., LERNMARK, Å., SEHLIN, J. and TÄLJEDAL, I.-B. (1973b): Role of thiol groups in insulin release: studies with poorly permeating disulphides. *Molec. Pharmacol., 9,* 792.

HELLMAN, B., IDAHL, L.-Å., LERNMARK, Å., SEHLIN, J. and TÄLJEDAL, I.-B. (1973c): Stimulation and inhibition of insulin release by a probe of plasma membrane. *J. Membrane Biol., 14,* 135.

HELLMAN, B., IDAHL, L.-Å., LERNMARK, Å., SEHLIN, J. and TÄLJEDAL, I.-B. (1973d): The pancreatic β-cell recognition of insulin secretagogues. VIII. Comparisons of glucose with glyceraldehyde isomers and dihydroxyacetone. *Arch. Biochem. Biophys.,* in press.

HELLMAN, B., LERNMARK, Å., SEHLIN, J., SODERBERG, M. and TÄLJEDAL, I.-B. (1973e): The pancreatic β-cell recognition of insulin secretagogues. VII. Binding and permeation of chloromercuribenzene-*P*-sulphonic acid into the plasma membrane of pancreatic β-cells. *Arch. Biochem. Biophys., 158,* 435.

HELLMAN, B., LERNMARK, Å., SEHLIN, J. and TÄLJEDAL, I.-B. (1972b): Effects of phlorizin on metabolism and function of pancreatic β-cell. *Metabolism, 21,* 60.

HELLMAN, B., LERNMARK, Å., SEHLIN, J. and TÄLJEDAL, I.-B. (1972c): The pancreatic β-cell recognition of insulin secretagogues. V. Binding and stimulatory action of phlorizin. *Molec. Pharmacol., 8,* 759.

HELLMAN, B., LERNMARK, Å., SEHLIN, J. and TÄLJEDAL, I.-B. (1973f): The pancreatic β-cell recognition of insulin secretagogues. VI. Inhibitory effects of a membrane probe on the islet uptake and insulin-releasing action of glibenclamide. *FEBS Letters, 34,* 347.

HELLMAN, B., LERNMARK, Å., SEHLIN, J., TÄLJEDAL, I.-B. and WHISTLER, R. L. (1973g): The pancreatic β-cell recognition of insulin secretagogues. III. Effects of substituting sulphur for oxygen in the D-glucose molecule. *Biochem. Pharmacol., 22,* 29.

HELLMAN, B., SEHLIN, J. and TÄLJEDAL, I.-B. (1971): The pancreatic β-cell recognition of insulin secretagogues. II. Site of action of tulbutamide. *Biochem. biophys. Res. Commun., 45,* 1384.

HELLMAN, B., SEHLIN, J. and TÄLJEDAL, I.-B. (1973h): Transport of 3-O-methyl-D-glucose into mammalian pancreatic β-cells. *Pflügers Arch. ges. Physiol., 340,* 51.

HELLMAN, B., SEHLIN, J. and TÄLJEDAL, I.-B. (1973i): The pancreatic β-cell recognition of insulin secretagogues. IV. Islet uptake of sulfonylureas. *Diabetologia, 9,* 210.

IDAHL, L.-Å. (1973): Dynamics of pancreatic β-cell responses to glucose. *Diabetologia, 9,* 403.

KNAUF, P. A. and ROTHSTEIN, A. (1971a): Chemical modification of membranes. I. Effects of sulfhydryl and amino reactive reagents on anion and cation permeability of the human red blood cell. *J. gen. Physiol., 58,* 190.

KNAUF, P. A. and ROTHSTEIN, A. (1971b): Chemical modification of membranes. II. Permeation paths for sulfhydryl agents. *J. gen. Physiol., 58,* 211.

MADDY, A. H. (1964): A fluorescent label for the outer components of the plasma membrane. *Biochim. biophys. Acta (Amst.), 88,* 390.

MARINETTI, G. V. and GRAY, G. M. (1967): A fluorescent chemical marker for the liver cell plasma membrane. *Biochim. biophys. Acta (Amst.), 135,* 580.

MATSCHINSKY, F. M., LANDGRAF, R., ELLERMAN, J. and KOTLER-BRAJTBURG, J. (1972): Glucoreceptor mechanisms in islets of Langerhans. *Diabetes, 21,* 555.

MATTHEWS, E. K. and DEAN, P. M. (1970): Electrical activity in islet cells. In: *The Structure and Metabolism of the Pancreatic Islets,* Vol. 2, pp. 305-313. Editors: S. Falkmer, B. Hellman and I.-B. Täliedal. Pergamon Press, Oxford.

PANTEN, U., DAL RI, H., POSER, W. and HASSELBLATT, A. (1971): Eine Methode der Gewebsumströmung für Fluoreszenzmessungen. *Pflügers Arch. ges. Physiol., 323,* 86.

ROTHSTEIN, A. (1970): Sulfhydryl groups in membrane structure and function. In: *Current Topies in Membranes and Transport, pp. 135–176. Editors: F. Bronner and A. Kleinzeller. Axademie Press, New York, N.Y.*

SCHWARTZ, I. L., RASMUSSEN, H., SCHOESSLER, M. A., SILVER, L. and FONG, C. T. O. (1960): Relation of chemical attachment to physiological action of vasopressin. *Proc. nat. Acad. Sci. U.S.A., 46,* 1288.

SEHLIN, J. (1973): Effects of mannoheptulose on the dynamics of glucose oxidation in the pancreatic β-cells. *FEBS Letters, 30,* 45.

THOMAS, L., KINNE, R. and FROHNERT, P. P. (1972): N-Ethylmaleimide labeling of a phlorizin-sensitive D-glucose binding site of brush border membrane from the rat kidney. *Biochim. biophys. Acta (Amst.), 290,* 125.

ROLE OF BETA CELL MEMBRANE IN INSULIN SECRETION*

ANDRÉ E. LAMBERT, JEAN-CLAUDE HENQUIN** and LELIO ORCI

Unité de Diabète et Croissance, University Hospital St Pierre, Louvain, Belgium, and Institutes of Histology and Clinical Biochemistry, University of Geneva, Switzerland

Whether insulinotropic agents initiate secretion by a direct effect or indirectly through changes in the level of a particular metabolite or cofactor remains an open question. The latter hypothesis has been widely accepted over the last few years. It seems, however, reasonable to assume that the beta cell is equipped with a system which recognizes and discriminates insulinotropic agents. This recognition would initiate a series of sequential reactions that finally lead to the extrusion of secretory granules. On the basis of experiments showing that glucose may stimulate insulin secretion prior to any detectable change in the level of its metabolites, Matschinsky et al. (1971) have recently proposed that the glucose molecule itself may exert its stimulant action by activating specific membrane receptors. On the other hand, Hales and Milner (1968) have postulated that exchanges of specific cations through the beta cell membrane might be involved in the facilitation of insulin secretion.

The present study attempts to evaluate further the role of beta cell membrane in the insulin-releasing mechanisms. We shall summarize the results of experiments dealing firstly with the effect of modifications in cell membrane structure induced by a proteolytic enzyme on insulin release, and secondly with the effects of extracellular sodium and potassium on the kinetics of insulin secretion.

MATERIAL AND METHODS

Isolated islets

All experiments were performed with isolated islets of Langerhans. They were obtained by collagenase digestion (Lacy and Kostianovsky, 1967; Lacy et al., 1972) of pancreas removed from fed male albino rats, weighing 225 to 300 g.

Incubation and perifusion media

All incubations and perifusions were carried out in a Krebs-Ringer bicarbonate buffer

* These studies were supported by grant 20029 from the Fonds de la Recherche Scientifique Médicale, Brussels (Belgium).

** Aspirant of the Fonds National de la Recherche Scientifique, Brussels, Belgium.

(KRB) supplemented with bovine serum albumin (0.5 and 1%, w/v, respectively for perifusions and incubations) and 50 mg glucose/100 ml. KRB was equilibrated against a mixture of O_2/CO_2 (94/6). Unless otherwise specified, the medium had the following ionic composition (in mM): Na^+ 143.3, K^+ 6.0, Ca^{++} 2.5, Mg^{++} 1.2, Cl^- 126.0, $PO_4H_2^{--}$ 1.2, SO_4^{--} 1.2 and CO_3H^- 24.6. Calcium-depleted medium was prepared by omitting calcium chloride; 1 mM EGTA (ethylene glycol bis tetra acetic acid) was also added for incubation experiments. Total calcium content measured in this medium was less than 0.03 mM. When the effect of an excess K^+ was studied, KCl was added and NaCl was decreased as required to maintain isotonicity. In experiments designed to study the effect of the absence of extracellular Na^+, this cation was totally replaced by choline$^+$. A residual amount of 1 mM Na^+ was measured; it was probably due to contamination by Na^+ of the preparation of albumin used.

Incubation experiments

Pools of islets were first preincubated at 37°C during 90 minutes in 5 ml KRB alone or with different concentrations (0.8 to 500 μg/ml) of pronase E (70,000 PUK/g, Merck A.G., Darmstadt). Thereafter, the islets were placed in a Petri dish containing prewarmed KRB and repeatedly washed. Groups of 5 islets were transferred into glass tubes containing 1.5 ml KRB with the appropriate concentration of glucose. The tubes were carefully gassed and stoppered before starting a 30–90 min. incubation period at 37°C.

Perifusion experiments

The perifusion system utilized for these experiments is similar to that previously described by Burr et al. (1970). Two groups of 27 islets were placed in the twin-perifusion chambers (volume 0.8 ml), through which a double-channel peristaltic pump conveyed KRB at a constant rate of 2.8 ml/min. The dead volume of the system was 2 ml. Temperature of the medium in reservoir flasks, connecting tubing and chambers, was constantly maintained at 38°C by thermostatic control of the temperature of surrounding water. Continuous gassing of the perifusate with a mixture of O_2/CO_2 (94/6) maintained pH at 7.4 (± 0.05) throughout the experiment. The effluent, collected at 30 to 180 seconds intervals, was rapidly frozen until assay. An equilibration period of 25 minutes preceded a stimulation period starting at minute 0, by a square-wave change in the concentration of glucose to 300 mg/100 ml and/or of the cation tested. In each experiment, one chamber served as a control for the other chamber where the experimental modification of the medium was studied.

Insulin secretion

Immunoreactive insulin (IRI) released in the medium was measured by a double antibody radioimmunoassay (Hales and Randle, 1963) against purified rat insulin (20 U/mg) as standard. Results are expressed as ng secreted IRI per 5 islets over the considered period of incubation or as ng per minute per 27 islets for perifusion experiments.

The total amount of IRI released by perifused islets was estimated during the early (min. 0.5–5.5) and late (min. 5.5–40) phases of glucose-induced secretion and during the response to 24 mM K^+ (min. 0.5–12); it was obtained by summation of all secretion rates (in ng/min.) measured in the successive fractions and multiplied by the time of collection (in min.). From each individual secretion rate the basal rate of IRI release was first subtracted, and determined as the mean of the 3 last measurements during the equilibration period. Negative values of total IRI output calculated in some experiments reflect the fact that IRI secretion rate continued to decline with time after the end of the equilibration period. Statistical significance of differences between means of experimental and control groups was assessed by Student's t test (for paired data in the case of perifusions).

RESULTS AND DISCUSSION

Effect of pronase upon IRI secretion

The rapid destruction of insulin by pronase required initial preincubation of the islets with the enzyme and its removal by careful washing, before studying its effects on IRI secretion. Preincubation of islets with pronase concentrations between 2 and 20 μg/ml enhanced IRI secretion induced by 300 mg glucose/100 ml without major effect upon basal IRI release (50 mg glucose/100 ml). Pronase concentrations equal to or higher than 100 μg/ml markedly increased basal IRI output and concomitantly diminished the net effect of glucose upon IRI secretion (Fig. 1).

A square-wave increase of glucose concentration from 50 to 300 mg/100 ml induced a biphasic pattern of IRI secretion from perifused control islets analogous to that described by Grodsky et al. (1968) in the perfused rat pancreas (Fig. 2). The amplitude of the first phase of release was always reduced in control islets preincubated for 90 minutes as compared with islets perifused immediately after isolation. When glucose concentration was decreased to 50 mg/100 ml, IRI release returned towards basal levels within 15 minutes. A second glucose stimulation induced a similar pattern of secretion though the early phase was clearly higher than that observed during the first stimulation.

Pretreatment of the islets with a *low pronase concentration* (4 μg/ml) slightly in-

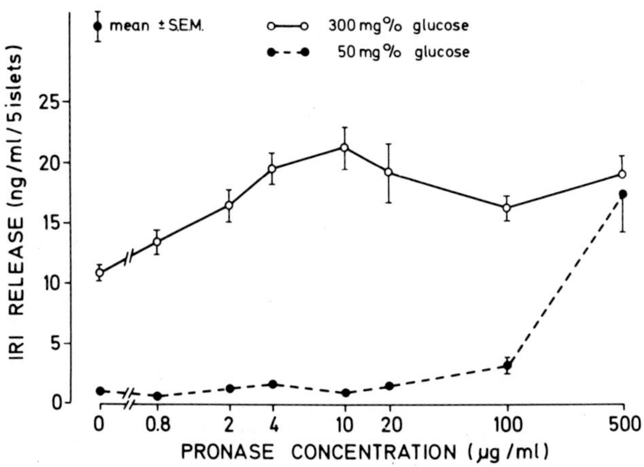

FIG. 1. IRI secretion by islets preincubated with different concentrations of pronase and incubated during 30 minutes in the presence of 50 or 300 mg glucose/100 ml. Each point represents the mean (± S.E.M.) of 14 or more determinations.

creased basal IRI output in the presence of 50 mg glucose/100 ml. It markedly enhanced both the early and late secretory responses to 300 mg glucose/100 ml (Fig. 2). Total IRI output during the early and late phases of secretion was increased by about 300 and 40%, respectively, after preincubation with pronase. Both phases were still enhanced during the second glucose stimulation (Fig. 2). Pretreatment with 4 μg pronase/ml potentiated the

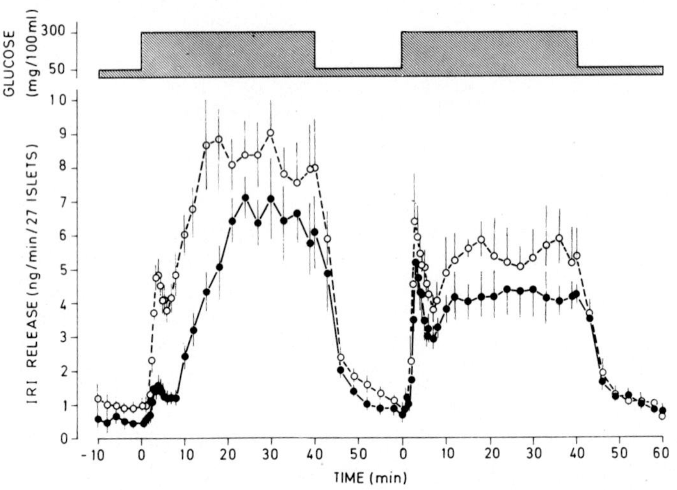

FIG. 2. Profiles of IRI release by control islets (●———●) and islets pretreated with 4 μg pronase/ml (○----○) in response to 2 successive square-wave stimulations with 300 mg glucose/100 ml, between minutes 0 and 40. Only the 10 last minutes of the equilibration period are shown. Each point represents the mean (± S.E.M.) of 6 and 4 experiments respectively for the 1st and 2nd stimulations.

stimulant action of glucose at concentrations between 100 and 400 mg/100 ml; it also rendered beta cells more sensitive to glucose since IRI release from pronase-treated islets was stimulated by 50 mg glucose/ml which had normally no effect (Lambert et al., 1974c).

When incubation was carried out in the absence of extracellular calcium, glucose failed to stimulate IRI secretion from pronase-treated islets as from control islets (Fig. 3). After preincubation in a calcium-depleted medium and incubation with calcium, the insulinotropic effect of glucose was unchanged in control islets whereas it was markedly inhibited in islets pretreated with 4 μg pronase/ml (Fig. 3).

As shown in Figure 4, basal secretion rate during the initial equilibration period was elevated in islets pretreated with a *high pronase concentration* (500 μg/ml). The rapid secretory response to 300 mg glucose/100 ml was present in pronase-treated islets whereas only a small secondary response was noted. When the glucose concentration of the medium was decreased to 50 mg/100 ml, IRI release from pronase-treated islets diminished to a low secretion rate comparable to that of the controls. A second glucose stimulation provoked a typical biphasic IRI response in islets pretreated with 500 μg pronase/ml, though both phases of secretion were markedly decreased.

After preincubation with 500 μg pronase/ml, IRI output during incubation in the presence of 50 or 300 mg glucose/ml was not inhibited in a calcium-free medium (Fig. 5).

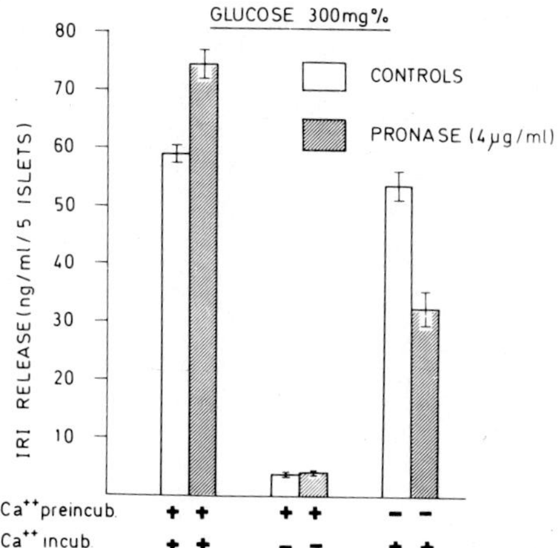

FIG. 3. Effect of the absence of Ca^{++} during preincubation or incubation upon IRI secretion, by control islets and islets pretreated with 4 μg pronase/ml. Mean values (± S.E.M.) of at least 9 determinations are shown. Incubation time: 90 min.

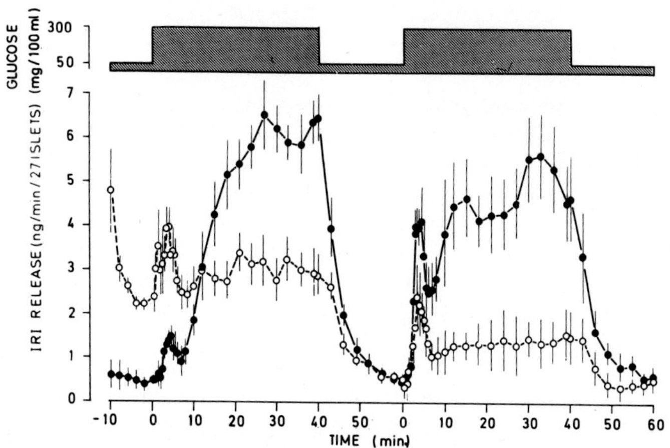

FIG. 4. Profiles of IRI release by control islets (●———●) and islets pretreated with 500 μg pronase/ml (○- - - -○) in response to 2 successive square-wave stimulations with 300 mg glucose/100 ml, between minutes 0 and 40. Only the 10 last minutes of the equilibration period are shown. Each point represents the mean (± S.E.M.) of 5 and 3 experiments respectively for the 1st and 2nd stimulations.

It may therefore represent a passive diffusion of IRI through damaged beta cell membranes. Time curve studies have shown that this leakage of IRI essentially occurred during the first 30 minutes of incubation (Lambert et al., 1974c). When pretreatment with 500 μg pronase/ml occurred in a calcium-depleted medium, basal IRI release was only slightly increased whereas glucose-induced IRI secretion was inhibited by approximately 65% as compared with the controls (Fig. 5).

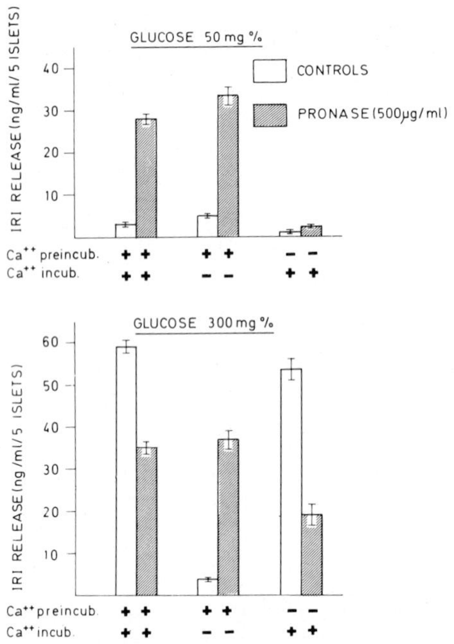

FIG. 5. Effect of the absence of Ca^{++} during preincubation or incubation upon IRI secretion, by control islets and islets pretreated with 500 μg pronase/ml. Mean values (± S.E.M.) of at least 9 determinations are shown. Incubation time: 90 min.

Pronase is a complex mixture of at least 11 different proteolytic enzymes, including both exo- and endopeptidases (Narahashi and Yanagita, 1967). Some of these enzymes are calcium-dependent, others are not (Narahashi et al., 1968). The action of pronase upon IRI secretion appears to be modulated by its concentration and the presence of calcium in the medium.

There is no evidence that preincubation with a *low pronase concentration* significantly damaged beta cells. Such pretreatment remarkably potentiated glucose-induced IRI release. These results are in agreement with studies in other tissues demonstrating that mild proteolysis may unmask a number of receptor sites which normally reside far enough within the plasma membrane to be inaccessible from the outside (Wallach, 1972). An alternative explanation would be that limited proteolytic treatment releases a small amount of glycopeptides from the most exposed portions of cell membrane glycoproteins. Such treatment by changing the electrical charges would lead to a redistribution or a clustering of these glycoproteins on the membrane surface. This would conceivably increase the probability of interactions between receptor sites and their specific activators (Singer and Nicolson, 1972). In this respect, it is interesting to note that sialic acid is probably an important component of this hypothetical glucoreceptor involved in insulin secretion. Indeed, neuraminidase treatment was recently reported to inhibit the effect of glucose upon IRI release but not the effect of some other insulinotropic agents (Maier et al., 1973). That pronase produced modifications of the beta cell membrane has been demonstrated by electron microscopy combined with the freeze-etching technique. After preincubation with 4 μg pronase/ml, a 5-fold increase in the number of tight junctions was noticed. The development of these membrane specializations was such that, after stimulation with 300 mg glucose/100 ml, it trapped secretory products within relatively closed areas of the extracellular space (Orci et al., 1973). When pretreatment with pronase was carried out in a calcium-free medium, the secretory response to glucose was decreased. These data suggest that Ca^{++}-independent enzymes present in pronase inhibited IRI secretion. This inhibitory effect could have been masked in the presence of extracellular calcium by the pronounced enhancing effect of calcium-dependent enzymes.

Pretreatment with a *high pronase concentration* has a deleterious effect upon beta cells which, however, appears reversible with time. We have elsewhere given arguments favouring the view that the effect of 500 μg pronase/ml upon the secretory response to glucose reflects the action of the enzyme on a critical step of IRI-releasing mechanisms rather than some non-specific alteration in beta cell function (Lambert et al., 1974c). The late secretory response to glucose was markedly inhibited in islets pretreated with a high pronase concentration. This correlates well with observations made in other cell types, showing that a pronounced protease action may inactivate, or even destroy, membrane receptor sites (Wallach, 1972). The early phase to a first glucose stimulation was, however, not inhibited after pronase treatment. These results indicate that the early and late phases of secretion in response to glucose might be dependent, at least in part, upon different mechanisms.

Effect of cations upon the kinetics of IRI secretion

Figure 6 shows that total removal of calcium from the perifusate completely abolished the rapid and late phases of IRI secretion induced by glucose (Table 1, lines 2 vs. 1). This corroborates the results of Grodsky and Bennett (1966), Milner and Hales (1967) and Curry et al. (1968), who demonstrated that the presence of extracellular calcium is a prerequisite for the stimulation of IRI release. In contrast, calcium is not required for glucose metabolism in islet cells (Ashcroft et al., 1970), nor for insulin synthesis (Lin and Haist, 1973; Pipeleers et al., 1973). As suggested by Malaisse (1973), the cytoplasmic concentration of Ca^{++} is thought to regulate the activity of the microtubular-microfilamentous system involved in the release of beta granules (Lacy, 1970; Orci et al., 1973). Glucose has been shown to decrease Ca^{++} efflux from the beta cell (Malaisse et al., 1973) whereas agents raising cyclic AMP levels might displace calcium from an organelle-bound pool into the cytosol (Brisson et al., 1972; Rasmussen, 1970).

As illustrated in Figure 7, total replacement of extracellular Na^+ by choline$^+$ in the presence of 50 mg glucose/100 ml provoked a rapid but transient rise in IRI secretion (Table 1, lines 4 vs. 3). When removal of Na^+ and stimulation with 300 mg glucose/100 ml occurred simultaneously (Fig. 8), the rapid secretory phase was not affected whereas the later phase was markedly diminished (Table 1, lines 6 vs. 5). This observation paralleled the electrical activity recorded in the islets under similar conditions; regular bursts of action potentials normally induced by a stimulatory concentration of glucose ceased approximately 15 minutes after removal of all extracellular Na^+ (Dean and Matthews, 1970). Equilibration of the islets in a medium deprived of Na^+ for 25 minutes reduced the effect of glucose to a small early phase (Fig. 9; Table 1, lines 8 vs. 7). This inhibition was reversible since, after restoring a normal Na^+ concentration, secretion rate returned to almost control values. However, this recuperation was not immediate but required a

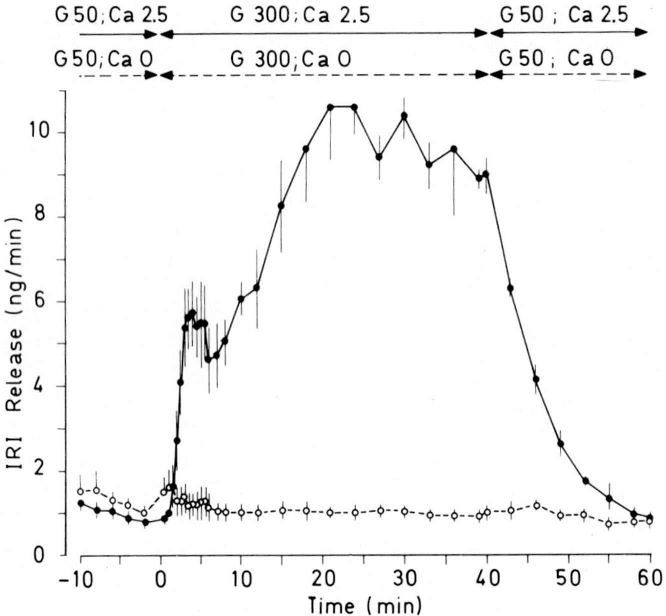

FIG. 6. Effect of the absence of calcium (Ca) on glucose (G) induced IRI secretion from perifused islets. Composition of the perifusate is shown in the upper part of the Figure. Concentrations are expressed in mg/100 ml and mM for glucose and ions respectively. Each value represents the mean (± S.E.M.) of 4 experiments.

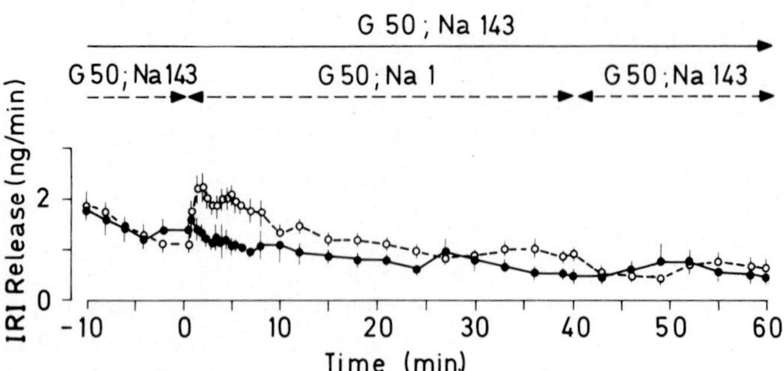

FIG. 7. Effect of the absence of sodium (Na) on IRI secretion from perifused islets. Composition of the perifusate is shown in the upper part of the Figure. Same expression of symbols as in Figure 6. Each value represents the mean (± S.E.M.) of 4 experiments. Na was replaced by choline.

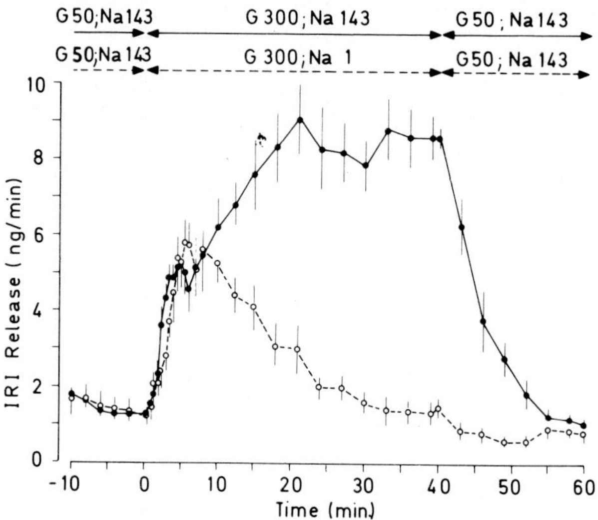

FIG. 8. Effect of the absence of sodium (Na) on glucose-induced IRI secretion from perifused islets. Composition of the perifusate is shown in the upper part of the Figure. Same expression of symbols as in Figure 6. Each value represents the mean (± S.E.M.) of 4 experiments. Na was replaced by choline.

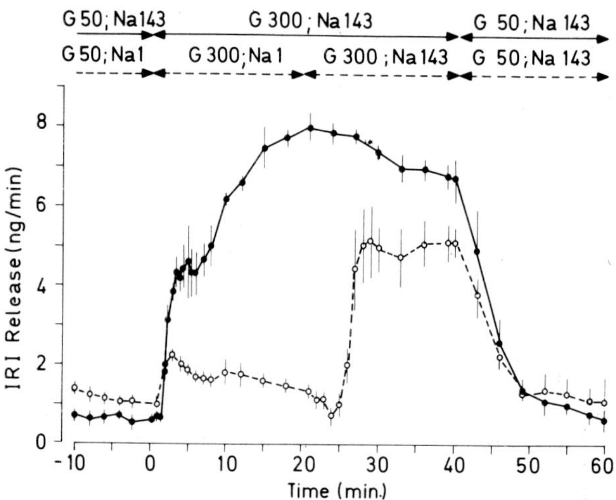

FIG. 9. Reversibility of the inhibition of glucose-induced IRI secretion observed in the absence of sodium (Na) in perifused islets. Composition of the perifusate is shown in the upper part of the Figure. Same expression of symbols as in Figure 6. Each value represents the mean (± S.E.M.) of 4 experiments. Na was replaced by choline.

TABLE 1
Effect of the absence of Ca^{++} and Na^{+} upon total IRI output during each phase of secretion

Line	Equilibration		Stimulation		IRI output (ng)			
	Glucose (mg/100 ml)	Modification (mM)	Glucose (mg/100 ml)	Modification (mM)	1st phase	P	2nd phase	P
1	50	Ca^{++} 2.5	300	Ca^{++} 2.5	17.04 ± 2.32	< 0.01	276.09 ± 20.90	< 0.005
2	50	Ca^{++} 0	300	Ca^{++} 0	0.49 ± 0.37		−7.19 ± 5.62	
3	50	Na^{+} 143	50	Na^{+} 143	−0.49 ± 0.43	< 0.005	−20.72 ± 2.44	< 0.05
4	50	Na^{+} 1	50	Na^{+} 143	4.17 ± 0.07		−1.89 ± 5.67	
5	50	Na^{+} 143	300	Na^{+} 143	12.81 ± 1.28	N.S.	228.06 ± 25.25	< 0.005
6	50	Na^{+} 1	300	Na^{+} 143	11.29 ± 1.15		48.49 ± 17.41	
7	50	Na^{+} 143	300	Na^{+} 143	17.82 ± 1.91	< 0.02	—	
8	50	Na^{+} 1	300	Na^{+} 1	4.61 ± 0.94		—	

IRI output was calculated from min. 0.5 to 5.5 and from min. 5.5 to 40, respectively for the 1st and 2nd phases of release. Each value represents the mean (± S.E.M.) of 4 experiments. P refers to statistical comparison of differences between control and experimental groups. N.S. = not significant. For details in calculation of IRI output, see under 'Material and Methods'.

delay of approximately 5 minutes (Fig. 9). A concentration of 24 mM Na^+, using choline$^+$ as substitute, did not affect either phase of glucose-induced IRI release. In contrast, replacement of Na^+ by lithium$^+$ completely abolished the effect of glucose; this inhibitory effect was, however, poorly reversible (Lambert et al., 1974a). These data indicate that an extracellular concentration of 24 mM Na^+ is sufficient for a normal secretory function of the beta cell.

Our results, showing an inhibition of IRI secretion in a Na^+-deprived medium, are in accordance with those of Hales and Milner (1968). The absence of Na^+ has also been reported to decrease glucose uptake (Hellman et al., 1971), glycolysis (Matschinsky and Ellerman, 1973), glucose oxidation (Ashcroft et al., 1972) and insulin synthesis (Pipeleers et al., 1973) in the beta cell. It seems unlikely that the partial inhibition of glucose uptake and metabolism alone accounts for the suppression of IRI release observed in the absence of Na^+. Moreover, if the only role of Na^+ was to enable glucose to enter the beta cell, one would expect an immediate IRI secretion upon restoration of a normal Na^+ concentration. The delay observed suggests that a threshold concentration of intracellular Na^+ must be regained to permit a normal secretory function. Taken as a whole, these results stressed the crucial role of intracellular Na^+ in many functions of the beta cell, and especially in insulin-releasing mechanisms.

From studies in other tissues, it was suggested that removal of Na^+ from the extracellular medium might lead to an increase in Ca^{++} influx by either of the 2 following mechanisms: a downhill efflux of Na^+ would be coupled with a pump-mediated influx of Ca^{++}; alternatively, the competitive inhibition of Ca^{++} entry, normally exerted by extracellular Na^+, could be suppressed (Baker et al., 1969). From their experiments with rabbit pancreatic slices, Hales and Milner (1968) postulated the existence of the former mechanism in the beta cell; the latter one was rather favoured by Dean and Matthews (1970) on the basis of their studies of the electrical activity measured in islet cells. Our results are compatible with either of these hypotheses and suggest that changes in Ca^{++} influx play some role in the regulation of insulin secretion.

The excess of K^+ in the extracellular fluid has been previously shown to stimulate IRI secretion (Grodsky and Bennett, 1966; Hales and Milner, 1968; Lambert et al., 1969). Figure 10 depicts the rapid burst of IRI release evoked by a square-wave increase of extracellular K^+ from 6 to 24 mM (Table 2, lines 2 vs. 1). This pattern is analogous to that recently reported by Gomez and Curry (1973) in the perfused rat pancreas. The presence of 50 mg glucose/100 ml in the perifusate increased both the amplitude and the duration of the response to 24 mM K^+ (Fig. 10; Table 2). A potentiating action of 24 mM K^+ on the rapid phase of IRI release induced by 300 mg glucose/100 ml was also noticed (Henquin and Lambert, 1974b). Blockade of the Na^+ pump by 0.1 mM ouabain (Howell and Taylor, 1968) inhibited the IRI output in response to 24 mM K^+ by about 45% (Fig. 11, Table 2, lines 6 vs. 5). The effect of K^+ was markedly reduced in the absence of Na^+ (Fig. 12, Table 2, lines 8 vs. 7) whereas it was totally abolished in a calcium-depleted medium (Fig. 12, Table 2, lines 10 vs. 9).

An elevation of extracellular K^+ to 23.5 mM in a medium containing 2.8 mM glucose was followed by depolarization in islet cells without induction of action potentials (Dean and Matthews, 1970). K^+-induced depolarization is known to increase membrane permeability to various cations, in particular to Ca^{++} and, perhaps, to Na^+ (Van Breemen et al., 1973). Such cationic movement might trigger IRI secretion in a medium containing Na^+ and Ca^{++}. The suppression of K^+-induced IRI release observed in the absence of Ca^{++} is in agreement with this hypothetical mechanism. The inhibition of the secretory

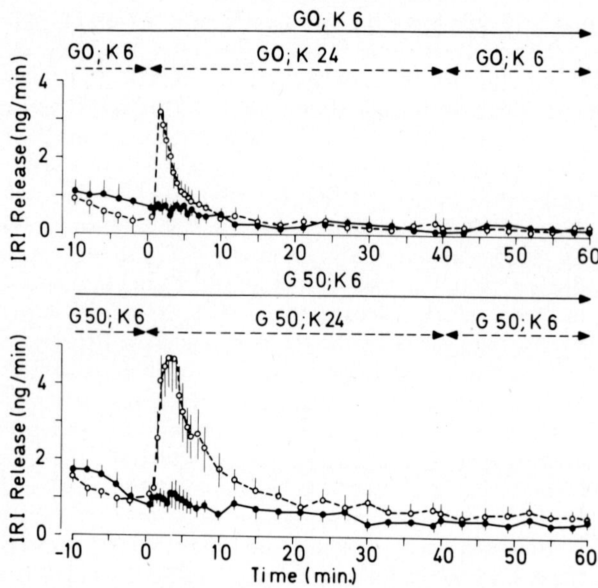

FIG. 10. Effect of 24 mM potassium (K) upon IRI secretion from perifused islets, in the absence of glucose (G0, upper panel) or in the presence of 50 mg glucose/100 ml (G50, lower panel). Composition of the perifusate is shown in the upper part of the Figure. Same expression of symbols as in Figure 6. Each value represents the mean (± S.E.M.) of 5 and 7 experiments.

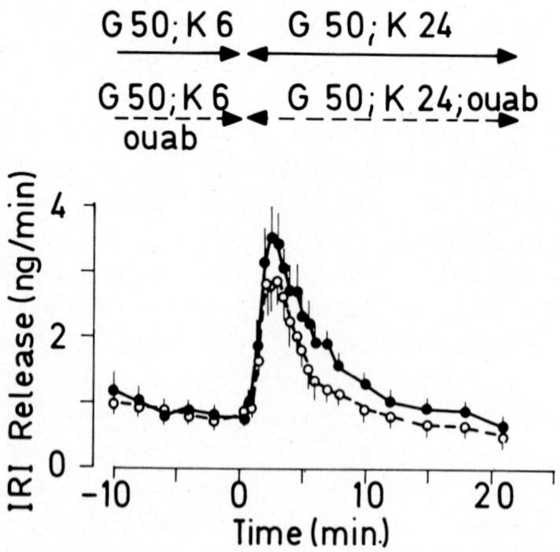

FIG. 11. Effect of 0.1 mM ouabain (ouab) on K-induced IRI secretion from perifused islets. Composition of the perifusate is shown in the upper part of the Figure. Same expression of symbols as in Figure 6. Each value represents the mean (± S.E.M.) of 5 experiments.

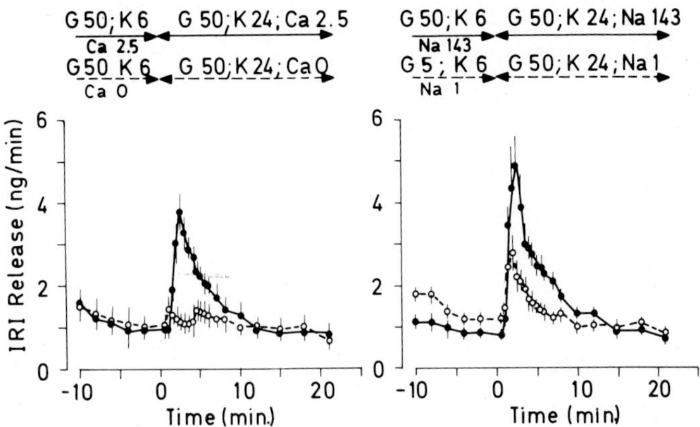

FIG. 12. Effect of the absence of calcium (Ca) or sodium (Na) on K-induced IRI secretion from perifused islets. Composition of the perifusate is shown in the upper part of the Figure. Same expression of symbols as in Figure 6. Each value represents the mean (± S.E.M.) of 5 and 4 experiments.

response to K^+ in a Na^+-free medium suggests that Ca^{++} entry is less efficient in promoting IRI secretion when intracellular Na^+ is decreased. The ionic and electrical modifications induced by a blockade of the Na^+-pump with ouabain might create a certain refractoriness to the effect of 24 mM K^+. This is in contrast with the slight enhancement of the rapid phase of glucose-induced IRI secretion observed in the presence of ouabain (Lambert et al., 1974b) or in the absence of extracellular K^+ (Henquin and Lambert, 1974a).

SUMMARY AND CONCLUSIONS

Alterations in the structure of beta cell membrane induced by pronase modified the responsiveness of insulin-releasing mechanisms to glucose. These experimental data support the concept that membrane receptor sites are implicated in an early step of the sequence of events leading to insulin secretion. Dynamic studies of insulin release from islets perifused with media of different Na^+ and K^+ concentrations emphasize the importance of intracellular Na^+ in the secretion process. They also favour the hypothesis that changes in Ca^{++} influx play a role in the stimulus-secretion coupling.

ACKNOWLEDGEMENTS

The skilful technical assistance of Mrs De Bie-Horemans, Miss J. Verniers and Mr. V. E. De Coster is acknowledged. We thank Mrs M. Verpoorten-Detaille for secretarial help.

TABLE 2

Total IRI output during K^+-induced IRI release

Line	n	Equilibration			Stimulation			IRI output (ng)	P
		Glucose (mg/100 ml)	K^+ (mM)	Modification (mM)	Glucose (mg/100 ml)	K^+ (mM)	Modification (mM)		
1	(5)	0	6	–	0	6	–	-2.75 ± 1.55	
2	(5)	0	6	–	0	24	–	7.65 ± 0.78	vs. 1 < 0.05
3	(7)	50	6	–	50	6	–	-0.90 ± 0.74	vs. 4 < 0.02
4	(7)	50	6	–	50	24	–	16.14 ± 4.58	vs. 2 N.S.
5	(5)	50	6	–	50	24	–	13.56 ± 2.32	vs. 2 < 0.05
6	(5)	50	6	Ouabain 0.1	50	24	Ouabain 0.1	7.53 ± 1.93	vs. 5 < 0.05
7	(5)	50	6	Na^+ 143	50	24	Na^+ 125	15.92 ± 3.01	vs. 2 < 0.05
8	(5)	50	6	Na^+ 1	50	24	Na^+ 1	2.21 ± 0.39	vs. 7 < 0.01
9	(4)	50	6	Ca^{++} 2.5	50	24	Ca^{++} 2.5	11.65 ± 0.60	vs. 2 < 0.01
10	(4)	50	6	Ca^{++} 0	50	24	Ca^{++} 0	1.42 ± 0.28	vs. 9 < 0.001

IRI output was calculated from min. 0.5 to 12. Each value represents the mean (± S.E.M.) of (n) experiments. Statistical comparison (P) of differences between 2 groups is indicated by vs. line No of the second group. N.S. = not significant. For details in calculation of IRI output, see under 'Material and Methods'.

REFERENCES

ASHCROFT, S. J. H., BASSETT, J. H. and RANDLE, P. J. (1972): Insulin secretion mechanisms and glucose metabolism in isolated islets. *Diabetes, 21/Suppl. 2,* 538.

ASHCROFT, S. J. H., HEDESKOV, C. J. and RANDLE, P. J. (1970): Glucose metabolism in mouse pancreatic islets. *Biochem. J., 118,* 143.

BAKER, P. F., BLAUSTEIN, M. P., HODGKIN, A. L. and STEINHARDT, R. A. (1969): The influence of calcium on sodium efflux in squid axons. *J. Physiol., 200,* 431.

BRISSON, G. R., MALAISSE-LAGAE, F. and MALAISSE, W. J. (1972): The stimulus-secretion coupling of glucose-induced insulin release. VII. A proposed site of action for adenosine-3′,5′-cyclic monophosphate. *J. clin. Invest., 51,* 232.

BURR, I. M., BALANT, L., STAUFFACHER, W. and RENOLD, A. E. (1970): Perifusion of rat pancreatic tissue in vitro: substrate modification of theophylline-induced biphasic insulin release. *J. clin. Invest., 49,* 2097.

CURRY, D. L., BENNETT, L. L. and GRODSKY, G. M. (1968): Requirement for calcium ion in insulin secretion by the perfused rat pancreas. *Amer. J. Physiol., 214,* 174.

DEAN, P. M. and MATTHEWS, E. K. (1970): Electrical activity in pancreatic islet cells: effect of ions. *J. Physiol., 210,* 265.

GOMEZ, M. and CURRY, D. L. (1973): Potassium stimulation of insulin release by the perfused rat pancreas. *Endocrinology, 92,* 1126.

GRODSKY, G. M. and BENNETT, L. L. (1966): Cation requirements for insulin secretion in the isolated perfused pancreas. *Diabetes, 15,* 910.

GRODSKY, G. M., CURRY, D. L., BENNETT, L. L. and RODRIGO, J. J. (1968): Factors influencing different rates of insulin release in vitro. *Acta diabet. lat., 5/Suppl. 1,* 140.

HALES, C. N. and MILNER, R. D. G. (1968): The role of sodium and potassium in insulin secretion from rabbit pancreas. *J. Physiol., 194,* 725.

HALES, C. N. and RANDLE, P. J. (1963): Immunoassay of insulin with insulin-antibody precipitate. *Biochem. J., 88,* 137.

HELLMAN, B., SEHLIN, J. and TÄLJEDAL, I. B. (1971): Stereospecific glucose uptake by pancreatic β cells. *Hormone metabol. Res., 3,* 219.

HENQUIN, J. C. and LAMBERT, A. E. (1974a): Cationic environment and dynamics of insulin secretion. II. Effect of the absence of potassium. Submitted for publication.

HENQUIN, J. C. and LAMBERT, A. E. (1974b): Cationic environment and dynamics of insulin secretions. III. Effect of a high concentration of potassium. Submitted for publication.

HOWELL, S. L. and TAYLOR, K. W. (1968): Potassium ions and the secretion of insulin by islets of Langerhans incubated in vitro. *Biochem. J., 108,* 17.

LACY, P. E. (1970): Beta cell secretion – from the standpoint of a pathobiologist. *Diabetes, 19,* 895.

LACY, P. E. and KOSTIANOVSKY, M. (1967): Method for the isolation of intact islets of Langerhans from the rat pancreas. *Diabetes, 16,* 35.

LACY, P. E., WALKER, M. M. and FINK, C. J. (1972): Perifusion of isolated rat islets in vitro. Participation of the microtubular system in the biphasic release of insulin. *Diabetes, 21,* 987.

LAMBERT, A. E., HENQUIN, J. C. and MALVAUX, P. (1974a): Cationic environment and dynamics of insulin secretion. I. Effect of low concentrations of sodium. Submitted for publication.

LAMBERT, A. E., HENQUIN, J. C. and MALVAUX, P. (1974b): Cationic environment and dynamics of insulin secretion. IV. Effect of ouabain. Submitted for publication.

LAMBERT, A. E., HENQUIN, J. C., ORCI, L. and RENOLD, A. E. (1974c): Enzyme-induced modifications of beta cell function. I. Effect of pronase on insulin secretion. Submitted for publication.

LAMBERT, A. E., JEANRENAUD, B., JUNOD, A. and RENOLD, A. E. (1969): Organ culture of fetal rat pancreas. II. Insulin release induced by amino and organic acids, by hormonal peptides, by cationic alterations of the medium and by other agents. *Biochim. biophys. Acta (Amst.), 174,* 540.

LIN, B. J. and HAIST, R. E. (1973): Effects of some modifiers of insulin secretion on insulin biosynthesis. *Endocrinology, 92,* 735.

MAIER, V., HINZ, M., SCHATZ, H., NIERLE, C. and PFEIFFER, E. F. (1973): Evidence for a specific glucose receptor by removal of sialic acid from isolated pancreatic islets of mice. *Diabetologia, 9,* 80.

MALAISSE, W. J. (1973): Insulin secretion: Multifactorial regulation for a single process of release. *Diabetologia, 9,* 167.

MALAISSE, W. J., BRISSON, G. R. and BAIRD, L. E. (1973): Stimulus-secretion coupling of glucose-induced insulin release. X. Effect of glucose on ^{45}Ca efflux from perifused islets. *Amer. J. Physiol., 224,* 389.

MATSCHINSKY, F. M. and ELLERMAN, J. (1973): Dissociation of the insulin releasing and the metabolic functions of hexoses in islets of Langerhans. *Biochem. biophys. Res. Commun., 50,* 193.

MATSCHINSKY, F. M., ELLERMAN, J. E., KRZANOWSKY, J., KOTLER-BRAJTBURG, J., LANDGRAF, R. and FERTEL, R. (1971): The dual function of glucose in islets of Langerhans. *J. biol. Chem., 246,* 1007.

MILNER, R. D. G. and HALES, C. N. (1967): The role of calcium and magnesium in insulin secretion from rabbit pancreas studied in vitro. *Diabetologia, 3,* 47.

NARAHASHI, Y., SHIBUYA, K. and YANAGITA, M. (1968): Studies on proteolytic enzymes (pronase) of *Streptomyces Griseus* K-1. II. Separation of exo- and endopeptidases of pronase. *J. Biochem., 64,* 427.

NARAHASHI, Y. and YANAGITA, M. (1967): Studies on proteolytic enzymes (pronase) of *Streptomyces Griseus* K-1. I. Nature and properties of the proteolytic enzyme system. *J. Biochem., 62,* 633.

ORCI, L., AMHERDT, M., HENQUIN, J. C., LAMBERT, A. E., UNGER, R. H. and RENOLD, A. E. (1973): Pronase effect on pancreatic beta cell secretion and morphology. *Science, 180,* 647.

ORCI, L., AMHERDT, M., MALAISSE-LAGAE, F., ROUILLER, C. and RENOLD, A. E. (1973): Insulin release by emiocytosis: Demonstration with freeze-etching technique. *Science, 179,* 82.

PIPELEERS, D. G., MARICHAL, M. and MALAISSE, W. J. (1973): Metabolic, cationic and pharmacological influences on insulin biosynthesis. *Diabetologia, 9,* 86.

RASMUSSEN, H. (1970): Cell communication, calcium ion and cyclic adenosine monophosphate. *Science, 170,* 404.

SINGER, S. J. and NICOLSON, G. L. (1972): The fluid mosaic model of the structure of cell membranes. *Science, 175,* 720.

VAN BREEMEN, C., FARINAS, B. R., CASTEELS, R., GERBA, P., WUYTACK, F. and DETH, R. (1973): Factors controlling cytoplasmic Ca^{2+} concentration. *Phil. Trans. B, 265,* 57.

WALLACH, D. F. H. (1972): The disposition of proteins in the plasma membranes of animal cells: Analytical approaches using controlled peptidolysis and protein labels. *Biochim. biophys. Acta (Amst.), 265,* 61.

THE ROLE OF CATIONS IN INSULIN SYNTHESIS AND RELEASE*

W. J. MALAISSE and D. G. PIPELEERS**

Laboratory of Experimental Medicine, Brussels University, Brussels, Belgium

The cationic composition of the extracellular medium bathing the beta cell exerts a marked influence on the magnitude of the insular biosynthetic and secretory response to various metabolic, hormonal and pharmacological agents. In this paper, we want to summarize some aspects of our present view on the role of cations in insulin biosynthesis and release.

MATERIAL AND METHODS

The methods used for measurement of insulin release by pieces of rat pancreatic tissue (Malaisse et al., 1967b) and rat isolated islets (Malaisse et al., 1967a), the uptake of ^{45}Ca by isolated islets (Malaisse-Lagae and Malaisse, 1971), the efflux of ^{45}Ca from perifused islets (Malaisse et al., 1973a), and the biosynthesis of proinsulin and insulin by islets (Pipeleers et al., 1973a) have all been described in detail in previous publications from our laboratory.

RESULTS AND COMMENTS

Participation of divalent cations in the release process

It has been known for the last 7 years that the presence of a sufficient amount of extracellular calcium is required for glucose and other insulinotropic agents to stimulate insulin release in the beta cell (Grodsky and Bennett, 1966; Milner and Hales, 1967). More or less severe depletion of the cellular and/or pericellular calcium capital might be required to abolish the secretory response, depending on the agent or association of agents used to stimulate the beta cell (Brisson et al., 1972; Malaisse et al., 1972). Only barium is able to stimulate insulin release, at least transiently, even after prolonged

* This work was supported in part by grants from the F.R.S.M. (Brussels, Belgium) and a contract of the Ministère de la Politique Scientifique within the framework of the association Euratom-Universities of Brussels and Pisa.

** D.G.P. is a Research Fellow of the N.F.W.O. (Brussels, Belgium).

deprivation of extracellular calcium (Hales, 1970; Malaisse et al., 1973a). However, the barium-induced release of insulin may well represent a rather unphysiological process, since exposure of islets to barium in the absence of calcium is associated with a marked inhibition of glucose-induced insulin biosynthesis (Pipeleers et al., 1973b).

The ubiquitous inhibition of insulin secretion under conditions of calcium depletion suggests that calcium participates in a late and essential event in the secretory sequence. Consistent with this view is the fact that glucose oxidation and glucose-induced insulin synthesis (Fig. 1) are not inhibited in islets incubated in the absence of calcium (Ashcroft and Randle, 1969; Pipeleers et al., 1973b). The concept that calcium accumulation in a critical site of the beta cell provokes insulin release has 2 major implications (Malaisse, 1973). First, agents which either stimulate or inhibit insulin secretion should do so by altering calcium handling by the beta cell. Second, calcium should in turn trigger insulin release through a single and invariable modality. A number of observations suggest that this is indeed the case.

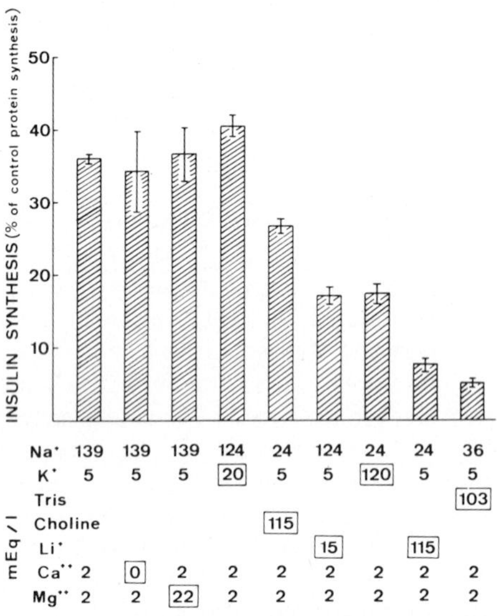

FIG. 1. Effect of cations on glucose-induced insulin synthesis by isolated islets. Mean values (± S.E.M.) are expressed as percentage of the mean value for total protein synthesis found in control media. The concentration of cations is shown as mEq/l in the lower part of the Figure, the first column corresponding to the control medium. All media contained glucose at a 16.7 mM concentration.

The influence of stimulators and inhibitors of insulin release on calcium handling by the beta cell is discussed in the next section of the present report. At this point, however, we wish to underline the fact that, if all these agents ultimately affect calcium movements in the beta cell, they may do so through a wide variety of primary mechanisms. For instance, the stimulant action of glucose on calcium net uptake by the beta cell being apparently dependent on the integrity of glucose metabolism, inhibition of glucose-induced calcium accumulation can be provoked by agents such as mannoheptulose, known to alter glucose metabolism in the islets (Malaisse-Lagae and Malaisse, 1971), but it is also possible to inhibit glucose-induced calcium accumulation without interfering with glucose metabolism. Thus, excess magnesium, which does not affect the stimulant action of glucose upon insulin biosynthesis (Fig. 1), a process itself highly sensitive to changes in glucose metabolism, abolishes glucose-induced calcium accumulation and subsequent insulin release, probably through a direct competition with calcium for a common carrier system (Malaisse-Lagae and Malaisse, 1971).

As far as the mode of action of calcium is concerned, we have previously suggested that intracellularly accumulated calcium triggers insulin secretion by activating a microtubular-microfilamentous system involved in the translocation and release of secretory granules (Malaisse and Malaisse-Lagae, 1970). Thus, there are reasons to believe that agents interfering with the structure and function of microtubules and microfilaments (e.g. colchicine, vincristine, deuterium oxide, and cytochalasin B) modify the secretory response of the beta cell to various insulinotropic agents by altering the sensitivity and/or responsiveness of the microtubular-microfilamentous system to the triggering action of intracellularly-accumulated calcium (Malaisse, 1972). A recent cinematographic study of monolayer-cultured beta cells has provided further evidence to support the participation of microtubules in the controlled movement of secretory granules (Kanazawa et al., 1973). Combined functional and ultrastructural studies with the isolated perfused rat pancreas or isolated islets have also documented the involvement of these primitive contractile structures in the multiphasic dynamics of insulin secretion (Devis et al., 1974; Lacy et al., 1972, 1973; Somers et al., 1973; Van Obberghen et al., 1973a, b). However, little is known concerning the mode of interaction of calcium with the microtubular cytoskeleton and microfilamentous web of the beta cell.

The regulation of calcium handling by the beta cell

Because of the key role played by calcium in the insulin-releasing process, the metabolism of this cation in insular tissue deserves some consideration. Most of our present knowledge concerning the handling of calcium by the beta cell is derived from radioisotopic measurements of ^{45}Ca net uptake, subcellular distribution and efflux in isolated islets (Malaisse-Lagae and Malaisse, 1971; Malaisse et al., 1973a). These 3 types of measurement are each to be considered with their own limitations in mind.

The net uptake of ^{45}Ca by incubated islets is a static measurement performed after a fixed period of incubation followed by extensive washings of the islets in order to remove most of the extracellular radioactivity. With this method, it is hardly possible to obtain a detailed time-related estimation of the kinetics of calcium uptake. No distinction can be made between increased influx or decreased efflux of calcium across the cell membrane. The residual ^{45}Ca measured in the islets after the washing period could reflect not only a change in the net uptake of calcium, but conceivably also a redistribution of ^{45}Ca among the various subcellular pools, each of which is characterized by its own transfer rate constant and, therefore, susceptible to more or less rapid depletion of its radioactivity during the washing procedure (Hellman et al., 1971).

The subcellular distribution of ^{45}Ca is open to even more severe criticisms. First, the presently available techniques for the isolation of cell organelles might not be adequate to preserve some components of the vacuolar system thought to be actively involved in the subcellular distribution of cations. Second, in view of the tendency of calcium to bind on different structures, the presence of ^{45}Ca in a given pellet of organelles does not necessarily imply that the cation was indeed taken up by these organelles in the intact tissue.

The measurement of ^{45}Ca efflux from islets which have been loaded with the radioactive cation prior to perifusion provides a dynamic view of calcium outward transport across the cell membrane. However, the radioactivity collected in the effluent perifusate does not correspond solely to cations transported across the intact membrane of the beta cell: indeed, the emiocytotic release of insulin is associated with a concomitant release of ^{45}Ca presumably within the secretory granules (Malaisse et al., 1973a). In order to distinguish between outward transport and emiocytotic release of ^{45}Ca, it is necessary to perform experiments under conditions known to abolish insulin release and yet supposed not to interfere with calcium handling by the beta cell. Even so, the effluent radioactivity is only representative of the outward transport and is unable to provide any information as to the rate of calcium influx into the beta cell.

With these limitations in mind, the experimental data have led us to postulate the following working hypotheses:

(1) Calcium is distributed in the beta cell among at least 2 pools: the first pool represents the calcium present in the cytosol; the second pool is likely to be heterogeneous and to correspond to the calcium taken up by or bound to various organelles; it is here quoted as the vacuolar pool. The rate of insulin release is controlled by the concentration of calcium in the cytosol of the beta cell, whatever agent is used to either stimulate or inhibit the secretory process (Malaisse, 1972, 1973).

(2) Glucose and those agents which simulate its insulinotropic modality (e.g. mannose and leucine) increase the cytosolic concentration of calcium by enhancing the net uptake of calcium by the beta cell (Malaisse-Lagae and Malaisse, 1971; Malaisse-Lagae et al., 1971). In the case of glucose, the increased net uptake appears to be due mostly, if not exclusively, to reduced outward transport of calcium across the cell membrane (Malaisse et al., 1973a). Incidentally, increased net uptake of calcium should theoretically lead to increased concentrations of calcium in both the cytosolic and vacuolar pools.

(3) Agents such as theophylline and the dibutyryl derivative of adenosine-3′,5′-cyclic monophosphate (db-cAMP), which are thought to cause an accumulation of cAMP in the beta cell, provoke a glucose-independent intracellular translocation of calcium from the vacuolar system into the cytosol (Brisson et al., 1972; Brisson and Malaisse, 1973). The term ‘glucose-independent’ is used to indicate that the effect of theophylline on calcium distribution in the beta cell does not require the presence of glucose. It is not meant to imply that the magnitude of the theophylline-induced increment in cAMP concentration and subsequent calcium translocation may not be regulated by the amount of glucose available to the beta cell, that the fate of the load of calcium initially translocated in the cytosol is not ultimately also affected by the concentration of glucose, and that cAMP, in addition to and independently of its effect on calcium distribution, may not also stimulate glucose metabolism and hence modify the net uptake of calcium by the beta cell. As a matter of fact, we have obtained data to suggest that, under appropriate experimental conditions, each of these 3 latter effects indeed occur in the beta cell (Brisson et al., 1972; Brisson and Malaisse, 1973; Malaisse, unpublished observations).

(4) Sulfonylureas could exert a dual effect upon calcium handling by the beta cell analogous to that of both glucose and theophylline (Malaisse et al., 1973b). Epinephrine antagonizes the effect of insulinotropic agents by facilitating both the outward transport and vacuolar uptake of calcium (Brisson and Malaisse, 1973).

The apparent complexity of calcium movements in the beta cell led us to design a model allowing for the computation of ^{45}Ca net uptake, subcellular distribution and efflux under different experimental conditions (Fig. 2). This work is still in progress. So far, the data suggest that the effects of glucose and theophylline on calcium handling by the beta cell can indeed be simulated by assuming that glucose inhibits the outward transport of calcium across the cell membrane and that theophylline increases the transfer rate constant for calcium translocation from the vacuolar system into the cytosol.

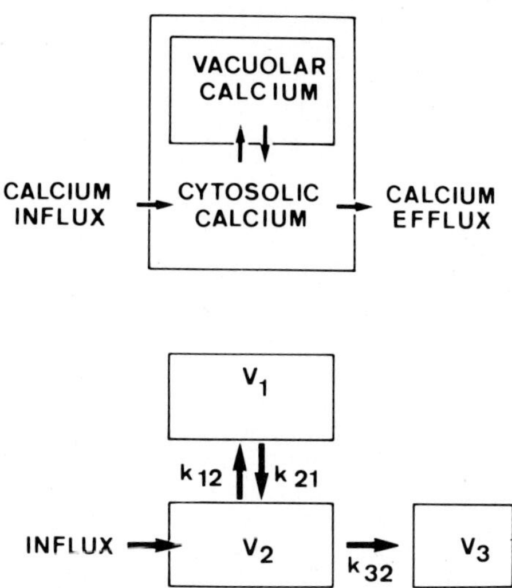

FIG. 2. Schematic and hypothetical view of calcium movements in the beta cell (top) and its mathematical modeling (bottom).

The bioelectrical data collected in impaled beta cells by Dean and Matthews (1970a, b) and Pace and Price (1972) are also compatible with though not conclusive of the concept that glucose inhibits the outward transport of calcium. Other approaches are now introduced for the study of calcium distribution and movements in the beta cell. They are based on the semiquantitative measurement and localization of calcium at the ultrastructural level in islets which have been incubated at various glucose concentrations or in the presence of other insulinotropic agents (Herman et al., 1973). The above-mentioned hypotheses concerning calcium handling by the beta cell might thus become amenable to direct testing in the not too distant future.

The influence of monovalent cations upon insular function

From the preceding remarks it is obvious that the regulation and mechanism of calcium transport across the plasma membrane of the beta cell represent a critical aspect of insular cytophysiology. Milner and Hales (1970) were the first to suggest that such a transport is mediated through a sodium-sensitive pump characterized by competition between calcium and sodium for the same carrier system and activated whenever sodium accumulates in the beta cell. This concept, which is illustrated in Figure 3, would explain why conditions likely to lower the sodium concentration in the beta cell are accompanied by depressed insulin release (Hales and Milner, 1968a, b; Malaisse et al., 1971). Although we

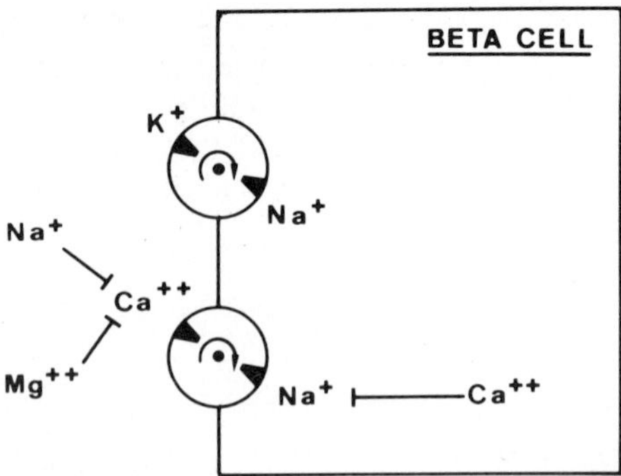

FIG. 3. Model for the movement of cations across the beta cell membrane. The classical ouabain-sensitive potassium-dependent sodium pump (top) and the calcium-dependent sodium pump (bottom) are shown together with the possible sites of competition between cations (T-shaped bars) for the same carrier.

do not deny the existence of such a process, we now suggest that the influence of monovalent cations upon insular function cannot be solely accounted for through concomitant changes in calcium handling by the beta cell.

As illustrated in Figure 1, the replacement of sodium by an amount of potassium likely to cause cell depolarization enhances glucose induced insulin biosynthesis, whereas the replacement of sodium by lithum, choline, tris-(hydroxymethyl)-aminomethane or larger amounts of potassium inhibits it. The latter inhibitory effects cannot be explained by a reduction in glucose-induced calcium uptake, since reduced availability of calcium to the beta cell does not impair its biosynthetic activity. Another explanation for these inhibitory effects could be that the recognition of glucose by the beta cell represents a sodium-sensitive process, as first suggested by Randle (1971). As outlined in greater detail elsewhere (Pipeleers et al., 1973b). 2 arguments can be advanced in support of such a concept.

First, the alteration induced by sodium replacement in the ratio of immunoreactive insulin-like to total protein synthesis by the isolated islets is identical to that normally seen at various glucose levels. This ratio, which is representative of the preferential stimulant action of glucose upon proinsulin synthesis, would not be affected in such a manner if the influence of sodium were to be due to poorly specific mechanisms (e.g. inhibition of leucine transport or ATP depletion) rather than to a specific alteration of the glucoreceptor system (Malaisse et al., 1973c; Pipeleers et al., 1973a, b).

Second, under most experimental conditions, the changes in glucose-induced insulin biosynthesis were parallelled by concomitant changes in glucose-induced calcium accumulation and subsequent insulin release by the isolated islets (Pipeleers et al., 1973b), suggesting that the recognition of glucose as a signal for both insulin biosynthesis and release is dependent on the same sodium-sensitive step of glucose handling by the beta cell.

In order to verify definitely whether the effect of sodium upon insulin biosynthesis is indeed specific to the process of glucose recognition by the beta cell, one should use an agent almost as potent as glucose to stimulate insulin biosynthesis, but yet strictly unrelated to glucose as far as its mode of action is concerned. Possibly, certain amino acids may provide the appropriate tool for such a study. Meanwhile, the present results are compatible with the idea that a sodium-dependent mechanism participates in the glucosensor device of the pancreatic beta cell.

CONCLUSION

It is concluded that calcium availability to the beta cell represents a specific requirement of the insulin-releasing mechanism, but does not interfere with the identification of insulinotropic agents by this cell, whereas sodium apparently participates in the recognition of glucose as a signal for both insulin synthesis and release.

REFERENCES

ASHCROFT, S. J. H. and RANDLE, P. J. (1969): Metabolism and insulin secretion in isolated islets. *Acta diabet. lat., 6/Suppl. 1,* 538.

BRISSON, G. R. and MALAISSE, W. J. (1973): The stimulus-secretion coupling of glucose-induced insulin release. XI. Effects of theophylline and epinephrine on ^{45}Ca efflux from perifused islets. *Metabolism, 22,* 455.

BRISSON, G. R., MALAISSE-LAGAE, F. and MALAISSE, W. J. (1972): The stimulus-secretion coupling of glucose-induced insulin release. VII. A proposed site of action for adenosine-3′,5′-cyclic monophosphate. *J. clin. Invest., 51,* 232.

DEAN, P. M. and MATTHEWS, E. K. (1970a): Glucose-induced electrical activity in pancreatic islet cells. *J. Physiol., 210,* 255.

DEAN, P. M. and MATTHEWS, E. K. (1970b): Electrical activity in pancreatic islet cells: effect of ions. *J. Physiol., 210,* 265.

DEVIS, G., VAN OBBERGHEN, E., SOMERS, G., MALAISSE-LAGAE, F., ORCI, L. and MALAISSE, W. J. (1974): Dynamics of insulin release and microtubular-microfilamentous system. II. Effect of vincristine. *Diabetologia, 10,* in press.

GRODSKY, G. M. and BENNETT, L. L. (1966): Cation requirements for insulin secretion in the isolated perfused pancreas. *Diabetes, 15,* 910.

HALES, C. N. (1970): Ion fluxes and membrane function in β-cells and adipocytes. *Acta diab. lat., 7/Suppl. 1,* 64.

HALES, C. N. and MILNER, R. D. G. (1968a): The role of sodium and potassium in insulin secretion from rabbit pancreas. *J. Physiol., 194,* 725.

HALES, C. N. and MILNER, R. D. G. (1968b): Cations and the secretion of insulin from rabbit pancreas in vitro. *J. Physiol., 199,* 177.

HELLMAN, B., SEHLIN, J. and TÄLJEDÄL, I.-B. (1971): Calcium uptake by pancreatic β-cells as measured with the aid of ^{45}Ca and mannitol-^{3}H. *Amer. J. Physiol., 221,* 1795.

HERMAN, L., SATO, T. and HALES, C. N. (1973): The electron microscopic localization of cations to pancreatic islets of Langerhans and their possible role in insulin secretion. *J. ultrastruct. Res., 42,* 298.

KANAZAWA, Y., HAYASHI, M., KUZUYA, T., IDE, T. and KOSAKA, K. (1973): Dynamic cytology of the pancreatic B-cell in monolayer culture. In: *Abstracts, VIII Congress of the International Diabetes Federation, Brussels, 1973,* p. 3. Editors: J. J. Hoet and P. Lefebvre. International Congress Series No. 280, Excerpta Medica, Amsterdam.

LACY, P. E., WALKER, M. M. and FINK, C. J. (1972): Perifusion of isolated rat islets in vitro. Participation of the microtubular system in the biphasic release of insulin. *Diabetes, 21,* 987.

LACY, P. E., KLEIN, N. J. and FINK, C. J. (1973): Effect of cytochalasin B on the biphasic release of insulin in perifused rat islets. *Endocrinology, 92,* 1458.

MALAISSE, W. J. (1972): Role of calcium in insulin secretion. *Israel J. med. Scis, 8,* 244.

MALAISSE, W. J. (1973): Insulin secretion: multifactorial regulation for a single process of release. The Minkowski Award Lecture. *Diabetologia, 9,* 167.

MALAISSE, W. J., BRISSON, G. R. and BAIRD, L. E. (1973a): Stimulus-secretion coupling of glucose-induced insulin release. X. Effect of glucose on ^{45}Ca efflux from perifused islets. *Amer. J. Physiol., 224,* 389.

MALAISSE, W. J., MAHY, M., BRISSON, G. R. and MALAISSE-LAGAE, F. (1972): The stimulus-secretion coupling of glucose-induced insulin release. VIII. Combined effects of glucose and sulfonylureas. *Europ. J. clin. Invest., 2,* 85.

MALAISSE, W. and MALAISSE-LAGAE, F. (1970): A possible role for calcium in the stimulus-secretion coupling for glucose-induced insulin secretion. *Acta diabet. lat., 7/Suppl. 1,* 264.

MALAISSE, W. J., MALAISSE-LAGAE, F. and BRISSON, G. (1971): The stimulus-secretion coupling of glucose-induced insulin release. II. Interaction of alkali and alkaline earth cations. *Hormone metabol. Res., 3,* 65.

MALAISSE, W. J., MALAISSE-LAGAE, F., LACY, P. E. and WRIGHT, P. H. (1967a): Insulin secretion by isolated islets in presence of glucose, insulin and anti-insulin serum. *Proc. Soc. exp. Biol. Med. (N.Y.), 124,* 497.

MALAISSE, W., MALAISSE-LAGAE, F. and WRIGHT, P. H. (1967b): A new method for the measurement in vitro of pancreatic insulin secretion. *Endocrinology, 80,* 99.

MALAISSE, W. J., PIPELEERS, D. G. and MAHY, M. (1973b): The stimulus-secretion coupling of glucose-induced insulin release. XII. Effects of diazoxide and gliclazide upon ^{45}calcium efflux from perifused islets. *Diabetologia, 9,* 1.

MALAISSE, W. J., PIPELEERS, D. G., VAN OBBERGHEN, E., SOMERS, G., DEVIS, G., MARICHAL, M. and MALAISSE-LAGAE, F. (1973c): The glucoreceptor mechanism in the pancreatic beta-cell. *Amer. Zoologist, 13,* 605.

MALAISSE-LAGAE, F., BRISSON, G. R. and MALAISSE, W. J. (1971): The stimulus-secretion coupling of glucose-induced insulin release. VI. Analogy between the insulinotropic mechanisms of sugars and amino acids. *Hormone metabol. Res., 3,* 374.

MALAISSE-LAGAE, F. and MALAISSE, W. J. (1971): Stimulus-secretion coupling of glucose-induced insulin release. III. Uptake of ^{45}calcium by isolated islets of Langerhans. *Endocrinology, 88,* 72.

MILNER, R. D. G. and HALES, C. N. (1967): The role of calcium and magnesium in insulin secretion from rabbit pancreas studied in vitro. *Diabetologia, 3,* 47.

MILNER, R. D. G. and HALES, C. N. (1970): Ionic mechanisms in the regulation of insulin secretion. In: *The Structure and Metabolism of the Pancreatic Islets,* pp. 489–493. Editors: S. Falkmer, B. Hellman and I.-B. Täljedal. Pergamon Press, Oxford.

PACE, C. S. and PRICE, S. (1972): Electrical response of pancreatic islet cells to secretory stimuli. *Biochem. biophys. Res. Commun., 46,* 1557.

PIPELEERS, D. G., MARICHAL, M. and MALAISSE, W. J. (1973a): The stimulus-secretion coupling of glucose-induced insulin release. XIV. Glucose regulation of insular biosynthetic activity. *Endocrinology, 93,* 1001.

PIPELEERS, D. G., MARICHAL, M. and MALAISSE, W. J. (1973b): The stimulus-secretion coupling of glucose-induced insulin release. XV. Participation of cations in the recognition of glucose by the β cell. *Endocrinology, 93,* 1012.

RANDLE, P. J. (1971): Islet metabolism and insulin secretion. In: *Proceedings, VII Congress of the International Diabetes Federation, Buenos Aires, 1970,* p. 232. Editor: R. R. Rodriguez. International Congress Series No. 231, Excerpta Medica, Amsterdam.

SOMERS, G., DEVIS, G., VAN OBBERGHEN, E., RAVAZZOLA, M., ORCI, L. and MALAISSE, W. J. (1973): Effect of deuterium oxide and cytochalasin B on the dynamics of insulin release by the isolated perfused rat pancreas. In: *Abstracts, VIII Con-*

gress of the International Diabetes Federation, Brussels, 1973, p. 27. Editors: J. J. Hoet and P. Lefebvre. International Congress Series No. 280, Excerpta Medica, Amsterdam.

VAN OBBERGHEN, E., SOMERS, G., DEVIS, G., RAVAZZOLA, M., ORCI, L. and MALAISSE, W. J. (1973a): Dual effect of colchicine upon the dynamics of insulin release by the isolated perfused rat pancreas. In: *Abstracts, VIII Congress of the International Diabetes Federation, Brussels, 1973,* p. 28. Editors: J. J. Hoet and P. Lefebvre. International Congress Series No. 280, Excerpta Medica, Amsterdam.

VAN OBBERGHEN, E., SOMERS, G., DEVIS, G., VAUGHAN, G. D., MALAISSE-LAGAE, F., ORCI, L. and MALAISSE, W. J. (1973b): Dynamics of insulin release and microtubular-microfilamentous system. I. Effect of cytochalasin B. *J. clin. Invest., 52,* 1041.

THE B CELL BOUNDARY*†

L. ORCI, M. RAVAZZOLA, M. AMHERDT and F. MALAISSE-LAGAE

Institut d'Histologie et d'Embryologie, Université de Genève,
Genève, Suisse

Over the last two decades, extensive investigations have been carried out on the influence of various metabolic, hormonal and pharmacological agents on the process of insulin biosynthesis and release. Confronted with such a wealth of data, a major difficulty remains in understanding the sequence of events leading to insulin secretion, and especially the role of the cell surface in the process. Obviously, basic information on cell surface organization is of the utmost importance with respect to this subject. With this in mind, the aim of this paper is to bring to the attention of diabetologists the fact that the selective, regulatory and protective properties of the B cell surface may depend on the integrated function of at least 3 structurally identifiable components:

a. an outermost layer of varying thickness, formed by carbohydrate-protein complexes and called *the cell coat,*

b. an innermost layer formed by a meshwork of actin-like microfilaments, *the cell web,* and

c. a middle layer, *the plasma membrane* or cell membrane, which has lipids and proteins as its main components.

THE CELL COAT

Numerous cytochemical and biochemical experiments (for review, see Martinez-Palomo, 1970; Rambourg, 1971) have led to the identification of a carbohydrate-rich layer, the cell coat, on the outer surface of most animal cells. It is known that in a variety of cell types the cell coat is composed of glycoproteins and mucopolysaccharides, and forms a system adapted to serve a variety of functions, including cell permeability, cell immunity, cell adhesion and intercellular contacts. It has been suggested that the cell coat may confer a high degree of specificity to the cell surface, and that its integrity is essential for the maintenance of important physiological activities occurring at this surface (Ito, 1969).

* This study was supported in part by grants No. 3.541.71, 3.553.71, 3.0310.73, and 3.8080.72 from Fonds National Suisse de la Recherche Scientifique, and by grant-in-aid from Hoechst Pharmaceutical Industry, Frankfurt-Hoechst, Federal Republic of Germany.

† Dedicated to Professor A. E. Renold for his 50th birthday.

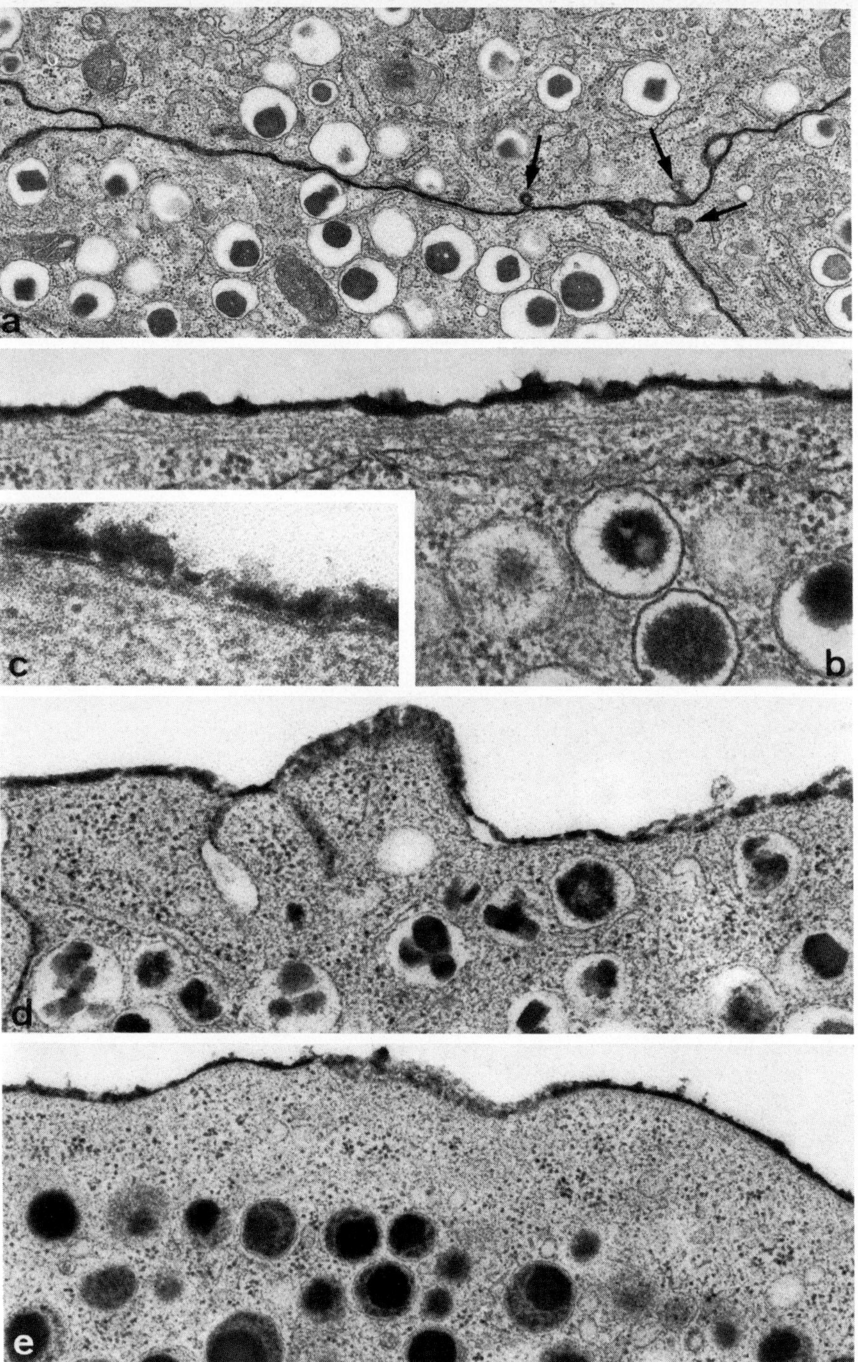

FIG. 1. *a*: B cells from isolated rat islet stained by the ruthenium red procedure (Luft, 1964). Ruthenium red positive material is present in intercellular spaces and in micropinocytotic invaginations along the plasma membrane (arrows). X 17,000. *b* and *c*: Monolayer culture prepared from newborn rat pancreatic cells (Orci et al., 1973b), and fixed in glutaraldehyde-Alcian blue (Behnke and Zelander, 1970). *b*: The free surface of a B cell is heavily coated with stained material. X 52,000. *c*: High magnification micrograph illustrating the close relationship of the densely stained cell coat with the outer leaflet of the plasma membrane. X 143,000. *d* and *e*: Insulin-producing cell and glucagon-producing cell from human isolated islet processed with the Alcian blue method. Both cells are coated with a dense layer. d: X 32,000; e: X 26,000.

In order to demonstrate whether a surface coat is also present on islet cells, we have used ruthenium red and Alcian blue (Luft, 1964; Behnke and Zelander, 1970). At the fine structural level these polycationic dyes reveal a material, presumably a polysaccharide-protein complex, which covers the plasma membrane. As shown in Figure 1, islet cells from both humans and laboratory rodents are coated with a layer of dense material of varying thickness and applied directly to the outer leaflet of the trilaminar unit plasma membrane. Whether this surface coating is essential for islet cell functions and how it could mediate these functions has not been established. However, being the first barrier between the environment and the islet cell, the cell coat may be supposed to play an initial and decisive role in controlling the interaction between the immediate external cell environment and the cell.

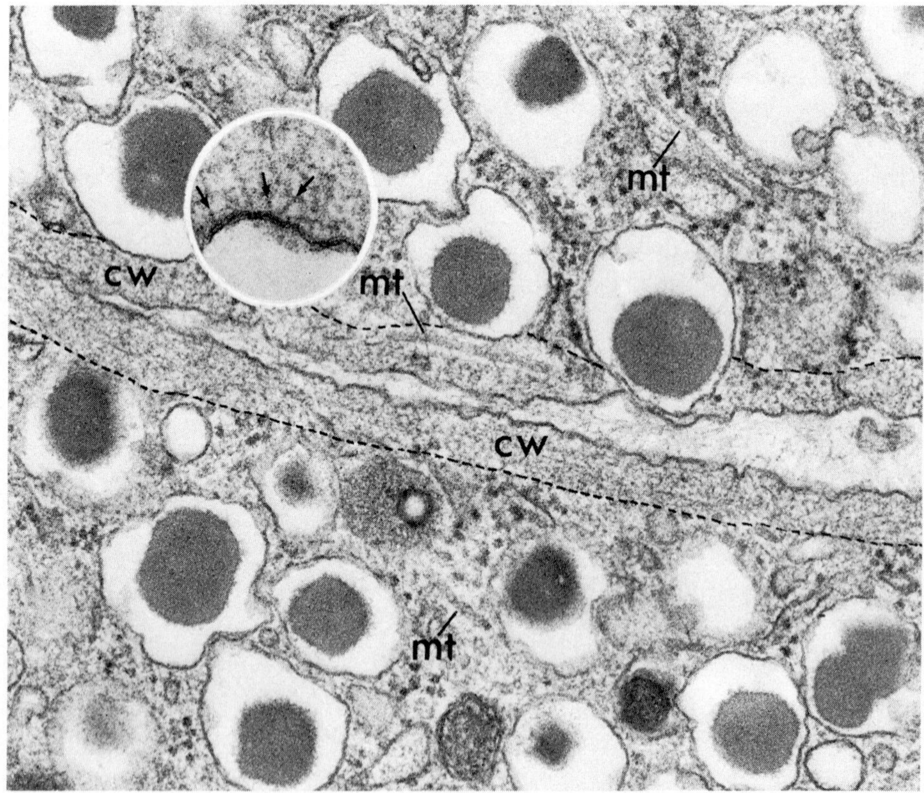

FIG. 2. Parts of 2 B cells of rat pancreatic islet. The cell web (cw) is roughly underlined by the dotted line. The insert shows at high magnification the relationship of individual elements of microfilamentous network with the inner leaflet of the cell membrane (arrows). mt: microtubules, × 52,000. Insert: × 100,000.

THE CELL WEB

The cell web (Fig. 2) is a layer of short, interconnected filaments, 40 to 70 Å in diameter, lying under the plasma membrane in the form of a network the distribution and function of which can be altered by a mold metabolite, cytochalasin B (Wessels et al., 1971; Orci et al., 1972b). Morphological evidence indicates that the filaments of the cell web may be in some manner attached to the inner surface of the plasma membrane (Fig. 2). Its presence creates a zone of exclusion, since, with the exception of granules undergoing extrusion, of pinocytotic vesicles and of ribosomes, other recognizable cytoplasmic structures are virtually absent from the area occupied by the cell web.

In 1968, Lacy et al. suggested that microtubules played a role in the intracellular translocation of secretory granules towards the cell membrane, and in their extrusion during the process of emiocytosis. Microtubules, however, have so far never been seen in direct contact with the plasma membrane, and, when they approach it, they are seen ending in the microfilamentous cell web (Fig. 2).

By establishing a link between the cell membrane and the microtubules, the cell web may thus form part of a 'cytoskeleton', responsible for or contributing to the polarity of movement of the secretory granules and endocytotic vesicles in the cytoplasm, as well as their relationship with the plasma membrane.

Biochemical and ultrastructural findings have been reported elsewhere in support of the conclusion that the microfilamentous cell web may control the access of secretory granules to the plasma membrane. It was suggested that the cell web might act as a sphincter, being both a barrier to and an effector of emiocytosis (Orci et al., 1972b; Malaisse et al., 1972). It is not known how this microfilamentous system works. In particular, it is not known whether the network should be visualized as a contractile system, or whether mechanisms such as reversible polymerization could account for its function. However, the microfilamentous appearance of the islet cell web might be indicative of its contractile nature, by analogy to other well-documented studies of microfilament-dependent contractility in a variety of systems (Buckley and Porter, 1967; Ishikawa et al., 1969; Schroeder, 1972). Indirect evidence supporting this finding may be found in a recent study using immunofluorescent technique and demonstrating the presence of actin in islet cells as well as its preferential location in the peripheral cytoplasm of the cells (Gabbiani et al., unpublished data).

THE PLASMA MEMBRANE

According to the classical Danielli-Davson model (Danielli and Davson, 1935) and the unit membrane concept (Robertson, 1959), the basic structure of membranes has been thought to consist of a lipid bilayer covered on both hydrophilic sides by proteins. Recently, the discussions on membrane structure have centered around the fluid mosaic model (Singer and Nicolson, 1972) which provides more flexibility in the orientation of membrane proteins.

In this model (Fig. 3), the proteins or glycoproteins of the membranes (most membrane-bound enzymes, histocompatibility antigens, drug and hormone receptors) are considered to be a heterogenous set of globular molecules that are partially or totally embedded in a matrix of fluid lipid bilayer, and that are capable of translational diffusion within the membrane plane.

This model accounts best for the results of freeze-etching experiments. The introduc-

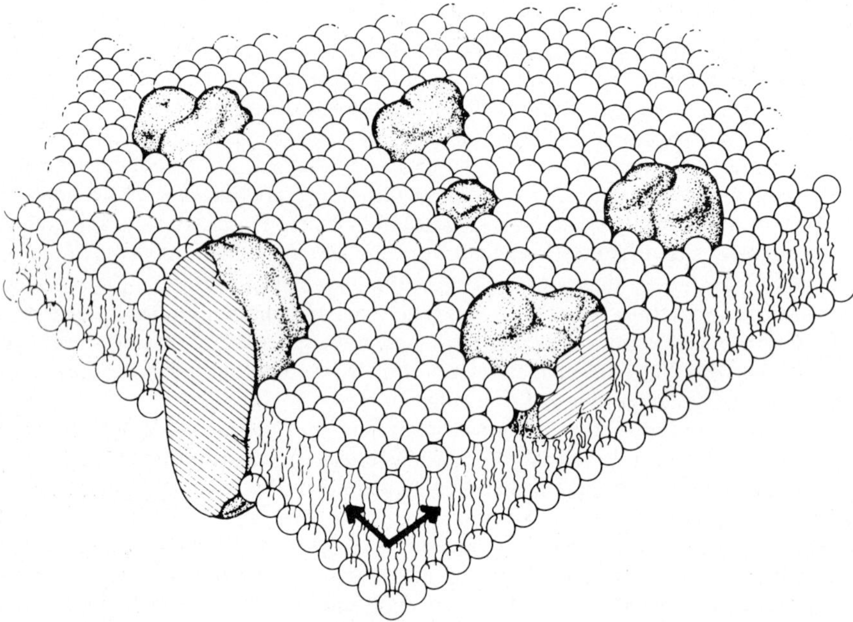

FIG. 3. The fluid mosaic model: schematic 3-dimensional and cross-sectional view. The solid bodies with stippled surfaces represent the globular integral proteins, while the balls and thin wavy lines represent the pole heads and the fatty acid chains, respectively, of the phospholipids. The surfaces of the integral proteins that are exposed to the aqueous solvent contain the ionic and highly polar residues of the proteins, whereas the portions of the proteins embedded in the membrane contain the non-ionic and mostly hydrophobic residues of the proteins. At long range, the integral proteins are randomly distributed in the plane of the membrane. At short range, some may form specific aggregates as shown. Some of the integral proteins may span the entire thickness of the membrane, while others are only partly embedded in the membrane. The bulk of the lipid is arranged as an interrupted bilayer. The arrows indicate the plane of cleavage in freeze-etch experiments (Singer and Nicolson, 1972).

tion of freeze-etching technique (Steere, 1957; Moor et al., 1961) has provided a valuable new approach to examine the ultrastructure of cell membranes (Moor and Mühlethaler, 1963; Branton, 1966). Its main advantages over conventional electron microscopy lie in the fact that tissues can be examined in a condition closer to the living state and that extensive 'en face' views of membranes, rather than sectional profiles, can be inspected.

Briefly outlined, the principle of the method is as follows: after cryoprotection with glycerol, the tissue is rapidly frozen to −180°C, fractured in vacuo, and then the exposed surface is replicated with platinum and carbon. The replica is separated from the thawed tissue, cleaned by washing and placed upon a grid for examination in the electron microscope.

According to Branton (1966), freeze-fracturing splits membranes so as to expose their inner, hydrophobic matrix (for explanation, see Fig. 4). A characteristic feature of the

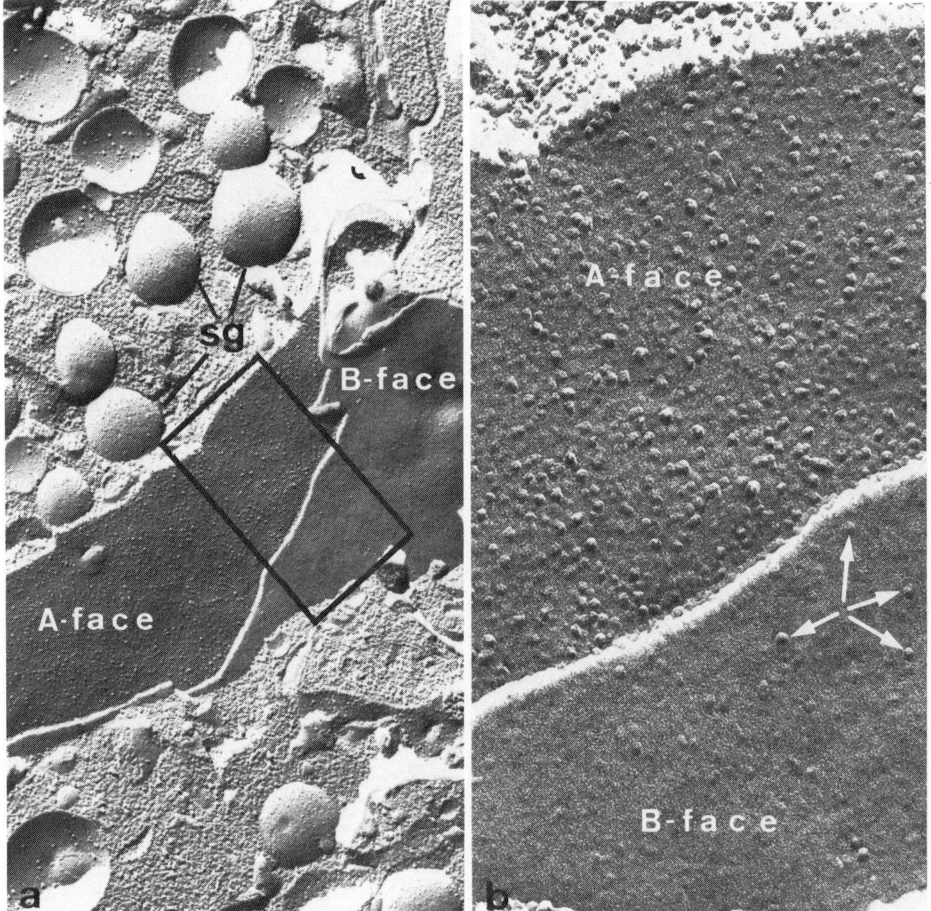

FIG. 4. Replica of freeze-etched islet cells. *a*: The fracture plane has passed through 2 cells, and exposed the adjacent cell membranes. Plasma membranes apparently fracture along planes within their interiors, exposing 2 complementary fracture faces, one facing the extracellular space (A-face), the other facing the interior of the cell (B-face). sg: secretory granules. × 38,000. *b*: Higher magnification of the area outlined by a rectangle in *a*. The exposed faces appear as smooth sheets (probably representing lamellar lipid regions) interrupted by particles of various sizes (protein-containing structures). A majority of particles usually are associated with the A-face, while only a few (arrows) are seen associated with the B-face. × 140,000.

exposed matrix of most functional membranes is a mosaic-like structure consisting of smooth areas interrupted by a varying number of particles averaging 85 Å in diameter (Branton, 1969). Available experimental data suggest that these particles are protein-containing sites (Branton, 1971; Tillack et al., 1972) and that their frequency somehow reflects the metabolic activity of the membrane (Branton, 1971). Indeed, the myelin sheath (Fig. 5) which is rather inert metabolically, has extremely few particles, whereas

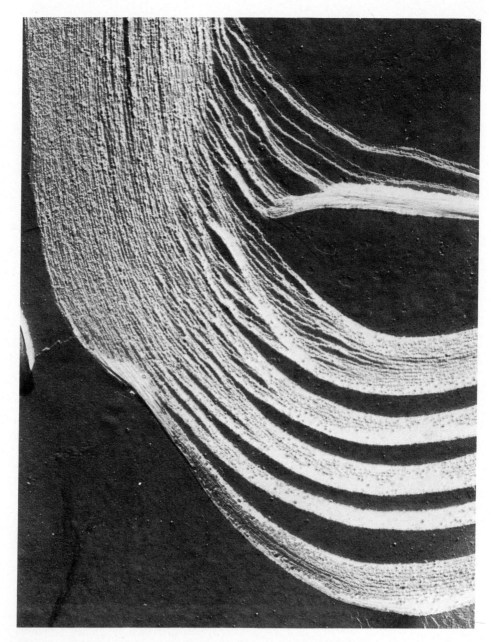

FIG. 5. Freeze-fracture of myelinated fiber from the sciatic nerve of the mouse. A few particles are seen on the exposed faces of myelin sheath. × 25,000.

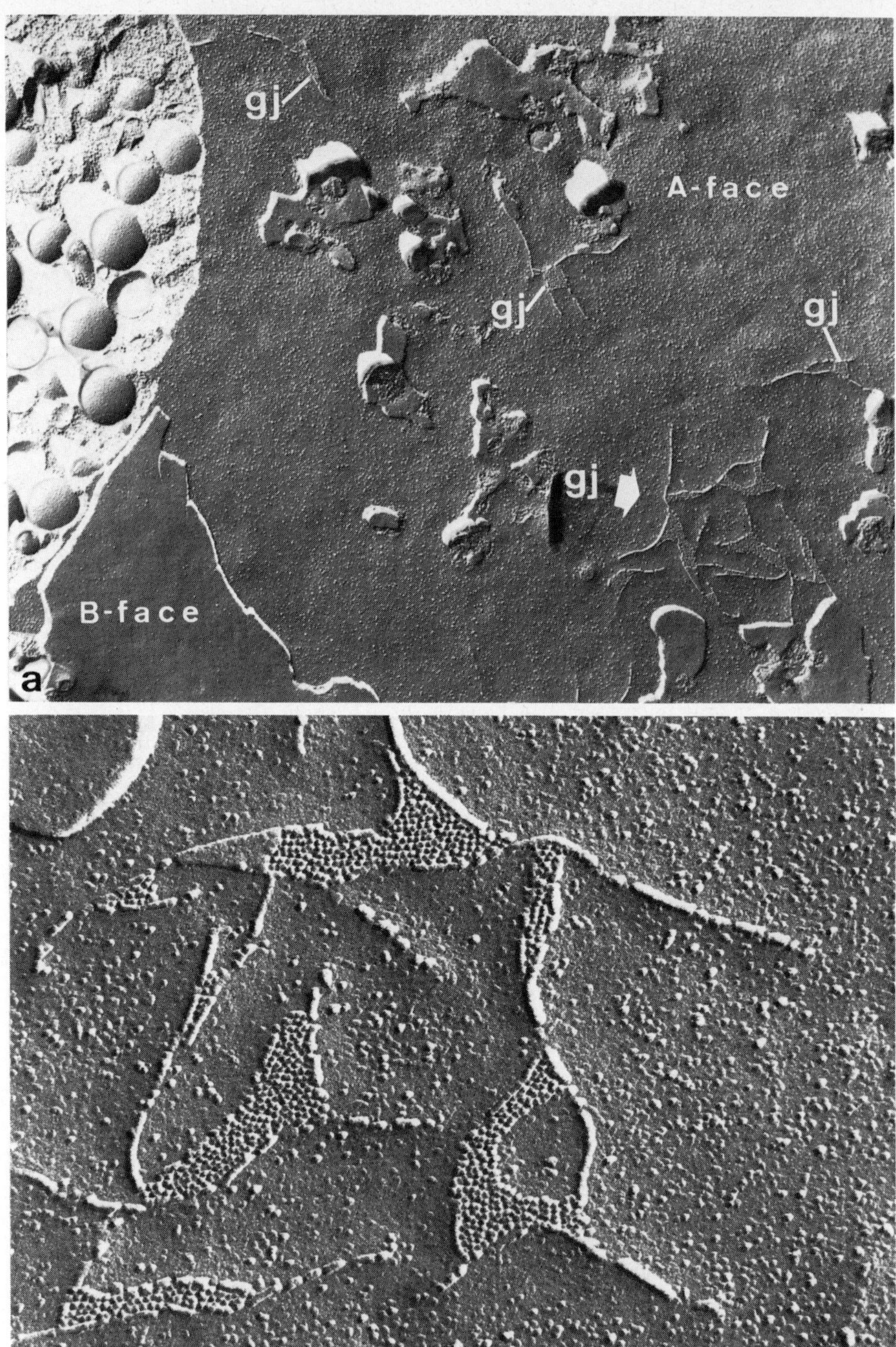

FIG. 6. *a*: Low magnification view of the central part of a freeze-etched rat islet. Several plaque-like membrane particles aggregates (gj) corresponding to gap junctions are present on the A-face of the exposed cell membrane. × 26,000. *b*: Higher magnification of the area indicated by the arrow in *a*. Gap junctions characteristically composed of well ordered arrays of particles are seen in proximity of tight junctional elements (linear ridges). Gap junctions are now widely implicated (Payton et al., 1969; Johnson and Sheridan, 1971) in cell-to-cell transfer of ions and in cell-to-cell transfer of cellular metabolites. × 83,000.

physiologically-active membranes, such as the plasma membrane (Fig. 4b), carry a large number of such particles.

Recent work has shown that particles might aggregate in specific manners on fracture faces, and that the resultant patterns could indicate the specific function in this particular area of the membrane. The most distinctive patterns described so far are the closely packed arrays of particles (Fig. 6) at the sites of gap junctions (Revel and Karnovsky, 1967; Kreutziger, 1968; Goodenough and Revel, 1970; McNutt and Weinstein, 1970; Friend and Gilula, 1972; Orci et al., 1973c), and the 'necklace' figures accompanying certain exoçytotic (Satir et al., 1973) and endocytotic (Orci and Perrelet, 1973; Fig. 7) processes. Along the same line of reasoning, another membrane differentiation, namely the tight junction (Kreutziger, 1968; Goodenough and Revel, 1970; Friend and Gilula, 1972; Orci et al., 1973a, c) (Fig. 8a) could be regarded as resulting from a particular form of membrane particle distribution. These junctions appear on A-face as a meshwork of branching and anastomosing ridges, some of which appear to be the result of linear fusion of particles (Friend and Gilula, 1972). We have recently been able to demonstrate the possibility of modifying these junctions (Orci et al., 1973a). Exposure of islet cells to proteolysis by low concentrations of either pronase (Fig. 8b) or pancreatic protease (Fig. 9) induces a major development of the normally very restricted tight junctional elements. The ability to stimulate the proliferation of tight junctions within a relatively short period of time underlines their labile nature. This lability, also apparent from the existence of the above-described membrane differentiations, tempts us to believe that their assembly and disassembly could be ascribed at least in part to the drifting of pre-existing particles to specific regions within the plane of the membrane*. In addition to this translational motion of particles we also have to take into account the possibility of a de novo addition of new particles at these specific sites.

So far, too little is known about the relationship between the type of aggregation of particles and membrane functions. However, it may be relevant that pronase, in addition to increasing the extent of tight junctions, also increases glucose-induced insulin release from B cells (Orci et al., 1973a), and it is tempting to speculate that any factor which interferes with the normal dispersion or aggregation of membrane particles might disturb the membrane's organization and properties. Furthermore, alloxan and streptozotocin, which ultimately cause B cell necrosis, have been observed in preliminary experiments by freeze-etching (Orci et al., 1972a) to produce irregular clumping and significant loss of membrane particles, at a time at which no structural change in the B cells can be detected by conventional electron microscopy. Whether this modification is indeed the first step in the sequence of events leading eventually to B cell necrosis remains to be firmly established.

It is hoped that a more direct experimental approach, involving selective removal or modification of membrane components and definition of the molecular mechanisms responsible for the translational movement of membrane particles (aggregation and redispersion), will explain the problem of a structure-function relationship in plasma membranes and in membranes in general.

* It must be noted that the capability of membrane particles to perform translational movements along the plane of the membrane has been demonstrated (Pinto da Silva, 1972).

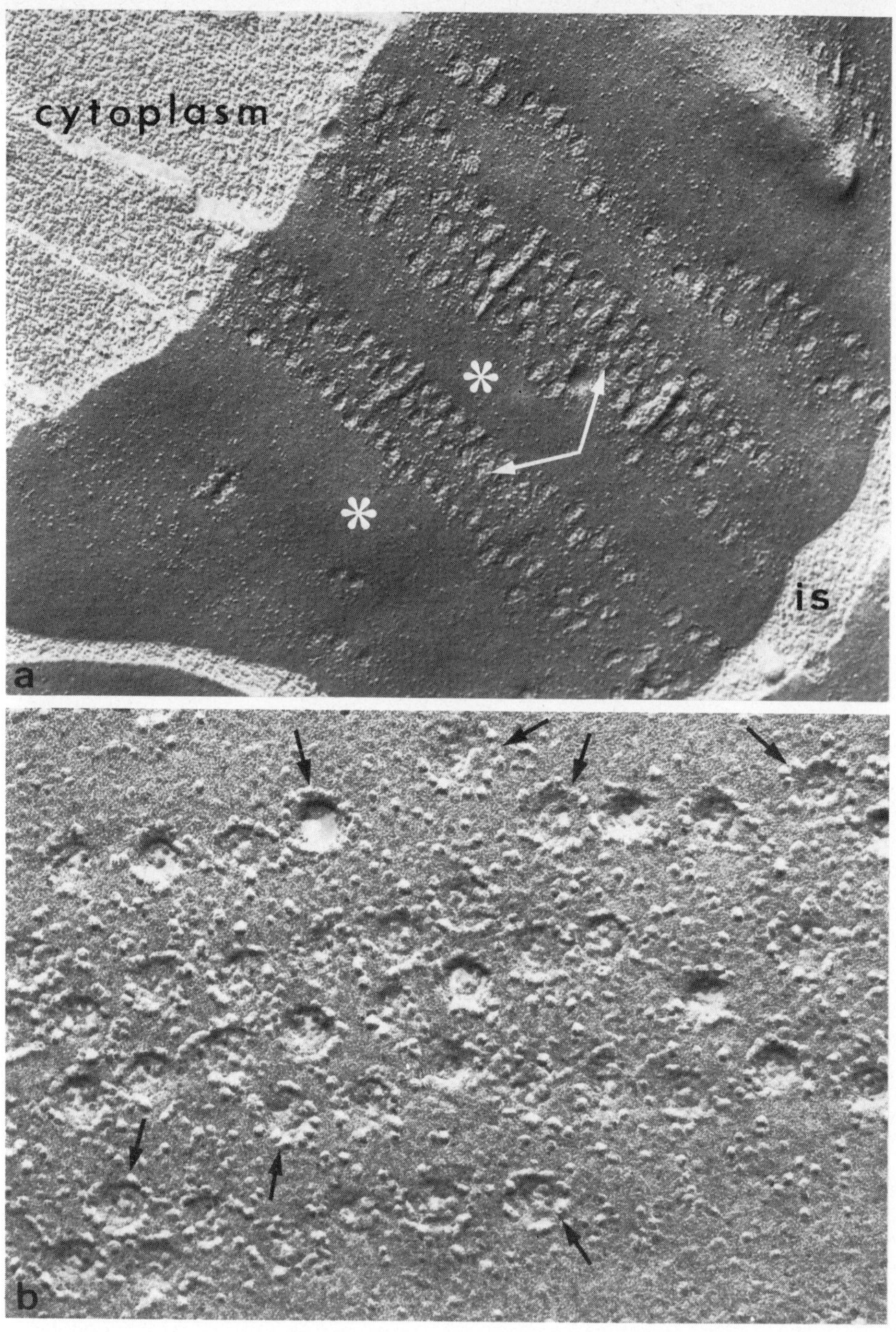

FIG. 7. Freeze-fracture replica through the intestinal smooth muscle cell of mouse. *a*: The fracture plane has exposed extensive areas of cell membrane, revealing the characteristic disposition of the pinocytotic rows (arrows), separated by bands of smooth surface (asterisks). The membrane-associated particles are more numerous inside the pinocytotic rows than outside. is: intercellular space. × 44,000. *b*: High magnification of a pinocytotic row. The membrane-associated particles are preferentially localized as necklaces around the caveolar craters (arrows). × 127,000.

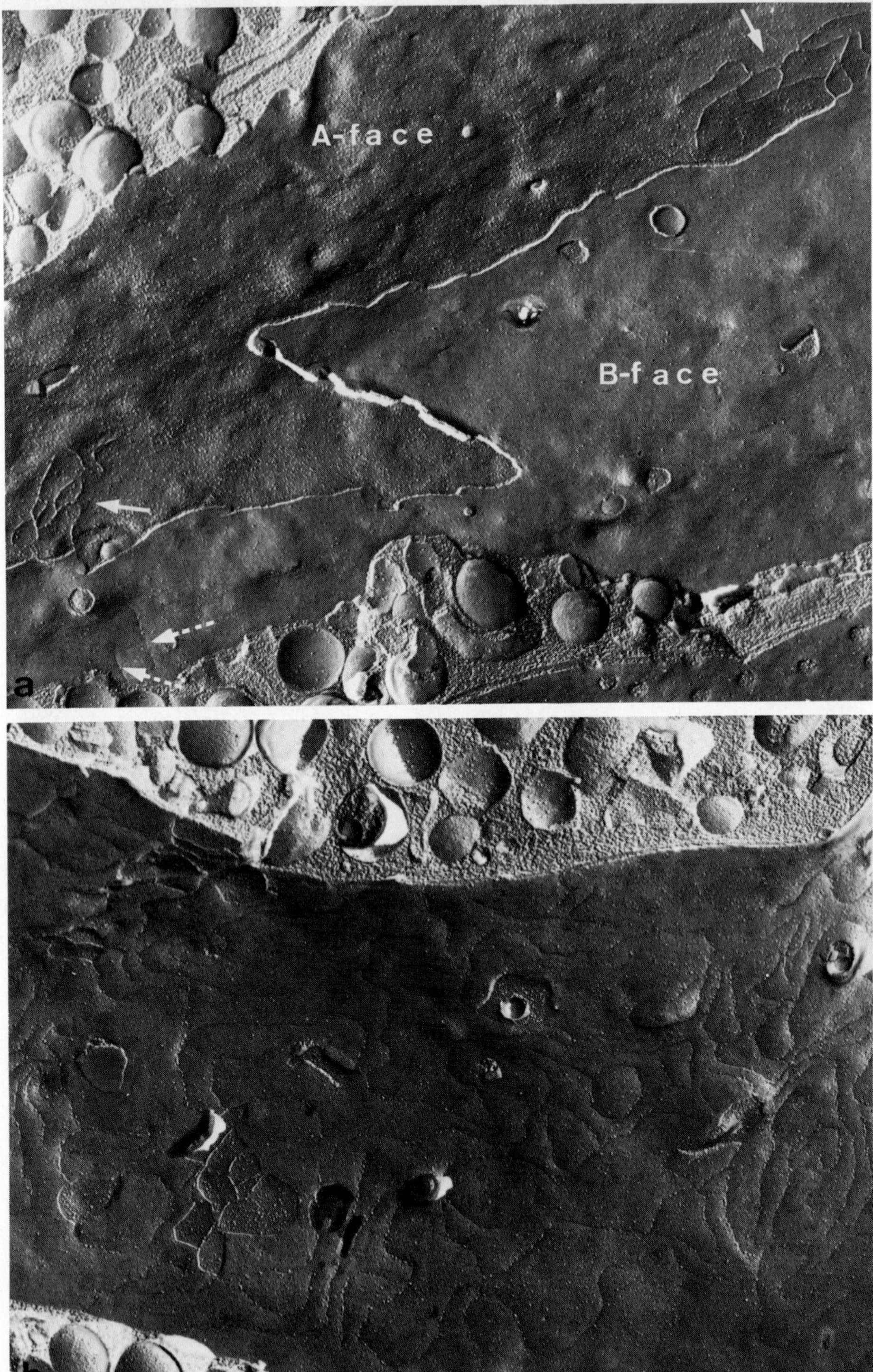

FIG. 8. Replicas of freeze-etched islet cells. *a*: Control islet. The solid arrows indicate 2 small tight junctions appearing as linear branching and anastomosing ridges on the A-face. The dotted arrows indicate 2 short tight junctional elements (linear furrows) as seen on the B-face. × 27,000. *b*: Islet treated with pronase (4 μg/ml) for 90 minutes. Note the complex pattern of highly developed tight junctional network on the B-face of the islet cell membrane. × 27,000.

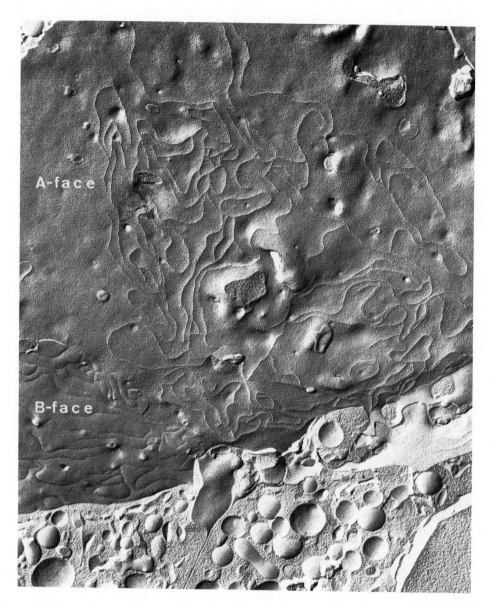

FIG. 9. Replica of freeze-etched islet cells treated with pancreatic protease (Sigma, Type I, 10 μg/ml) for 90 minutes. The tight junctional network (linear and anastomosing ridges on the A-face and linear branching and anastomosing furrows on the B-face) appears highly developed. × 17,000.

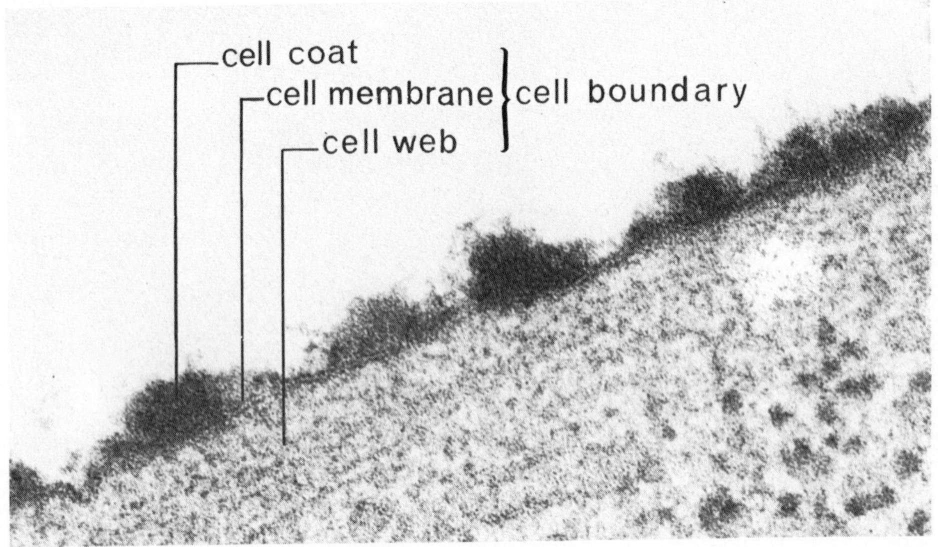

FIG. 10. High magnification micrograph illustrating the 3 components of an islet cell boundary. × 110,000.

CELL BOUNDARY

On the basis of the foregoing observations, the cell coat and the cell web should be considered together with the plasma membrane as parts of a large functioning complex, here defined as the cell boundary (Fig. 10). We believe that such a set of components provides the structural framework mediating and regulating a series of metabolic events such as the recognition of circulating stimuli, the active and passive movements of material between the inside and the outside of the cell, the coupling of exocytotic and endocytotic processes, and intercellular communication. Extensive work, mainly correlating morphology and chemistry, is needed in order to obtain the basic information which might be of significant importance regarding the etiology and pathogenesis of certain forms of diabetes mellitus.

ACKNOWLEDGEMENTS

We thank A. Perrelet and J. G. Schofield for suggestions, and M. Sidler-Ansermet and M. Bernard for technical assistance.

REFERENCES

BEHNKE, O. and ZELANDER, T. (1970): Preservation of intercellular substances by the cationic dye Alcian blue in preparative procedures for electron microscopy. *J. Ultrastruc. Res., 31,* 424.

BRANTON, D. (1966): Fracture faces of frozen membranes. *Proc. nat. Acad. Sci. U.S.A., 55,* 1048.

BRANTON, D. (1969): Membrane structure. *Ann. Rev. Plant Physiol., 20,* 209.

BRANTON, D. (1971): Freeze-etching studies of membrane structure. *Phil. Trans. B, 261,* 133.

BUCKLEY, I. K. and PORTER, K. R. (1967): Cytoplasmic fibrils in living culture cells. A light and electron microscope study. *Protoplasma, 64,* 349.

DANIELLI, J. R. and DAVSON, H. A. (1935): A contribution to the theory of permeability of thin films. *J. cell. comp. Physiol., 5,* 495.

FRIEND, D. S. and GILULA, N. B. (1972): Variations in tight and gap junctions in mammalian tissues. *J. Cell Biol., 53,* 758.

GOODENOUGH, D. A. and REVEL, J. P. (1970): A fine structural analysis of intercellular junctions in the mouse liver. *J. Cell Biol., 45,* 272.

ISHIKAWA, H., BISCHOFF, R. and HOLTZER, H. (1969): Formation of arrowhead complexes with heavy meromyosin in a variety of cell types. *J. Cell Biol., 43,* 312.

ITO, S. (1969): Structure and function of the glycocalyx. *Fed. Proc., 28,* 12.

JOHNSON, R. G. and SHERIDAN, J. D. (1971): Junctions between cancer cells in culture: ultrastructure and permeability. *Science, 174,* 717.

KREUTZIGER, G. O. (1968): Freeze-etching of intercellular junctions of mouse liver. In: *Proceedings of the 26th Meeting of the Electron Microscopy Society of America,* pp. 234–235. Claitor's Publishing Division, Baton Rouge, La.

LACY, P. E., HOWELL, S. L., YOUNG, D. A. and FINK, C. J. (1968): New hypothesis of insulin secretion. *Nature (Lond.), 219,* 1177.

LUFT, J. H. (1964): Electron microscopy of cell extraneous coats as revealed by ruthenium red staining. *J. Cell Biol., 23,* 54A.

MALAISSE, W. J., HAGER, D. L. and ORCI, L. (1972): The stimulus-secretion coupling of glucose-induced insulin release. IX. The participation of the beta cell web. *Diabetes, 21,* 594.

MARTINEZ-PALOMO, A. (1970): The surface coat of animal cells. *Int. Rev. Cytol., 29,* 29.

McNUTT, N. S. and WEINSTEIN, R. S. (1970): The ultrastructure of the nexus. A correlated thin-section and freeze-cleave study. *J. Cell Biol., 47,* 666.

MOOR, H. and MÜHLETHALER, K. (1963): Fine structure in frozen-etched yeast cells. *J. Cell Biol., 17,* 609.

MOOR, H., MÜHLETHALER, K., WALDNER, H. and FREY-WYSSLING, A. (1961): A new freezing-ultramicrotome. *J. biophys. biochem. Cytol., 10,* 1.

ORCI, L., AMHERDT, M., HENQUIN, J. C., LAMBERT, A. E., UNGER, R. H. and RENOLD, A. E. (1973a): Pronase effect on pancreatic beta cell secretion and morphology. *Science, 180,* 647.

ORCI, L., AMHERDT, M., STAUFFACHER, W., LIKE, A. A., ROUILLER, C. and RENOLD, A. E. (1972a): Structural changes in membranes of beta cells exposed to alloxan and streptozotocin demonstrated by freeze-etching. *Diabetes, 21/Suppl. 1,* 326.

ORCI, L., GABBAY, K. H. and MALAISSE, W. J. (1972b): Pancreatic β-cell web: its possible role in insulin secretion. *Science, 175,* 1128.

ORCI, L., LIKE, A. A., AMHERDT, M., BLONDEL, B., KANAZAWA, Y., MARLISS, E. B., LAMBERT, A. E., WOLLHEIM, C. B. and RENOLD, A. E. (1973b): Monolayer cell culture of neonatal rat pancreas: an ultrastructural and biochemical study of functioning endocrine cells. *J. Ultrastruct. Res., 43,* 270.

ORCI, L. and PERRELET, A. (1973): Membrane-associated particles: increase at sites of pinocytosis demonstrated by freeze-etching. *Science, 181,* 868.

ORCI, L., UNGER, R. H. and RENOLD, A. E. (1973c): Structural coupling between pancreatic islet cells. *Experientia (Basel), 29,* 1015.

PAYTON, B. W., BENNETT, M. V. L. and PAPPAS, G. D. (1969): Permeability and structure of junctional membranes at an electronic synapse. *Science, 166,* 1641.

PINTO DA SILVA, P. (1972): Translational motility of the membrane intercalated particles of human erythrocyte ghosts. pH-dependent, reversible aggregation. *J. Cell Biol., 53,* 777.

RAMBOURG, A. (1971): Morphological and histochemical aspects of glycoproteins at the surface of animal cells. *Int. Rev. Cytol., 31,* 57.

REVEL, J. P. and KARNOVSKY, M. J. (1967): Hexagonal array of subunits in intercellular junctions of the mouse heart and liver. *J. Cell Biol., 33,* C7.

ROBERTSON, J. D. (1959): The ultrastructure of cell membranes and their derivatives. *Biochem. Soc. Symposia, 16,* 3.

SATIR, B., SCHOOLEY, C. and SATIR, P. (1973): Membrane fusion in a model system. Mucocyst secretion in *Tetrahymena. J. Cell Biol., 56,* 153.

SCHROEDER, T. E. (1972): The contractile ring. II. Determining its brief existence, volumetric changes, and vital role in cleaving *Arbacia* eggs. *J. Cell Biol., 53,* 419.

SINGER, S. J. and NICOLSON, G. L. (1972): The fluid mosaic model of the structure of cell membranes. *Science, 175,* 720.

STEERE, R. L. (1957): Electron microscopy of structural detail in frozen biological specimens. *J. biophys. biochem. Cytol., 3,* 45.

TILLACK, T. W., SCOTT, R. E. and MARCHESI, V. T. (1972): The structure of erythrocyte membranes studied by freeze-etching. II. Localization of receptors for phytohemagglutinin and influenza virus to the intramembranous particles. *J. exp. Med., 135,* 1209.

WESSELS, N. K., SPOONER, B. S., ASH, J. F., BRADLEY, M. O., LUDUENA, M. O., TAYLOR, E. L., WRENN, J. T. and YAMADA, K. M. (1971): Microfilaments in cellular developmental processes. *Science, 171,* 135.

COMPARATIVE ASPECTS OF PROINSULIN AND INSULIN STRUCTURE AND BIOSYNTHESIS*+

D. F. STEINER†, J. D. PETERSON†, H. S. TAGER†,
S. O. EMDIN☆, Y. OSTBERG☆ and S. FALKMER☆

†Department of Biochemistry, The University of Chicago, Chicago, Ill., U.S.A., and ☆Institute of Pathology, University of Umeå, Umeå, Sweden

SYNOPSIS

This review summarizes the available information on the composition and structure of vertebrate insulins and proinsulins with emphasis on the important structural features of these molecules that are involved in the formation and function of the active hormone. Studies in several teleost fishes have demonstrated the existence of larger single-chain precursors similar to the mammalian proinsulins. Preliminary results of experiments on insulin biosynthesis in the primitive hagfish (*Myxine glutinosa*) also indicate the existence of a similar precursor form. Insulin, however, appears to be the major storage product in the beta cells in all the vertebrate species studied thus far. In most fishes an intracellular trypsin-like enzyme may suffice to convert proinsulin to insulin, while in mammals a more complex mechanism involving both an endopeptidase and an exopeptidase is probably required. These reactions occur within the Golgi apparatus and newly formed secretory granules in the beta cells.

The preservation of many important biosynthetic and structural aspects of insulin throughout the vertebrate phylum indicates that the properties and biological role of this hormone have remained fairly constant throughout at least 500 million years, or that its evolution has followed a similar pattern in most extant organisms despite considerable differences in their origin and living conditions. A possible mode of evolution of insulin and of beta cells based on proinsulin and its conversion to insulin is proposed.

INTRODUCTION

Endocrine systems provide fruitful areas for comparative studies because changing life conditions have necessitated continual modification and diversification of the cellular and hormonal regulatory mechanisms which serve to integrate and modulate the various metabolic processes occurring in the organism. The hormonal molecules, their cells of origin, their biosynthetic mechanisms, and their cullular receptor sites have all evolved parallel to these changing regulatory demands. The reconstruction of this progression in hormone

* This work has been supported in part by grants from the U.S.P.H.S. (AM 13914), the Kroc Research Foundation, the Swedish Medical Research Council (Project No. B73-12X-718-08B), and the Nordic Insulin Fund.

+ This paper represents a condensed and updated version of an earlier review of this subject (Steiner et al., 1973, *Amer. Zool., 13,* 591–604).

structure and function offers many possibilities for broadening our understanding of metabolic regulation and the molecular mechanisms of action of hormones, as well as of the developmental and functional disorders which occur in endocrine systems and give rise to distinctive diseases.

Our purpose here is to provide an overview of the evolution of insulin in the vertebrates. After reviewing the present state of knowledge concerning insulin and proinsulin structure and biosynthesis in mammals and some teleost fishes, we shall describe some preliminary observations on the insulin and proinsulin of the Atlantic hagfish, *Myxine glutinosa.* The hagfish is one of the two extant orders of the cyclostomes which represent a sister group of all the other vertebrates, viz. the gnathostomes. The other order of cyclostomes is the lampreys. The hagfishes and the lampreys are of particular interest in the comparative endocrinology of the endocrine pancreas as they may represent an evolutionary link between the gut-connected insulin-producing parenchyma of Deuterostomian invertebrates and the pancreatic islets of vertebrates (Falkmer and Patent, 1972). The cyclostomes have attracted the attention of comparative endocrinologists in general, and that of scientists working in the field of diabetes research in particular, since the hagfish and the lamprey are the highly specialized survivors of the earliest vertebrates, the Ostracoderms (Falkmer et al., 1973) and may possibly have some precambrian ancestor in common with the Gnathostomes (Jarvik, 1964). Thus, we may anticipate that these organisms produce an insulin with some 'primitive' features.

INSULIN STRUCTURE

The primary structures of insulins isolated from a variety of vertebrate species have been determined in the interval since the pioneering studies of Sanger and coworkers (Ryle et al., 1955; Smith, 1966). These results, shown in Figure 1, indicate that amino acid substitutions can occur at many positions within either chain without greatly altering the biological effectiveness of the hormone as measured in various bioassay systems. On the other hand, certain structural features are conserved throughout vertebrate evolution including the positions of the 3 disulfide bonds, the N-terminal and C-terminal regions of the A chain and the hydrophobic residues in the C-terminal regions of the B chain, as well as others (Smith, 1966; Humbel et al., 1972). Since chemical modifications in any of these regions tend to markedly reduce or abolish biological activity, these evidently play important roles in maintaining important secondary and tertiary structural features needed for biological activity (Humbel et al., 1972; Carpenter, 1966). The C-terminal hydrophobic sequence of the B chain (residues 23–27) also plays an important role in the formation of insulin dimers (*vide infra*). As might be anticipated from the extensive amino acid substitutions that occur between mammalian and piscine insulins, it is not surprising that the immunological cross-reactivity between these proteins is rather weak. Generally some weak cross-reactivity can be detected by means of conventional immunoassays, especially when the heterologous insulin is used as the labeled tracer. For detailed considerations of insulin antigenicity in relation to structure several recent reviews may be consulted (Humbel et al., 1972; Arquilla et al., 1972).

Preliminary results in the characterization and amino acid sequence of hagfish (*Myxine glutinosa*) insulin in our laboratories (Peterson et al., 1973) indicate that, although more than half the amino acid residues differ from those found in the mammalian insulins, structural conservation is found in the important regions of the molecule described above

```
A Chains
                       1           5                 10                15                   20 21
Hagfish                Gly-Ilu-Val-Glu-Gln-Cys-Cys-His-Lys-Arg-Cys-Ser-Ilu-Tyr-Asn-Leu-Gln-Asn-Tyr-Cys-Asn
Porcine                Gly-Ilu-Val-Glu-Gln-Cys-Cys-Thr-Ser-Ilu-Cys-Ser-Leu-Tyr-Gln-Leu-Glu-Asn-Tyr-Cys-Asn
Other Residues                 His Asp             Ala Gly Pro Asp Arg Phe Asp         Ser
                                                       Arg Val Asn Lys His
                                                       Asn Thr Thr

B Chains
                     0     1           5                 10                15                20
Hagfish                    Arg-Thr-Thr-Gly-His-Leu-Cys-Gly-Lys-Asp-Leu-Val-Asn-Ala-Leu-Tyr-Ilu -Ala-Cys-Gly-
Porcine                    Phe-Val-Asn-Gln-His-Leu-Cys-Gly-Ser- His -Leu-Val-Glu-Ala-Leu-Tyr-Leu-Val-Cys-Gly-
Other Residues       Val   Ala Pro Pro Arg                 Pro Asn         Asp Thr                   Gln
                     Met       Ala Lys Pro
                     Del           Ser
                                   Ala

                       21          25                30  31
Hagfish                -Val-Arg-Gly-Phe-Phe-Tyr-Asx-Pro-Thr-Lys-Met
Porcine                -Glu-Arg-Gly-Phe-Phe-Tyr-Thr-Pro-Lys-Ala
Other Residues          Asp Asp                 Ser Ser Met Ser(Arg)
                                                Ilu         Thr
                                                Gln  Del    Asp
```

FIG. 1. Compilation of known amino acid substitutions in the insulin molecule, including sequences of the A and B chains of hagfish insulin (Peterson et al., 1973). Invariant positions are indicated by dashes. Del = assumed deletion (After Smith, 1966; and Humbel et al., 1972).

(Fig. 1). One interesting difference is the substitution of aspartic acid for histidine at position 10 of the B chain, an important residue for zinc binding in the formation of insulin hexamers as described below. Hagfish insulin crystallizes under conditions similar to those required for the crystallization of mammalian insulin but zinc or other divalent metal ions are not needed (Coulter et al., 1973). The biological activity of hagfish insulin (Falkmer and Wilson, 1967) has been reported to be 2. I.U./mg (i.e. 8% of mammalian insulin) as determined by the fat pad assay (Weitzel et al., 1967). Further activity studies with other bioassay systems would, however, be desirable.

Within the last 3 years the 3-dimensional structure of crystalline porcine insulin at a high resolution has been determined successfully by means of X-ray diffraction analysis (Blundell et al., 1971). The results have proven invaluable in interpreting much of the available chemical data on the properties of insulin. Detailed knowledge of the spatial organization of the molecule also promises to provide further insight into the mechanism of action of insulin at a molecular level. The hexameric unit cell of crystalline zinc insulin (Fig. 2) consists of 3 dimers arranged around a major 3-fold axis which passes through 2 zinc atoms each of which is coordinated with three B10 histidine side chains located just above or below the plane of the hexamer (Blundell et al., 1971). The insulin dimers are held together in the crystals by hydrogen bonds between the peptide groups of residues 24 and 26 within the C-terminal segments of the B chain forming an antiparallel pleated-sheet structure, as well as by interactions between the hydrophobic side chains of residues B11 and B12. The locations in space of the known invariant amino acids within the insulin monomer are shown in Figure 3 (Blundell et al., 1971).

INSULIN BIOSYNTHESIS IN MAMMALS

Recent studies on proinsulin and insulin biosynthesis in mammalian islet tissues have been reviewed in detail elsewhere (Steiner et al., 1969, 1970, 1972). When islets of Langerhans isolated from rat pancreas are incubated with labeled amino acids, proinsulin (Fig. 4) is synthesized first and is subsequently transformed to insulin by proteolysis within the beta cells (Steiner and Oyer, 1967; Steiner et al., 1967; Clark and Steiner, 1969). During biosynthesis proinsulin ensures the efficient formation of insulin by providing the stoichiometrically correct proportions of A and B chains as well as the necessary chemical determinants for appropriate folding of the polypeptide chain in a configuration that is conducive to the formation of the correct disulfide bonds and tertiary structure (Steiner and Clark, 1968). Several kinds of evidence indicate that newly synthesized proinsulin is transferred from the cisternal spaces of the rough endoplasmic reticulum to secretory granules via the Golgi apparatus in a sequence similar to that known to occur in many other secretory cells (Steiner et al., 1972, 1970; Kemmler et al., 1971, 1972). The conversion of proinsulin to insulin is a slow process having a half-time of about 1 hour in rat islets in vitro (Steiner et al., 1969). Conversion appears to begin at about the same time that the newly synthesized proinsulin reaches the Golgi apparatus and it continues for a relatively long time after new secretion granules have been formed. The general features of the biosynthesis, conversion and intracellular transport of proinsulin and insulin in the beta cell are summarized in Figure 5.

Although about 95% of the proinsulin is converted to insulin in the beta granules before secretion occurs, small amounts escape conversion and are secreted into the blood under normal conditions in man and other species. Additional physiologic roles for this

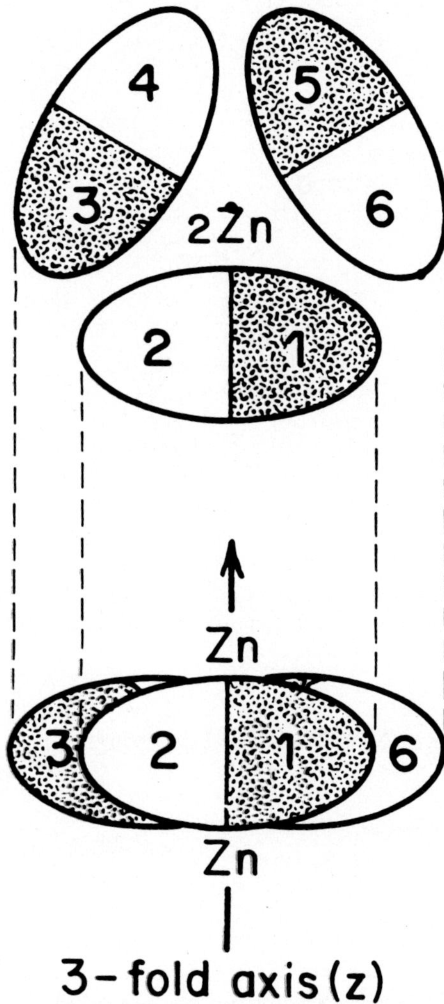

FIG. 2. Diagrammatic representation of the zinc insulin hexamer showing the 3-fold crystallographic axis with 3 dimers arranged around 2 zinc atoms which lie along the 3-fold axis. Upper view is oriented along the 3-fold axis.

secreted proinsulin are not known (Rubenstein et al., 1972). Likewise, as a consequence of the sequestration of the proinsulin conversion process within the secretion granules of the beta cells, the C-peptide (see Fig. 4) also is retained in the secretory granules of the beta cells and discharged along with insulin in essentially equivalent amounts during granule exocytosis (Rubenstein et al., 1969). The amino acid sequences of the 9 mammalian C-peptides that have been isolated thus far are shown in Figure 6. This region of the proinsulin molecule is far more variable than the insulin portion. Thus, while accepted point mutations occur at a rate of approximately 4 per 100 residues per million years in

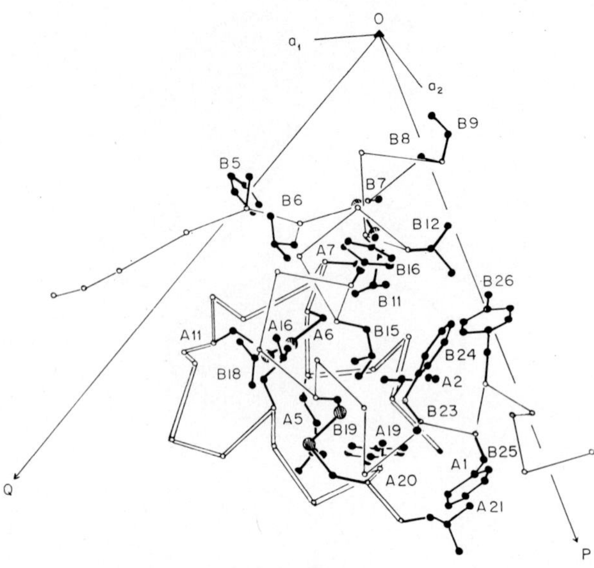

FIG. 3. Locations of invariant side chains in the insulin monomer. This view is oriented along the 3-fold axis. (Reproduced with permission from Blundell et al., 1971.)

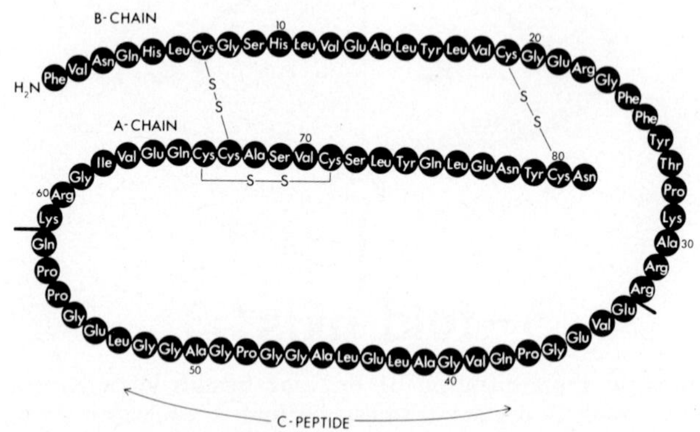

FIG. 4. Structure of bovine proinsulin (reproduced from Nolan et al., 1971).

insulin (Dayhoff, 1972), this figure for the C-peptide is about 60. Only the fibrinopeptides have undergone as rapid evolutionary change, and these results thus suggest that the C-peptide portion of the proinsulin molecule has fewer highly specific structural requirements that must be conserved. This large degree of variability also implies that the C-peptide probably does not function as an endocrine substance in a physiological sense, even though it is secreted into the bloodstream with insulin (Rubenstein et al., 1972). Nevertheless, from a comparison of the available C-peptide structures as well as the

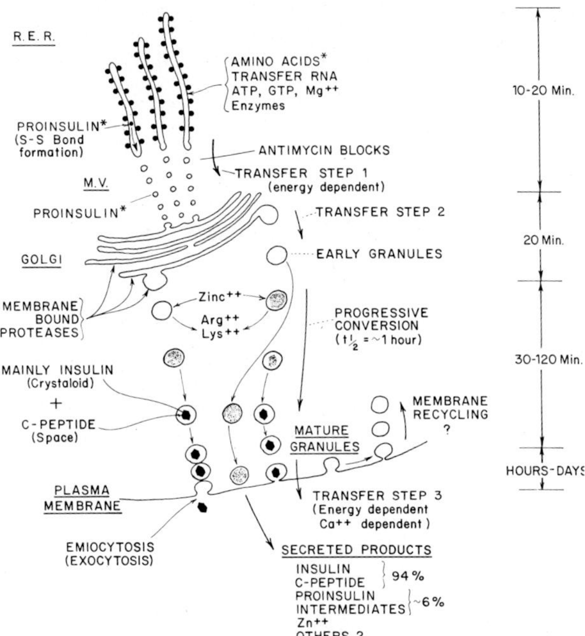

FIG. 5. Diagrammatic representation of the insulin biosynthetic mechanism of the beta cell. R.E.R. = rough endoplasmic reticulum; M.V. = microvesicles.

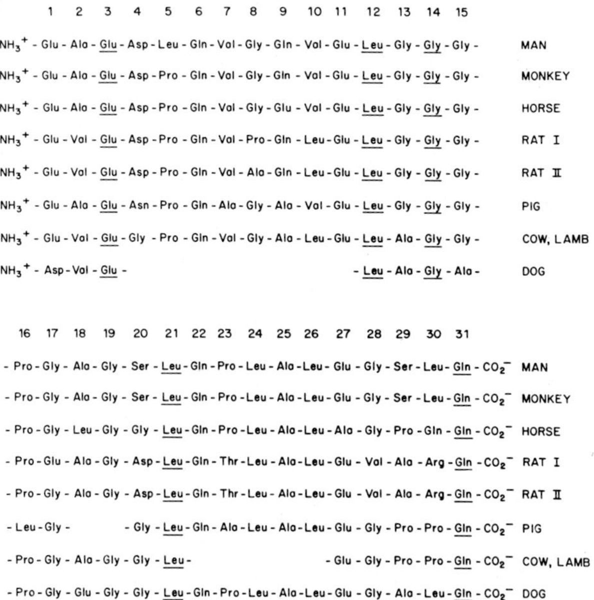

FIG. 6. Amino acid sequences of several mammalian C peptides. These sequences do not include the basic residues at each end that link the C peptide to the insulin chains in the proinsulins of these species.

known compositions of the C-peptides of the anglerfish and codfish (Table 1), it is clear that considerable structural conservatism has occurred. This is reflected in the unusual and restricted composition of these peptides, in the presence of a glycine rich central region surrounded by hydrophobic regions and in the presence of more hydrophilic character in the regions near the cleavage sites (Fig. 6). These features may play important roles in dictating the folding of the peptide chain necessary for correct disulfide bond formation, and they also may provide conformations that serve to direct the specific cleavage of proinsulin by the converting enzymes. The properties and probable conformation of the mammalian proinsulins have been discussed elsewhere (Steiner et al., 1972, 1973; Steiner, 1973).

Recent studies on several peptide hormones which do not contain disulfide bonds have indicated the existence of larger precursor forms (Cohn et al., 1972; Gregory and Tracy, 1972; Noe and Bauer, 1971; Tager and Steiner, 1973). Clearly in these instances other explanations must exist for the occurrence of these precursors, and we may anticipate that additional reasons for the existence of proinsulin also will emerge as more information accumulates regarding these other biosynthetic systems.

TABLE 1

Amino acid composition of cod and anglerfish proinsulin connecting polypeptides

	Cod*	Anglerfish†
Asp	1	
Thr	2	4
Ser	3	3
Glu	9	5
Gly	1	2
Ala	4	3
Val		
Met	1	
Leu	3	2
Ile		1
Pro		
Lys	4	7
Arg	2	6
Total	30	33

* Data from Grant and Reid (1968).

† Data from Trakatellis and Schwartz (1970).

COMPARATIVE ASPECTS OF INSULIN BIOSYNTHESIS

Several studies indicate that insulin biosynthesis in teleost fishes (Trakatellis and Schwartz, 1970; Grant and Reid, 1968; Grant and Coombs, 1971) as well as in cyclostomes (Emdin et al., 1973), proceeds via a precursor that is similar to mammalian proinsulin. Labeled amino acids were incorporated into proinsulin in incubated principal islets from the cod and anglerfish (Grant and Reid, 1968; Trakatellis and Schwartz, 1970). Insulin began to appear later during incubation, and several intermediate forms also could be identified. In the hagfish the rate of incorporation of [^{3}H]leucine into proinsulin and insulin was found to be a slow process, requiring 12–15 times more time at 11°C than for rat islets at 37°C. Also the rate of proinsulin synthesis and conversion was shown to be temperature-dependent; at 30° essentially no incorporation into proinsulin occurred. The approximate half-time of conversion of proinsulin to insulin was 12 hours at 11°C and 9 hours at 18°C. The corresponding half-time for conversion in the rat is approximately 1 hour at 37°C.

An interesting intermediate protein has been isolated in the anglerfish. It consists of anglerfish insulin bearing an additional tripeptide sequence, Gly•Thr•Lys, at the aminoterminus of the A chain. This region presumably represents a residuum of the connecting region of anglerfish proinsulin (Yamaji et al., 1972). These workers also have shown that this intermediate can be transformed to insulin by trypsin treatment. Grant and coworkers have presented evidence suggesting that tryptic activity alone can account for the conversion of codfish proinsulin to insulin (Grant and Coombs, 1971; Grant et al., 1971). They have identified a trypsin-like enzyme in codfish islets which also appears to exist in a zymogen or inactive form and which can be inhibited by NEP (O-ethyl-O-(p-nitrophenyl)-phenylpropylphosphonate), an inhibitor of trypsin-like enzymes and by DFP (Reid et al., 1968). In many of the fish insulins, including the cod and the anglerfish, a C-terminal basic residue is present on the B chain which corresponds to the penultimate lysine residue at position B29 in most mammalian insulins (Reid et al., 1968; Humbel et al., 1972). These lysine residues evidently provide the necessary basic sites for tryptic cleavage of the fish proinsulins. However, the lack of any data on residual proinsulin connecting peptide fragments arising from the conversion of proinsulin to insulin in these fishes makes it difficult to draw definite conclusions regarding the nature and specificity of the converting proteases.

Biosynthetic studies with rat islets indicate that a further cleavage of the C-peptide at or near position 22 occurs in about 20% of the proinsulin, giving rise to a shortened C-peptide fragment (Tager et al., 1973). Cleavage at this position in the C-peptide (Gln•Thr) would most likely be due to an endopeptidase with chymotryptic rather than tryptic specificity. Kinetic data suggest that this cleavage may occur only in intact proinsulin, suggesting that a particular conformation in this region also may be required for cleavage susceptibility.

The presence of an additional C-terminal residue of alanine, threonine or serine in the mammalian insulins beyond the lysine residue at B29 (Fig. 1) requires a more complex cleavage mechanism for conversion of the mammalian proinsulins. Similarly, in the hagfish the C-terminus of the B chain is methionine. The mammalian converting system cleaves the proinsulin at pairs of basic residues at either end of the connecting segment, releasing these basic residues as free amino acids, and giving rise to insulin and the free C-peptide as the major products of conversion (Fig. 7). The situation in the hagfish remains to be clarified. We have shown that pancreatic trypsin combined with an excess

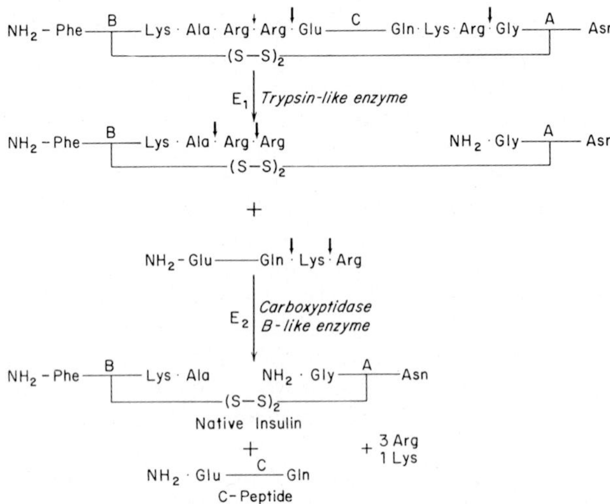

FIG. 7. The cleavage of a mammalian proinsulin to insulin and C-peptide by the combined action of trypsin-like and carboxypeptidase B-like proteases.

of carboxypeptidase B, an exopeptidase that cleaves C-terminal basic residues from peptides, can quantitatively convert bovine proinsulin to insulin and C-peptide in vitro (Kemmler et al., 1971). No degradation of the insulin occurred under the conditions used in these model experiments. Moreover, studies with isolated crude secretion granule fractions from rat islets have provided evidence for the existence of trypsin-like and carboxypeptidase B-like activities in these particles (Kemmler et al., 1972), but the enzymes have not yet been isolated or characterized. These results suggest that trypsin or a similar enzyme may have constituted the primitive 'converting enzyme' and that in the evolution of terrestrial forms modifications in insulin structure and in the converting enzyme system were gradually added. In some species carboxypeptidase B-like enzymes, and possibly others having chymotrypsin-like activity as described earlier in the case of the rat (Tager et al., 1973) may complement the tryptic cleavage. These results raise the interesting possibility that the secretion granules may contain small amounts of a variety of proteases. Thus, the kinds of cleavage that occur may be determined to a greater extent by the structural peculiarities of the substrates than by unusual adaptations of the proteases, although both factors obviously could play important roles.

It is possible that the pairs of basic residues found at the cleavage sites in the mammalian proinsulins allow for greater specificity and for more rapid rates of cleavage by the trypsin-like enzyme in the beta granules. The product of this kind of cleavage alone would be insulin bearing 2 additional residues of arginine at the C-terminus of the B chain. This form has somewhat lower biological activity than insulin (Chance, 1970) and is less soluble near neutral pH due to its higher isoelectric point. Removal of the arginine residues by a carboxypeptidase B-like enzyme may thus help to circumvent difficulties in storage or secretion that may arise from these altered properties.

It may be concluded that, despite some differences in the details, the major biochemical pathways involved in insulin biosynthesis, as well as the molecular structure of insulin in a wide sampling of the vertebrates, ranging from the hagfish through man, are strikingly similar. It is tempting to speculate that some of the protein hormones, perhaps especially those associated with the gastrointestinal tract and certain basic metabolic functions, can remain remarkably constant even though evolution over several hundred million years has evoked extensive changes in many other processes and organ systems.

SOME SPECULATIONS ON THE EVOLUTION OF INSULIN AND THE BETA CELLS

Evidence has been presented elsewhere that insulin-producing cells are located in the intestinal mucosa in certain invertebrate species and that these cells possibly were arranged similarly in the ancestral vertebrates (Falkmer et al., 1973). Likewise, during the development of the pancreas in mammals, beta cells first appear in the endoderm of the gut in the region of the pancreatic anlage (Pictet and Rutter, 1972). Whether these cells indeed arise from the endoderm of the gut has been questioned (Epple and Lewis, 1973); however, a definitive answer to this question is not as yet available.

The existence of a zymogen-like proinsulin and the presence in the beta cells of a proteolytic converting enzyme system which has components having modes of cleavage similar to certain exocrine pancreatic proteases is consistent with a close evolutionary relationship between the acinar and beta cells. These relationships prompt the hypothesis that in the most primitive form the secretory cells forming the mucosa of the intestine discharged a number of digestive hydrolytic enzymes into the gut, among which was a protein resembling proinsulin (Steiner et al., 1973, 1972, 1969). This primitive proinsulin, or protoproinsulin, may have had some kind of hydrolytic activity that has since been lost, or occurs only when it is combined with its receptor. In the gut during the digestion of food, the protoproinsulin may have been degraded by the digestive proteases with the intermediate production of small amounts of insulin-like proteins that could be absorbed into the blood (Fig. 8). The close temporal association between the appearance of this insulin-like protein in the blood and the influx of nutrients such as amino acids

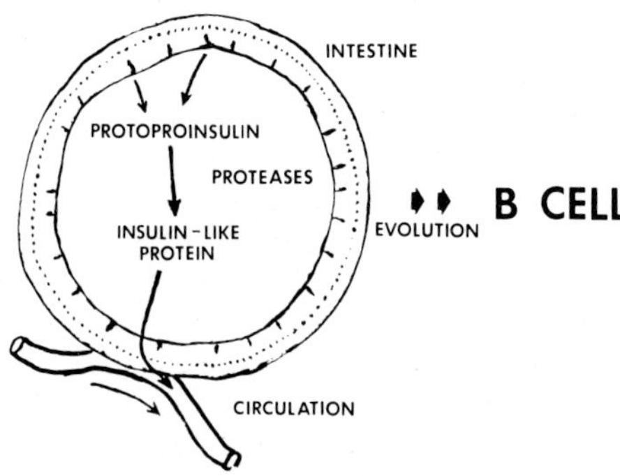

FIG. 8. Hypothetical mode of evolution of insulin and the beta cell system. The primitive mucosal cells of the digestive tract may have elaborated a proinsulin-like protein along with other digestive hydrolases. During digestion this protoproinsulin could be degraded to give rise to fragments having insulin-like properties. This process might then have been internalized in specialized cells (beta cells) restricted to this function in order to provide more precise regulation of the synthesis, storage and release of the hormone.

and sugars would have enhanced the possible evolution of an endocrine role for this protein. This would, of course, be especially likely if the insulin-like protein enhanced the utilization of these nutrients by the tissues of the organism in some way, perhaps by interacting in a favorable manner with the plasma membranes of the tissue cells, perhaps even by hydrolyzing certain critical bonds in the membranes. This cyclic absorption and interaction could have constituted the basis for a rudimentary regulatory system which conferred a selective advantage to these organisms. In the course of time this primitive endocrine system may have been refined by the gradual specialization of some of the mucosal cells for the unique role of making and storing the insulin-like protein and releasing it in judicious amounts at appropriate times. These specialized cells also eventually began to discharge the finished hormone directly into the bloodstream, and thus retained a close association with the vascular system even though their direct association with the intestinal cells was lost.

Although this is an attractive hypothesis, many gaps in our knowledge of the origin and function of the beta cells must be filled in before we can determine whether it is correct. Information is especially needed regarding the existence of proinsulin-like proteins in invertebrates and in more primitive vertebrates. Modern methods of protein purification and the use of powerful immunological tools should enable us to carry out these studies in the near future. As more structural information on many different classes of proteins accumulates, unsuspected relationships may suddenly emerge. Thus a recent study of the salivary gland nerve growth factor has suggested that this protein is closely related to proinsulin and that its gene may have arisen from the gene for proinsulin by the process of gene duplication (Frazier et al., 1972). This observation is especially interesting in view of the many developmental and functional similarities between the salivary glands and the pancreas. Likewise, secretin from the intestine and glucagon from the pancreatic alpha cells clearly are closely related proteins derived from a common ancestral gene (Mutt et al., 1970). Further study of many exocrine pancreatic and intestinal protein sequences may reveal important evolutionary relationships between these and some of the proteins of the beta cells. Only time and much more patient study can slowly fill in the gaps in this fascinating but incomplete picture, but these efforts will surely be richly rewarded, both in terms of practical and of theoretical gains.

REFERENCES

ARQUILLA, E. R., MILES, P. V. and MORRIS, J. W. (1972): Immunochemistry of insulin. In: *Handbook of Physiology – Endocrinology I, Chapter 9,* pp. 159–173. Editors: D. F. Steiner and N. Freinkel. American Physiological Society, Washington, D.C.

BLUNDELL, T. L., DODSON, G. G., DODSON, E., HODGKIN, D. C. and VIJAYAN, M. (1971): X-ray analysis and the structure of insulin. *Rec. Progr. Hormone Res., 27,* 1.

CARPENTER, F. H. (1966): Relationship of structure to biological activity of insulin as revealed by degradative studies. *Amer. J. Med., 40,* 750.

CHANCE, R. E. (1970): Chemical, physical, biological and immunological studies on porcine proinsulin and related polypeptides. In: *Proceedings of the 7th Congress of the International Diabetes Federation, Buenos Aires, 1970,* pp. 292–305. International Congress Series No. 231, Excerpta Medica, Amsterdam.

CLARK, J. L. and STEINER, D. F. (1969): Insulin biosynthesis in the rat: demonstration of two proinsulins. *Proc. nat. Acad. Sci. U.S.A., 62,* 278.

COHN, D. V., MacGREGOR, R. R., CHU, L. L., KIMMEL, J. R. and HAMILTON, J. W. (1972): Calcemic fraction-A: Biosynthetic peptide precursor of parathyroid hormones. *Proc. nat. Acad. Sci. U.S.A., 69,* 1521.

COULTER, C. L., PETERSON, J. D., STEINER, D. F., EMDIN, S. O. and FALKMER, S. (1973): Hagfish insulin: structural and crystallographic observations on a primitive protein hormone. In preparation.

DAYHOFF, M. O. (1972): Editor of: *Atlas of Protein Sequence and Structure, Vol. 5,* p. 50. National Biomedical Research Foundation, Washington, D.C.

EMDIN, S., PETERSON, J. D., COULTER, C. L., OSTBERG, Y., FALKMER, S. and STEINER, D. F. (1973): The structure and biosynthesis of insulin in a primitive vertebrate, the cyclostome, *Myxine glutinosa.* In: *Abstracts, 9th International Congress of Biochemistry, Stockholm,* in press.

EPPLE, A. and LEWIS, T. L. (1973): Comparative histophysiology of the pancreatic islets. *Amer. Zool.,* in press.

FALKMER, S., EMDIN, S., HAVU, N., LUNDGREN, G., MARQUES, M., OSTBERG, Y., STEINER, D. F. and THOMAS, N. W. (1973): Insulin in invertebrates and cyclostomes. *Amer. Zool.,* in press.

FALKMER, S. and PATENT, G. J. (1972): Comparative and embryological aspects of the pancreatic islets. In: *Handbook of Physiology – Endocrinology I, Chapter 1,* pp. 1–23. Editors: D. F. Steiner and N. Freinkel. Williams and Wilkins Company, Baltimore, Md.

FALKMER, S. and WILSON, S. (1967): Comparative aspects of the immunology and biology of insulin. *Diabetologia, 3,* 519.

FRAZIER, W. A., ANGELETTI, R. H. and BRADSHAW, R. A. (1972): Nerve growth factor and insulin. *Science, 176,* 482.

GRANT, P. T. and COOMBS, T. L. (1971): Proinsulin, a biosynthetic precursor of insulin. In: *Essays in Biochemistry, Vol. 6,* pp. 69–92. Editors: P. N. Campbell and G. D. Greville. Academic Press, London, England.

GRANT, P. T., COOMBS, T. L., THOMAS, N. W. and SARGENT, J. R. (1971): The conversion of [^{14}C] proinsulin to insulin in isolated subcellular fractions of fish islet preparations. In: *Subcellular Organization and Function in Endocrine Tissues. Memoirs of the Society for Endocrinology, London, Vol. 19,* pp. 481–495. Editors: H. Heller and K. Lederis. Cambridge University Press, Cambridge, Mass.

GRANT, P. T. and REID, K. B. M. (1968): Biosynthesis of an insulin precursor by islet tissue of cod (*Gadus callarias*). *Biochem. J., 110,* 281.

GREGORY, R. A. and TRACY, H. J. (1972): Isolation of two 'big gastrins' from Zollinger-Ellison tumour tissue. *Lancet, II,* 797.

HUMBEL, R. E., BOSSHARD, H. R. and ZAHN, R. (1972): Chemistry of insulin. In: *Handbook of Physiology – Endocrinology I, Chapter 6,* pp. 111–132. Editors: D. F. Steiner and N. Freinkel. Williams and Wilkins Company, Baltimore, Md.

JARVIK, E. (1964): Specializations in early vertebrates. *Ann. Soc. Roy. Zool. Belg., 94,* 11–95.

KEMMLER, W., PETERSON, J. D., RUBENSTEIN, A. H. and STEINER, D. F. (1972): On the biosynthesis, intracellular transport and mechanism of conversion of proinsulin to insulin and C-peptide. *Diabetes, 21,* 572.

KEMMLER, W., PETERSON, J. D. and STEINER, D. F. (1971): Studies on the conversion of proinsulin to insulin. I. Conversion in vitro with trypsin and carboxypeptidase B. *J. biol. Chem., 246,* 6786.

MUTT, V., JORPES, J. E. and MAGNUSSEN, S. (1970): Structure of porcine secretin. *Europ. J. Biochem., 15,* 513.

NOE, B. D. and BAUER, G. E. (1971): Evidence for glucagon biosynthesis involving a protein intermediate in islets of the anglerfish (Lophius Americanus). *Endocrinology, 89,* 642.

NOLAN, C., MARGOLIASH, E., PETERSON, J. D. and STEINER, D. F. (1971): The structure of bovine proinsulin. *J. biol. Chem., 246,* 2780.

PETERSON, J. D., STEINER, D. F., EMDIN, S. O., OSTBERG, Y. and FALKMER, S. (1973): Isolation, composition and amino acid sequence of the insulin from a primitive vertebrate (Hagfish; *Myxine glutinosa*). *Fed. Proc., 32,* 577.

PICTET, R. and RUTTER, W. J. (1972): Development of the embryonic endocrine pancreas. In: *Handbook of Physiology – Endocrinology I, Chapter 2,* pp. 25–66. Editors: D. F. Steiner and N. Freinkel, Williams and Wilkins Company, Baltimore, Md.

REID, K. B. M., GRANT, P. T. and YOUNGSON, A. (1968): The sequence of amino acids in insulin isolated from the islet tissue of the cod (*Gadus callarias*). *Biochem. J., 110,* 289.

RUBENSTEIN, A. H., CLARK, J. L., MELANI, F. and STEINER, D. F. (1969): Secretion of proinsulin C-peptide by pancreatic β cells and its circulation in blood. *Nature (Lond.), 224,* 697.

RUBENSTEIN, A. H., MELANI, F. and STEINER, D. F. (1972): Circulating proinsulin: Immunology, measurement, and biological activity. In: *Handbook of Physiology – Endocrinology I, Chapter 33,* pp. 515–528. Editors: D. F. Steiner and N. Freinkel. Williams and Wilkins Company, Baltimore, Md.

RYLE, A. P., SANGER, F., SMITH, L. F. and KITAI, R. (1955): The disulfide bonds of insulin. *Biochem. J., 60,* 541.

SMITH, L. F. (1966): Species variation in the amino acid sequence of insulin. *Amer. J. Med., 40,* 662.

STEINER, D. F. (1973): Cocrystallization of proinsulin and insulin. *Nature (Lond.), 243,* 528.

STEINER, D. F. and CLARK, J. L. (1968): The spontaneous reoxidation of reduced beef and rat proinsulins. *Proc. nat. Acad. Sci. U.S.A., 60,* 662.

STEINER, D. F., CLARK, J. L., NOLAN, C., RUBENSTEIN, A. H., MARGOLIASH, E., ATEN, B. and OYER, P. E. (1969): Proinsulin and the biosynthesis of insulin. In: *Recent Progress in Hormone Research, Vol. 25,* pp. 207–282. Editor: E. B. Astwood. Academic Press, New York, N.Y.

STEINER, D. F., CLARK, J. L., NOLAN, C., RUBENSTEIN, A. H., MARGOLIASH, E., MELANI, F. and OYER, P. E. (1970): The biosynthesis of insulin and some speculations regarding the pathogenesis of human diabetes. In: *The Pathogenesis of Diabetes Mellitus. Proceedings of the Thirteenth Nobel Symposium,* pp. 123–132. Editors: E. Cerasi and R. Luft. Almqvist and Wiksell, Stockholm.

STEINER, D. F., CUNNINGHAM, D. D., SPIGELMAN, L. and ATEN, B. (1967): Insulin biosynthesis: evidence for a precursor. *Science, 157,* 697.

STEINER, D. F., KEMMLER, W., CLARK, J. L., OYER, P. E. and RUBENSTEIN, A. H. (1972): The biosynthesis of insulin. In: *Handbook of Physiology – Endocrinology I, Chapter 10,* pp. 175–198. Editors: D. F. Steiner and N. Freinkel. Williams and Wilkins Company, Baltimore, Md.

STEINER, D. F. and OYER, P. E. (1967): The biosynthesis of insulin and a probable precursor of insulin by a human islet cell adenoma. *Proc. nat. Acad. Sci. U.S.A., 57,* 473.

STEINER, D. F., PETERSON, J. D., TAGER, H., EMDIN, S., ÖSTBERG, Y. and FALKMER, S. (1973): Comparative aspects of proinsulin and insulin structure and biosynthesis. *Amer. Zool.,* in press.

TAGER, H. S., EMDIN, S. O., CLARK, J. L. and STEINER, D. F. (1973): Studies on the conversion of proinsulin to insulin. II. Evidence for a chymotrypsin-like cleavage in the connecting peptide region of insulin precursors in the rat. *J. biol. Chem., 248,* 3476.

TAGER, H. S. and STEINER, D. F. (1973): Isolation of a glucagon-containing peptide: primary structure of a possible fragment of proglucagon. *Proc. nat. Acad. Sci. U.S.A.,* in press.

TRAKATELLIS, A. C. and SCHWARTZ, G. P. (1970): Biosynthesis of insulin in anglerfish islets. *Nature (Lond.)*, *225*, 473.

WEITZEL, V., STRATLING, W., HAHN, J. and MARTINI, O. (1967): Insulin vom Schleimfisch (*Myxine glutinosa; Cyclostomata*). *Hoppe-Seyler's Z. physiol. Chem.*, *348*, 525.

YAMAJI, K., TADA, K. and TRAKATELLIS, A. C. (1972): On the biosynthesis of insulin in anglerfish islets. *J. biol. Chem.*, *247*, 4080.

THE ROLE OF GLUCAGON IN HEALTH AND DIABETES

NEW ASPECTS OF GLUCAGON PATHOLOGY AND PATHOPHYSIOLOGY

ROGER H. UNGER

Department of Internal Medicine, The University of Texas Southwestern Medical School and Veterans Administration, Dallas, Tex., U.S.A.

1973 marks the 50th anniversary of the hormone, glucagon, discovered in 1923 by Murlin and Kimbell. Throughout the entire half century, glucagon has been the center of controversy. However, whereas little more than a decade ago most authorities in the field regarded with scepticism its role as a hormone, today its status as an important, if not vital, regulating force in nutrient homeostasis is unquestioned, and its importance in a broad spectrum of pathophysiologic states is now being recognized.

The present review will consider 3 relatively new areas relating to alpha cell function in health and disease: first, the alpha cell response to fat ingestion, second, the alpha-beta cell relationship, and third, their function in catabolic diseases.

ISLET CELL RESPONSE TO A FAT MEAL

There is very little information concerning the islet cell response to a fat meal. Pi-Sunyer et al. (1969) reported a small rise in insulin, but Ooms and Ballasse (1968) found no rise. Böttger et al. (1973) have observed that in conscious dogs the ingestion of fat evokes a most dramatic secretory response from the pancreatic alpha cell, in addition to the small rise in insulin first noted by others. A very large intraduodenal fat meal given to conscious dogs in unemulsified form elicits a rise in glucagon and a very minor, more short-lived increase in insulin (Fig. 1). Hyperglucagonemia persists throughout the experimental period. A smaller, more physiologic dose of 3 g of fat per kilo emulsified in egg yolk evokes an even more dramatic increase in glucagon, again accompanied by a small rise in insulin which is not statistically significant.

The islet cell response to carbohydrate and protein is under the primary control of the nutrients themselves, modified by anticipatory and augmenting signals from the gut. A fat meal, however, differs in that the absorbed nutrient circulates as chylomicrons which are devoid of any influence on either insulin or glucagon secretion. As shown in Figure 2, chyle harvested from dogs with thoracic duct fistulae following the intraduodenal administration of fat failed to induce a rise in glucagon when infused in intact, conscious recipient animals, despite chylomicronemia exceeding that which occurs after the ingestion of fat. The small early rise in the insulin was not noted either. It can be concluded that chylomicronemia does not account for the islet cell response to a fat meal, which suggests that the entire response is a consequence of a signal arising from the gut. This suspicion is further supported by studies shown in Figure 3, in which dogs with thoracic

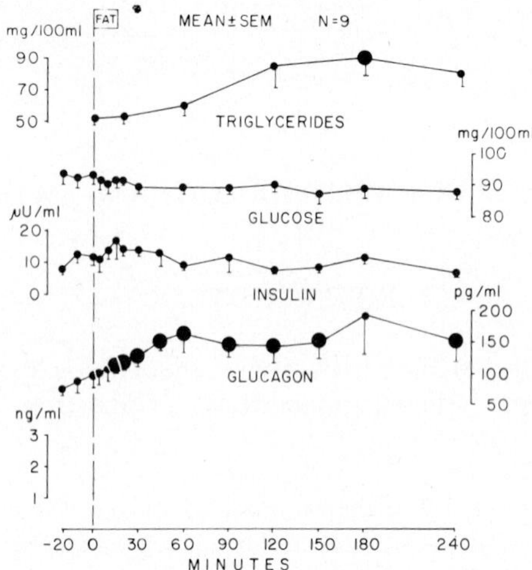

FIG. 1. The effect of intraduodenal administration of 10 g/kg of peanut oil on glucagon and insulin in a group of 9 conscious dogs. Large circles signify points which differ statistically ($P < 0.02$) from the mean of the 3 base-line values. (Reprinted with permission of the Journal of clinical Investigation.)

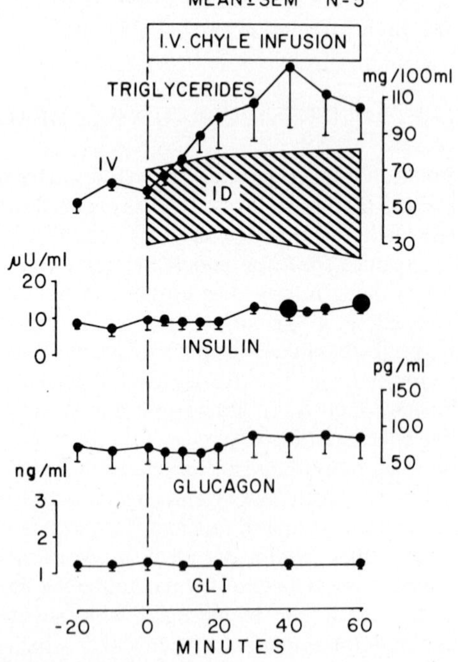

FIG. 2. The effect of canine chyle, infused intravenously at a rate of 1.2–2.1 mg/min. for 60 minutes, on glucagon, insulin, and GLI in a group of 5 conscious dogs. The large circles represent points which differ statistically ($P < 0.02$) from the mean of the 3 base-line values. (Reprinted with permission of the Journal of clinical Investigation.)

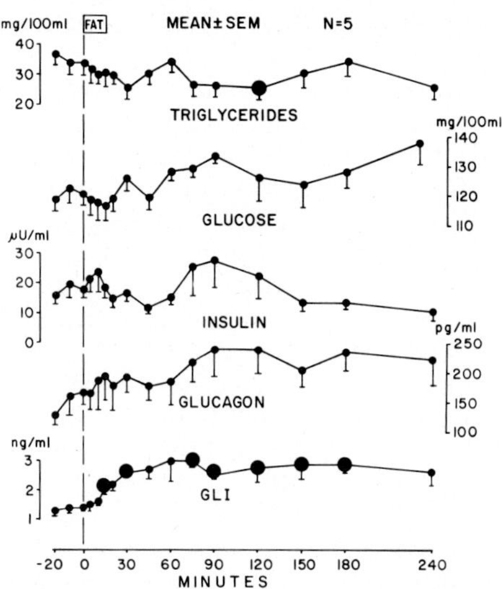

FIG. 3. The effect of intraduodenal administration of 10 g/kg of peanut oil in a group of 5 conscious dogs with a thoracic duct fistula. The large circles signify points which differ statistically ($P < 0.02$) from the mean of the 3 base-line values. (Reprinted with permission of the Journal of clinical Investigation.)

duct fistulae were given an intraduodenal fat meal during which chyle flowed out of the thoracic duct fistulae rather than into the circulation. Virtually complete exclusion of chyle from the circulation is verified by the absence of a rise in triglycerides during these experiments. Despite this, the secretory response of the alpha and beta cells to a fat meal appears to be intact. In other words, the islet cell response to fat absorption must be attributed to a signal originating either from the gut or from some point between the gut and the thoracic duct fistulae.

The nature of the signal is obscure. Pancreozymin, known to be released during the absorption of fat, stimulates glucagon secretion, and remains a strong candidate for this role.

It is well established that alpha cell stimulation can be completely blocked by hyperglycemia, reduced by a high carbohydrate diet, and exaggerated by a low carbohydrate diet. In other words, the response of alpha and beta cells is greatly influenced by the present and past availability of exogenous carbohydrate. It is not surprising, therefore, that fat-induced hyperglucagonemia is totally abolished when glucose is infused, while the insulin response to fat ingestion is enormously increased. If, as has been suggested by many workers, glucagon diminishes lipoprotein secretion by the liver and insulin increases it, it may well be that the phenomenon of carbohydrate induction of hyperlipoproteinemia is mediated by this altered response of the alpha and beta cells to the absorption of fat (Eaton and Kipnis, 1969). Since the complete absorption of a fat meal requires hours, the gut and its contents may well exert an influence upon the islet cell response for a large portion of a given day. If so, these observations may have important physiologic and pathophysiologic implications with respect to blood lipid homeostasis.

ALPHA-BETA CELL RELATIONSHIPS

The alpha and beta cells are believed to operate as a bicellular, bihormonal unit functioning in tightly coordinated fashion for the purpose of regulating the disposition of key nutrients in cells throughout the body in a manner appropriate to their needs for and availability of exogenous fuels in the environment. When they function in appropriate fashion, the alpha-beta cell couple can achieve a remarkably efficient utilization of exogenous nutrients, storing them rapidly irrespective of the magnitude of the presented load, and thus avoiding wastage. This efficient storage capability may be of potential significance with respect to the number of organisms that can be sustained on the earth by the available planetary food supply. The proper function of the islet cells in time of famine makes possible the most judicious allocation of these stored fuels as required to meet energy needs, minimizing use of precious nitrogen-containing substrates for glucagoneogenesis (Cahill et al., 1966). This remarkable regulation of nutrient economy is believed to be controlled on a moment-to-moment basis by the relative perfusing concentrations of the anabolic hormone insulin and the catabolic hormone glucagon in the portal blood. Thus, a high concentration of insulin relative to glucagon would be appropriate only during an influx of exogenous fuels and would promote their prompt storage in macromolecular forms of glycogen, triglycerides, or proteins. A low concentration of insulin relative to glucagon would be appropriate only when exogenous fuels are not available, and would promote the release of stored fuels for energy needs. Hepatic glycogen provides immediate glucose for cerebral requirements, adipose tissue furnishes free fatty acids and glycerol, and, when necessary, proteins of muscle and other tissues can donate amino acids for hepatic glucagoneogenesis.

The molar ratio of insulin to glucagon has been proposed as a crude, semi-quantitative, but nevertheless convenient means of expressing in integrated form the bihormonal concentration (Unger, 1971). It is clear that, whenever there is maximal need for endogenous glucose production, as in total starvation, violent exercise, and shock, the ratio in these circumstances declines to well below 1.0; at the opposite extreme, as during abundance of exogenous carbohydrate, the ratio may be as high as 70. After an overnight fast, it ranges between 2 and 4.

As pointed out earlier, it is clear that the response of the alpha and beta cells to a given circumstance is influenced not only by the levels of nutrients which perfuse them at that moment, but also by the nutrient availability within the recent past, suggesting a 'memory' for the recent nutritional events and needs. In normal subjects this islet cell memory permits a highly appropriate disposition of circulating nutrients, particularly precious amino acids. For example, in a normal, well-fed individual, after an overnight fast an influx of amino acids, whether from a beef meal or an amino acid infusion, stimulates both insulin and glucagon; but in this situation the insulin rise is always greater than the glucagon rise, causing a 90% increase in the molar insulin-glucagon ratio, a change which predictably would permit utilization of a substantial fraction of the exogenous amino acids for protein synthesis. However, the same amino acid load given to the same individuals after a week of starvation does not stimulate an increase in insulin but causes an exaggerated increase in glucagon; instead of an anabolic rise in response to amino acids, there is a catabolic decline in the insulin-glucagon ratio. This predictably would pre-empt a substantial share of exogenous amino acids for gluconeogenesis at the expense of protein synthesis. Thus, the bi-hormonal response to the same amino acid load can be either anabolic or catabolic, depending on the present and/or previous availability of carbohydrates. If, for example, protein is ingested during a glucose infusion, the anabolic rise in the bihormonal ratio is greatly exaggerated, rising 600%, a response which must completely block gluconeogenesis from the ingested amino acids. This may explain the well-known protein-sparing effect of glucose and the efficacy of hyperalimentation regimens in reversing a negative nitrogen balance.

The mechanism by which these appropriate islet cell responses come about is not clear. Certainly nutrients, particularly glucose, seem to have overriding control, with important modifications by hormones from the gut, the adrenal medulla and cortex, and the autonomic nervous system. More recently, however, the studies of Orci et al. (1973) have revealed the existence of intercellular communications between alpha and beta cells, as well as between beta and beta cells and alpha and alpha cells. It is thus possible that the islets of Langerhans function as a synctitium through membrane specializations which are the sites of electrical and metabolic coupling; at least, the morphologic basis for the existence of such a system has been established.

It is proposed that the proper operation of this bihormonal islet cell unit is essential for health, and, when it fails to respond appropriately to the wide changes in fuel availability and need which must be endured as part of life, optimal health is not long maintained. As will be pointed out below, virtually every catabolic disorder thus far studied is associated with an inappropriate response of the islets of Langerhans.

ISLET CELL FUNCTION IN CATABOLIC DISEASES

Genetic diabetes mellitus appears to constitute a primary disorder of the alpha-beta cell couple in which the insulin-glucagon ratio is fixed at a basal or sub-basal level, comparable to that of starvation, irrespective of the availability of nutrients. Thus, an anabolic increase in the ratio is never possible and ingested nutrients are inefficiently and wastefully handled. It appears that in certain non-diabetic states similarly characterized by wasteful handling of the nutrients, particularly amino acids, the insulin-glucagon ratio is also similarly fixed. In patients with severe and moderately severe infection (Fig. 4), hyperglucagonemia was present; even when glucose was provided in abundance, glucagon levels remained high and insulin failed to rise in normal fashion, although none of these individuals were known to be diabetic before or after their illness. During their illness, however, they undoubtedly had abnormal glucose tolerance, weight loss and negative nitrogen balance. As shown in Figure 5, hyperglucagonemia of the magnitude encountered in non-diabetics with severe infection is sufficient to worsen the state of metabolic control; it is therefore possible that infection-induced hyperglucagonemia is a major factor in the worsening of the diabetes which characteristically accompanies infection in diabetics.

Patients with severe trauma exhibit similar hyperglucagonemia at the time of their hospitalization and, irrespective of the availability of exogenous glucose, glucagon is not suppressed, nor is insulin adequately stimulated. Patients with severe burns also exhibit this abnormality, despite constant glucose infusion, precisely during the period of nitrogen loss.

While the mechanism of these abnormalities has not been established, it is reasonable to link them to hormonal changes already known to occur in such disorders, changes which tend to increase glucagon secretion. Increased corticosteroids have been reported by Marco et al. (1973) to cause increased plasma glucagon. Increased catecholamines have been shown by many workers to stimulate glucagon, while inhibiting stimulated insulin

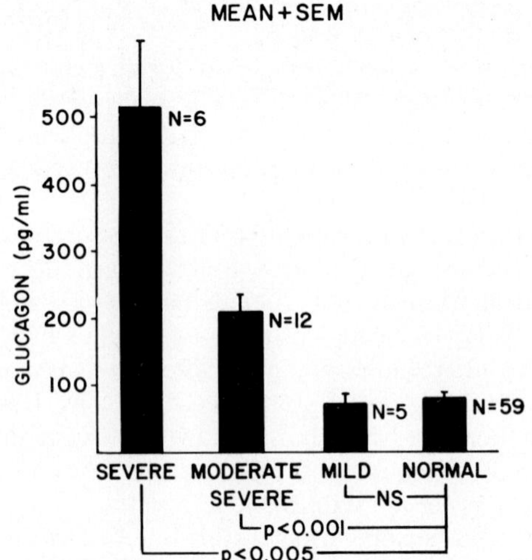

FIG. 4. Mean glucagon levels in non-diabetic patients with acute infection.

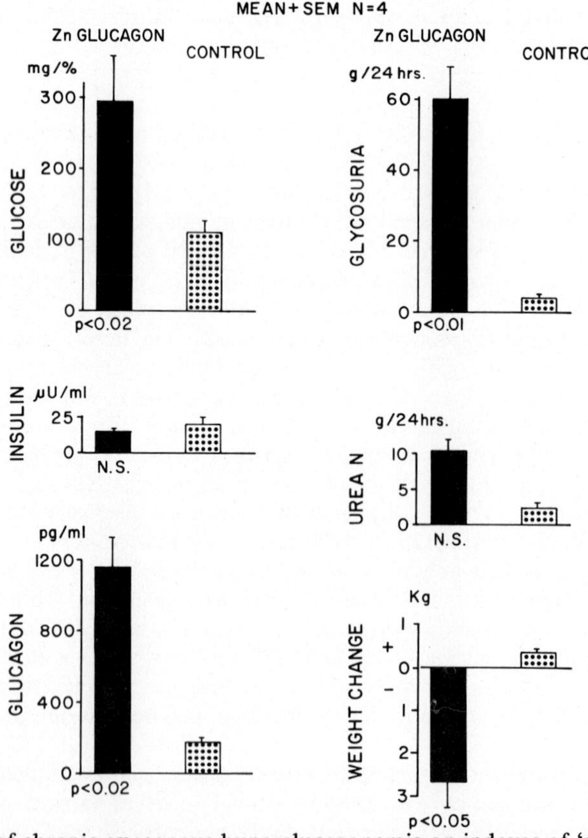

FIG. 5. Effect of chronic exogenous hyperglucagonemia on indexes of 'diabetic control' in 4 alloxan-diabetic dogs (bars denote means ± S.E.M.). (Reprinted with permission of the New England Journal of Medicine.)

secretion, and increased sympathetic tone has a similar effect on the islets of Langerhans. Whatever the cause, it seems likely that the inappropriate 'fixing' of the insulin-glucagon ratio in a low catabolic range would permit unnecessary use of amino acids for glucose and urea production at a time when protein synthesis is needed for healing and immunologic response.

Amherdt et al. (1973) have recently reported that hepatic lysosomes are significantly increased during hyperglucagonemia when the insulin-glucagon ratio is low. Glucagon is also believed to interfere with hepatic regeneration in vivo and DNA synthesis in cultured liver cells (Leffert, 1973). The implications of a prolonged and fixed reduction of the insulin-glucagon ratio could conceivably transcend the important issues of amino acid disposition, and actually influence the intracellular anatomy of various cells and possibly their ability to reproduce themselves.

REFERENCES

AMHERDT, M., HARRIS, V., RENOLD, A., ORCI, L. and UNGER, R. H. (1973): Hepatic autophagy and the insulin/glucagon ratio (I/G) in severe diabetic ketoacidosis (DKA). *Diabetes, 22/Suppl. 1,* 302.

BALASSE, E. and OOMS, H. A. (1968): Effet d'une élévation aiguë du taux des acides gras libres (NEFA) sur la tolérance glucidique et la réponse insulinique à l'hyperglycémie chez l'homme normal. *Rev. franç. Ètud. clin. biol., 13,* 62.

BÖTTGER, I., DOBBS, R., FALOONA, G. R. and UNGER, R. H. (1973): The effects of triglyceride absorption upon glucagon, insulin and gut glucagon-like immunoreactivity. *J. clin. Invest., 52,* 10.

CAHILL Jr., G. F., HERRERA, M. G., MORGAN, A. P., SOELDNER, J. S., STEINKE, J., LEVY, P. L., REICHARD Jr., G. A. and KIPNIS, D. M. (1966): Hormone fuel interrelationships during fasting. *J. clin. Invest., 45,* 1751.

EATON, P. P. and KIPNIS, D. M. (1969): Effect of glucose feeding on lipoprotein synthesis in the rat. *Amer. J. Physiol., 217,* 1153.

LEFFERT, H. L. (1973): Growth control of primary cultured fetal rat hepatocytes. VI. Hormonal control of DNA synthesis and its possible significance to the problem of linear regeneration. In preparation.

MARCO, J., CALLE, C., RAMON, D., DIAZ-FIERROS, M., VILLANUEVA, M. L. and VALVERDE, I. (1973): Hyperglucagonism induced by glucocorticoid treatment in man. *New Engl. J. Med., 288,* 128.

MURLIN, J. R., PIPER, H. A. and ALLEN, R. S. (1923): Aqueous extracts of pancreas: physical and chemical behavior of insulin. *J. biol. Chem., 58,* 321.

ORCI, L., UNGER, R. H. and RENOLD, A. E. (1973): Structural basis for intercellular communications between cells of the islets of Langerhans. *Experientia (Basel), 29,* 777.

PI-SUNYER, F. X., HASHIM, S. A. and VAN ITALLIE, T. B. (1969): Insulin and ketone responses to ingestion of medium and long-chain triglycerides in man. *Diabetes, 18,* 96.

UNGER, R. H., MÜLLER, W. A. and FALOONA, G. R. (1971): Insulin/glucagon ratio. *Trans. Ass. Amer. Phycns, 84,* 122.

SOME ASPECTS OF THE PHYSIOLOGY OF GLUCAGON*

R. ASSAN[1], J. R. ATTALI[1], G. BALLERIO[2], J. R. GIRARD[3], M. HAUTECOUVERTURE[1], A. KERVRAN[3], P. F. PLOUIN[1], G. SLAMA[1], E. SOUFFLET[3], G. TCHOBROUTSKY[1] and A. TIENGO[4]

[1] Department of Diabetology, Hôtel Dieu, Paris, France; [2] University of Parma, Italy; [3] Faculté des Sciences, Paris, France; [4] University of Padova, Italy

That the A_2 cells play an actual role in fuel regulation in daily conditions progressively appears from multiple recent studies. The physiological factors responsible for this secretion are not limited to a simple blood glucose level/glucagon response regulatory mechanism.

Hyperaminoacidemia, diabetes mellitus (or any impairment of glucose utilization) and the neonatal period (in some species at least), are three physiological or physiopathological conditions where hyperglucagonemia is detected. The following presentation deals with the data found in the literature, as well as the results of personal investigations concerning these three conditions, in each of which very different metabolic patterns are associated with a common final hyperglucagonemia. It may be fruitful to compare these situations, if one bears in mind not only the teleological significance but also the analytical explanatory mechanisms of A_2 cell function.

INFLUENCE OF AMINO ACIDS ON GLUCAGON SECRETION

An increase in the plasma concentration of some amino acids is associated with a rise in the plasma level of pancreatic glucagon; this response occurs in man and in several animal species, under a wide variety of experimental conditions. The glucagon secretion observed after a protein meal illustrates the physiology of this process, when A_2 cells are faced with an exogenous amino acid load. Among the best stimulators of glucagon secretion is arginine, providing a convenient test for A_2 cell function in vivo and in vitro. The significance of the aminogenic glucagon secretion is unequivocal in such cases, the glucagon secreted prevents the hypoglycemia which would occur as a consequence of the aminogenic insulin release; it also enhances the uptake by the liver of the amino acid presented.

Whether endogenous amino acidemia can also rise enough to stimulate glucagon secretion in some physiological or pathological circumstances remains a point for discussion.

* This work was supported by grants from the Institut National de la Santé et de la Recherche Médicale (INSERM), the Fondation Nationale pour la Recherche Médicale, the Université Paris VI (U.E.R. Broussais-Hôtel-Dieu), and from the Délégation Générale de la Recherche Scientifique et Technique (No 71-7-3250-01).

In some catabolic situations with a high level of amino acids, glucagon may be secreted, stimulating then their utilization by the liver.

The exquisite sensitivity of A_2 cells to amino acids, and the early appearance in fetal life of this glucagon responsiveness suggest that this function may play an actual role in the fuel-regulatory mechanism.

Little is known about the intimate mechanism of the aminogenic glucagon secretion. The respective glucagon-stimulating potencies of natural amino acids are not correlated with their metabolic fate; the stimulatory effect of some non-metabolized artificial amino acids supports the hypothesis associating the membrane transport system with the triggering of glucagon secretion. The regulatory effect of glucose concentration on the response to arginine and the disappearance of this effect in diabetes, suggest that metabolic processes inside the A_2 cell are also involved.

OCCURRENCE OF THE AMINOGENIC GLUCAGON SECRETION

In vivo aminogenic glucagon secretion

In man the simple ingestion of a protein meal (500 g of beef meat) is rapidly followed by a brisk rise in glucagon concentration (Assan et al., 1967; Assan, 1971). Beginning from the first minutes of the meal, it reaches a peak at 150 minutes after the start of the meal, with a maximum peak of 120 pg/ml above the fasting level (Müller et al., 1970). Together with this rise in glucagon there is an increase in insulin concentration and in alpha-amino-nitrogen but the blood glucose concentration is unchanged or even slightly reduced (Pek et al., 1968, 1969).

The intraduodenal administration of a mixture of 10 amino acids in the dog induces similar changes; glucagon from pancreatic origin electively rises (Ohneda et al., 1969a; Unger et al., 1969).

The intravenous infusion of a mixture of 10 amino acids in dogs also induces a rise of glucagon in plasma, most of the rise occurring during the first 5 minutes; a uniform increase of insulin and a slight blood glucose increment simultaneously occur (Unger et al., 1969).

Intravenous infusion of arginine in man provides a convenient test for alpha cell function; doses of 25 g during 30 minutes (Assan et al., 1967) or nearly 12 mg/min./kg body weight (Pek et al., 1968, 1969) have been used. Such doses induce a rise of at least 100 pg/ml in every normal individual. A dose response proportionality can be measured for doses between 2.5 and 15 mg/kg/min. (Assan et al., unpublished results), and a significant glucagon response was detected for the lowest of these doses.

Among other amino acids tested in man, mainly the glucogenic amino acids, glycine and alanine have been studied because of the possible physiological significance of their glucagon-stimulating activities: doubling the basal alanine concentration in plasma has no effect, but tripling this concentration induces a significant glucagon response; only high doses of exogenous glycine induce an effect in men fasted for 2 weeks (Müller et al., 1973a).

Histidine and arginine infused into the pancreatic artery of dogs are glucagon-stimulatory (Kaneto and Kosaka, 1971).

Twenty natural amino acids have been tested in the dog by intravenous infusion (Marreiro et al., 1972): particularly the most glycogenic amino acids were found to be stimulators, and among these particularly those entering the gluconeogenic pathway at the pyruvate level (alanine, serine, threonine, glycine, cysteine); those entering at the level of alpha-ketoglutarate or of succinyl-CoA were less active and those with an aliphatic branched structure were inactive.

Glucagon-stimulating and insulin-stimulating potencies were unrelated. The non-glucogenic amino acid leucine was usually non-stimulating (Pek et al., 1968; Unger et al., 1969). Tryptophan, which blocks the gluconeogenesis, was a stimulator in the adult rat (Assan et al., 1972a) and in the neonate rat (Girard et al., unpublished results).

In vitro studies

An arginine-induced glucagon secretion was also obtained in vitro with incubated rat and mice islets (Buchanan et al., 1972; Chesney and Schofield, 1969), with isolated perfused canine pancreas (Iversen, 1971) and with rat pancreas (Assan et al., 1972a). The aminogenic glucagon response can be detected early in pancreases from newborn and fetal animals and from man.

The techniques of perfusion and, to a less extent, of perifusion, have allowed dynamic studies to be carried out: a diphasic pattern of release is induced by a square-wave arginine stimulation (Iversen, 1971; Assan et al., 1972a; Hautecouverture et al., unpublished results), as illustrated by Figures 1 and 2. As occurs for insulin release, the kinetics

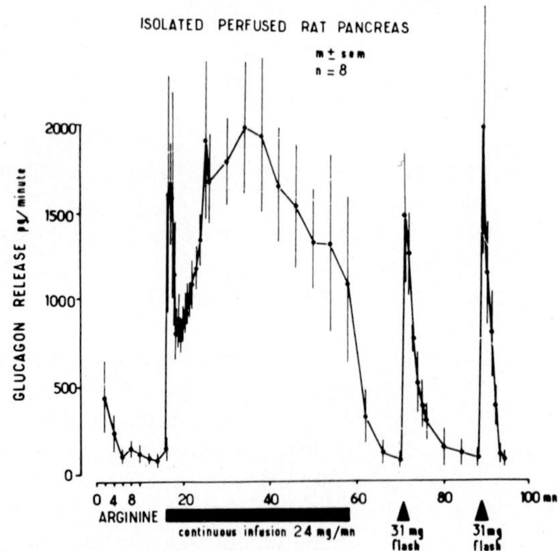

FIG. 1. Diphasic glucagon response to arginine in the perfused rat pancreas (from Nature New Biol., 1972, 239, 125, with permission of the editor).

of this diphasic glucagon secretion can be altered by poisons (colchicine, vincristine, cytochalazine) known to interfere with the microtubular microfilamentous system (Soufflet et al., 1973).

Some other natural amino acids stimulate glucagon release from the isolated perfused pancreas, according to a similar diphasic pattern (Fig. 3).

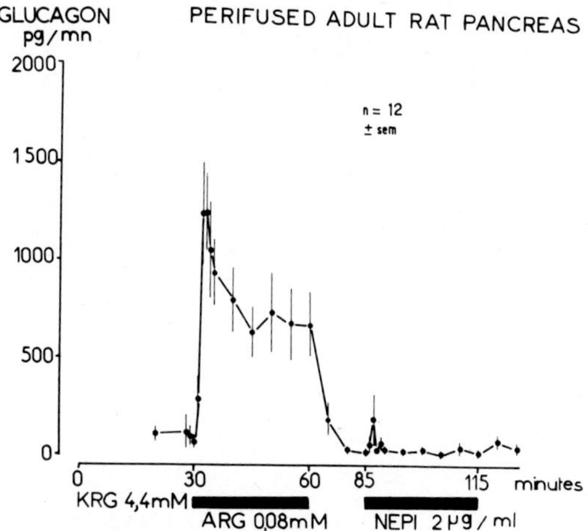

FIG. 2. Response to arginine of rat pancreas (adult) in the perifusion system (from Hautecouverture et al., unpublished results).

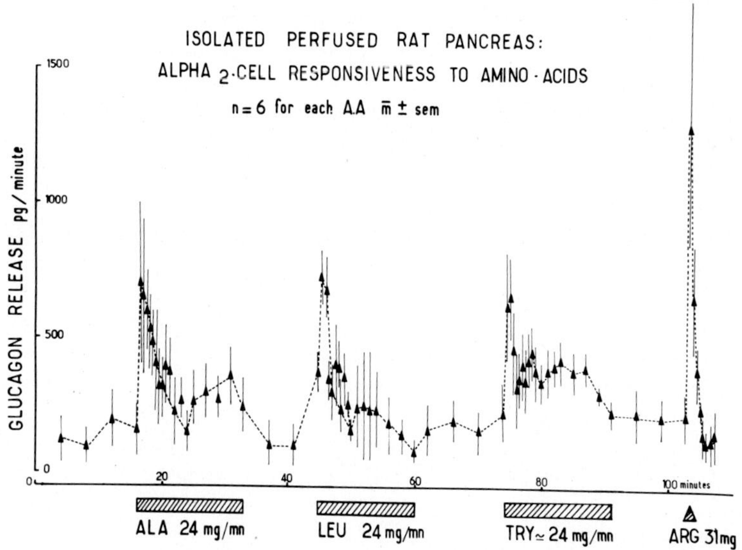

FIG. 3. Glucagon responses to various amino acids in the perfused isolated rat pancreas.

Moreover, some artificial amino acids, homoarginine and guanyl piperidine, carboxylic acid (G.P.A.), were found to be strong glucagon stimulators on the same preparation (Fig. 4). These artificial amino acids are not metabolized but are transported through the plasma membrane (Christensen et al., 1971); they are structurally closely related to arginine. Two other artificial amino acids, unrelated to arginine (cycloleucine and amino-isobutyric acid) were found to be poor glucagon stimulators (Assan et al., unpublished results).

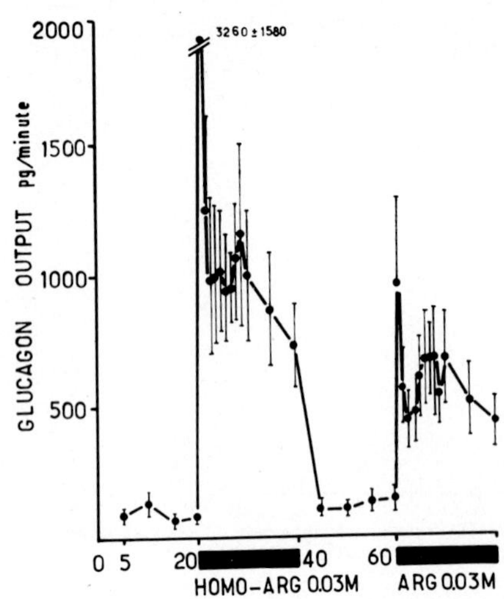

FIG. 4. Glucagon responses to artificial amino acid homo-arginine in the isolated perfused rat pancreas.

FACTORS INFLUENCING THE AMINOGENIC GLUCAGON SECRETION

Situations of fuel abundance and fuel need

Fuel abundance depresses the aminogenic glucagon secretion: An intravenous infusion of glucose, in non-diabetic human subjects, inhibits glucagon response to a meal; a sharp glucagon rebound occurs at the end of the glucose infusion (Ohneda et al., 1969b). Similarly a slow intravenous glucose infusion inhibits the glucagon secretion induced by amino acids in dogs (Ohneda et al., 1969b). The arginine-induced glucagon secretion in normal man is similarly inhibited by intravenous glucose and a dose-inhibition proportionality can be established.

In vitro, the arginine-induced glucagon secretion (Fig. 5) and the alanine-induced glucagon secretion (Luyckx, 1973) in the isolated perfused rat pancreas are strongly inhibited by a high glucose concentration in the perfusate.

Conversely, fuel need enhances the aminogenic response of A_2 cells: Glucagon response to a protein meal is enhanced by fasting, or by an antecedent carbohydrate-free diet (Müller et al., 1971b); fasting also enhances the response to 2 other glucogenic amino acids (Müller et al., 1973a). A 3-day fast is sufficient to enhance significantly the glucagon response to arginine (Assan et al., 1972a). After restoration of a normal blood glucose level by a short i.v. glucose infusion, the glucagon response to a subsequent arginine stimulation returns to normal, thus suggesting that the fast-induced decrease of

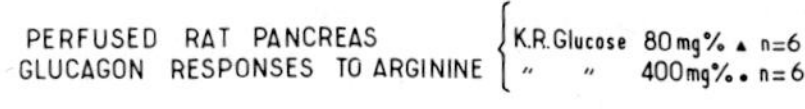

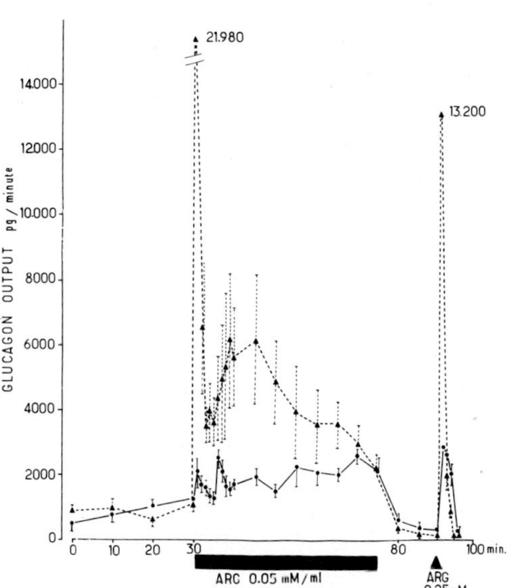

FIG. 5. Influence of glucose concentration on the glucagon response to arginine in the perfused rat pancreas (from Assan et al., unpublished results).

circulating glucose was the important factor in this fast-induced glucagon hyperresponsiveness (Assan et al., 1972a). Incidentally pancreases from rats fasted for 3 days, once isolated and perfused at a 80 mg% glucose concentration, failed to exhibit any hyperresponsiveness to a standard arginine stimulation (Assan et al., unpublished results).

Glucagon response to amino acids in diabetes mellitus is that observed in situations of fuel need when a hyperresponsiveness to arginine infusion is present. Moreover, it is not blunted by supranormal blood glucose levels, unless insulin is also administered (see this Volume, 'The role of glucagon in health and diabetes', pp. 137–216)'

In hyperlipemic patients high glucagon levels and hyperresponsiveness to arginine have been recently documented in normoglycemic subjects with endogenous hypertriglyceridemia (Tiengo et al., 1973).

In non-diabetic obese patients glucagon response to arginine has been found to be diminished (Wise et al., 1972).

The effect of prior dietary intake

Not only does the relative glucose and amino acid content of a meal influence the glucagon (and insulin) response to a meal, but the composition of the antecedent diet may also modify the bihormonal response. After one week of a low carbohydrate diet, the glucagon response to a protein meal was higher (and the insulin response weaker) than after a balanced diet (Müller et al., 1971a, b).

Potentiations by intestinal hormones

Pancreozymin, or a factor present in pancreozymin preparations, stimulates glucagon secretion by itself in vivo (Unger et al., 1967) and in the perfused rat pancreas in vitro (Iversen, 1971; Fussgänger et al., 1969). It is presumed that in physiological circumstances this factor potentiates the glucagon response following ingestion of a protein meal.

Caerulein, a gastrin-related hormone from lower vertebrates, can, in experimental conditions, stimulate glucagon release (De Caro et al., 1971; Fallucca et al., 1972). On perifused fragments of rat pancreas, these 2 hormones enhanced the glucagon release induced by arginine, as shown in Figure 6 (Hautecouverture et al., unpublished results). Secretin, which can suppress glucagon secretion when infused in vivo (Santeusiano et al., 1972), did not modify the arginine-induced glucagon release in the perifused fragments of rat pancreas.

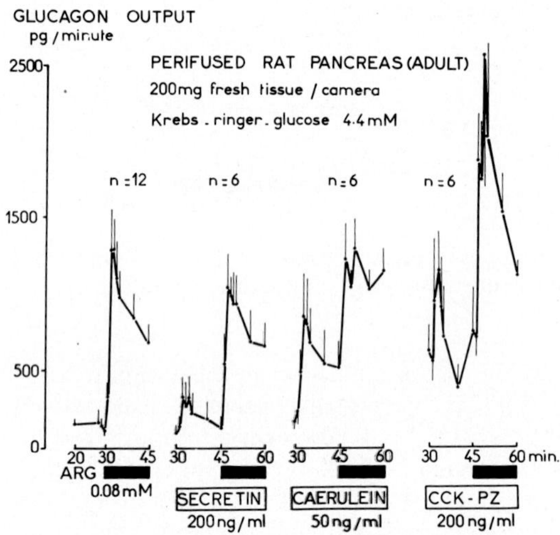

FIG. 6. Responses of perifused rat pancreas fragments to secretin, caerulein, and partially purified pancreozymin alone and associated with arginine (from Hautecouverture et al., unpublished results).

Influence of pharmacological agents

Sulfonylurea administration, in most studies, did not modify the arginine-induced glucagon secretion (see this Volume, pp. 137–216).

The addition of drugs affecting the cyclic AMP system has been variously appreciated: theophylline infusion in humans significantly reduced the arginine-induced glucagon secretion (Marco et al., 1972); in vitro, theophylline, cyclic AMP and dibutyryl cyclic AMP depressed the glucagon release in pancreatic monolayer cultures (Wollheim et al., 1973). In vitro, however, theophylline potentiated the aminogenic glucagon secretion from newborn rat pancreas (Rosselin et al., 1973). Thus the intervention of cAMP or a mediator in arginine-induced glucagon secretion is still a matter for discussion.

Glucocorticoid treatment enhanced the glucagon response to arginine in normal human subjects provided that the administration lasted for several days before the test (Marco et al., 1973).

PHYSIOLOGICAL ROLE OF THE AMINOGENIC GLUCAGON SECRETION

The glucagon response to exogenous amino acid loads occurs in daily physiological life during protein meals. The teleology of this glucagon rise has been discussed and developed (Unger et al., 1969); it prevents the hypoglycemia which would occur as a consequence of aminogenic insulin secretion. The slight elevation of blood glucose during arginine infusion is directly related to the glucagon response, the turnover of glucose during the test being enhanced (Cherrington and Vranic, 1973), while the direct contribution to gluconeogenesis of the infused arginine is poor, as demonstrated with labelled arginine (Felig and Marliss, 1972).

After a protein meal, the increased amino acid uptake by the liver (under the influence of glucagon) may contribute to spare these substrates, in situations of protein abundance. The decisive role of the aminogenic glucagon response in the maintenance of blood glucose level is illustrated by clinical situations where hypoglycemic episodes have been precipitated by arginine infusion, no glucagon rise being observed at the same time (Bleicher et al., 1970; Nonaka et al., 1973).

Can the aminogenic glucagon response and its variations during a prolonged fast play a role in adaptation to fasting?

Some evidence gives support to the possibility that glucagon might mediate the glucose-alanine cycle, which has been suggested to be an important gluconeogenic system during the first week of starvation (Felig et al., 1970). Alanine extraction by the liver is considerably enhanced by the administration of physiologic quantities of crystalline glucagon (Marliss et al., 1970).

In the dog, glucagon rises after administration of alanine at infusion rates well within the physiologic limits for this amino acid. In these fasted dogs no change in peripheral insulin level was detected, so that a large decline of the insulin:glucagon ratio occurred, presumably promoting gluconeogenesis. When glucose need was abolished by a prior infusion of glucose, an entirely different hormonal pattern was observed, i.e. no rise of glucagon and a rise of insulin (Müller et al., 1971).

These observations suggest that glucagon secretion may be regulated during fasting by both glucose and endogenous amino acid concentrations.

GLUCAGON SECRETION IN HUMAN AND EXPERIMENTAL DIABETES MELLITUS

An increased glucagon secretion has been documented in human diabetes mellitus, characterized by high plasma glucagon levels during acute metabolic episodes, inappropriately high levels in the basal state, absence of suppressibility by glucose and excessive response to amino acids. Similarly, in several animal species with experimental or spontaneous diabetes, evidence of A_2 cell hyperfunction has been found.

The mechanism of this diabetic hyperglucagonemia is still under discussion. Because it can be experimentally reproduced in animals, it appears to depend on some metabolic disturbance secondary to the diabetic state, e.g. insulin lack or its consequences. The disappearance of the normal regulatory role of glucose on glucagon secretion strongly suggests that A_2 cells need adequate amounts of insulin to be normally sensitive to glucose. Other factors may be superimposed during acute episodes, e.g. hyperaminoacidemia or the excessive release of some neurotransmitters.

On the other hand, the sluggish and incomplete return of plasma glucagon to normal levels when insulin is acutely administered to human patients, and the glucagon hyperresponsiveness which occurs even when glucose intolerance is mild, have prompted the hypothesis that a primary A_2 cell abnormality is present in human genetic diabetes. However, an early A_2 cell hyperfunction in genetic prediabetic subjects with normal glucose tolerance has yet to be demonstrated.

GENETIC HUMAN DIABETES MELLITUS

The most obviously elevated glucagon levels were first detected in severe diabetic ketoacidosis and in other acute metabolic disturbances occurring in diabetic patients: lactic acidosis and non-ketotic hyperosmolar coma. High glucagon levels, however, absolute or relative to the concomitant blood glucose concentrations, and A_2 cell hyperresponsiveness have also been demonstrated in the absence of these acute conditions, in juvenile, ketosis-prone diabetes, and in mild, maturity-onset diabetes mellitus.

Acute metabolic conditions

In several groups of severely ketoacidotic patients, high plasma glucagon levels on admission have been documented (Assan et al., 1969; Müller et al., 1973b); the levels vary widely, from 120 to 1290 pg/ml among individual patients in each group studied. The use of highly specific assay systems demonstrates the pancreatic origin of this material; the higher values, with a parallel evolution in time and yielded by less specific systems (cross-reacting with fragments of the glucagon molecule) suggest that a substantial amount of partially degraded glucagon circulates in plasma besides intact pancreatic glucagon (Assan, 1970). The hyperglucagonemia can be correlated to some symptoms of severity: blood glucose level (Fig. 7), breathing frequency (expressing the depth of acidosis), and the insulin requirement for the reversal of ketosis (Müller et al., 1973b). No correlation could be established between glucagon and free fatty acid or free glycerol levels, nor with the concomitant growth hormone level (Assan et al., 1969); no correlation has been published to date with amino acidemia or plasma catecholamine levels.

Thus, initial elevated glucagon values can coincide with high blood glucose and free fatty acid levels, which normally are expected to inhibit glucagon secretion. But a profound impairment of glucose utilization is present before treatment, associated with high levels of amino acids (Felig et al., 1970), catecholamine hypersecretion (Christensen et al., 1971; Assan et al., 1973), high levels of cortisol, and frequently of growth hormone (Assan et al., 1969). Later glucagon levels decrease rather slowly while the other parameters measured come back to normal, and glucose utilization improves (Fig. 8).

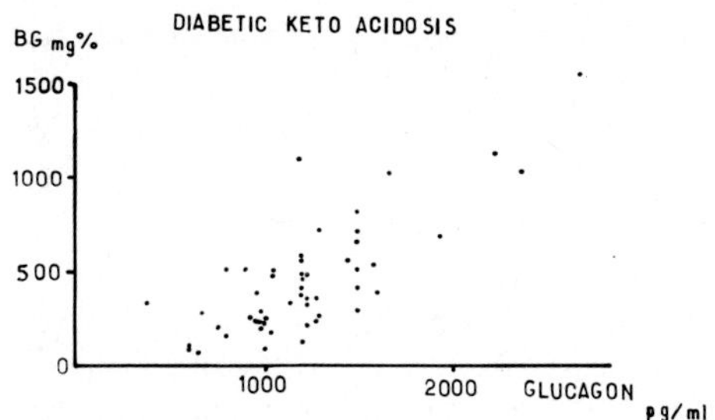

FIG. 7. Correlation of blood glucose and glucagon levels in human ketoacidotic patients.

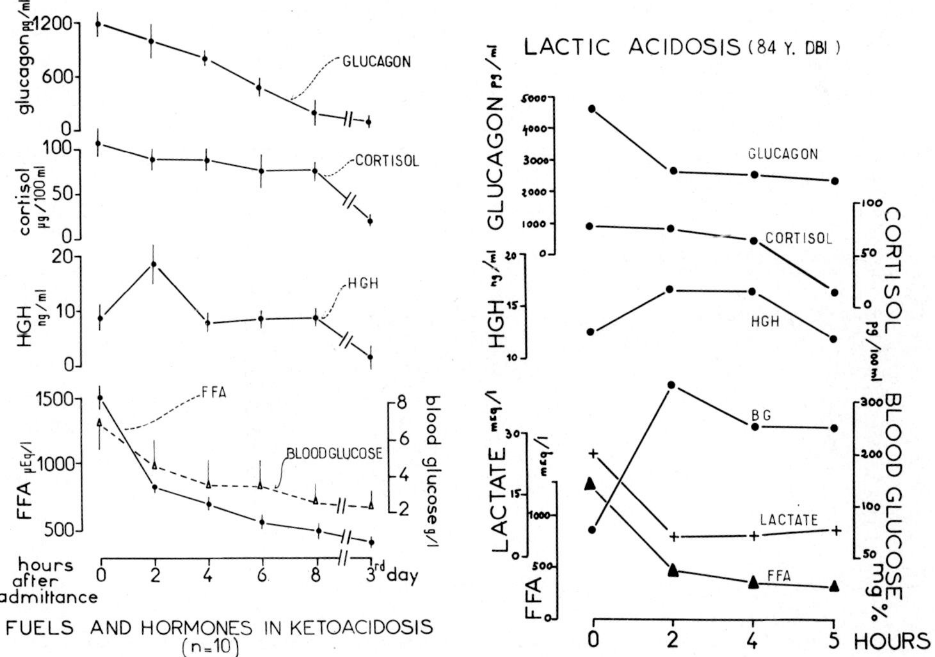

FIG. 8. Evolution in time of plasma hormones and fuels during treatment of ketoacidosis.

FIG. 9. Evolution in time of plasma hormones and fuels during lactic acidosis in a diabetic patient.

In several cases of lactic acidosis, sustained elevations of glucagon levels have been measured (Fig. 9); severe shock, and in some cases low blood glucose levels, were present; these low blood glucose levels, high lactate levels, as well as the hyperamino acidemia documented by others (Marliss et al., 1972) were interpreted as expressions of a gluconeogenic block, a consequence of phenformin overdosage or accumulation (Assan et al., unpublished results).

During hyperosmolar non-ketotic coma hyperglucagonemia has been found (Assan,

1971; Unger et al., 1972) associated with an abundance of extracellular fuels and the absence of overt ketosis and hyperlactatemia, but also with severe shock and cerebral involvement.

Fasting glucagon levels in diabetic patients

After an overnight fast, glucagon levels of diabetic subjects fall within the normal range of 50–250 pg/ml and average approximately 110 pg/ml (Unger et al., 1972); in obese patients with chemical diabetes we found basal glucagon values slightly but not significantly higher than in normal subjects (Assan et al., 1972b). Thus, in the absolute sense, 'normal' fasting glucagon values were found in diabetic subjects. However, it has been stressed that these were excessive, relative to the concomitant blood glucose levels; normal glucagon levels around 100 pg/ml were measured in patients with a Bg level of 200 mg%, while control subjects in whom a comparable hyperglycemia had been induced exhibited glucagon levels around 75 pg/ml. Twice as high values (150 pg/ml) were obtained in diabetic subjects with therapeutically induced normoglycemia (Unger et al., 1972). One may speculate whether the sharp normalization of blood glucose by therapeutic means is comparable to a strict (and long-lasting) correction of glucose utilization. However, it appears clear that in acutely studied diabetic subjects, fasting glucagon levels are unappropriately high.

Glucagon response to carbohydrate meal

This non-suppressibility by glucose of diabetic glucagon secretion, studied in the fasting state, appears even more obvious when glucose is ingested. Normal subjects respond to a carbohydrate meal by a reduction of plasma glucagon, as a consequence of hyperglycemia (Müller et al., 1970; Heding et al., 1972) possibly potentiated by secretin (Santeusiano et al., 1972). Neither adult-type nor juvenile-type diabetics exhibit this decline in plasma glucagon (Müller et al., 1970; Heding et al., 1972), and a paradoxical increase in glucagon is in fact sometimes observed in the diabetic human (Day and Anderson, 1973) and in the diabetic dog (Braaten et al., 1973).

Glucagon responses to protein meal and arginine i.v. infusion

Diabetic subjects exhibit a normal rise in glucagon, following ingestion of beef meat (Müller et al., 1970). When the glucagon levels are related to the glucose levels they are much higher than those measured in normal subjects. When control subjects were made similarly hyperglycemic by means of a glucose i.v. infusion, ingestion of the protein meal induced no rise of glucagon in plasma.

Arginine infusion test The glucagon rise induced by i.v. infusion of arginine is excessive, not only 'relatively', with respect to the concomitant glucose levels, but absolutely. This greater than normal glucagon response occurs in juvenile, insulin-dependent, diabetic subjects (Unger et al., 1970), in mild maturity-onset diabetic patients, and even in diabetics with very mild elevations of basal blood glucose levels. Figure 10 illustrates that when obese diabetic patients (with very mild diabetes) are compared with non-diabetic obese subjects (of comparable weight) the glucagon response to arginine is significantly

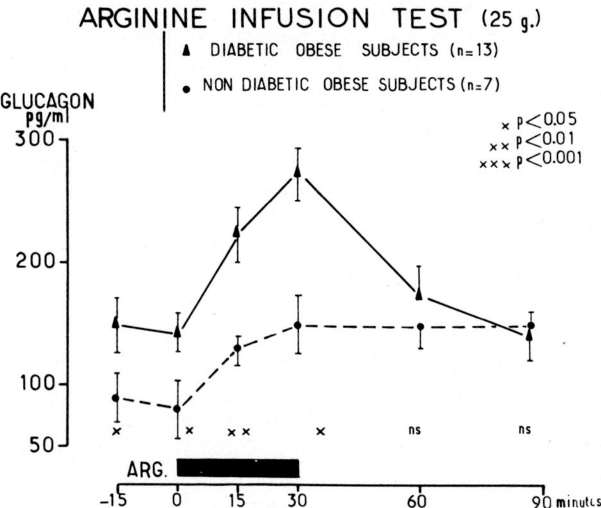

FIG. 10. Glucagon response to arginine (25 g i.v. over 30 min.) in obese non-diabetic and in obese diabetic patients.

higher in the diabetic group (Assan et al., 1972b), despite the higher blood glucose rise in these patients.

Recently it has been possible to distinguish between the rapid glucagon response to an arginine pulse, which was found in the normal range, and the secondary response to arginine infusion, found to be higher in diabetic than in normal subjects (Palmer et al., 1973).

Effects of sulfonylureas on glucagon level

Suppression of glucagon secretion by sulfonylureas had been reported in man and some other animal species (Samols et al., 1970), and this has been proposed as an important mechanism for the hypoglycemic effect of the drugs. Further studies did not confirm these findings: in man, no suppressive effect was obtained by tolbutamide or chlorpropamide on basal glucagon levels and the response to arginine and hypoglycemia (Pek et al., 1972). Similarly no effect on glucagon release was observed after glibenclamide in dogs (Buchanan et al., 1969a; Aguilar-Parada et al., 1969a, b). Discordant effects were observed on various animal systems in vitro (Buchanan et al., 1969a, b; Chesney and Schofield, 1969; Iversen, 1970; Pfeiffer et al., 1972).

ACQUIRED PANCREATIC HUMAN DIABETES MELLITUS

Even if initially surprising and rather provocative, glucagon hypersecretion in genetic diabetes, once detected, has raised little discussion; but some discrepancies exist for glucagon level in pancreatic (acquired) diabetes.

When diabetes is related to anatomic lesions of the pancreas, and not to a selective alteration of beta cells, one can expect a defective secretion of both A_2 and B cells. The abolished or decreased glucagon responses to arginine and hypoglycemia after partial or subtotal pancreatectomy confirm the specificity of the assay system used; a significant reduction of glucagon responses in patients with a calcifying pancreatitis was also observed (Figs 11 and 12). Similar observations have been made by others with arginine (Aguilar-Parada et al., 1969a, b; Persson et al., 1971) and with alanine (Wise et al., 1973a, b), while others found occasionally increased glucagon values (Paloyan et al., 1967). In hemochromatosis, when the patients had been regularly treated by bleeding, intact or non-significantly reduced glucagon responses were measured (Gay et al., 1968; Assan and Tiengo, 1972), as illustrated in Figures 11 and 12.

GLUCAGON SECRETION IN DIABETIC ANIMALS

The diabetic A_2 cell hyperfunction can be detected in a wide variety of conditions, provided that pancreatic A_2 cells are present and relatively intact. This hyperfunction is not specific of genetic diabetes; it can appear in a brief interval of time after creation of the diabetic state. It can be still manifest in vitro, after isolation of pancreas (or islets) from the diabetic organism. A further analysis, however, will show serious differences between the respective A_2 cell hyperfunctions in genetic and in acutely acquired diabetes.

Acute, experimentally induced insulin deficiency

This is rapidly followed by a rise in glucagon: in alloxan-treated dogs extremely high values were reached, up to 14,000 pg/ml, with a mean of 5,000 pg/ml (Müller et al., 1971c). The administration of insulin promptly lowered the high glucagon level, even when a modest quantity of insulin was given. The glucagon rise can be extremely rapid: in rats treated by anti-insulin serum, a two-fold increase of glucagon level occurred within 120 minutes (Müller et al., 1971c). Administration of streptozotocin to rats similarly increased glucagon secretion (Pfeiffer et al., 1972). Morphological evidence of A_2 cell hyperfunction was observed in the pancreas of diabetic hamsters (Orci et al., 1970b).

Partial pancreatectomy in ducks, with selective ablation of the beta cells-rich portions of the pancreas, and conservation of the A_2 cells-rich lobe, induced diabetes mellitus associated with hyperglucagonemia (Karman and Mialhe, 1973).

In vitro glucagon release, effects of glucose and insulin

Islets from streptozotocin-treated mice (Chesney and Schofield, 1969) and rats (Buchanan and Mawhinney, 1973) released exaggerated amounts of glucagon; for rat islets, glucagon release was increased only in severely insulin-deficient rats, but not in rats showing a moderate insulin deficiency (Buchanan and Mawhinney, 1973).

In contrast, in guinea pigs treated with streptozotocin 5 days earlier and exhibiting no hyperglycemia at death, Howell et al. (1971) were unable to detect abnormal glucagon release.

Exposure to a high glucose concentration did not reduce the excessive glucagon release, and, in some cases, enhanced it rather unexpectedly (Buchanan and Mawhinney, 1973) as was also observed in the perfused rat pancreas preparation (Pfeiffer et al., 1972).

Administration of insulin was capable of restoring the ability of glucose to suppress glucagon release, only when large amounts of insulin were added (Buchanan and Mawhinney, 1973).

Spontaneous diabetes in the chinese hamster

A 'diabetic-type' of glucagon hypersecretion has been recently observed in spontaneously diabetic chinese hamsters; the pancreas from such animals, isolated and perfused in vitro, exhibits an exaggerated glucagon response to arginine, in the presence of a glucose concentration of 100 mg% and an insulin concentration described as 'subnormal' (Frankel et al., 1973).

WHY IS GLUCAGON ELEVATED IN DIABETES MELLITUS?

This question has not received a definitive answer at this time: differences between genetic human diabetes and acutely induced experimental diabetes have led to the 'bihormonal pancreatic disease' hypothesis (Unger et al., 1972).

Some strong arguments substantiate a prominent role for insulin lack and the impairment of glucose metabolism

Among the most striking features of A_2 cell hyperfunction in diabetes is the disappearance of the suppressive effect of glucose. Impairment of glucose metabolism by poisons of the oxidation-phosphorylations pathway and of the subsequent generation of ATP (cyanide – malonate – iodacetate . . .), enhances glucagon secretion (Edwards et al., 1970). Mannoheptulose and 2-deoxyglucose, which block the intracellular metabolism of glucose, act similarly on glucagon secretion (Müller et al., 1971c). The correction of experimentally-induced diabetic hyperglucagonemia (by insulin) makes it probable that A_2 cells require insulin for the uptake and/or metabolism of glucose, and for the subsequent inhibitory effect of glucose on glucagon secretion.

Is A_2 cell abnormal in genetic human diabetes?

There are serious differences between the A_2 cell hyperfunction in genetic and in acutely acquired diabetes: in experimental animals with insulin deficiency the administration of insulin promptly lowered the high glucagon level, even when a modest quantity of insulin was available. In vitro (islets from streptozotocin-treated rats) higher amounts were necessary. In human genetic diabetes, the 'blindness to glucose' of A_2 cells appears much more difficult to correct. In ketoacidosis, glucagon levels decrease slowly despite the huge amounts of insulin administered. Even more striking is the glucagon hyperresponsiveness in mild maturity-onset diabetes despite appreciable insulin concentrations in plasma; the simple restoration of the plasma insulin concentrations to normal or supernormal levels did not restore the normal suppressibility of A_2 cell secretion by glucose. From these observations and experiments it was suggested that 'glucose blindness' of the genetically human diabetic may involve a factor (or factors?) other than simple insulin lack alone. The possibility of a primary bihormonal abnormality in diabetes mellitus has been considered (Unger et al., 1972).

The differences between human and animal diabetes, regarding A_2 cell sensitivity to insulin therapy can, however, be explained by simple arguments, and the definite demonstration of a genetic abnormality of A_2 cells in human diabetic subjects is still lacking.

As for human ketosis, many factors may contribute to enhance glucagon secretion before and during treatment by insulin: catecholamine hypersecretion, stress, the high aminoacidemia, and later the sharp decrease of metabolic fuels in plasma. Similarly, for growth hormone a secondary rise occurs during the therapeutic period, when glucose utilization is restored, presumably attributable to the decrease of blood glucose and FFA levels (Assan et al., 1972b). On recovery from ketosis, the acute or episodic normalization of blood glucose cannot be considered to be equivalent to strict long-term normalization of glucose utilization; here again the situation of glucagon may be parallelled to that of growth hormone: the exercise-induced growth hormone secretion is normal in diabetic subjects when these are perfectly controlled for several days (Hansen, 1972); similarly the exercise-induced glucagon secretion was normal in some perfectly controlled diabetic patients (Tchobroutsky et al., unpublished results).

Obese diabetic patients, even if hyperinsulinemic, still have impaired glucose tolerance which may be sufficient to explain their abnormal glucagon release, while non-diabetic obese subjects exhibit a normal glucagon response to amino acids (Assan et al., 1972b; Wise et al., 1973a).

As for the prediabetic subjects, their decreased liver glucose output, compared to normal (Wahren et al., 1973) makes glucagon hypersecretion rather improbable, unless a decreased responsiveness of liver cells to glucagon is present (which has not been demonstrated). A decisive point is the behaviour of A_2 cells in the genetically prediabetic subject: during an oral glucose tolerance test, the inhibition by glucose has been found slightly less efficient than normal in the non-diabetic siblings of diabetic subjects (Day and Tattersall, 1972). In contrast, in several low insulin responders to glucose, we have up to now been unable to detect either an enhanced glucagon response to arginine, or a less efficient inhibitory effect of i.v. glucose (Assan et al., unpublished results).

INFLUENCE OF A_2 HYPERFUNCTION ON DIABETES

An important contribution of this hyperglucagonemia to the metabolic disturbances present in diabetes is highly probable. As long as the hepatic glucose output is regulated by the insulin:glucagon ratio, the inappropriately high glucagon concentrations encountered in diabetic patients contribute (with the insulin deficiency) to elevate the blood glucose levels. The immunoassayable glucagon in plasma has been demonstrated as biologically active (Marco et al., 1971); the selectively decreased level of glucogenic amino acids during ketoacidosis (Felig et al., 1971) has been interpreted as reflecting the increased uptake by the liver of these substrates, possibly under the influence of glucagon.

Exogenous glucagon, injected to diabetic patients, increases protein catabolism and azoturia (see this Volume, pp. 137–143).

More questionable is the role of the exaggerated lipolysis of hyperglucagonemia during ketoacidosis, but even this cannot be excluded, since glucagon and some glucagon fragments exhibit a lipolytic effect in the human, under some experimental conditions (Guy-Grand and Assan, 1973). In contrast, the reduced or absent glucagon secretion demonstrated in human pancreatic diabetes is correlated with the more profound hypoglycemia induced by insulin, and the attenuated blood glucose rise induced by arginine in such patients. This may contribute (together with the malnutrition frequently associated) to the brittleness of pancreatic diabetes.

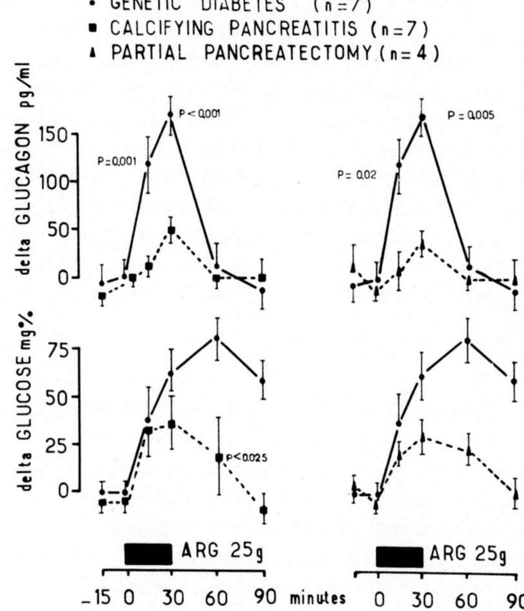

FIG. 11. Glucagon response to arginine in pancreatic diabetic and genetic diabetic subjects.

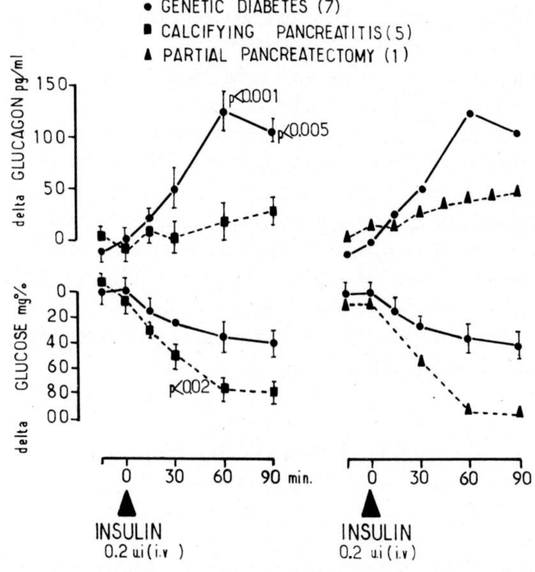

FIG. 12. Glucagon response to the insulin-induced hypoglycemia in pancreatic and in genetic diabetic subjects.

Conclusions

Glucagon hypersecretion appears to be present in most diabetic conditions (genetic or not) provided that A_2 cells are present. This glucagon hypersecretion has an important effect on blood glucose levels (as demonstrated by the hypoglycemic-prone pancreatic diabetes) and probably contributes to the hyperglycemia and enhanced lipolysis in diabetic ketoacidosis. Insulin lack and impaired glucose metabolism are probably responsible for the main part of the A_2 cell hyperfunction in diabetes. Some recent results make a genetic hyperfunction of the A_2 cells in genetic diabetes improbable. The resistance of the A_2 cell to exogenous insulin in human diabetes may reflect the need for long-term metabolic normalization, rather than for rapid attainment of normal insulin concentrations.

GLUCAGON IN THE FETUS AND THE NEWBORN

It is only recently, with the development of electron microscopic techniques, and of a sensitive radioimmunoassay for glucagon, that A_2 cells and glucagon have been positively identified in the fetal pancreas of several animal species. Glucagon appears in the pancreas early in intra-uterine life. It can also be detected in fetal plasma, and its fetal origin is rendered highly likely by the placental impermeability to exogenous glucagon. Some variations of fetal glucagon levels have been measured during the last few days of gestation in rat and rabbit. The causes and the possible effects of these variations remain unclear. Only few results are now available about the responsiveness of fetal A_2 cells to some possible stimulators.

During the first hours of extra-uterine life, an elevation of plasma glucagon level occurs in some mammal species: rat, rabbit, and human. Several factors appear as possible candidates for the triggering of this glucagon secretion, for instance cataglycemia and the stress-induced stimulation of the autonomic nervous system.

The data from recent literature, and the results of personal investigations, will be presented successively on the ontogenetic development of A_2 cell function in several mammal species. The effects of experimental stimulation in vivo and in vitro on the variations of plasma glucagon in the fetus and the newborn will also be analyzed.

The physiological significance of glucagon secretion in the newborn will be discussed, in the light of the acute variations of fuels that occur in plasma at birth. The rise of glucagon associated with a fall of insulin is highly appropriate for the appearance of hepatic gluconeogenesis and glycogenolysis and for provision of glucose to the newborn.

Whether the presence of glucagon contributes to some metabolic adaptation during intra-uterine life remains unanswered.

GLUCAGON IN THE FETUS

Fetal rat pancreas

Islets were detected by conventional light microscopy as early as the 13th day of gestation, but the granules of A_2 cells were not visible before birth (Hard, 1944). However, Schweisthal and Frost (1973), using a modification of the Grimelius silver nitrate technique, demonstrated the presence of A_2 cells in 18-days-old fetal rat pancreas. Using electron microscopic technique, typical A_2 cells were identified in rat fetuses 18-days-old (Orci et al., 1969), 16-days-old (Perrier et al., 1969) and even 11-days-old (Pictet and Rutter, 1972). On day 20 of gestation, the granules of A_2 cells became more numerous, bigger, and were frequently close to the plasma membranes (Perrier, 1970). In the fetal rat at term (21 days gestation), nerve fibers were visible in contact with the islets of Langerhans (Perrier, 1970; Orci et al., 1970a).

The presence of glucagon in fetal rat pancreas was first noted by bioassay (Okuno et al., 1964) and later by radioimmunoassay (Orci et al., 1969; Rutter, 1969; Pictet and Rutter, 1972; Blazquez et al., 1972; Jarousse et al., 1973a). Immunoreactive glucagon was present as early as the 11th day of gestation, and the total amount rose rapidly to a 500-fold increase at the end of gestation; the concentration of glucagon (reported to protein amount or to DNA) varied according to a bell-shaped curve, with maximal concentration at 14 days (Pictet and Rutter, 1972). We have measured, during the last 4 days of gestation, pancreatic glucagon concentrations varying from 2.4 μg/g wet weight at 18 days to 3.7 μg/g at 21 days (Girard et al., 1973a).

Human fetus

Until recent years only morphologic descriptions, by light microscopic techniques, have been available: silver-stained A cells were detected in 12 human fetuses (gestational age 3 to 4 months) by Ferner and Stoeckenius (1951), and as early as the 11th week of gestation in a study of 37 fetuses aged 10 to 42 weeks (Robb, 1961). Similarly A cells, stained by Gomori's technique, were found at the end of the 2nd month of gestation by Lin and Potter (1962), analyzing 130 fetuses aged 4 to 42 weeks. Electron microscopic studies of fetal human islets have also recently appeared (Bjorkman et al., 1966; Wellman et al., 1971; Like and Orci, 1972). From this later study, no endocrine cells were identified at 8.5 weeks of gestation, A cells were observed at 9 weeks while the B cells only appeared at 10.5 weeks gestation. Morphometry also suggested several successive generations of islets (at least 2) in the human fetus (Lin and Potter, 1962). A predominance of A or B cells at the beginning of embryonic life followed by a progressive decrease in the number of A cells (Ferner and Stoeckenius, 1951; Schultze-Jenna, 1953; Lin and Potter, 1962) have been described. An explanation is that degeneration of A cells takes place in the last 3 months of intra-uterine life (Emery and Bury, 1964). Our personal findings concerning 65 human fetuses (between 6 and 26 weeks after last menses) are shown in Figure 13.

Glucagon was undetectable at 6 weeks, but was present at 8 weeks; then it sharply increased over the period studied, reaching a plateau level at about 26 weeks when the glucagon concentration was higher than that commonly measured in the adult human pancreas, i.e. 2 to 5 μg/g (Assan and Boillot, 1971, 1973). The evidence of extractable glucagon in the fetal human pancreas of 7 weeks to 20 weeks gestation has also appeared recently (Schaeffer et al., 1973).

Rabbit fetus

Ultrastructural studies of fetal rabbit pancreas have shown that A cells were present from day 24 of gestation to term (Bencosme et al., 1970). Immunoreactive glucagon in the pancreas was detectable as soon as 13 days, a maximal concentration was reached at 26

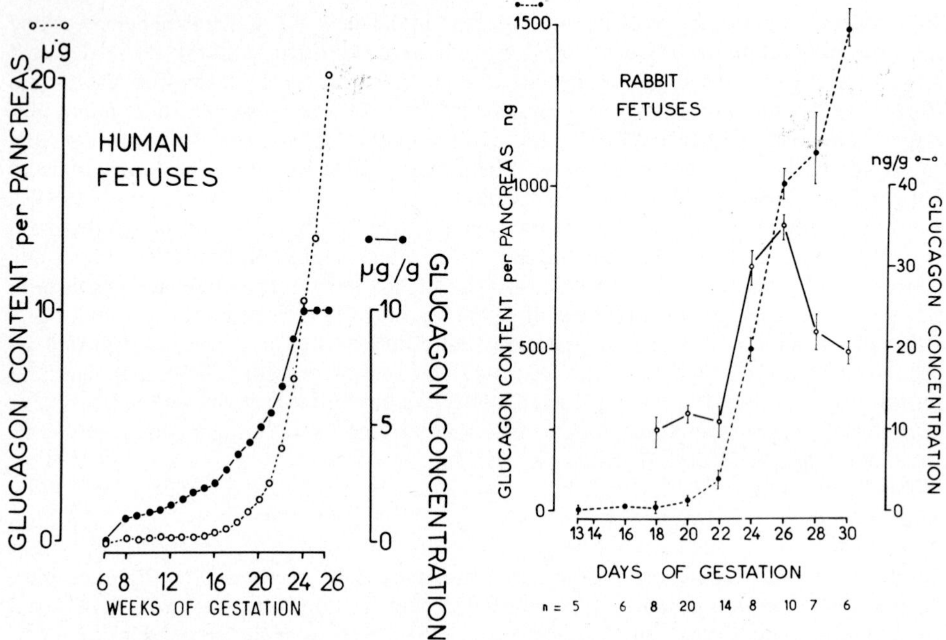

FIG. 13. Glucagon content and concentration of human fetal pancreas (from Assan and Boilot, 1971, by courtesy).

FIG. 14. Glucagon content and concentration of rabbit fetal pancreas.

days; then the concentration decreased until the end of gestation (Kervran and Assan, unpublished results) as is shown in Figure 14.

Mouse fetus

Recent immunofluorescence, cytochemical and ultrastructural studies of fetal mouse pancreas (Pearce et al., 1973) have shown that A cells and glucagon were detectable at the 14th day of gestation (term 20 days). Glucagon-like immunoreactivity has also been found in 18-days-old mouse embryos (Lernmark and Wenngren, 1972).

Sheep fetus

Glucagon could also be detected in the fetal pancreas of sheep at a relatively early stage of gestation. Higher glucagon concentrations were found in the pancreas of fetuses aged 100–117 days than in fetuses near term i.e. of 130–143 days (Alexander et al., 1971a).

Thus the early appearance of glucagon in fetal pancreas is well documented; A cells and glucagon appear earlier than B cells and insulin in human and rat. The initial low concentrations of hormone in the pancreas, and the relatively low sensitivity of histochemical techniques (compared to electron microscopic technique or radioimmunoassay) must account for the discrepancy in the earlier studies. The evolution of concentration with time is similar in the several species studied – the highest concentrations being reached before the end of gestation; this recalls the morphometric observation relating to the respective numbers of A and B cells.

Glucagon-like immunoreactivity in the fetal gastroenteric tract

It should be noted that besides glucagon in fetal pancreas, a glucagon-like immunoreactive material (GLI) was detected in gastrointestinal tissues of human (Assan and Boillot, 1971, 1973), rat (Blazquez et al., 1972) and rabbit fetuses (Kervran and Assan, unpublished results). The time of appearance of GLI in the gut closely followed that of glucagon in the pancreas but the amount and concentration estimated in glucagon equivalents, was low.

Glucagon and glucagon-like immunoreactivity in fetal plasma and other biological fluids

Glucagon in fetal plasma Pancreatic glucagon can be detected in plasma of rat fetuses aged 18.5 to 21.5 days (Girard et al., 1971, 1973a; Blazquez et al., 1972), of sheep fetuses aged 59 to 143 days (Alexander et al., 1971a) and of human fetuses 15 to 26 weeks old (Assan and Boillot, 1971, 1973). At term the plasma glucagon levels in the umbilical vessels and in maternal blood were similar (Johnston et al., 1972a; Milner et al., 1973) and the fetal glucagon concentration was unrelated to either glucose or insulin levels.

Glucagon level in rat fetal plasma increased from 18.5 to 20.5 days of gestation, where the maximal values were observed (423 ± 34 pg/ml); thereafter it decreased on day 21.5 of gestation (Girard et al., 1971, 1973a). No variations of plasma glucagon level (about 500 to 560 pg/ml) were reported by Blazquez et al. (1972) for 19 to 22 day fetal rats. In rabbit fetuses (Fig. 15), plasma glucagon rose between 24 and 28 days of gestation, then

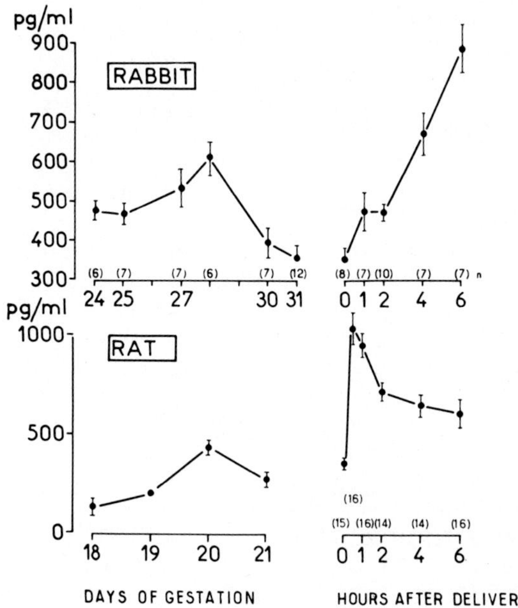

FIG. 15. Plasma glucagon levels in fetal and newborn rat and rabbit (for rat, data come from Girard et al., 1973a, b).

decreased during the last 2 days of intra-uterine life (Kervran, Girard and Assan, unpublished results). The significance of these variations in fetal rat or rabbit remains unanswered.

Glucagon-like material in plasma, amniotic fluid, allantoic fluid Glucagon-like immunoreactivity can be detected in fetal plasma using less specific antisera (cross-reacting with fragments of the glucagon molecule, or gastroenteric extracts): this cross-reacting material was detected in plasma of rat fetus (Girard et al., 1971; Blazquez et al., 1972), of human fetuses (Assan and Boillot, 1971, 1973) and sheep fetuses (Alexander et al., 1971a). It has also been detected in rat amniotic fluid (Blazquez et al., 1972) and, in substantial amounts, in the sheep allantoic fluid (Alexander et al., 1971b).

Absence of transplacental transfer of glucagon

The absence of placental transfer of glucagon strongly suggests that the hormone detected in fetal plasma and fluids is released by the fetal pancreas; the fetal origin of the glucagon circulating in fetal plasma is substantiated by the absence of transplacental transfer in experimental conditions. Exogenous glucagon injected into the mother could not be detected in the fetal blood in the various species studied: rat (Girard et al., 1971, 1973a; Blazquez et al., 1972), human (Johnston et al., 1972b; Adam et al., 1972a) and sheep (Alexander et al., 1971b) as illustrated in Figure 16.

These results suggest that the increases in fetal glucagon observed on day 20 in the rat and on day 28 in the rabbit result from increased release by the fetal pancreas.

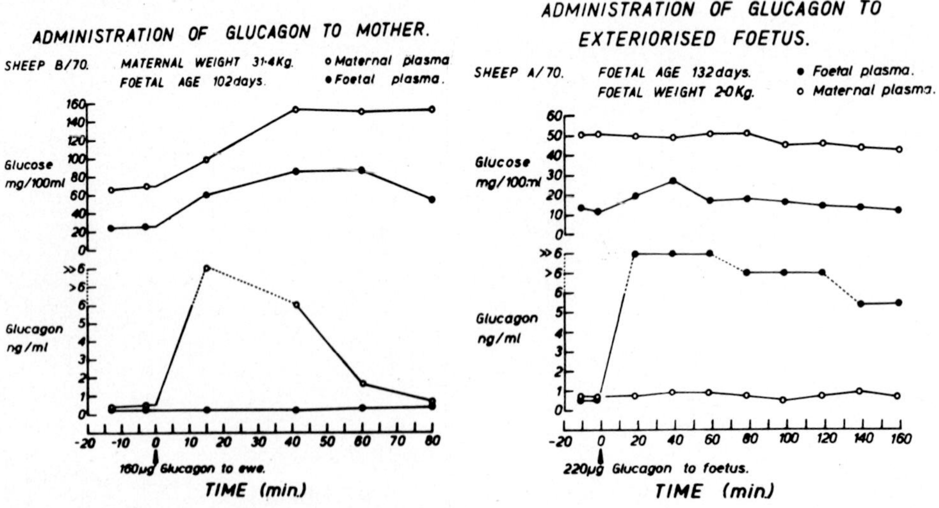

FIG. 16. Absence of transplacental transfer of glucagon in the sheep (from Alexander et al., 1971b, by courtesy).

SPONTANEOUS VARIATIONS OF PLASMA GLUCAGON IN THE NEWBORN

In the newborn rat a four-fold increase of plasma glucagon occurs within 30 minutes following birth by caesarian section (Girard et al., 1971, 1972, 1973b). Then plasma glucagon decreases from 1 to 2 hours and remains at a plateau value, higher than the level observed at birth, for 6 hours. Similar results have been obtained in rats born by vaginal delivery (Blazquez et al., 1972).

In the newborn rabbit a three-fold increase of plasma glucagon similarly occurs, from zero time to the sixth hour of extra-uterine life, as shown in Figure 15 (Kervran, Girard and Assan, unpublished results).

In the newborn calf plasma glucagon was not elevated 24 hours after birth but a rise occurred during the following days (Bloom et al., 1973a).

In the newborn lamb plasma glucagon did not rise in the 2 hours following birth (Alexander et al., unpublished results).

In the human newborn an unequivocal rise of plasma glucagon occurs in the normal infant (Bloom and Johnston 1972; Luyckx et al., 1972) but it is of smaller magnitude than in the rat. Newborn infants suffering from hypoxia during delivery (Johnston and Bloom, 1973) or from erythroblastosis fetalis (Milner et al., 1972) had higher plasma glucagon levels than normal infants at birth. A failure of glucagon release has been reported in the newborn infants of diabetic mothers (Bloom and Johnston, 1972) despite a greater fall in blood glucose levels. Small for dates newborns who have suffered intra-uterine malnutrition have a greater rise in plasma glucagon than normal newborns (Bloom and Johnston, 1972).

The variations in magnitude and occurrence in time of the neonatal glucagon release may be related to specific difference in the forms of energy storage and metabolism (for instance between newborn rat and newborn ruminant). An attractive working hypothesis is that acute glucose need triggers glucagon release; but the exact mechanism is not clear, and other factors, such as the stressful situation occurring at birth, may also influence glucagon release.

In order to clarify the responsiveness of fetal and neonatal A_2 cell, some factors known to stimulate glucagon secretion in adult were investigated in vivo and in vitro.

EXPERIMENTAL STIMULATION OF FETAL ALPHA 2 CELL

Fetal and neonatal glucagon secretion in vivo

In 21.5-days-old rat fetuses, acute hypoglycemia (induced by a one-hour insulin infusion into the mother) does not significantly stimulate fetal glucagon release, but a significant increase occurs after prolonged fetal hypoglycemia (mothers fasted for 4 days, or intra-uterine growth retardation produced by ligating the artery supplying the uterus on day 17 of gestation). During acute fetal hyperglycemia (glucose infusion to mother for 1 hour) no decrease of fetal plasma glucagon occurs (Figs 17 and 18; Girard et al., 1973a, c). Intraperitoneal injection of some amino acids also induced a glucagon secretion in vivo; arginine appeared as the most potent for glucagon stimulation in the fetus (Fig. 19) but tryptophan has also a clear-cut effect; alanine and leucine were weak stimulators of A cells.

These experiments do not rule out the possible intervention of nerve stimulation

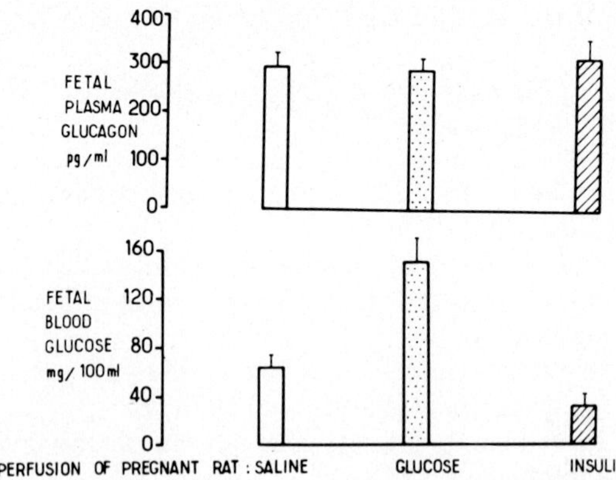

FIG. 17. Effect of acute blood glucose variations on plasma glucagon levels in fetal rats at term (from Girard et al., 1973c).

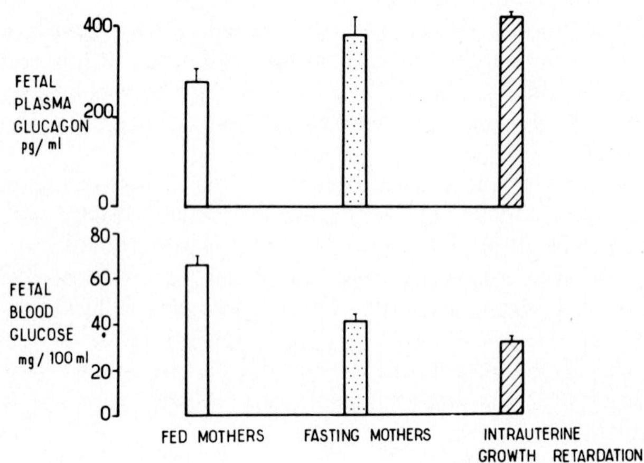

FIG. 18. Effect of prolonged hypoglycemia on plasma glucagon levels in fetal rats at term (from Girard et al., 1973c).

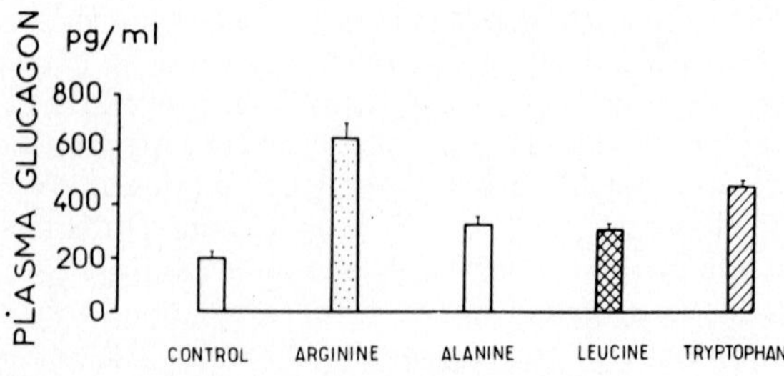

FIG. 19. Effect of amino acids on plasma glucagon level in fetal rats at term.

interfering with the metabolic factor investigated, since norepinephrine injected into fetal rat at term (10 μg) acted as a fast and potent stimulus for glucagon secretion (Fig. 20) and acetylcholine also increased plasma glucagon levels.

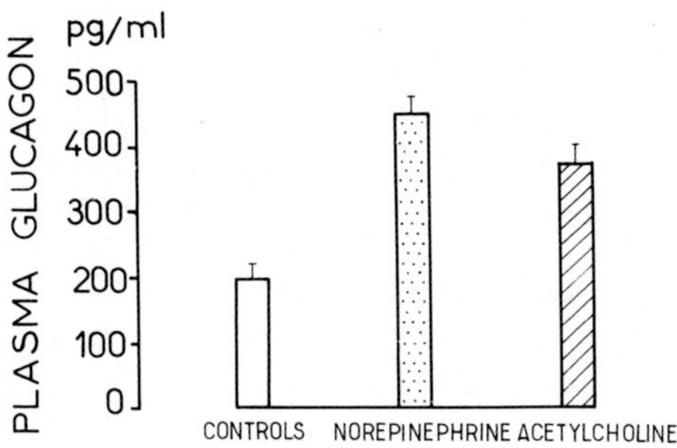

FIG. 20. Effect of neurotransmitters on plasma glucagon level in fetal rats at term (from Girard et al., 1973b).

In sheep fetuses, plasma glucagon levels were unchanged after glucose infusion, or alanine infusion (Fiser et al., 1973). There is no obvious relationship between glucagon and blood glucose levels in the fetal lamb, but a definite rise in glucagon was observed in hypoxic fetal lambs (Shelley and Girard, unpublished results).

In the normal newborn infant an intravenous glucose load did not decrease plasma glucagon. By contrast, glucose load decreased plasma glucagon in newborn infants of diabetic mothers (Luyckx et al., 1972). If normal infants were infused with glucose plus insulin, plasma glucagon fell (Massi-Bennedetti et al., 1973).

In view of the recent data suggesting that the entry of glucose in A cells is an insulin-dependent process (Unger et al., 1970), the difference in glucagon suppression by glucose seen in normal newborns and in newborns from diabetic mothers might be the result of the well known hyperinsulinemia present in the infant of diabetic mothers.

Infusion of arginine at full term (Sperling et al., 1973), preterm and small for dates newborn infants (Falorni et al., 1973) produced an increase in plasma glucagon levels. Similarly, alanine infused into normal women during labor, resulted in an elevation of plasma glucagon in the human fetus by 150% (Wise et al., 1973b).

In newborn calves tested within 24 hours following birth, insulin-induced hypoglycemia (Bloom et al., 1973a) or stimulation of splanchnic nerves (Bloom et al., 1973b) produced a rise in plasma glucagon. Greater responses were obtained in calves tested 30 days after birth.

Fetal and neonatal glucagon secretion in vitro

Arginine stimulated the release of glucagon by fetal (18 days of gestation) mouse pancreas incubated in vitro and high glucose levels did not inhibit arginine-induced glucagon secretion (Lernmark and Wengrenn, 1972). On the first postnatal day, glucose depressed arginine-induced glucagon secretion.

Glucagon release by newborn rat pancreas in vitro was stimulated by arginine and inhibited by octanoic acid but was not modified by modifying the glucose concentrations (Edwards et al., 1972). In 3-days-old newborn rat, the secretion from the pancreas incubated in vitro was not affected by changes in glucose concentrations but was increased by cyclic AMP and by a mixture of amino acids (Jarousse et al., 1973b; Rosselin et al., 1973).

In monolayer cultures of newborn rat pancreas, glucagon release was stimulated by alanine, arginine, lactate, pyruvate and epinephrine and decreased by beta hydroxybutyrate (Marliss et al., 1973). High glucose concentrations (Marliss et al., 1973; Orci et al., 1973) and cyclic AMP (Wollheim et al., 1973) decreased glucagon release in monolayer culture of newborn rat pancreas. The discrepancies between the results obtained with the monolayer cultures or with pieces of newborn rat pancreas remain unanswered.

We have recently used the in vitro perifusion technique (Burr et al., 1970) to study glucagon secretion by fetal rat pancreas pieces at term (Girard et al., unpublished results). Arginine induced a strong and biphasic glucagon output in the presence of glucose 3.3 mM (Fig. 21). This response is enhanced by lowering glucose concentration in perfusion

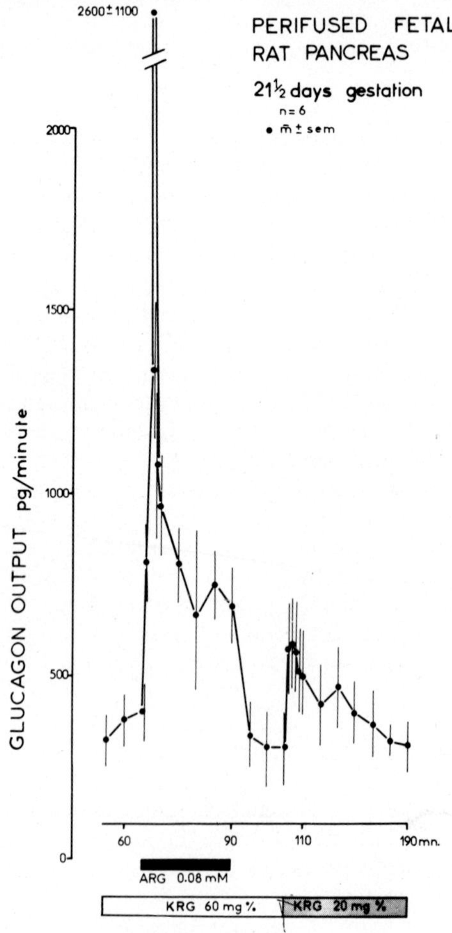

FIG. 21. Effect of arginine and abrupt change in glucose concentration on glucagon output from the perifused pancreas of fetal rat at term.

medium to 2.2 mM. In absence of arginine an abrupt fall of glucose in perfusion medium from 3.3 to 2.2 mM was accompanied by a transient but significant rise in glucagon output (Fig. 21). Norepinephrine also increases glucagon output with a biphasic pattern in this in vitro system.

The same perifusion technique could be applied to the pancreases of 6 human fetuses (Hautecouverture et al., unpublished results), obtained by hysterotomy (the pregnancy had been interrupted because of carcinologic or severe psychiatric reasons, and the mothers were free of overt metabolic disease). All 6 fetuses (15–19 weeks old) responded to arginine stimulation, while the decrease of glucose in perifusate was not followed by glucagon secretion (Fig. 22).

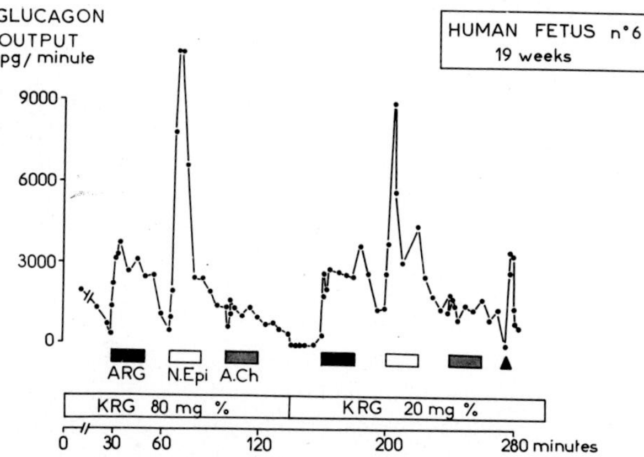

FIG. 22. Effect of arginine, change in glucose concentration, norepinephrine and acetylcholine on glucagon output from perifused human fetal pancreas.

Norepinephrine (20 μg/ml) induced a strong response. Responses to arginine and to norepinephrine were not potentiated by lowering the glucose concentration. No response was observed during acetylcholine perfusion. Arginine also produced a significant increase in the secretion of glucagon from slices of human fetal pancreas while glucose did not affect glucagon release (Schaeffer et al., 1973).

Thus A_2 cell responsiveness to arginine can be demonstrated early in fetal life. It appears from a survey of the various studies that arginine is, among the various experimental stimulators, the most constant and one of the most potent and the possible physiological significance of this arginine-stimulatory effect needs further investigation. The effect of glucose concentration appears more clearly through potentiation (by low glucose) or suppression (by high glucose) of the effect of arginine, than by a direct effect of low glucose on the A_2 cell. The latter effect does not exclude an indirect influence of hypoglycemia in vivo through the stimulation of glucose-dependent nervous centers.

The efficiency of neurotransmitters on fetal glucagon secretion is supported by the experimental responses induced by norepinephrine (in vitro and in vivo) and acetylcholine (in vivo), but much more investigation is necessary to demonstrate the factor(s) actually responsible for the neonatal glucagon secretion, and to ascertain whether an active, regulated, glucagon secretion occurs before birth and contributes to the development of fetal homeostasis.

PHYSIOLOGICAL SIGNIFICANCE OF GLUCAGON IN THE FETUSES AND THE NEWBORNS

Rat

Several lines of evidence support a role of glucagon in metabolic adaptations observed at birth in the rat. This has been reviewed recently by Girard et al. (1973d) and can be summarized as follows: (1) The rise of plasma glucagon at birth is concomitant with a dramatic fall in plasma gluconeogenic substrates and precedes the appearance of glycogenolysis and gluconeogenesis in the newborn rat liver. (2) Exogenous glucagon injected into a fetal rat in utero at term or added to fetal liver explant in vitro is capable of provoking premature liver glycogenolysis and gluconeogenesis. (3) Exogenous glucagon also increases hepatic uptake of amino acid and stimulates the conversion of lactate and amino acids to glucose in newborn rats.

Several of the hepatic effects of glucagon can be antagonized by insulin and it is probable that the concurrent fall of plasma insulin which occurs at birth with the rise of plasma glucagon greatly favors the expression of hepatic effects of glucagon. The very low insulin:glucagon molar ratio in plasma of newborn rats which is characteristic of an organism in a catabolic state is appropriate for provision of glucose to the newborn. Glycogenolysis and gluconeogenesis occur in the liver and some plasma amino acids contribute to the maintenance of normal blood glucose in fasting newborn rats through hepatic gluconeogenesis.

By contrast, during fetal life, the very elevated insulin:glucagon molar ratio is entirely appropriate for a metabolic situation where no endogenous glucose is required, since glucose is supplied by the mother through the placenta. It cannot, however, be excluded that glucagon can play a role in the early differentiation of the pancreas in the rat since the ontogenic studies have shown that the A cells are the first differentiated endocrine cells in the rat embryo (Pictet and Rutter, 1972). The closely parallel evolution of insulin and glucagon in plasma of fetal rat at the end of gestation (Girard et al., 1973c) might result from the well established insulinotropic effect of glucagon on fetal rat pancreas (Vecchio et al., 1966).

Other species

Observations concerning the metabolic adaptations of the rat at birth may not be directly extrapolated to other mammals since there are several peculiar features of this species: an absence of white adipose tissue, primary energy fuel in form of glucose and a very high basal metabolism.

Sheep

Recent observations challenge the current dogma that glucose is the primary fetal fuel in the lamb (review by Battaglia and Meschia, 1973). Glucose accounts for only 45% of fetal oxygen consumption or CO_2 production. The high rate of fetal urea production suggests an amino acid oxidation which accounts for 25% of fetal O_2 consumption. Free fatty acids, glycerol, lactate and pyruvate are not significant fetal fuels and, as commentated by Cahill (1972), ketone bodies oxidation may provide the remaining 30% of O_2 consumption of the fetus. The finding of active gluconeogenesis in fetal ruminants (Ballard et al.,

1969) is not surprising since the pregnant ruminant obtains very little carbohydrate from the diet. The fetus must have the potential to convert all gluconeogenic substrates to glucose, particularly during maternal starvation when 80% of the fetal O_2 consumption can be accounted for by protein catabolism (Simmons et al., 1973). In this situation a stable fetal glucose concentration results probably from increased gluconeogenesis from amino acids and a role of glucagon in this adaptation cannot be withheld.

However, at birth the presence of a well developed adipose tissue and of an active gluconeogenesis may render the newborn ruminant less dependent upon glucose as an energy fuel. It can immediately use ketone bodies and amino acids for energy and thus spares glucose, so that neonatal hypoglycemia does not occur in newborn ruminants. It is conceivable that glucagon has a minor role in this situation, which is in agreement with the absence of increase in plasma glucagon in the newborn lamb (Alexander et al., unpublished results) and calf (Bloom et al., 1973a).

Human

In full-term human fetuses, glucose can supply approximately 80% of energetic requirement (Morris et al., 1973), but they are also capable of oxidizing amino acids and producing urea (Gresham et al., 1971); the fetal brain has the ability to use ketone bodies as energetic substrate (Page and Williamson, 1971; Adam et al., 1973). So the human fetus is in a metabolic situation intermediate between fetal rat and fetal ruminant. The capacity for gluconeogenesis in the human fetus is probably limited since the activity of key regulatory enzymes is about 1/10 of that observed in human adults (Raiha and Lindros, 1969) and the rate of gluconeogenesis from labelled lactate or alanine was negligible in isolated perfused human fetal liver (Adam et al., 1972b). The unequivocal increase in plasma glucagon in newborn infants (Luyckx et al., 1972; Bloom and Johnston, 1972), although of a smaller magnitude than in the rat, may also play a regulatory role in gluconeogenesis and glycogenolysis. Neonatal hypoglycemia is a frequent occurrence in some pathological situations such as in the infant of a diabetic mother or in a newborn child small for gestational age. Failure of glucagon secretion has been reported in the newborn infant of a diabetic mother (Bloom and Johnston, 1972) which, associated with the well known increased plasma insulin level, probably delays the onset of gluconeogenesis and glycogenolysis and may be a significant factor in their hypoglycemia. By contrast, infants born small for dates had a larger rise of pancreatic glucagon than normal children at birth (Bloom and Johnston, 1972). Hypoglycemia in those born small for dates may reflect in part defective gluconeogenesis (Haymond et al., 1973) superimposed upon limited hepatic glycogen stores (Shelley and Neligan, 1966) rather than upon disturbed glucagon secretion.

ACKNOWLEDGEMENTS

We wish to thank Mrs. A. Delage, J. Boillot and C. Labeta-Caballier for their helpful technical assistance. We are indebted to Professor P. Lefebvre and Dr. A. Luyckx for help in setting up the perifusion technique, and to Drs. E. Marliss and M. Kikuchi for introducing us to the perifusion technique as it was currently practised in the laboratory of Professor A. E. Renold in Geneva.

REFERENCES

ADAM, P. A. J., KING, K. C., SCHWARTZ, R. and TERDMO, K. (1972a): Human placental barrier to ^{125}I. Glucagon early in gestation. *J. clin. Endocr., 34,* 772.

ADAM, P. A. J., KEKOMAKI, M., RAHIALA, E. L. and SCHWARTZ, A. L. (1972b): Autoregulation of glucose production by the isolated perfused human fetal liver (abstract). *Pediat. Res., 6,* 396.

ADAM, P. A. J., RAIHA, N., RAHIALA, E. L. and KEKOMAKI, M. (1973): Cerebral oxidation of glucose and D. BOH. butyrate by the isolated perfused human fetal head (abstract). *Pediat. Res., 7,* 309.

AGUILAR-PARADA, E., EISENTRAUT, A. M. and UNGER, R. H. (1969a): Pancreatic glucagon secretion in normal and diabetic subjects. *Amer. J. med. Sci., 257,* 415.

AGUILAR-PARADA, E., EISENTRAUT, A. M. and UNGER, R. H. (1969b): Effect of HB-419-induced hypoglycemia on pancreatic glucagon secretion. *Hormone metabol. Res., Suppl. 1,* 48.

ALEXANDER, D. P., ASSAN, R., BRITTON, H. G. and NIXON, D. A. (1971a): Glucagon in the foetal sheep. *J. Endocr., 51,* 597.

ALEXANDER, D. P., ASSAN, R., BRITTON, H. G. and NIXON, D. A. (1971b): Glucagon permeability of the sheep placenta. *J. Physiol., 216,* 63P.

ASSAN, R. (1971): Contribution to the study of glucagon secretion and catabolism in vivo. In: *Diabetes, Proceedings of the VIIth Congress of the International Diabetes Federation, Buenos Aires, August 1970,* pp. 610–624. Editors: R. R. Rodriguez and J. Vallance-Owen. International Congress Series No. 231, Excerpta Medica, Amsterdam.

ASSAN, R. and BOILLOT, J. (1971): Pancreatic glucagon and glucagon like material in tissues and plasma from human foetuses 6–26 weeks old. In: *Metabolic Processes in the foetus and newborn infant,* pp. 210–219. Editors: J. M. P. Jonxis, H. K. A. Visser and J. A. Troelstra. Stenfert Kroese, Leiden.

ASSAN, R. and BOILLOT, J. (1973): Pancreatic glucagon and glucagon like material in tissues and plasma from human fetuses 6–26 weeks old. *Pathol. Biol., 21,* 149.

ASSAN, R., BOILLOT, J., ATTALI, J. R., SOUFFLET, E. and BALLERIO, G. (1972a): Diphasic glucagon release induced by arginine in the perfused rat pancreas. *Nature New Biol., 239,* 125.

ASSAN, R., HAUTECOUVERTURE, G., GUILLEMANT, S., DAUCHY, F., PROTIN, P. and DEROT, M. (1969): Evolution de paramètres hormonaux (glucagon – cortisol – hormone somatotrope) et énergétiques (glucose – acides gras – glycérol libre) dans 10 acidocétoses graves traitées. *Pathol. Biol., 17,* 1095.

ASSAN, R., ROSSELIN, G. and DOLAIS, J. (1967): Effet sur la glucagonémie des perfusions et ingestions d'acides aminés. In: *Journées Annuelles de Diabétologie de l'Hôtel-Dieu, 1 vol.,* pp. 25–41. Flammarion, Paris.

ASSAN, R., TCHOBROUTSKY, G. and TIENGO, A. (1972b): Influence of some nutrients and metabolic substrates on glucagon secretion. In: *Nutrition and Diabetes Mellitus, VI Capri Conference, July 1972, Vol. 1.* Editors: E. R. Froesch and J. Yudkin. Il Ponte, Milano. Also in: *Acta diabet. lat., IX/Suppl. 1.*

ASSAN, R. and TIENGO, A. (1972): Comparaisons des sécrétions de glucagon dans les diabètes sucrés avec ou sans pancréatopathie organique acquise. *Pathol. Biol., 21,* 17.

BALLARD, F. J., HANSON, R. W. and KRONFELD, D. S. (1969): Gluconeogenesis and lipogenesis in tissue from ruminant and non ruminant animals. *Fed. Proc., 28,* 218.

BATTAGLIA, F. C. and MESCHIA, G. (1973): Foetal metabolism and substrate utilization. In: *Foetal and Neonatal Physiology,* pp. 382–397. Editors: K. S. Combine, K. W. Cross, G. S. Dawes and P. W. Nathanielsz. Cambridge University Press, Cambridge.

BENCOSME, S. A., WILSON, M. B., ALEYASSINE, H., De BOLD, A. J. and De BOLD, M. L. (1970): Rabbit pancreatic B cell. Morphological and functional studies during embryonal and post natal development. *Diabetologia, 6,* 399.

BJORKMAN, N., HELLERSTRÖM, C., HELLMAN, B. and PETTERSON, B. (1966): The cell types in the endocrine pancreas of the human fetus. *Z. Zellforsch., 72,* 425.

BLAZQUEZ, E., SUGASE, T., BLAZQUEZ, M. and FOA, P. P. (1972): The ontogeny of metabolic regulation in the rat, with special reference to the development of insular function. *Acta diabet. lat., 9/Suppl. 1,* 13.

BLEICHER, S. J., SPERGEL, G., LEVY, L. and ZAROWITZ, H. (1970): Aglucagonemic man. A model for analysis of the arginine infusion test. *Clin. Res., 18,* 355.

BLOOM, S. R. and JOHNSTON, D. I. (1972): Failure of glucagon release in infants of diabetic mothers. *Brit. med. J., 4,* 453.

BLOOM, S. R., VAUGHAN, N. J. A. and EDWARDS, A. V. (1973a): Pancreatic glucagon levels in the calf (abstract). *Diabetologia, 9,* 61.

BLOOM, S. R., EDWARDS, A. V. and VAUGHAN, N. J. A. (1973b): The role of the sympathetic innervation in the control of plasma glucagon concentration in the calf. *J. Physiol.,* in press.

BRAATEN, J. T., FALOONA, G. R. and UNGER, R. H. (1973): Comparison of alpha cell dysfunction in acquired and inherited diabetes mellitus. *Diabetes, 22/Suppl. 1,* 302.

BUCHANAN, K. D., VANCE, J. E. and WILLIAMS, R. H. (1969a): Effect of blood glucose on glucagon secretion in anesthetized dogs. *Diabetes, 18,* 11.

BUCHANAN, K. D., VANCE, J. E. and WILLIAMS, R. H. (1969b): Insulin and glucagon release from isolated islets of Langerhans. *Diabetes, 18,* 381.

BURR, I. M., BALANT, L., STAUFFACHER, W. and RENOLD, A. E. (1970): Perifusion of rat pancreatic tissue in vitro: Substrate modification of theophylline-induced biphasic insulin release. *J. clin. Invest., 49,* 2097.

CAHILL, G. F. (1972): Prenatal nutrition of lambs, bears and babies? *Pediatrics, 50,* 357.

CHERRINGTON, A. D. and VRANIC, M. (1973): Effect of arginine on glucose turnover and plasma free fatty acids in normal dogs. *Diabetes,* in press.

CHESNEY, T. McC. and SCHOFIELD, J. G. (1969): Studies on the secretion of pancreatic glucagon. *Diabetes, 18,* 627.

CHRISTENSEN, H. N., CULLEN, A. M., HARRISSON, L. I., FAJANS, S. S. and PEK, S. (1971): Stimulation of glucagon and insulin release by non-metabolizable amino-acid derivatives: their use to identify transport systems responsible to glucagon. In: *Physiology and Pharmacology of Cyclic AMP, Proceedings of the International Conference, Milan, July 1971,* p. 81.

DAY, J. L. and TATTERSALL, R. (1972): Abnormalities of glucagon metabolism in unaffected twices of diabetic subjects. In: *Abstracts, Proceedings of the British Diabetic Association Meeting, Brighton, September 1972.*

DAY, J. L. and ANDERSON, J. (1973): Abnormalities of glucagon metabolism in diabetes mellitus. In preparation.

DE CARO, G., IMPROTA, G. and MELCHIORRI, P. (1970): Effect of caerulein infusion on glucagon secretion in the dog. *Experientia (Basel), 26,* 1145.

EDWARDS, J. C., ASPLUND, K. and LUNDQVIST, G. (1972): Glucagon release from the pancreas of the newborn rat. *J. Endocr., 54,* 493.

EDWARDS, J. C., HOWELL, S. L. and TAYLOR, K. W. (1970): Effects of metabolic inhibitors on glucagon release of isolated guinea pigs islets of Langerhans. *Biochem. J., 117,* 32P.

EMERY, J. L. and BURY, H. P. R. (1964): Involutionary changes in the islets of Langerhans. *Biol. Neonat. (Basel), 6,* 15.

FAJANS, S. S., FLOYD, J. C., KNOPF, R. F. and CONN, J. N. (1967): Effect of amino acids and proteins on insulin secretion in man. *Rec. Progr. Hormone Res., 23,* 617.

FALLUCCA, F., CARRATU, R., TAMBURRANO, G., JAVICOLI, M., MENZINGER, G. and ANDREANI, D. (1972): Effects of caerulein and pancreozymin on insulin secretion in normal subjects and in patients with insuloma. *Hormone metabol. Res., 4,* 55.

FALORNI, A., GALLO, G. and MASSI-BENEDETTI, F. (1973): Effect of arginine infusion on blood glucose and plasma insulin and glucagon in low birth weight infants. In: *Abstracts, 8th Congress of the International Diabetes Federation, Brussels, 1973,* p. 143. International Congress Series No. 280, Excerpta Medica, Amsterdam.

FELIG, P. (1972): Interaction of insulin and amino-acid metabolism in the regulation of gluconeogenesis. *Israel J. med. Sci., 8,* 262.

FELIG, P., POZEFSKY, T., MARLISS, E. B. and CAHILL Jr., G. F. (1970): Alanine: key role in gluconeogenesis. *Science, 167,* 1003.

FELIG, P. and MARLISS, E. (1972): The glycemic response to arginine in man. *Diabetes, 21,* 308.

FERNER, H. and STOECKENIUS Jr., W. (1951): Die Zytogenese des Inselsystems beim Menschen. *Z. Zellforsch., 35,* 147.

FISER, R. H., PHELPS, D. L., ERENBERG, A., SPERLING, M. A., OH, W. and FISHER, D. A. (1973): Pancreatic alpha and beta cell responsiveness in fetal and newborn lambs (abstract). *Pediat. Res., 7,* 311.

FRANKEL, B. J., GERICH, J. E., FANSKA, R. E. and GRODSKI, G. M. (1973): Subnormal insulin and excessive glucagon release from in vitro perfused pancreases of non obese, genetically diabetic chinese hamsters. *Diabetes, 22/Suppl. 1,* 307.

FUSSGÄNGER, R., STRAUB, K., GOBERNA, R., JARDS, P., SCHRÖDER, K. E., RAPTIS, S. and PFEIFFER, E. F. (1969): Primary secretion of insulin and secondary release of glucagon from the isolated perfused rat pancreas following stimulation with pancreozymin. *Hormone metabol. Res., 1,* 224.

GAY, J., TCHOBROUTSKY, G., ROSSELIN, G., ASSAN, R., DOLAIS, J., FREYCHET, P. and DEROT, M. (1968): Etude de 8 cas d'hémochromatoses primitives: dosages de H.G.H., F.S.H., glucagon. *Pathol. Biol., 16,* 53.

GIRARD, J., ASSAN, R. and JOST, A. (1973a): Glucagon in the rat fetus. In: *Foetal and Neonatal Physiology,* pp. 456–461. Editors: K. S. Comline, K. W. Cross, G. S. Dawes and P. W. Nathanielsz. Cambridge University Press, Cambridge.

GIRARD, J., BAL, D. and ASSAN, R. (1971): Rat plasma glucagon during the perinatal period. *Diabetologia, 7,* 481.

GIRARD, J., BAL, D. and ASSAN, R. (1972): Glucagon secretion during the early postnatal period in the rat. *Hormone metabol. Res., 4,* 168.

GIRARD, J. R., CUENDET, G. S., MARLISS, E. B., KERVRAN, A., RIEUTORT, M. and ASSAN, R. (1973b): Hormones, fuels and liver metabolism at term and during the early postnatal period in the rat. *J. clin. Invest.,* in press.

GIRARD, J. R., KERVRAN, A., SOUFFLET, E. and ASSAN, R. (1973c): Factors affecting the secretion of insulin and glucagon by the rat fetuses in utero. *Diabetes,* in press.

GIRARD, J. R., MARLISS, E. B. and ASSAN, R. (1973d): Glucagon and perinatal metabolism in the rat. *Advanc. Biosci., 13,* in press.

GRESHAM, E. L., SIMMONS, P. S. and BATTAGLIA, F. C. (1971): Maternal-fetal urea concentration difference in man -- metabolic significance. *J. Pediat., 79,* 809.

GUY-GRAND, B. and ASSAN, R. (1973): Lipolytic activity of synthetic (1–23) glucagon in vitro. *Hormone metabol. Res., 5,* 60.

HANSEN, A. P. (1971): Normalization of growth hormone hyperresponse to exercise in juvenile diabetics after normalization of blood sugar. *J. clin. Invest., 50,* 1806.

HARD, W. L. (1944): The origin and differentiation of the alpha and beta cells in the pancreatic islets of the rat. *Amer. J. Anat., 75,* 369.

HAYMOND, M., KARL, I. and PAGLIARA, A. (1973): Defective gluconeogenesis in small for gestational age infants (abstract). *Pediat. Res., 7,* 381.

HEDING, L. G. and RASMUSSEN, S. M. (1972): Determination of pancreatic and gut glucagon-like immuno-reactivity (G.L.I.) in normal and diabetic subjects. *Diabetologia, 8,* 408.

HOWELL, S. L., EDWARDS, J. C. and WHITFIELD, M. (1971): Preparation of insulin deficient guinea pigs islets of Langerhans. *Hormone metabol. Res., 3,* 37.

IVERSEN, J. (1970): Secretion of immunoreactive insulin and glucagon from the isolated perfused canine pancreas following stimulation with glucose, pancreozymin, arginine, and tolbutamide. In: *Abstracts, 7th Congress of the International Diabetes Federation, Buenos Aires, 1970,* p. 11. International Congress Series No. 209, Excerpta Medica, Amsterdam.

IVERSEN, J. (1971): Secretion of glucagon and insulin from the isolated perfused canine pancreas. *J. clin. Invest., 50,* 2123.

JAROUSSE, C., RANCON, F. and ROSSELIN, G. (1973a): Hormonogenèse périnatale de l'insuline et du glucagon chez le rat. *C.R. Acad. Sci. (Paris), 276,* 585.

JAROUSSE, C., RANCON, F., ROSSELIN, G. and FREYCHET, P. (1973b): Sécrétion de l'insuline et du glucagon par le pancréas du rat nouveau-né: effet du glucose et de l'adénosine 3′5′ cyclique monophosphate. *C.R. Acad. Sci. (Paris), 276,* 797.

JOHNSTON, D. I., BLOOM, S. R., GREENE, K. R. and BEARD, R. W. (1972a): Plasma pancreatic glucagon relationship between mother and fetus at term (abstract). *J. Endocrinol., 55,* XXV.

JOHNSTON, D. I., BLOOM, S. R., GREENE, K. R. and BEARD, R. W. (1972b): Failure of the human placenta to transfer pancreatic glucagon. *Biol. Neonate, 21,* 375.

JOHNSTON, D. I. and BLOOM, S. R. (1973): Plasma glucagon levels in the term human infant and effect of hypoxia. *Arch. Dis. Childh., 48,* 451.

KANETO, A. and KOSAKA, K. (1971): Stimulation of glucagon secretion by arginine and histidine infused intra-pancreatically. *Endocrinology, 88,* 1239.

KARMAN, H. and MIALHE, P. (1973): Glucose-glucagon feed-back mechanism in normal and diabetic geese and ducks. In: *EASD 8th Annual Meeting, Madrid, September 1972.* Abstract No. 142.

LEFEBVRE, P. J. and UNGER, R. H. (1972): *Glucagon, Molecular Physiology, Clinical and Therapeutic Implication, Vol. 1.* Editors: P. J. Lefebvre and R. H. Unger. Pergamon, Oxford.

LERNMARK, A. and WENNGREN, B. I. (1972): Insulin and glucagon release from the isolated pancreas of foetal and newborn mice. *J. Embryol. exp. Morphol., 28,* 607.

LIKE, A. A. and ORCI, L. (1972): Embryogenesis of the human pancreatic islets: A light and electron microscopic study. *Diabetes, 21/Suppl. 2,* 511.

LIN, H. M. and POTTER, E. L. (1962): Development of human pancreas. *Arch. Pathol., 74,* 439.

LUYCKX, A. (1973): *Le Contrôle de la Sécrétion de Glucagon à Hormones et Régulations Métaboliques, Vol. 1.* Masson, Paris.

LUYCKX, A. S., MASSI-BENEDETTI, F., FALORNI, A. and LEFEBVRE, P. (1972): Presence of pancreatic glucagon in the portal plasma of human neonates. Differences in the insulin and glucagon responses to glucose between normal infants and infants from diabetic mothers. *Diabetologia, 8,* 296.

MARCO, J., CALLE, C., ROMAN, O., DIAZ-FIERROS, M., VILLANUEVA, M. L. and VALVERDE, I. (1973): Hyperglucagonism induced by glucocorticoid treatment in man. *New Engl. J. Med.,* in press.

MARCO, J., DIAZ-FIERROS, M., BAROJA, I. M., VILLANUEVA, M. L. and VALVERDE, I. (1972): Opposite effects of aminophylline on arginine-induced glucagon and insulin secretion in humans. *Diabetes, 21,* 289.

MARCO, J., FALOONA, G. R. and UNGER, R. H. (1971): The glycogenolytic activity of immunoreactive glucagon in plasma. *J. clin. Invest., 50,* 1650.

MARLISS, E. B., AOKI, T. T., TOEWS, C. J., FELIG, P., CONNON, J. J., KYNER, J., HUCKABEE, W. E. and CAHILL Jr., G. F. (1972): Amino-acid metabolism in lactic acidosis. *Amer. J. Med., 52,* 474.

MARLISS, E. B., AOKI, T. T., UNGER, R. H., SOELDNER, J. S. and CAHILL Jr., G. F. (1970): Glucagon levels and metabolic effects in fasting man. *J. clin. Invest., 49,* 2256.

MARLISS, E. B., WOLLHEIM, C. B., BLONDEL, B., ORCI, L., LAMBERT, A. E., STAUFFACHER, W., LIKE, A. A. and RENOLD, A. E. (1973): Insulin and glucagon release from monolayer cell cultures of pancreas from newborn rats. *Europ. J. clin. Invest., 3,* 16.

MARREIRO, D. R., FALOONA, G. R. and UNGER, R. H. (1972): Glucagon-stimulating activity of 20 amino-acids in dogs. *J. clin. Invest., 51,* 2346.

MASSI-BENEDETTI, F., LUYCKX, A., FRACASSINI, F., LEFEBVRE, P. and FALORNI, A. (1973): Glucose metabolism and insulin-glucagon relationship in newborn infants of normal and diabetic mothers (abstract). *Diabetologia, 9,* 81.

MILNER, R. D. G., FEKETE, M. and ASSAN, R. (1972a): Glucagon, insulin and growth hormone response to exchange transfusion in premature and term infants. *Arch. Dis. Childh., 47,* 186.

MILNER, R. D. G., FEKETE, M., ASSAN, R. and HODGE, J. S. (1972b): Effect of glucose on plasma glucagon, growth hormone and insulin in exchange transfusion. *Arch. Dis. Childh., 47,* 179.

MILNER, R. D. G., CHOUKSEY, S. K., MICKLESON, K. N. P. and ASSAN, R. (1973): Plasma pancreatic glucagon and insulin:glucagon ratio at birth. *Arch. Dis. Childh., 48,* 241.

MORRIS, F. H., MESCHIA, G., MAKOWSKI, E. L. and BATTAGLIA, F. C. (1973): Umbilical glucose/O_2 quotient of the human fetus (abstract). *Pediat. Res., 7,* 314.

MÜLLER, W. A., AOKI, T. T. and CAHILL Jr., G. F. (1973a): Pancreatic glucagon stimulation by alanine and glycine in humans. In: *Abstracts, 8th Congress of the International Diabetes Federation, Brussels, July 1973,* no. 107. International Congress Series No. 280, Excerpta Medica, Amsterdam.

MÜLLER, W. A., FALOONA, G. R. and UNGER, R. H. (1970): Abnormal alpha cell function in diabetes: response to carbohydrate and protein ingestion. *New Engl. J. Med., 283,* 109.

MÜLLER, W. A., FALOONA, G. R. and UNGER, R. H. (1971a): The effect of alanine on glucagon secretion. *J. clin. Invest., 50,* 2215.

MÜLLER, W. A., FALOONA, G. R. and UNGER, R. H. (1971b): The influence of the antecedent diet upon glucagon and insulin secretion. *New Engl. J. Med., 285,* 1450.

MÜLLER, W. A., FALOONA, G. R. and UNGER, R. H. (1971c): The effect of experimental insulin deficiency on glucagon secretion. *J. clin. Invest., 50,* 1992.

MÜLLER, W. A., FALOONA, G. R. and UNGER, R. H. (1973b): Hyperglucagonemia in diabetic keto-acidosis, its prevalence and significance. *Amer. J. Med., 54,* 52.

NONAKA, K., YOSHIDA, T., ICHIHARA, K., SHIMA, K., TARVI, S. and NISHIKAWA, M. (1973): Spontaneous hypoglycemia associated with low pancreatic glucagon response to arginine load. In: *Abstracts, 8th Congress of the International Diabetes Federation, Brussels, July 1973,* No. 491. International Congress Series No. 280, Excerpta Medica, Amsterdam.

OHNEDA, A., AGUILAR-PARADA, E., EISENTRAUT, A. M. and UNGER, R. H. (1969a): Control of pancreatic glucagon secretion by glucose. *Diabetes, 18,* 1.

OHNEDA, A., PARADA, E., EISENTRAUT, A. M. and UNGER, R. H. (1969b): Characterization of response of circulating glucagon to intraduodenal and intravenous administration of amino-acids. *J. clin. Invest., 47,* 2305.

OKUNO, G., PRICE, S., GRILLS, T. A. I. and FOA, P. P. (1964): Development of phosphorylase and phosphorylase-activating (glucagon-like) substances in the rat embryo. *Gen. comp. Endocr., 4,* 446.

ORCI, L., LAMBERT, A. E., ROUILLER, C., RENOLD, A. E. and SAMOLS, E. (1969): Evidence for the presence of A cells in the endocrine fetal pancreas of the rat. *Hormone metabol. Res., 1,* 108.

ORCI, L., LAMBERT, A. E., AMHERDT, M., CAMERON, D., KANAZAWA, Y. and STAUFFACHER, W. (1970a): The autonomic nervous system and the B cell: metabolic and morphological observations made in spiny mice and in cultured fetal rat pancreas. *Acta diabet. lat., 7/Suppl. 1,* 184.

ORCI, L., LIKE, A. A., AMHERDT, M., BLONDEL, B., KANAZAWA, Y., MARLISS, E. B., LAMBERT, A. E., WOLLHEIM, C. B. and RENOLD, A. E. (1973): Monolayer cell culture of neonatal rat pancreas: an ultrastructural and biochemical study of functioning endocrine cells. *J. ultrastruct. Res., 43,* 270.

ORCI, L., STAUFFACHER, W., DULIN, W. E., RENOLD, A. E. and ROVILLER, C. (1970b): Ultrastructural changes in A cells exposed to diabetic hyperglycemia. Observations made on pancreas of chinese hamsters. *Diabetologia, 6,* 199.

PAGE, M. A. and WILLIAMSON, D. H. (1971): Enzymes of ketone body utilization in human brain. *Lancet, 2,* 66.

PALMER, J. P., WALTER, R. M. and ENSINCK, J. W. (1973): Acute phase of glucagon release in normal and diabetic man. *Diabetes, 22/Suppl. 1,* 302.

PALOYAN, E., LAWRENCE, A., STRAUS, F. H., PALOYAN, D., HARPER, P. V. and CUMMINGS, D. (1967): Alpha-cell hyperplasia in calcified pancreatitis associated with hyperparathyroidism. *J. Amer. med. Ass., 200,* 757.

PEARCE, A. G. E., POLAK, J. M. and HEATH, C. M. (1973): Development, differentiation and derivation of the endocrine polypeptide cells of the mouse pancreas. Immunofluorescence, cytochemical and ultrastructural studies. *Diabetologia, 9,* 120.

PEK, S., FAJANS, S. S., FLOYD Jr., J. C., KNOPF, R. F. and CONN, J. W. (1968): Effect of amino-acids on plasma glucagon in man. *J. lab. clin. Med., 72,* 1003.

PEK, S., FAJANS, S. S., FLOYD Jr., J. C., KNOPF, R. H. and CONN, J. W. (1969): Effects upon plasma glucagon of infused and ingested amino-acids and of protein meals in man. *Diabetes, 18,* 328.

PEK, S., FAJANS, S. S., FLOYD Jr., J. C., KNOPF, R. F. and CONN, J. W. (1972): Failure of sulfonylureas to suppress plasma glucagon in man. *Diabetes, 21,* 216.

PERRIER, H., PORTE, A. and JACQUOT, R. (1969): Présence de cellules A dans le pancréas foetal de rat. *C.R. Acad. Sci. (Paris), 269,* 841.

PERRIER, H. (1970): Evolution de l'ultrastructure du pancréas chez le foetus de rat. *Diabetologia, 6,* 605.

PERSSON, I., GYNTELBERG, F., HEDING, L. G., BOSS-NIELSEN, J. (1971): Pancreatic glucagon-like immunoreactivity after i.v. insulin in normals and chronic-pancreatitis patients. *Acta Endocr. (Kbh.), 67,* 401.

PFEIFFER, E. F., FUSSGÄNGER, R. and RAPTIS, S. (1972): Gastro intestinal hormones and islet functions. In: *'Nutrition and Diabetes Mellitus', VIth Capri Conference, July 1972, Vol. 1.* Editors: E. R. Froesch and J. Yudkin. Il Ponte, Milan.

PICTET, R. and RUTTER, W. J. (1972): Development of the embryonic endocrine pancreas. In: *Endocrine Pancreas,* pp. 25–66. Editors: D. F. Steiner and N. Freinkel. American Physiological Society, Washington, D.C.

RAIHA, N. C. R. and LINDROS, K. O. (1969): Development of some enzymes involved in gluconeogenesis human liver. *Ann. Med. Exp. Fenn., 47,* 146.

ROBB, P. (1961): The development of the islets of Langerhans in the human foetus. *Quart. J. exp. Physiol., 46,* 335.

ROSSELIN, G., JAROUSSE, C., RANCON, F. and PORTHA, B. (1973): L'AMP cyclique médiateur de la sécrétion du glucagon due aux acides aminés. *C.R. Acad. Sci. (Paris), 276,* 1017.

RUTTER, W. J. (1969): Independently regulated synthetic transitions in foetal tissues. In: *Foetal Autonomy,* pp. 59–76. Editors: G. E. W. Wolstenholme and M. O'Connor. Churchill, London.
SAMOLS, E., TYLER, J. and MIALHE, P. (1969): Suppression of pancreatic glucagon release by the hypoglycemic sulfonylureas. *Lancet, I,* 174.
SANTEUSANIO, F., FALOONA, G. R. and UNGER, R. H. (1972): Suppressive effect of secretion upon pancreatic alpha cell function. *J. clin. Invest., 51,* 1743.
SCHAEFFER, L. D., WILDER, M. L. and WILLIAMS, R. H. (1973): Secretion and content of insulin and glucagon in human fetal pancreas slices in vitro. *Proc. Soc. exp. Biol. Med. (N.Y.), 143,* 314.
SCHULTZE-JENNA, B. S. (1953): Das quantitative und qualitative Inselbild menschlicher Foeten und Neugeborener. *Virchows Arch. Path. Anat., 323,* 653.
SCHWEISTHAL, M. R. and FROST, C. C. (1973): Differentiation of alpha cells in the fetal rat pancreas grown in organ culture. *Amer. J. Anat., 136,* 527.
SHELLEY, H. J. and NELIGAN, G. A. (1966): Neonatal hypoglycemia. *Brit. med. Bull., 22,* 34.
SIMMONS, M. A., MESCHIA, G., MAKOWSKI, E. L. and BATTAGLIA, F. C. (1973): Phases of fetal metabolic adjustment to maternal starvation (abstract). *Pediat. Res., 7,* 309.
SOUFFLET, E., BALLERIO, G., ATTALI, J. R., BOILLOT, J., GIRARD, J. R. and ASSAN, R. (1973): Effects of cycloheximide, colchicine, vincristine, on the arginine-induced glucagon secretion, in isolated perfused rat pancreas. In: *Abstracts, 8th Congress of the International Diabetes Federation, Brussels, July 1973,* No. 109. International Congress Series No. 280, Excerpta Medica, Amsterdam.
SPERLING, M. A., PHELPS, D., DELAMATER, P. V., FISER, R. H. and FISHER, D. A. (1973): Islet cell function in the human newborn (abstract). *Pediat. Res., 7,* 407.
TIENGO, A., FEDELE, D., MUGGEO, M. and CREPALDI, G. (1973): Diabetic-like behaviour of glucagon secretion in primary endogenous hypertriglyceridemia. In: *Abstracts, 8th Congress of the International Diabetes Federation, Brussels, July 1973,* No. 110. International Congress Series No. 280, Excerpta Medica, Amsterdam.
UNGER, R. H., AGUILAR-PARADA, E., MÜLLER, W. and EISENTRAUT, A. M. (1970): Studies of pancreatic alpha cell function in normal and diabetic subjects. *J. clin. Invest., 49,* 837.
UNGER, R. H., KETTERER, H., DUPRE, J. and EISENTRAUT, A. (1967): The effects of secretion, pancreozymin and gastrin on insulin and glucagon secretion in anaesthetized dogs. *J. clin. Invest., 46,* 630.
UNGER, R. H., MADISON, L. L. and MÜLLER, W. A. (1972): Abnormal alpha cell function in diabetics. Response to insulin. *Diabetes, 21,* 301.
UNGER, R. H., OHNEDA, E., AGUILAR-PARADA, E. and EISENTRAUT, A. M. (1969): The role of aminogenic glucagon secretion in blood glucose homeostasis. *J. clin. Invest., 48,* 810.
VECCHIO, D., LUYCKX, A., ZAHND, G. R. and RENOLD, A. E. (1966): Insulin release induced by glucagon in organ culture of fetal rat pancreas. *Metabolism, 15,* 577.
WAHREN, J., FELIG, P., CERASI, E., LUFT, R. and HENDLER, R. (1973): Splanchnic glucose production and its regulation in healthy monozygotic twins of diabetics. *Clin. Sci., 44,* 493.
WELLMAN, K. F., VOLK, B. W. and BRANCATO, P. (1971): Ultrastructure and insulin content of the endocrine pancreas in the human fetus. *Lab. Invest., 25,* 97.
WISE, J. K., HENDLER, R. and FELIG, P. (1972): Obesity: evidence of decreased glucagon secretion. *Science, 178,* 513.
WISE, J. K., HENDLER, R. and FELIG, P. (1973a): Evaluation of alpha-cell function by infusion of alanine in normal, diabetic, and obese subjects. *New Engl. J. Med., 288,* 484.

WISE, J. K., LYALL, S. S., HENDLER, R. and FELIG, P. (1973b): Evidence of stimulation of glucagon secretion by alanine in the human fetus at term. *J. clin. Endocr., 37,* 345.

WOLLHEIM, C. B., BLONDEL, B., RABINOVITCH, A. and RENOLD, A. E. (1973): Insulin and glucagon release in pancreatic monolayer cultures: effects of cyclic nucleotides. In: *Abstracts, 8th Congress of the International Diabetes Federation, Brussels, July 1973,* p. 48. International Congress Series No. 280, Excerpta Medica, Amsterdam.

HYPOGLUCAGONEMIC STATES

LISE G. HEDING

Novo Research Institute, Novo Alle, Bagsvaerd, Denmark

The purpose of this paper is to give a review of the various types of hypoglucagonemia. including obesity, hyperlipoproteinemia, chronic pancreatitis and isolated glucagon deficiency. Determinations of plasma glucagon by radioimmunoassay play an important role in the diagnosis of some hypoglucagonemic states. For this reason, the first part of the paper gives a brief outline of current glucagon immunoassay techniques with special reference to the type of immunoreactivity which is being measured.

RADIOIMMUNOLOGICAL GLUCAGON DETERMINATIONS

The determination of plasma glucagon by radioimmunoassay has been complicated by several methodological and immunological problems. Table 1 shows the principal factors that determine the amount and type of the immunoreactivity.

The standard glucagon solutions should be prepared using buffer without proteolytic

TABLE 1
Factors that determine the amount and type of glucagon immunoreactivity measured in an immunoassay

Reagents:
- Standard glucagon solutions
- ^{125}I-glucagon preparations
- Glucagon antibodies

Technical problems:
- Temperature, time, pH, separation method, etc.

Blood sampling:
- Plasma preparation (time, temperature, inhibition of proteolytic inhibition)
- Extraction procedure

activity; otherwise apparently too high results will occur. The use of a purified albumin can eliminate this problem.

The quality of the labelled glucagon may give more serious problems. A low-quality tracer containing several different labelled compounds shows a reduced binding to antibodies and gives less steep standard curves as compared to monoiodoglucagon (Jørgensen and Larsen, 1972). In addition it must be assumed that the various labelled components have a different affinity towards the antibodies. Plasma samples which most likely contain several immunological fragments will then compete differently with the labelled compounds – compared to the pure standard – for the antibodies.

The antibody is the most important reagent in an immunoassay as it determines the sensitivity and specificity of the assay. For many years these 2 characteristics were unsatisfactory and delayed the development of a valuable immunoassay. Although it is still quite difficult to produce high affinity glucagon antibodies, this problem has been nearly solved. Increasing the immunogenicity of the glucagon by various coupling techniques is now a routine. Thus we are left with the serious problem of the specificity. The more technical problems will not be dealt with here.

The recovery of pancreatic glucagon and pork gut glucagon-like immunoreactivity (GLI) that had been added to blood prior to the preparation of plasma at low temperature was found to vary from 15 to 80% (Heding, 1971). When 500 KIE of trasylol was added per ml blood, the recovery was in the range of 80 and 100% except in one case. Endogenous pancreatic glucagon and gut GLI from normal persons were likewise degraded to a great extent, unless protected, and it must be concluded that glucagon determinations in plasma prepared without trasylol are of dubious value. Having established that both pancreatic and gut GLI are degraded during the short period of plasma preparation, the next question to examine was: does the blood contain fragments of glucagon or gut GLI that react with the antibodies? As the antibodies are specific only for a small part of the molecule, it seems likely that some fragments could retain immunological activity, a phenomenon that is well-known from radioimmunoassay of other peptide hormones. The many synthetic, tryptic and chymotryptic fragments that have been prepared provided no information on the type and reactivity of the natural fragments. However, the high immunological activity observed for some synthetic peptides suggests the probability of the natural fragments reacting with the antibodies. Gel filtration on Sephadex G-15 of serum to which ^{125}I-glucagon was added showed that several radioactive fragments were formed and furthermore that some of these could react with glucagon antibodies (Heding, 1972).

In addition to this, we have found that unlabelled glucagon can be degraded into fragments that can react with up to 30% activity with one antiserum while others show no reaction. The reaction with the fragments is not dependent on the reaction with gut GLI. Some 'specific' sera show reaction, some do not.

Besides the fragments formed by enzymatic degradation, other substances in the plasma may react with glucagon antibodies (Table 2). Gut GLI reacts to varying degrees with different antisera (Heding, 1971), and it has become a routine procedure in most laboratories to test the antisera using a crude gut extract, thereby selecting the non-reacting sera. This criterion has greatly improved the quality of the assay. On the other hand, an antiserum that does not react with gut GLI cannot be considered specific for pancreatic glucagon unless further characterized.

The inactive modified glucagon which leaves the receptor sites after activation of cAMP has been described as behaving similarly to intact glucagon in several chromato-

TABLE 2
Substances in plasma which may react with glucagon antibodies

Fragments of pancreatic glucagon
Gut GLI
Fragments of gut GLI
modified glucagon, leaving the receptor sites
Human γ-globulin
Fragments of other hormones
Large GLI

graphic systems (Rodbell, 1972), and cannot consist of degraded small fragments. It is to be expected that this modified glucagon will react with the antibodies to a greater or lesser degree, although nothing is known about it.

Finally, it has been shown (Fig. 1) that crude gut GLI is degraded when incubated in plasma determined by a gut GLI reacting antiserum. Simultaneously a rise was observed in pancreatic GLI using an antiserum which showed only a few per cent reaction with the gut GLI. Similarly, after i.v. injection of pork gut GLI extracts in dogs a rise in plasma pancreatic GLI was observed (personal observations).

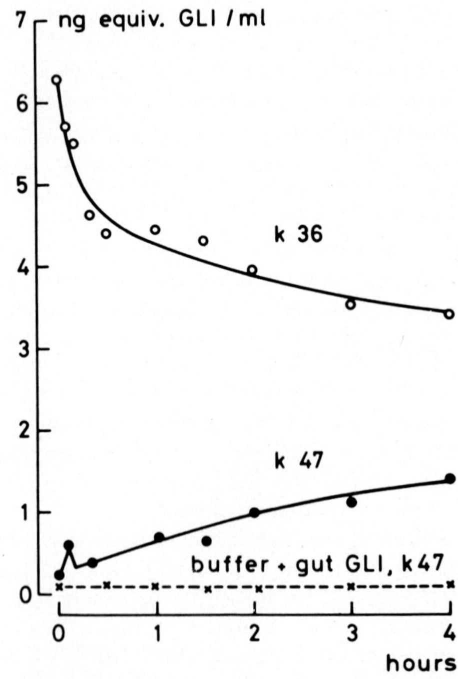

FIG. 1. Addition of crude gut GLI to plasma without trasylol. The GLI was determined at various intervals using a linear gut GLI cross-reacting antiserum, K36, and another serum, K47, only reacting a few per cent with gut GLI as compared to K36.

These results, which may be found for other antisera, add another confusing brick to the glucagon immunoassay and may explain the positive values found with many so-called specific sera in pancreatectomized individuals. Furthermore, this finding stresses the necessity of preparing plasma quickly and at low temperature.

A correlation between glycogenolytic activity and immunoreactive glucagon of plasma extracts has been described (Marco et al., 1971). As other components influence the glycogenolytic activity, the most convincing evidence of identity between immunoreactivity and biological activity was the suppression of the glucogenolytic activity by glucagon antibodies shown for 3 sera. Such comparisons will greatly increase the faith in glucagon immunoassay. However, Guy-Grand and Assan (1973) have shown that the N-terminal 1-23 peptide which does not react with the so-called pancreatic specific antisera but with the gut GLI cross-reactive, has full lipolytic activity compared to the intact glucagon. Thus no correlation can be expected between lipolytic activity and immunoreactivity using non-gut GLI reacting antisera, but probably between lipolytic activity and GLI using cross-reactive antisera. In this connection, it is interesting that turkey glucagon, which deviates from pork glucagon in position 28 only (serine instead of asparagine), behaves like low molecular weight gut GLI in immunoassays. Only a few per cent reactivity was obtained with antisera not reacting with gut GLI, whereas nearly 100% reactivity was seen with gut GLI reacting antisera (Markussen et al., 1972; personal observations).

TABLE 3

Characterization of glucagon antibodies to be used for plasma pancreatic glucagon determinations

1. No reaction with gut GLI
2. No reaction with pancreatic glucagon fragments
3. No reaction with gut GLI fragments
4. Zero glucagon in pancreatectomized persons
5. Close correlation between biological and immunological activities

In conclusion (Table 3), glucagon antisera should be carefully characterized before being used in plasma analyses. The correlation between biological (either glycogenolytic or lipolytic) and immunological activities would give information as to which activity is being measured and to what extent. It is evident that basal levels as well as fluctuations in plasma pancreatic glucagon immunoreactivity should at present be interpreted with caution.

HYPOGLUCAGONEMIC STATES

Definition

The very first problem encountered when talking about hypoglucagonemia is the definition of this condition. It seems reasonable to introduce the concept of relative hypoglucagonemia to describe conditions where endogenous glucagon secretion is inadequate to maintain a normal metabolic state, and where administration of exogenous glucagon exerts a normalizing effect.

Table 4 shows some of the various conditions of glucagon deficiency which, in the following, will be regarded as hypoglucagonemic.

TABLE 4

Criteria used to characterize absolute or relative hypoglucagonemia

1. Reduced number or lack of alpha cells (pancreatectomy, chronic pancreatitis, congenital)
2. Reduced glucagon release to various stimuli
   Elimination of symptoms by exogenous glucagon
3. Increased glucagon release to various stimuli
   Normalization by exogenous glucagon

Three criteria were used in this classification:

Patients with a verified lack, or reduced number, of alpha cells. This group includes the few pancreatectomized persons, severe chronic pancreatitis cases and patients in whom histologic examination of the islets has revealed a reduction in the percentage of the alpha cells. All 3 groups suffer from episodes of hypoglycemia.

The next group comprises conditions where glucagon release is either nil or reduced to physiological or test conditions. The possibility of the low glucagon response being due to a reduced number of alpha cells cannot be ruled out. Some cases of reactive hypoglycemia, obesity and unstable diabetes may have this type of hypoglucagonemia.

The third group – the most normal of the 3 from the point of view of plasma glucagon determinations – comprises clinical disorders such as some cases of hypoglycemia and hyperlipoproteinemia, where glucagon secretion seems to be normal or exaggerated. On the other hand, these disorders can be more or less normalized by exogenous glucagon administration.

Reduced number or lack of alpha cells

Pancreatectomy
Chronic pancreatitis
Spontaneous hypoglycemia
Hypopituitarism

Total pancreatectomy is the only condition with a known complete lack of pancreatic glucagon. Because of the insulin therapy, hypoglycemic episodes cannot be regarded simply as symptoms of glucagon deficiency. However, it is well-known that the diabetes that follows pancreatectomy in man is extremely labile, or insulin-sensitive, with daily episodes of severe hypoglycemia (Schultis et al., 1967; Brunner et al., 1968; Zarowitz, 1972). Schultis et al. (1967) demonstrated that hypoglycemia was particularly pronounced in connection with physical and psychic stress, and in the morning. They found that these disturbing symptoms could be relieved by the combined therapy of Zn-glucagon and insulin.

Patients with pancreatitis were reported to have increased glucagon levels in a non-specific assay (Paloyan et al., 1966; 1967a, b). Day et al. (1972) subsequently reproduced the findings of hyperglucagonemia in patients with moderately damaged alpha cells, using an antiserum not reacting with crude gut extract. Moreover, they found low glucagon in cases with severe damage to the pancreas, which has also been described by others (Aguilar-Parada et al., 1969).

Patients with diabetes caused by pancreatitis were observed either totally to lack, or to have a reduced glucagon response to insulin-induced hypoglycemia (Persson et al., 1971; Assan and Tiengo, 1973). This probably explains the more frequent and pronounced hypoglycemia recorded in this type of patient. In hypopituitary patients, low glucagon levels have been ascribed to reduced alpha cell function as a consequence of growth hormone deficiency (Lawrence, 1972).

The next group of patients is supposed to have too few alpha cells and to show symptoms of spontaneous hypoglycemia. Contrary to the groups mentioned before, the beta cell function in these patients is normal. McQuarrie et al. (1950) and McQuarrie (1954) found either total or next to total absence of alpha cells in some patients with spontaneous hypoglycemia, and similar findings were later reported by others (Bierich and Kornatz-Stegmann, 1954; Grollman et al., 1964). Severe spontaneous hypoglycemia in a small child was treated with Zn-glucagon, which practically eliminated the attacks, but, unfortunately, this therapy was instituted too late to avoid brain damage; a post mortem histological examination of the pacreas revealed total absence of the alpha cells (Wagner et al., 1969)

Reduced glucagon secretion to various stimuli

Spontaneous hypoglycemia
Newborn babies of diabetic mothers
Obesity
Labile diabetes

Relative rather than absolute hypoglucagonemia may be applicable to those hypoglycemic patients who show normal or decreased glucagon response to various stimuli (Nonaka et al., 1973; Rehfeld et al., 1973; Bleicher et al., 1970). In these cases, the symptoms could be eliminated by exogenous glucagon, but other pathogenetic factors may be involved (Rehfeld et al., 1973; Bataille et al., 1973). The hypoglycemia of the newborn may be due to the fact that the alpha cells respond poorly to low glucose (Sperling et al., 1973). In babies of diabetic mothers, the situation is complicated by the presence of insulin antibody complexes, which may release insulin. Higher IRI was reported in these babies by Luyckx et al. (1972) and related to a more effective suppression of the alpha cell. In accordance with this, Bloom and Johnston (1972) demonstrated that the increments in glucagon response to hypoglycemia were smaller in the newborns of diabetic mothers compared to normal babies. Hence, these children may be considered hypoglucagonemic. In the same article, Bloom and Johnston reported that small-for-dates infants responded to a fall in blood glucose with a larger than normal glucagon rise. This is consistent with the findings of Le Dune (1972) who demonstrated glycogen depletion in some children. Consequently, glucagon therapy is contraindicated in these children.

In obesity, a series of complex results have been reported. The anorexigenic effect of glucagon has been long recognized, and daily glucagon injections led to reduced calorie intake and weight loss (Schulman et al., 1957; Stunkard et al., 1955; Davidson et al.,

1957; Penick and Hinkle, 1961 and 1963). Nevertheless, glucagon hypersecretion has been reported in obese children (Paulsen and Lawrence, 1968), but, unfortunately, the assay used in this study determined the sum of pancreatic and gut GLI. Kalkhoff et al. (1972) found that glucagon response to i.v. arginine in 6 obese women was higher in the obese state than it was following weight reduction. However, their report lacked a comparison with normal persons, and the same can be pointed out in respect to the glucagon rise observed in obese persons during fasting by Marliss et al. (1970). Recently, evidence of reduced glucagon secretion in obese persons in response to i.v. alanine or an 84-hour fast has been presented by Wise et al. (1972, 1973) and to some extent by Floyd et al. (1972). The glucagon response to fasting was higher in normal persons, and the response to alanine was also enhanced in the normal subjects compared with the obese.

Wise et al. (1973) confirmed the finding of Unger's group (1972) that diabetics have higher than normal glucagon levels considering their hyperglycemia. However, the juvenile-type diabetic often suffers from hypoglycemic episodes. This could primarily be induced by hyperinsulinemia, due either to overdose or release of insulin from antibodies. It is important to note that the hypoglycemia of these patients can be treated with exogenous glucagon (Schubert, 1969). Reynolds et al. (1973) demonstrated that the glucagon response to insulin-induced hypoglycemia was markedly reduced in unstable diabetics compared with normal subjects. Each subject's ability to augment glucagon was documented by arginine infusion. Thus, in some cases of diabetes, hypoglycemia does not induce an adequate rise in glucagon, although hyperglucagonemia may be found in other situations.

Increased glucagon release to various stimuli

Hyperlipoproteinemia

The final group, with possible hypoglucagonemia, are people with hyperlipoproteinemia. It has been observed that insulin-treated pancreatectomized dogs with hyperlipemia could be normalized by administration of glucagon (Paloyan and Harper, 1961). Pancreatitis patients with hyperlipemia also exhibited a fall in total lipids after glucagon (Paloyan et al., 1962; Amatuzio et al., 1962), but this could not be demonstrated in hyperlipemic subjects with hyperprebetalipoproteinemia (Friedman et al., 1968). Glucagon determinations in patients with hyperlipoproteinemia are very few but Eaton and Schade (1973) reported raised plasma glucagon levels in some patients with hyperlipemia and enhanced release after i.v. arginine. This finding made the authors postulate the existence of resistance to glucagon, and their hypothesis was supported by the finding that exogenous glucagon suppresses hepatic lipoprotein synthesis, reduces serum triglycerides and lowers lipoprotein in rats in which hyperlipoproteinemia has been induced by $CoCl_2$.

SUMMARY

Table 5 shows a survey of the possible hypoglucagonemic states mentioned. It should be borne in mind that information about plasma glucagon is scarce in all these conditions and, furthermore, that the specificity of the various assays is still open to discussion as shown in the first part of this paper, for which reason the results should be interpreted with caution. But it appears that during the past few years evidence has been accumulating to suggest that hypoglucagonemia may play an important role in several clinical disorders.

TABLE 5
Possible hypoglucagonemic states

Clinical characterization	Evidence	Glucagon therapy
Pancreatectomy	No alpha cells	Relief of symptoms
Pancreatitis	Damaged alpha cells	Relief of symptoms
Spontaneous hypoglycemia	Reduced alpha cells and/or reduced IRG release	Relief of symptoms
Hypopituitary patients	Reduced IRG release	
'Diabetic' babies	Reduced IRG release	?
Obesity	Reduced IRG release	Weight loss
Labile diabetes	Reduced IRG release	Relief of symptoms
Hyperlipoproteinemia	Increased IRG release	Normalization

REFERENCES

AGUILAR-PARADA, E., EISENTRAUT, A. M. and UNGER, R. H. (1969): Pancreatic glucagon secretion in normal and diabetic subjects. *Amer. J. med. Scis, 257,* 415.

AMATUZIO, D. S., GRANDE, F. and WADA, S. (1962): Effect of glucagon on the serum lipids in essential hyperlipemia and in hypercholesterolemia. *Metabolism, 11,* 124.

ASSAN, R. and TIENGO, A. (1973): Comparaison des sécrétions de glucagon dans les diabetes sucrés avec ou sans pancréatopathie organique acquise. *Pathol.-Biol., 21,* 17.

BATAILLE, D. P., FREYCHET, P., KITABGI, P. E. and ROSSELIN, G. E. (1973): Gut glucagon: A common receptor site with pancreatic glucagon in liver cell plasma membranes. *FEBS Letters (Amst.), 30,* 215.

BIERICH, J. R. and KORNATZ-STEGMANN, B. (1954): Zur Entstehung der spontanhypoglykämischen Krämpfe. *Mschr. Kinderheilk., 102,* 49.

BLEICHER, S. J., LEVY, L. J., ZAROWITZ, H. and SPERGEL, G. (1970): Glucagon-deficiency hypoglycemia: A new syndrome. *Clin. Res., 18,* 355.

BLOOM, S. R. and JOHNSTON, D. I. (1972): Failure of glucagon release in infants of diabetic mothers. *Brit. med. J., 4,* 453.

BRUNNER, E., FRISCHAUF, H. and KÜHLMAYER, R. (1968): Stoffwechseluntersuchungen bei einem Fall nach totaler Pankreatektomie. *Wien. klin. Wschr., 80,* 805.

DAVIDSON, J. W., SALTER, J. M. and BEST, C. H. (1957): Calorigenic action of glucagon. *Nature (Lond.), 180,* 1124.

DAY, J. L., KNIGHT, M. and CONDON, J. R. (1972): The role of pancreatic glucagon in the pathogenesis of acute pancreatitis. *Clin. Sci., 43,* 597.

LE DUNE, M. A. (1972): Response to glucagon in small-for-dates hypoglycaemic and non-hypoglycaemic newborn infants. *Arch. Dis. Childh., 47,* 754.

EATON, R. P. and SCHADE, D. S. (1973): Glucagon resistance as a hormonal basis for endogenous hyperlipaemia. *Lancet, I/7810,* 973.

FLOYD Jr., J. C., PEK, S., FAJANS, S. S., SCHTEINGART, D. E. and CONN, J. W. (1972): Effect upon plasma glucagon of severe and prolonged restriction of food intake in obese and nonobese subjects. *Diabetes, 21/Suppl. 1,* 331.

FRIEDMAN, M., ROSENMAN, R. H. and BYERS, S. O. (1968): Response of hyperlipemic subjects to carbohydrates, pancreatic hormones and prolonged fasting. *J. clin. Endocr., 28,* 1773.

GROLLMAN, A., McCALEB, W. E. and WHITE, F. N. (1964): Glucagon deficiency as a cause of hypoglycemia. *Metabolism, 13,* 686.

GUY-GRAND, B. and ASSAN, R. (1973): Lipolytic activity of synthetic (1-23) glucagon in vitro. *Hormone metabol. Res., 5/1,* 60.

HEDING, L. G. (1971): Radioimmunological determination of pancreatic and gut glucagon in plasma. *Diabetologia, 7/1,* 10.

HEDING, L. G. (1972): Immunological properties of pancreatic glucagon: antigenicity and antibody characteristics. In: *Glucagon,* pp. 187–200. Editors: P. J. Lefebvre and R. H. Unger. Pergamon Press, Oxford and New York.

JØRGENSEN, K. H. and LARSEN, U. D. (1972): Purification of ^{125}I-glucagon by anion exchange chromatography. *Hormone metabol. Res., 4/3,* 223.

KALKHOFF, R., MATUTE, M. and GOSSAIN, V. (1972): Plasma glucagon in obesity. *Clin. Res., 20,* 802.

LAWRENCE, A. M. (1972): Pancreatic alpha-cell function in miscellaneous clinical disorders. In: *Glucagon,* pp. 259–274. Editors: P. J. Lefebvre and R. H. Unger. Pergamon Press, Oxford and New York.

LUYCKX, A. S., MASSI-BENEDETTI, F., FALONI, A. and LEFEBVRE, P. J. (1972): Presence of pancreatic glucagon in the portal plasma of human neonates. Differences in the insulin and glucagon responses to glucose between normal infants and infants from diabetic mothers. *Diabetologia, 8,* 296.

MARCO, J., FALOONA, G. R. and UNGER, R. H. (1971): The glycogenolytic activity of immunoreactive pancreatic glucagon in plasma. *J. clin. Invest., 50,* 1650.

MARKUSSEN, J., FRANDSEN, E., HEDING, L. G. and SUNDBY, F. (1972): Turkey glucagon. Crystallization, amino acid composition and immunology. *Hormone metabol. Res., 4/5,* 360.

MARLISS, E. B., AOKI, T. T., UNGER, R. H., SOELDNER, J. S. and CAHILL, G. F. (1970): Glucagon levels and metabolic effects in fasting man. *J. clin. Invest., 49,* 2256.

McQUARRIE, I., BELL, E. T., ZIMMERMANN, B. and WRIGHT, W. S. (1950): Deficiency of alpha cells of pancreas as possible etiological factor in familial hypoglycemosis. *Fed. Proc., 9,* 337.

McQUARRIE, I. (1954): Idiopathic spontaneously occurring hypoglycemia in infants. *Amer. J. Dis. Child., 87,* 399.

NONAKA, K., YOSHIDA, T., ICHIHARA, K., SHIMA, K., TARUI, S. and NISHIKAWA, M. (1973): Spontaneous hypoglycemia associated with low pancreatic glucagon response to arginine load. In: *Abstracts, VIII Congress of the International Diabetes Federation,* p. 222. Editors: J. J. Hoet and P. Lefebvre. International Congress Series No. 280, Excerpta Medica, Amsterdam.

PALOYAN, E. and HARPER, P. V. (1961): Glucagon as a regulating factor of plasma lipids. *Metabolism, 10,* 315.

PALOYAN, E., DUMBRYS, N., GALLAGHER, T. F., RODGERS, R. E. and HARPER, P. V. (1962): The effect of glucagon on hyperlipemic states. *Fed. Proc., 21,* 200.

PALOYAN, D., PALOYAN, E., WOROBEC, R., ERNST, K., DEMINGER, E. and HARPER, P. V. (1966): Serum glucagon levels in experimental acute pancreatitis in the dog. *Surg. Forum, 7,* 348.

PALOYAN, E., PALOYAN, D. and HARPER, P. V. (1967a): The role of glucagon hypersecretion in the relationship of pancreatitis and hyperparathyroidism. *Surgery, 62,* 167.

PALOYAN, E., LAWRENCE, A. M. STRAUS, F. H., PALOYAN, D., HARPER, P. V. and CUMMINGS, D. (1967b): Alpha cell hyperplasia in calcific pancreatitis associated with hyperparathyroidism. *J. Amer. med. Ass., 200,* 97.

PAULSEN, E. P. and LAWRENCE, A. M. (1968): Glucagon hypersecretion in obese children. *Lancet, II,* 110.

PENICK, S. B. and HINKLE Jr., L. E. (1961): Depression of food intake induced in healthy subjects by glucagon. *New Engl. J. Med., 264,* 893.

PENICK, S. B. and HINKLE Jr., L. E. (1963): The effect of glucagon, phenmetrazine and epinephrine on hunger, food intake and plasma nonesterified fatty acids. *Amer. J. clin. Nutr., 13,* 110.

PERSSON, I., GYNTELBERG, F., HEDING, L. G. and BOSS-NIELSEN, J. (1971): Pancreatic-glucagon-like immunoreactivity after intravenous insulin in normals and chronic pancreatitis patients. *Acta endocr., 67,* 401.

REHFELD, J. F., HEDING, L. G. and HOLST, J. J. (1973): Increased gut glucagon release as pathogenetic factor in reactive hypoglycaemia. *Lancet, I,* 116.

REYNOLDS, C., MOLNAR, G. D., JIANG, N., JONES, J. D. and TAYLOR, W. F. (1973): Abnormal glucagon response to hypoglycemia in unstable diabetics (Abstract). *Diabetes, 22/Suppl. 1,* 327.

RODBELL, M. (1972): Regulation of glucagon action at its receptors. In: *Glucagon,* pp. 61–75. Editors: P. J. Lefebvre and R. H. Unger. Pergamon Press, Oxford and New York.

SCHUBERT, P. U. (1969): Glucagon, ein neues Behandlungsprinzip zur Beseitigung hypoglykämischer Reaktionen nach ambulanter Diabetestherapie. *Med. Welt, 20,* 1878.

SCHULMAN, J. L., CARLETON, J. L., WHITNEY, G. and WHITEHORN, J. C. (1957): Effect of glucagon on food intake and body weight in man. *J. appl. Physiol., 11,* 419.

SCHULTIS, K., WILDBERGER, J. E. and WAGNER, E. (1967): Beobachtungen zur Substitution mit Depot-Glucagon nach totaler Pankreatektomie. *Klin. Wschr., 45,* 956.

SPERLING, M., FISER, R., DELAMATAR, P., ERENBERG, A., FISCHER, P. and PHELPS (1973): The significance of glucagon in perinatal glucose homeostasis (Abstract). *Diabetes, 22/Suppl. 1,* 303.

STUNKARD, A. J., ITALIE, T. B. and REIS, B. B. (1955): The mechanism of satiety: Effect of glucagon on gastric hunger contractions in man. *Proc. Soc. exp. Biol. Med. (N.Y.), 89,* 258.

UNGER, R. H., MADISON, L. L. and MÜLLER, W. A. (1972): Abnormal alpha cell function in diabetics. Response to insulin. *Diabetes, 21,* 301.

WAGNER, T., SPANGER, J. and BRUNCK, H. J. (1969): Kongenitaler alpha-Zellmangel als Ursache einer chronischen infantilen Hypoglykämie. *Mschr. Kinderheilk., 117,* 236.

WISE, J. K., HENDLER, R. and FELIG, P. (1972): Obesity: Evidence of decreased secretion of glucagon. *Science, 178,* 513.

WISE, J. K., HENDLER, R. and FELIG, P. (1973): Evaluation of alpha-cell function by infusion of alanine in normal, diabetic and obese subjects. *New Engl. J. Med., 288,* 487.

ZAROWITZ, H. (1972): Postpancreatectomy insulin-resistant diabetes mellitus. *N.Y. State J. Med., 72,* 3005.

THE ROLE OF ENERGY SUBSTRATES IN CONTROLLING GLUCAGON SECRETION. EXPERIMENTAL STUDIES

A. LUYCKX* and P. LEFEBVRE

Secteur Diabétologie, Institut de Médecine, Université de Liège, Belgique

The isolated perfused rat pancreas has been utilized by several groups for the study of insulin secretion (Grodsky and Bennett, 1966; Sussman et al., 1966; Loubatieres et al., 1967; Penhos et al., 1969; Fussganger et al., 1969; Basabe et al., 1971). Results obtained with this experimental model have generally confirmed, or have been confirmed, by those obtained in vivo or in vitro with incubated islets or pieces of pancreatic tissue (Grodsky, 1970). It should, however, be pointed out that the isolated perfused pancreas has permitted the study of the kinetics of the insulin response to glucose and other stimuli (Grodsky et al., 1968), providing conclusive evidence in favor of the existence of several pools of insulin within the β cell.

The regulation of pancreatic glucagon secretion has been studied in vivo in man and in experimental animals (review in Lefebvre and Unger, 1972). The results of these investigations have led to the concept that glucagon is a hormone of glucose need (Unger and Eisentraut, 1970), since glucagon secretion is stimulated markedly by a fall in blood glucose ('cataglycemia'). This concept has been extended to glucagon which is considered as a hormone of 'fuel need' (Lefebvre and Luyckx, 1971) in view of the stimulation of a_2 cell secretion by a decrease in plasma free fatty acid levels (Luyckx and Lefebvre, 1970) and the decrease in glucagon secretion in response to a rise in plasma FFA (Seyffert and Madison, 1967; Luyckx and Lefebvre, 1970). Studies on isolated islets of Langerhans incubated in vitro have shown that glucagon release is reduced in the presence of very high glucose concentrations and increased at hypoglycemic levels (Vance et al., 1968; Chesney and Schofield, 1969; Nonaka and Foa, 1969). A comparison of the amounts of glucagon released by isolated rat or guinea pig islets incubated with glucose concentrations varying from 150 to 30 mg% failed, however, to demonstrate significant differences (Vance et al., 1968; Buchanan et al., 1969; Edwards and Taylor, 1970; Leclercq-Meyer and Brisson, 1970). On the contrary, in vivo studies in the dog by Ohneda et al. (1969) have demonstrated that insulin-induced hypoglycemia (100 $\rightarrow$ 50 mg%) is uniformly associated with a rise in pancreaticoduodenal vein glucagon concentrations. In man, a significant rise in peripheral venous glucagon has also been observed with a plasma glucose decrease of about 40 mg% (Heding et al., 1970; Persson et al., 1971; Luyckx, 1973).

The lack of response of incubated islets to variations in glucose concentrations (known to affect glucagon release in vivo) is an important reason why this experimental preparation should not be used in physiologic studies. In contrast, the isolated perfused rat

* Chargé de Recherches du Fonds National de la Recherche Scientifique (Belgique).

pancreas (IPRP) offers the following theoretical advantages: (1) The supply of energetic substrates *via* the *usual capillary route* is certainly preferable in order to minimize diffusion problems. (2) The IPRP makes it possible to study the selective modification of a single substrate concentration in the perfusion medium *without simultaneously affecting* the concentrations of other substrates, capable of influencing a_2 cell secretion. (3) The IPRP used without recirculation enables one to isolate the *direct* effect of changes in the concentration of one substrate on the a_2 and β cell secretion rate, avoiding indirect effects mediated through changes in hormone concentrations reaching the islets after passing through the systemic circulation. This preparation is also suitable for demonstrating the presence or absence of a 'cell to cell' mechanism linking the a_2 and β cells. (4) The IPRP has the advantage that one can study the *kinetics* of the glucagon response to various stimuli. (5) *Antiserum cross-reacting* with gut GLI may be utilized for determinations in the perfusion medium since the duodenum, which is left attached in most preparations, has a very low level of gut glucagon-like immunoreactivity (Unger et al., 1966). (6) The IPRP permits precise measurement of the glucagon secretion rate since the *flow rate* is recorded continuously throughout the experiment.

These advantages led us to develop the isolated perfused rat pancreas technique as an experimental model for the study of glucagon and insulin secretion rate in response to variations in glucose, free fatty acid and amino acid concentrations in the perfusate.

MATERIAL AND METHODS

Male Wistar rats weighing 235–520 g (mean: 356 g) and fasted for 5 hours were utilized throughout the study. The in vitro pancreas preparation consisted of the rat pancreas with the duodenum attached, as previously described by Sussman et al. (1966) with minor modifications (Luyckx and Lefebvre, 1972b). The duodenum-pancreas preparation was transferred to the perfusion chamber of an AMBEC perfusion apparatus and immersed in a bath of normal saline maintained at a constant temperature of 37.5°. The flow rate was kept constant for each perfusion at values ranging from 2.0–3.2 ml/min. The corresponding arterial pressures were 25–85 (mean 55) mm Hg. Unless otherwise stated, the perfusate was a Krebs-Ringer bicarbonate buffer containing (in mEq/l) Na 146, K 5, Cl 117, Ca 2, Mg 1 and 4% bovine crystallized albumin. The basic medium contained about 750 μEq/l of FFA bound to the albumin and had a glucose concentration of 100 mg%. Various concentrations of palmitate, octanoate or alanine were added to the perfusate in the different experiments. In the alanine experiments, the glucose concentration in the medium was 75 or 150 mg% (see below). After removal, the pancreas was perfused for a 45-minute equilibration period with the selected medium. The measurements performed during the last 5 minutes of this equilibration period were used as basal values for the experiment itself, which followed immediately and lasted 40–60 minutes. Acute changes in the concentration of glucose or alanine were obtained by turning on or off a slow infusion (0.2 ml/min.) branched (very near the organ) on to the main perfusion circuit. The perfusate was collected from the portal vein catheter into chilled graduated cylinders during 2–5 minute periods. Sufficient Trasylol to reach a final concentration of 500 U/ml was added to an aliquot of each fraction, which was immediately deep frozen until the time for insulin and glucagon determinations. Insulin was assayed by a modification of the double antibody immunoassay of Hales and Randle (1963) using rat insulin as standard. Glucagon was assayed by our radioimmunoassay

(Luyckx, 1972), the standard curve being performed in an aliquot of the perfusion medium in order to avoid any difference in immunologic behavior between unknown samples and hormone standards. Glucose was measured by the glucose-oxidase method of Huggett and Nixon (1957) and free fatty acids by the micromethod of Dole and Meinertz (1960) using a palmitate reference curve for all experiments except when octanoate was added to the medium. In these cases, a reference curve was established with octanoate.

RESULTS

A. Basal insulin and glucagon production

Basel insulin and glucagon secretion rates were measured at the end of a 40-minute equilibration period. Insulin secretion rate is very low (18 ± 7 μU/g/min., n = 11) when the perfusate contains 100 mg% glucose and free fatty acid (200–1080, mean 550 μEq/1) concentrations similar to those of plasma under basal conditions. The addition of 2.4 mM octanoate or 2.2 mM palmitate does not significantly stimulate the insulin secretion rate in the limited number of experiments hitherto performed. Mean glucagon production under 'basal conditions' is 858 ± 242 pg/g/minute. A moderate and non-significant decrease in basal glucagon release occurs in the presence of high concentrations of palmitate and octanoate.

B. Control perfusions

In control perfusions in which glucose and free fatty acid concentrations in the perfusate are kept constant and close to their concentrations in plasma under basal conditions, the insulin secretion rate remains low and shows no systematic variations. In contrast, glucagon production declines gradually, ceasing almost completely by the end of the 60 minute period (Fig. 1).

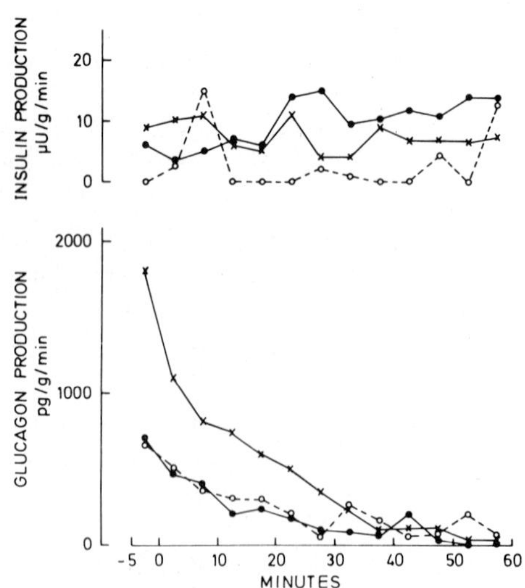

FIG. 1. Insulin and glucagon secretion rates in 3 perfusions during which glucose (100 mg%) and free fatty acids (750 μEq/l) concentrations in the perfusate are kept constant.

C. Acute hypoglycemia

As shown in Figure 2, acute hypoglycemia is accompanied by a multiphasic increase in glucagon production. A first peak occurs almost immediately and lasts 10–12 minutes after the onset of hypoglycemia; this corresponds to a 2–6 fold increase in the glucagon secretion rate. A second peak is often observed around the 20th minute. From the 25th to the 60th minute after the induction of hypoglycemia, glucagon production remains

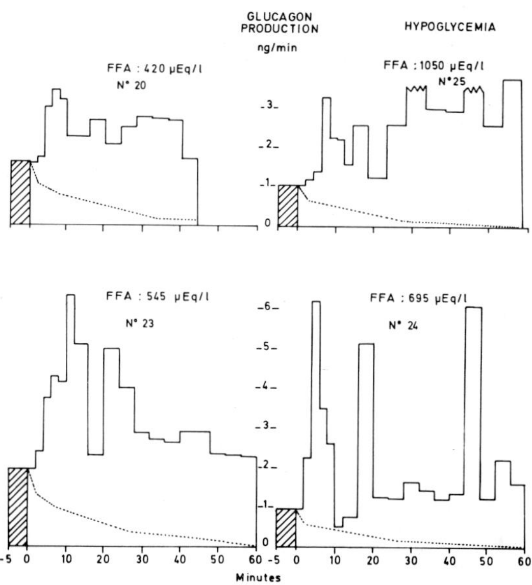

FIG. 2. Multiphasic increase in glucagon secretion rate after acute hypoglycemia in 4 perfusions. The dotted line corresponds to the glucagon production in the presence of normal and constant glucose concentration (see Fig. 1). The hatched column represents the glucagon secretion rate immediately before the induction of hypoglycemia.

elevated and far higher than in control perfusions. The general pattern of glucagon production remains much the same after hypoglycemia is induced, but important quantitative differences may be seen from one experiment to the next (Fig. 2). The induction of hypoglycemia is followed by a clear-cut reduction in insulin production which falls to zero within 10 minutes (Fig. 3).

D. Modification of the glucagonogenic effect of acute hypoglycemia by circulating free fatty acids

A cataglycemia from 100 mg to 25 mg% was used as an a_2 cell stimulatory test in the presence of several perfusate concentrations of octanoate and palmitate. Figure 4 shows that the glucagonogenic effect of cataglycemia is markedly reduced by *octanoate.* When the perfusate is supplemented with *palmitate* at concentrations corresponding to a molar

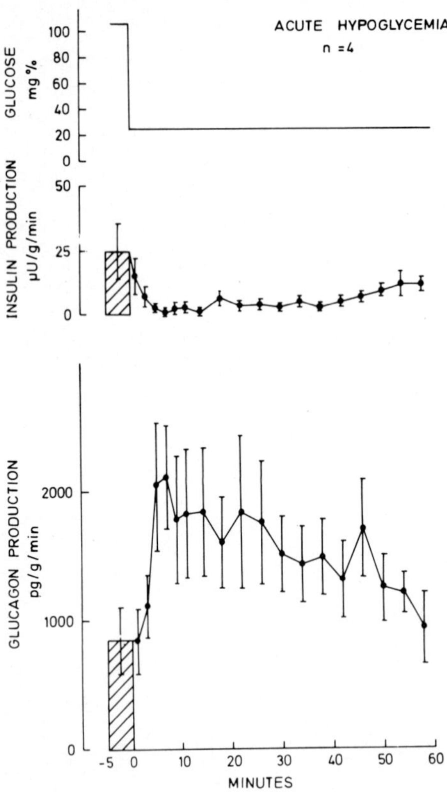

FIG. 3. Effect of acute hypoglycemia (100 → 25 mg%) on insulin and glucagon secretion rate in 4 perfusions. Results are expressed as mean ± S.E.M.

FFA/albumin ratio of about 4, acute hypoglycemia is still able to stimulate glucagon secretion slightly (Fig. 5). The a_2 cell response is, however, clearly decreased (Table 1).

E. Influence of the glucose concentration on the alanine-induced insulin and glucagon release

As shown in Figure 6, the isolated perfused rat pancreas responds to a 10 mM alanine stimulus by a clear-cut diphasic increase in glucagon and insulin release. The glucagonogenic effect of alanine is markedly reduced in the presence of a glucose concentration of 150 mg%, when compared with the one observed at 75 mg% glucose. Opposite results are obtained as far as the insulin response to alanine is concerned (Fig. 6 and Table 2). In addition, as shown in Table 2, during the 15-minute period preceding the initiation of the alanine infusion, basal glucagon release is significantly lower and basal insulin release significantly higher in the experiments perfomed with the highest concentration of glucose (150 mg%).

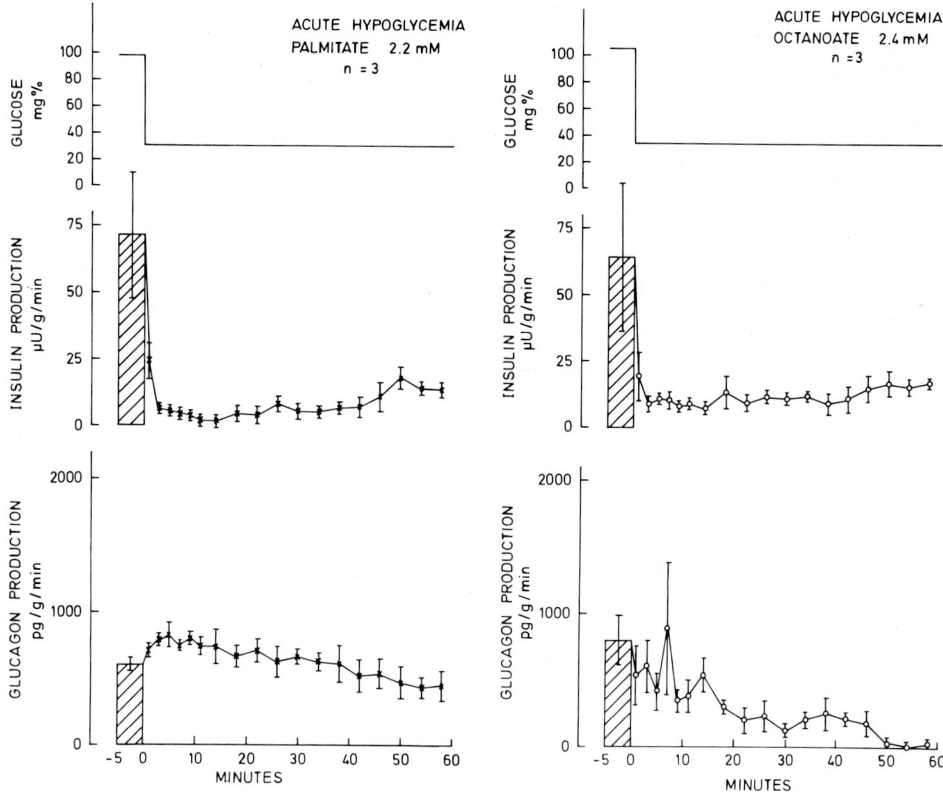

FIG. 4. Inhibition by octanoate of the stimulatory effect of acute hypoglycemia on glucagon secretion rate in 3 experiments. Results are expressed as mean ± S.E.M.

FIG. 5. Marked reduction by palmitate of the stimulatory effect of acute hypoglycemia on glucagon secretion rate in 3 experiments. Results are expressed as mean ± S.E.M.

DISCUSSION

Unger and Eisentraut (1970) have demonstrated a negative relationship between blood glucose concentration and pancreatic glucagon secretion in studies conducted in conscious dogs. These findings led Unger's group to suggest that glucose utilization within the a_2 cell is the signal for 'turning off' glucagon secretion. Furthermore, it has been demonstrated by Muller et al. (1971a, b) that glucose is unable to suppress a_2 cell secretion in the absence of insulin. The amount of glucose available to the a_2 cell is thus a critical factor in Unger's hypothesis. In contrast, glucagon release from the incubated islets of various species has been found to be poorly responsive to changes in glucose concentrations in the range of 30–150 mg%, whereas free fatty acids and ketone bodies have been shown by Edwards et al. (1969) and Edwards and Taylor (1970) to be potent

TABLE 1

Glucagon production (ng/g) during the successive periods of the perfusion of the isolated rat pancreas

		$\Sigma^{P}_{0 \to 12\ min.}$		$\Sigma^{P}_{12 \to 28\ min.}$		$\Sigma^{P}_{28 \to 60\ min.}$		$\Sigma^{P}_{0 \to 60\ min.}$	
	Control perfusions Glucose: 100 mg% FFA: 748 ± 166 μEq/l	4.8 5.0 11.1	7.0 ± 2.1	2.9 3.6 8.8	5.1 ± 1.9	2.1 4.2 3.6	3.3 ± 0.6	9.9 12.8 23.5	15.4 ± 4.2
									P < 0.02
Hypoglycemia 100 → 25 mg%	FFA 678 ± 136 μEq/l	22.0 32.7 13.7 18.8	21.8 ± 4.0	27.5 50.3 14.8 38.2	32.7 ± 7.6	47.3 58.9 28.6 76.0	52.7 ± 9.9	96.8 141.8 57.0 133.0	107.2 ± 19.3
									P < 0.05
Hypoglycemia 100 → 25 mg%	Palmitate 2190–2450 μEq/l	9.0 9.9 8.6	9.2 ± 0.4	13.0 11.7 7.9	10.9 ± 1.5	20.9 11.2 19.4	17.2 ± 3.0	43.0 32.8 35.8	37.2 ± 3.0
Hypoglycemia 100 → 25 mg%	FFA 400 μEq/l + Octanoate 2400 μEq/l	3.6 7.0 8.5	6.4 ± 1.4	6.5 6.3 2.4	5.1 ± 1.3	4.3 4.0 4.6	4.3 ± 0.2	14.4 17.4 15.4	15.7 ± 0.9

P < 0.02 (107.2 ± 19.3 vs. 15.7 ± 0.9)

$\Sigma^{P}_{0 \to 12\ min.}$: sum of glucagon productions (ng/g of pancreas) between 0 and 12 min.

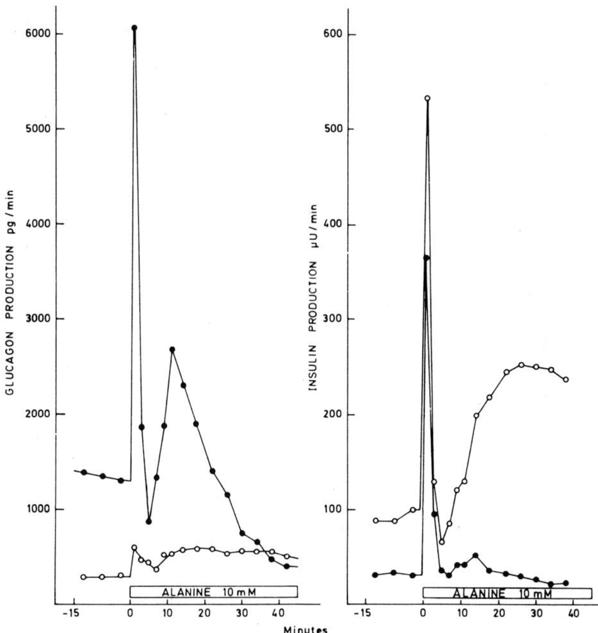

FIG. 6. Stimulation of glucagon (left panel) and insulin (right panel) release by 10 mM alanine. Mean of 4 experiments in the presence of 150 mg% glucose (○——○) and of 4 experiments in the presence of 75 mg% glucose (●——●). For statistical comparison, see Table 2.

inhibitors of glucagon release. In view of these observations, these authors have suggested that free fatty acids are more important than glucose in the control of glucagon secretion. Although we have provided evidence in favor of the role of free fatty acids in the regulation of glucagon secretion, we were intrigued by the lack of effect of glucose in vitro. We therefore wished to re-examine the respective roles of glucose and free fatty acids with another preparation, namely the IPRP. The observations reported herein demonstrate that the IPRP responds to acute hypoglycemia with an immediate, significant and multiphasic increase in the glucagon secretion rate. This pattern might correspond to the existence of several pools of glucagon within the α_2 cell. The simultaneous fall in insulin production permits us to conclude that endogenous glucagon does not stimulate β cell secretion under these conditions. The stimulatory effect of hypoglycemia on glucagon secretion is greatly reduced, or even completely abolished, in the presence of high free fatty acid concentrations in the perfusate. This suggests that, although hypoglycemia is a potent stimulus to glucagon secretion, the circulating level of free fatty acids modulates the response of the α_2 cells to hypoglycemia. This in turn supports the concept that glucagon mobilization depends upon the concentrations of energetic substrates available to the α_2 cell and might explain the observation that a spontaneous cessation of glucagon production is observed when the perfusate contains 100 mg% glucose throughout the experiment. Amino acids stimulate glucagon secretion in man (Assan et

TABLE 2

Glucagon and insulin production (per min. and per pancreas) in response to alanine at 2 glucose concentrations (75 and 150 mg/100 ml) in the perfusate

	Glucose mg%	Control Period Min. −15–0	Alanine 10 mM 0–2	2–10	10–16	16–24	24–32	32–40
Glucagon pg/min.	75	1316 ± 148 (12)	6057 ± 1486 (4)	1482 ± 267 (16)	2492 ± 483 (8)	1650 ± 331 (8)	952 ± 16 (8)	561 ± 68 (8)
	150	289 ± 12 (12)	600 ± 68 (4)	445 ± 21 (16)	537 ± 34 (8)	583 ± 34 (8)	546 ± 61 (8)	564 ± 79 (8)
	P	< 0.001	< 0.02	< 0.001	< 0.01	< 0.02	< 0.05	N.S.
Insulin μU/min.	75	32 ± 7 (12)	367 ± 70 (4)	52 ± 10 (16)	45 ± 6 (8)	35 ± 4 (8)	29 ± 3 (8)	24 ± 4 (8)
	150	91 ± 15 (12)	535 ± 242 (4)	101 ± 12 (16)	165 ± 55 (8)	233 ± 82 (8)	252 ± 94 (8)	244 ± 95 (8)
	P	< 0.01	N.S.	< 0.01	N.S.	< 0.05	< 0.05	< 0.05

al., 1967; Pek et al., 1969; Unger et al., 1970), in dogs (Ohneda et al., 1968; Rocha et al., 1972), as well as in rats (Assan et al., 1971). Most often, experiments were carried out using an amino acid mixture or an infusion of arginine. Since alanine appears as the main endogenous precursor for hepatic gluconeogenesis (Mallette et al., 1969; Felig et al., 1970) and since alanine has been implicated as a mediator for exercise-induced glucagon release (Felig et al., 1972), we have been interested in studying, in our preparation, the effect of this amino acid on glucagon release at normal or slightly elevated glucose concentrations. As previously demonstrated (Luyckx and Lefebvre, 1972b), alanine induces a biphasic glucagon release, a result which has been confirmed by Assan et al. (1972) for arginine using the same method. The present study clearly demonstrates that the glucagon response to alanine is modulated by the level of circulating glucose, a modest increase in glucose concentration inhibiting both phases of the response. The results, which are in agreement with those reported in dogs by Muller et al. (1972a, b), do not support the concept, proposed by Samols et al. (1972) that endogenous glucagon might be involved in the insulinogenic effect of amino acids.

CONCLUSION

Glucagon secretion, as studied in the isolated perfused rat pancreas, appears to be exquisitely regulated by the levels of circulating metabolic substrates. The effects induced by changes in the concentrations of one of these substrates are modulated by the levels of the others. This has been demonstrated here for the glucagonogenic effect of hypoglycemia which is affected by the level of circulating free fatty acids as well as for the glucagonogenic effect of alanine which is dependent upon the level of circulating glucose. This integrated regulation, of probable physiological relevance, does not exclude other mechanisms such as a nervous control of glucagon secretion as evidenced in dogs by Iversen (1971) and Marliss et al. (1973) or in exercised rats by Luyckx and Lefebvre (1972a).

REFERENCES

ASSAN, R., ROSSELIN, G. and DOLAIS, J. (1967): Effets sur la glucagonémie des perfusions et ingestions d'acides aminés. In: *Journées Annuelles de Diabétologie de* l'Hôtel-Dieu, *pp. 24–41.* Editor: M. Rathéry. *Flammarion, Paris.*

ASSAN, R., HANOUNE, J. and ATTALI, J. R. (1971): Effects on rat plasma glucagon of 6 sugars, 8 amino acids, lactate load and induced hyperlactacidemia. *Abstract, European Association for the Study of Diabetes. 7th Annual Meeting, Southampton, Sept. 15–17.* Novo Service, Copenhagen.

ASSAN, R., BOILLOT, J., ATTALI, J. R., SOUFFLET, E. and BALLERIO, G. (1972): Diphasic glucagon release induced by arginine in the perfused rat pancreas. *Nature (Lond.), 239,* 125.

BASABE, J. C., LOPEZ, N. L., VIKTORA, J. K. and WOLFF, F. W. (1971): Insulin secretion studied in the perfused rat pancreas. I. Effect of tolbutamide, leucine and arginine: their interaction with diazoxide and relation to glucose. *Diabetes, 20,* 449.

BOTTGER, I., FALOONA, G. R. and UNGER, R. H. (1971): The effect of intensive physical exercise on pancreatic glucagon secretion. *Abstract, 31st Annual Meeting of the American Diabetes Association. San Francisco, June. Diabetes, 20,* 339.

BUCHANAN, K., VANCE, J. E., DINSTL, K. and WILLIAMS, R. H. (1969): Effect of blood glucose on glucagon secretion in anesthetized dogs. *Diabetes, 18,* 11.

CHESNEY, T. McC. and SCHOFIELD, J. G. (1969): Studies on the secretion of pancreatic glucagon. *Diabetes, 18,* 627.

DOLE, V. P. and MEINERTZ, H. (1960): Microdetermination of long-chain fatty acids in plasma and tissues. *J. biol. Chem., 235,* 2395.

EDWARDS, J. C., HOWELL, S. L. and TAYLOR, K. W. (1969): Fatty acids as regulators of glucagon secretion. *Nature (Lond.), 224,* 808.

EDWARDS, J. C. and TAYLOR, K. W. (1970): Fatty acids and the release of glucagon from isolated guinea-pig islets of Langerhans incubated in vitro. *Biochim. biophys. Acta (Amst.), 215,* 310.

FELIG, P., POZEFSKY, T., MARLISS, E. and CAHILL Jr., G. F. (1970): Alanine: Key role in gluconeogenesis. *Science, 167,* 1003.

FELIG, P., WAHREN, J., HENDLER, R. and AHLBORG, G. (1972): Plasma glucagon levels in exercising man. *New Engl. J. Med., 287,* 184.

FUSSGANGER, R. D., HINZ, M., GOBERNA, R., JAROS, P., KARSTEN, C., PFEIFFER, E. F. and RAPTIS, S. (1969): Comparative studies on the dynamics of insulin secretion following HB419 and tolbutamide on the perfused isolated rat pancreas and the perifused islets of Langerhans. *Hormone Metabol. Res., Suppl. I,* 34.

GRODSKY, G. M. and BENNETT, L. L. (1966): Cation requirements for insulin secretion in the isolated perfused pancreas. *Diabetes, 15,* 910.

GRODSKY, G.M., CURRY, D. L., BENNETT, L. L. and RODRIGO, J. J. (1968): Factors influencing different rates of insulin release in vitro. *Acta diab. lat., 5/Suppl. 1,* 140.

GRODSKY, G. M. (1970): Insulin and the pancreas. In: *Vitamins and hormones, vol. 28,* pp. 37–101. Editors: R. S. Harris, I. G. Wool and J. A. Loraine. Academic Press, New York.

HALES, C. N. and RANDLE, P. J. (1963): Immunoassay of insulin with insulin-antibody precipitate. *Biochem. J., 88,* 137.

HEDING, E., GYNTELBERG, F., BOSS-NIELSEN, J. and PERSSON, I. (1970): Serum glucagon and chronic pancreatitis (abstract). *Diabetologia, 6,* 630.

HUGGETT, A. and NIXON, D. A. (1957): Enzymatic determinations of blood glucose. *Biochem. J., 66,* 12.

IVERSEN, J. (1971): Adrenergic receptors for the secretion of immunoreactive glucagon and insulin from the isolated perfused canine pancreas (abstract). *Diabetologia, 7,* 485.

LECLERCQ-MEYER, V. and BRISSON, G. R. (1970): In vitro release of glucagon (IRG) and insulin (IRI) from pancreatic tissue of duct-ligated rats (abstract). *Diabetologia, 6,* 636.

LEFEBVRE, P. J. and LUYCKX, A. S. (1971): The role of glucagon in clinical medicine. In: *The Action of Hormones, Genes to Population,* pp. 315–351. Editor P. P. Foà. Charles C. Thomas, Springfield.

LEFEBVRE, P. J. and UNGER, R. H. (1972): *Glucagon. Molecular Physiology. Clinical and Therapeutic Implications.* Pergamon Press, Oxford.

LOUBATIERES, A., MARIANI, M. M., ALRIC, R. and CHAPAL, J. (1967): Antagonistic mechanism of actions of tolbutamide and diazoxide on insulin secretion. In: *Tolbutamide after ten years.* Brook Lodge Symposium, Augusta, Michigan, March 6–7, pp. 100–114. International Congress Series No. 149, Excerpta Medica, Amsterdam.

LUYCKX, A. S. and LEFEBVRE, P. J. (1970): Arguments for a regulation of pancreatic glucagon secretion by circulating plasma free fatty acids. *Proc. Soc. exp. Biol. Med. (N.Y.), 133,* 524.

LUYCKX, A. S. (1972): Immunoassays for glucagon. In: *Glucagon. Molecular Physiology. Clinical and Therapeutic Implications,* pp. 285–298. Editors: P. Lefebvre and R. H. Unger. Pergamon Press, Oxford.

LUYCKX, A. S. and LEFEBVRE, P. J. (1972a): Role of catecholamines in exercise-induced glucagon secretion (abstract). *Diabetes, 21,* 334.

LUYCKX, A. S. and LEFEBVRE, P. J. (1972b): Changes in insulin and glucagon secretion related to concentrations of metabolic substractes in the isolated perfused pancreas. In: *Hormones pancréatiques, Hormones de l'eau et des électrolytes,* pp. 99–127. INSERM, Paris.

LUYCKX, A. S. (1973): Le contrôle de la sécrétion du glucagon. In: *Hormones et Régulations Métaboliques,* pp. 169–182. Masson, Paris.

MALLETTE, L. E., EXTON, J. H. and PARK, C. A. (1969): Effects of glucagon on amino acid transport and utilization in the perfused rat liver. *J. biol. Chem., 244,* 5724.

MARLISS, E. B., GIRARDIER, L., SEYDOUX, J., WOLLHEIM, C. B., KANAZAWA, Y., ORCI, L., RENOLD, A. E. and PORTE Jr., D. (1973): Glucagon release induced by pancreatic nerve stimulation in the dog. *J. clin. Invest., 52,* 1246.

MULLER, W. A., FALOONA, G. R. and UNGER, R. H. (1971a): The effect of alanine on glucagon secretion. *J. clin. Invest., 50,* 2215.

MULLER, W. A., FALOONA, G. R. and UNGER, R. H. (1971b): The effect of experimental insulin deficiency on glucagon secretion. *J. clin. Invest., 50,* 1992.

NONAKA, K. and FOA, P. P. (1969): A simplified glucagon immunoassay and its use in a study of incubated pancreatic islets. *Proc. Soc. exp. Biol. Med. (N.Y.), 130,* 330.

OHNEDA, A., AGUILAR-PARADA, E., EISENTRAUT, A. M. and UNGER, R. H. (1968): Characterization of response of circulating glucagon to intraduodenal and intravenous administration of amino acid. *J. clin. Invest., 47,* 2305.

OHNEDA, A., AGUILAR-PARADA, E., EISENTRAUT, A. M. and UNGER, R. H. (1969): Control of pancreatic glucagon secretion by glucose. *Diabetes, 18,* 1.

PEK, S., FAJANS, S. S., FLOYD Jr., J. C., KNOPF, R. F. and CONN, J. W. (1969): Effects upon plasma glucagon of infused and ingested amino acids and of protein meals in man (abstract). *Diabetes, 18,* 328.

PENHOS, J., WU, C. H., BASABE, J., LOPEZ, N. and WOLFF, F. (1969): A rat pancreas-small gut preparation for the study of intestinal factor(s) and insulin release. *Diabetes, 18,* 733.

PERSSON, I., GYNTELBERG, E., HEDING, L. H. and BOSS NIELSEN, J. (1971): Pancreatic-glucagon-like immunoreactivity after intravenous insulin in normals and chronic pancreatitis patients. *Acta endocr. (Kbh.), 67,* 401.

ROCHA, D. M., FALOONA, G. R. and UNGER, R. H. (1972): Glucagon stimulating activity of 20 amino acids in dogs. *J. clin. Invest., 51,* 2346.

SAMOLS, E., TYLER, J. M. and MARKS, V. (1972): Glucagon-insulin interrelationships. In: *Glucagon. Molecular Physiology. Clinical and Therapeutic Implications,* pp. 151–173. Editors: P. Lefebvre and R. H. Unger. Pergamon Press, Oxford.

SEYFFERT, W. A. and MADISON, L. L. (1967): Physiologic effects of metabolic fuels on carbohydrate metabolism. I. Acute effect of elevation of plasma free fatty acids on hepatic glucose output, peripheral glucose utilization, serum insulin and plasma glucagon levels. *Diabetes, 16,* 765.

SUSSMAN, K. E., VAUGHAN, G. D. and TIMMER, R. F. (1966): An in vitro method for studying insulin secretion in the perfused isolated rat pancreas. *Metabolism, 15,* 466.

UNGER, R. H., KETTERER, H. and EISENTRAUT, A. M. (1966): Distribution of immunoassayable glucagon in gastro-intestinal tissues. *Metabolism, 15,* 865.

UNGER, R. H., OHNEDA, A., AGUILAR-PARADA, E. and EISENTRAUT, A. M. (1969): The role of aminogenic glucagon secretion in blood glucose homeostasis. *J. clin. Invest., 48,* 810.

UNGER, R. H., AGUILAR-PARADA, E., MULLER, W. A. and EISENTRAUT, A. M. (1970): Studies of pancreatic alpha-cell function in normal and diabetic subjects. *J. clin. Invest., 49,* 837.

UNGER, R. H. and EISENTRAUT, A. M. (1970): Regulation of glucagon release in vivo. In: *The structure and metabolism of the pancreatic islets. A centennial of Paul Langerhans' discovery,* Vol 16, Umea, February 1969. Editors: S. Falkmer, B. Hellman and I. B. Täljedal. Wenner Gren International Symposium Series. Pergamon Press, Oxford.
VANCE, J. E., BUCHANAN, K. D., CHALLONER, D. R. and WILLIAMS, R. H. (1968): Effect of glucose concentration on insulin and glucagon release from isolated islets of Langerhans of the rat. *Diabetes, 17,* 187.

EFFECT OF ENTERIC FACTORS ON PANCREATIC ALPHA CELL FUNCTION*

SUMER PEK

Department of Medicine, Division of Endocrinology and Metabolism, University of Alabama in Birmingham, and Metabolism Research Laboratory, U.S. Veterans Administration Hospital, Birmingham, Ala.; and Department of Internal Medicine, Division of Endocrinology and Metabolism and the Metabolism Research Unit, The University of Michigan, Ann Arbor, Mich., U.S.A.

Demonstration of greater increases in plasma insulin in response to ingested glucose than to intravenously administered glucose (McIntyre et al., 1964; Perley and Kipnis, 1967) has revived the interest in possible effects of enteric factors upon the function of the pancreatic islets. During the recent years, considerable evidence has been accumulated which indicates that certain gastrointestinal hormones may influence the release of insulin as well as glucagon. Among various humoral factors which are released from the gut during absorption of nutrients, gastrin, pancreozymin and secretin have been studied in relation to pancreatic islet function. The interrelationships of these factors and glucagon will be the subject of this discussion.

Gastrin is released from the antrum of the pylorus in response to contact with all types of nutrients. Unger et al. (1967) administered endoportally to dogs a crude acetone extract of hog antrum. A minor and transitory rise in pancreatic venous levels of glucagon was observed which may have been the consequence of the glucagon contaminant in the crude extract. In healthy subjects, intravenous administration of synthetic human gastrin II failed to alter plasma levels of glucagon-like immunoreactivity (Dupre et al., 1969). Thus, an effect of gastrin on glucagon release could not be demonstrated.

Pancreozymin, which is identical to cholecystokinin, is secreted from the mucosa of the proximal small intestine. In man, sustained release of pancreozymin in response to intraduodenal administration of amino acids and of fatty acids has been demonstrated (Go et al., 1970). Essential amino acids are by far the most potent stimuli for pancreozymin release; individual amino acids differ in their ability to evoke this response (Go et al., 1970). The effect of glucose is minor and short-lived. Unger et al. (1967) have shown that endoportal injection of a highly purified preparation of pancreozymin induces a rapid and siginificant increase in pancreatic venous levels of glucagon in dogs. Similar observations in dogs were made by Buchanan et al. (1968). Ohneda et al. (1968) have shown that pancreozymin augments amino acid-induced glucagon release in dogs. Raptis et al. (1972) reported that intravenous injection of pancreozymin caused significant increases in plasma glucagon in healthy subjects as well as in patients with diabetes. Using an in vitro perfusion technique, Fussgänger et al. (1969) showed that pulse-injection of pancreo-

* Supported in part by an institutional research grant, The U.S. Veterans Administration Hospital in Birmingham, and by U.S. Public Health Service Grants AM-02244, National Institutes of Arthritis and Metabolic Diseases; and RR-32, General Clinical Research Program.

zymin into the pancreatic artery of the isolated rat pancreas stimulated the release of glucagon. Absence of glucose in the perfusion medium augmented this response. These in vitro experiments also presented evidence that pancreozymin can influence the islet function in a gland devoid of its nervous supply. In all these experiments, pancreozymin had been administered in pharmacological amounts. A recent report indicates that a preparation of cholecystokinin-pancreozymin of a much greater purity than that used by previous investigators failed to stimulate glucagon or insulin release in vivo or in vitro (Rabinovitch and Dupre, 1972). This observation raises the question as to whether enteric effects upon islet function attributed to pancreozymin may have been induced by other yet to be identified gastrointestinal hormones. Sufficient evidence is lacking for the stimulation of glucagon secretion by pancreozymin released endogenously during the absorptive process. In experiments of Ohneda et al. (1968) in dogs, the magnitude of glucagon release in response to intraduodenally or intravenously administered mixture of essential amino acids was similar. Our own observations in man indicate that the magnitude of the increases in plasma glucagon-like immunoreactivity is smaller when equimolar amounts of the amino acid mixture or of arginine are administered orally than when they are infused intravenously (Pek et al., 1969). On the other hand, Böttger et al. (1972) have reported recently that in dogs and in healthy subjects plasma glucagon rose following intraduodenal administration of peanut oil and not with intravenous infusion of triglycerides. This observation was interpreted as evidence for the activation during fat absorption of an enteric signal which is likely to be the release of pancreozymin.

Secretin originates from the upper small intestine. The major stimulus for its secretion is the influx of acid to the duodenum. Ingestion of glucose and, to a lesser degree, of amino acids also evokes secretin release. Earlier studies of Unger et al. (1967) had not suggested that secretin has an effect on the alpha cell function. A more recent report from the same laboratory indicates that endoportal infusion of purified secretin evokes decreases in pancreatic venous levels of glucagon in healthy and in alloxan-diabetic dogs (Santeusanio et al., 1972). Administered secretin augments the inhibition of glucagon release induced by intravenous glucose (Santeusanio et al., 1972). On the other hand, Raptis et al. (1972) observed no changes in peripheral plasma glucagon in response to administration of secretin in healthy subjects or in diabetic patients. The experiments of Santeusanio et al. in dogs demonstrated further that intraduodenal instillation of hydrochloric acid evoked a suppression of glucagon secretion which was thought to be mediated through the release of endogenous secretin. The physiological implications of these observations are not readily apparent. As shown in Figure 1, we have administered 30 grams of glucose intravenously over 60 minutes to 11 healthy subjects. Standard oral glucose tolerance tests (1.75 g/kg ideal body weight) were performed in another group of 11 healthy subjects. With intravenous glucose, the mean of maximal increments (± SEM) in plasma glucose was 114 ± 7 mg/100 ml, which was significantly greater than that which occurred during oral glucose tolerance tests, 62 ± 7 mg/100 ml ($P < 0.001$). Mean plasma glucagon decreased promptly and significantly in both series of experiments. The means of maximal decrements in plasma glucagon were similar (50 ± 8 pg/ml with intravenous and 44 ± 7 pg/ml with oral glucose, N.S.). With ingested glucose the suppression of glucagon release appeared to be more persistent than that which occurred with intravenous glucose. With oral glucose, mean plasma glucagon remained significantly below the basal level throughout the 3-hour test period, while with intravenous glucose mean glucagon had returned toward basal levels by the second hour. These observations suggest that the release of glucagon may be inhibited more effectively when hyperglycemia is induced

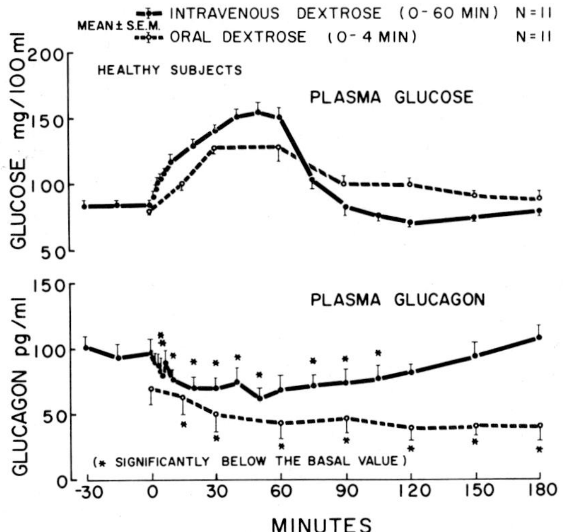

FIG. 1. Effect upon plasma glucose and glucagon of glucose administered orally (1.75 g/kg ideal body weight) or intravenously (30 g, 0–60 min.) in 11 healthy subjects.

by ingestion rather than by intravenous infusion of glucose. Similar observations were made also by Santeusanio et al. The release of secretin which occurs during absorption of glucose may possibly account for this phenomenon (Chisholm et al., 1969).

In summary, among the humoral factors released from the gastrointestinal tract during absorption of nutrients, pancreozymin appears to stimulate and secretin to inhibit the release of glucagon. The available information offers certain clues that this relationship between the enteric factors and the pancreatic alpha cells may be of physiological significance. Thus, the concept that the gastrointestinal hormones could serve as modifiers of islet cell response to nutrients becomes even more attractive. Pancreozymin would provide for an additional and early stimulus for glucagon and insulin release during absorption of amino acids, preparing the grounds for efficient utilization of the amino acids and moderating their blood levels. Similarly, secretin-induced inhibition of glucagon and stimulation of insulin release could improve the efficiency of glucose homeostatic mechanisms. To implicate pancreozymin and secretin exclusively in this regulatory system would be too simplistic. Further studies may show that the effects of the absorptive process upon the islet cells are mediated by a fine interplay of several intestinal factors.

REFERENCES

BÖTTGER, I., FALOONA, G. and UNGER, R. (1972): Response of islet cell and gut hormones to fat absorption: an 'entero-insular axis' for fat. *Clin. Res., 20,* 542.

BUCHANAN, K. D., VANCE, J. E., MORGAN, A. and WILLIAMS, R. H. (1968): Effect of pancreozymin on insulin and glucagon levels in blood and bile. *Amer. J. Physiol., 215,* 1293.

CHISHOLM, D. J., YOUNG, J. D. and LAZARUS, L. (1969): The gastrointestinal stimulus to insulin release. I. Secretin. *J. clin. Invest., 48,* 1453.

DUPRE, J., CURTIS, J. D., UNGER, R. H., WADDELL, R. W. and BECK, J. C. (1969): Effects of secretin, pancreozymin, or gastrin on the response of the endocrine pancreas to administration of glucose or arginine in man. *J. clin. Invest., 48,* 745.

FUSSGÄNGER, R. D., STRAUB, K., GOBERNA, R., JAROS, P., SCHRÖDER, K. E., RAPTIS, S. and PFEIFFER, E. F. (1969): Primary secretion of insulin and secondary release of glucagon from isolated perfused rat pancreas following stimulation with pancreozymin. *Hormone Metabol. Res., 1,* 224.

GO, V. L. W., HOFMANN, A. F. and SUMMERSKILL, W. H. J. (1970): Pancreozymin bioassay in man based on pancreatic enzyme secretion: potency of specific amino acids and other digestive products. *J. clin. Invest., 49,* 1558.

McINTYRE, N., HOLDSWORTH, C. D. and TURNER, S. (1964): New interpretation of oral glucose tolerance. *Lancet, 2,* 20.

OHNEDA, A., PARADA, E., EISENTRAUT, A. M. and UNGER, R. H. (1968): Characterization of response of circulating glucagon to intraduodenal and intravenous administration of amino acids. *J. clin. Invest., 47,* 2305.

PEK, S., FAJANS, S. S., FLOYD Jr., J. C., KNOPF, R. F. and CONN, J. W. (1969): Effects upon plasma glucagon of infused and ingested amino acids and of protein meals in man. *Diabetes, 18,* 328.

PERLEY, M. J. and KIPNIS, D. M. (1967): Plasma insulin responses to oral and intravenous glucose: studies in normal and diabetic subjects. *J. clin. Invest., 46,* 1954.

RABINOVITCH, A. and DUPRE, J. (1972): Insulinotropic and glucagonotropic activities in crude preparations of cholecystokinin-pancreozymin. *Clin. Res., 20,* 945.

RAPTIS, S., SCHRÖDER, K. E., ROTHENBUCHNER, G. and PFEIFFER, E. F. (1972): Effect of the gastrointestinal hormones, secretin and cholecystokinin-pancreozymin on insulin and glucagon release in healthy and diabetic subjects. *Israel J. med. Sci., 8,* 769.

SANTEUSANIO, F., FALOONA, G. R. and UNGER, R. H. (1972): Suppressive effect of secretin upon pancreatic alpha cell function. *J. clin. Invest., 51,* 1743.

UNGER, R. H., KETTERER, H., DUPRE, J. and EISENTRAUT, A. M. (1967): The effect of secretin, pancreozymin, and gastrin on insulin and glucagon secretion in anesthetized dogs. *J. clin. Invest., 46,* 630.

CLINICAL CONDITIONS ASSOCIATED WITH ELEVATED PLASMA LEVELS OF GLUCAGON*

SUMER PEK, STEFAN S. FAJANS, JOHN C. FLOYD, Jr. and R. F. KNOPF

Department of Internal Medicine, Division of Endocrinology and Metabolism and the Metabolism Research Unit, the University of Michigan, Ann Arbor, Mich.; and Department of Medicine, Division of Endocrinology and Metabolism, University of Alabama in Birmingham, and the Metabolism Research Laboratory, U.S. Veterans Administration Hospital, Birmingham, Ala., U.S.A.

Dr. Assan and Dr. Unger have reviewed the association of elevated plasma levels of glucagon with diabetes mellitus and with certain stressful illnesses, respectively (this Volume, pp. 144–179 and 137–143). Limited information is available on other clinical disorders associated with hyperglucagonemia. The failure to recognize abnormalities in dynamics of glucagon secretion more frequently may be due to paucity of symptoms induced by glucagon excess and to limited availability of sufficiently sensitive and specific methods for the determination of plasma levels of glucagon.

GLUCAGON-PRODUCING TUMORS

Reports on pancreatic islet cell tumors with the histological picture of alphacytomas have appeared in the literature since 1946 (Hess, 1946). In some of these cases, excessive glucagon-like biological activity has been found in extracts of plasma or tumor tissue. These early reports have been reviewed by Unger and Eisentraut (1967). More recently, several additional cases of glucagon-producing pancreatic tumors were identified by radioimmunological means (McGavran et al., 1966; Vance et al., 1969; Croughs et al., 1972; Walter et al., 1972). Most of these tumors were malignant. Interestingly, all benign tumors were observed as a part of the syndrome of multiple endocrine adenomatosis. Recently, we have observed 3 patients with pancreatic islet tumors who had persistently elevated plasma levels of glucagon (400–1500 pg/ml) (Pek et al., 1973). One of these patients had large hepatic metastases and markedly elevated plasma levels of insulin; hypoglycemia was observed only rarely. The second patient was a member of a large family with multiple endocrine adenomatosis. In addition to hyperglucagonemia, hyperinsulinemia was present, again without appreciable hypoglycemia. After the removal of multiple islet tumors, plasma glucagon and insulin returned to normal. The third patient had benign microadenomatosis of pancreatic islets, marked hyperinsulinemia and persistent and profound hypoglycemia. In this case, hyperglucagonemia may have been secondary to hypoglycemia. Thus, in patients with insulin-producing islet tumors, a co-

* Supported in part by U.S. Public Health Service Grants AM-02244 and AM-0888, National Institutes of Arthritis and Metabolic Diseases; RR-32, General Clinical Research Program; 5P11-GM15559, National Institutes of General Medical Sciences, and by an institutional grant, the U.S. Veterans Administration Hospital in Birmingham.

existing alpha cell tumor may moderate or mask the hypoglycemia. Conversely, in patients with glucagon-producing tumors, adequate or excessive production of insulin could prevent the development of hyperglycemia. We have very limited information on the dynamics of secretion of glucagon in our patients. In 2 patients, the increases in plasma glucagon in response to administered arginine were blunted; no suppression of glucagon release occurred with oral or intravenous administration of glucose.

ACUTE PANCREATITIS

Paloyan et al. (1967) have reported markedly elevated plasma glucagon-like immunoreactivity in patients with acute and chronic pancreatitis. The omission of plasmin-trypsin inhibitors in their assay may have resulted in spuriously high values. Recently, Day et al. (1972) have reported that in 26 patients with acute pancreatitis, plasma levels of glucagon were in the normal range, but inappropriately high for the prevailing levels of plasma glucose. In patients with chronic pancreatitis, Aguilar-Parada et al. (1969) observed diminished or absent glucagon responses to arginine.

HYPERPARATHYROIDISM

Paloyan (1967) has reported 9 patients with parathyroid adenomas, 8 of whom had elevated plasma glucagon-like immunoreactivity. He proposed that hyperglucagonemia may have contributed to the development of hyperparathyroidism. We had the opportunity to study 2 patients with primary hyperparathyroidism. In both cases, fasting levels and arginine-induced increases in plasma glucagon were normal before and after the removal of their tumors. The possible relationship between glucagon, calcium homeostasis and parathyroid hormone deserves further study.

DISEASES ASSOCIATED WITH CARBOHYDRATE INTOLERANCE

A search for abnormalities of glucagon release may be more rewarding among patients with diseases in which the prevalence of carbohydrate intolerance is high.

Acromegaly

We have studied the effects of administered human growth hormone upon plasma levels of glucagon in 7 healthy subjects (Pek et al., 1971a). As depicted in Figure 1, basal levels and arginine-induced increases in plasma glucagon were augmented significantly. Subsequently, Goldfine et al. (1972) have reported that in patients with active acromegaly, plasma glucagon responses to arginine were excessive. More recently, in 22 patients with acromegaly, Gerich et al. (1973a) have observed elevated fasting plasma levels of glucagon, exaggerated glucagon responses to arginine and normal suppression of glucagon with induced hyperglycemia. Hyperglucagonemia associated with acromegaly may be the result of a direct effect of growth hormone upon the alpha cells, which would be in line with its effect upon the beta cells of the pancreas.

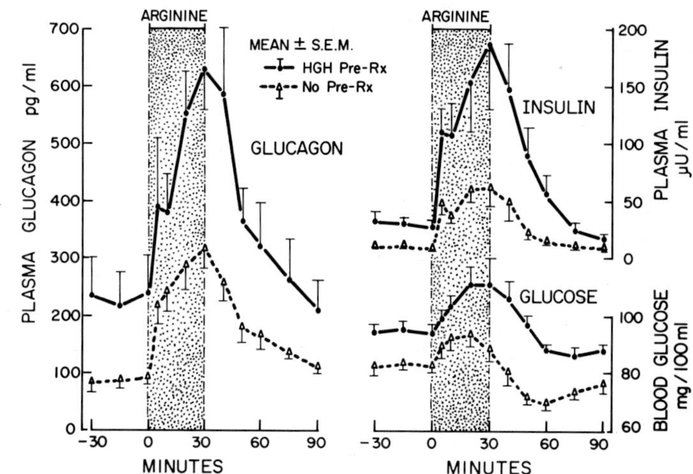

FIG. 1. Effect of pretreatment with human growth hormone (10 mg i.m. daily for 3 days) upon plasma levels of glucagon, insulin, and glucose in the fasting state and with the administration of arginine (0.41 g/kg body weight; i.v. 0–30 minutes) in 7 healthy subjects. Control experiments without pretreatment were done in the same subjects.

Pheochromocytoma

Using an assay not specific for pancreatic glucagon, Lawrence (1966) observed elevated plasma levels of glucagon in several patients with pheochromocytoma. No data are available on the dynamics of glucagon secretion in such patients in whom plasma glucagon has been measured by specific assays before and after removal of the tumors. Adrenergic receptor mechanisms influence the release of glucagon in vivo and in vitro (Leclercq-Meyer et al., 1971; Iversen, 1971; Pek et al., 1971b; Eaton et al., 1972; Dudl et al., 1972; Tyler and Kajinuma, 1972; Gerich et al., 1972; Luyckx and Lefebvre, 1972; Harvey et al., 1972; Lindsey and Faloona, 1973; Walter et al., 1973; Gerich et al., 1973b; Weir et al., 1973; Tyler, 1973). Controversy exists as to whether catecholamine-induced glucagon release is mediated through alpha- or beta-adrenergic receptors. Depending upon the preponderance of the type of catecholamines which is in excess, certain patients with pheochromocytoma may be expected to have altered dynamics of secretion of glucagon.

Glucocorticoid excess

Sufficient information is lacking on possible abnormalities of glucagon secretion in patients with Cushing's disease. Data on experimentally-induced glucocorticoid excess in man are controversial. Marco et al. (1973a) have observed augmentation of fasting levels and of arginine-induced increases of plasma glucagon in healthy subjects in response to pretreatment with prednisolone for 3–4 days. We have administered dexamethasone, 8 mg/day for 3 days to 7 healthy subjects (Fig. 2) (Pek et al., 1971a). No significant changes were observed in plasma glucagon in the fasting state. The increases in plasma glucagon in response to arginine were not altered.

In another series of experiments, standard oral glucose tolerance tests and cortisone-

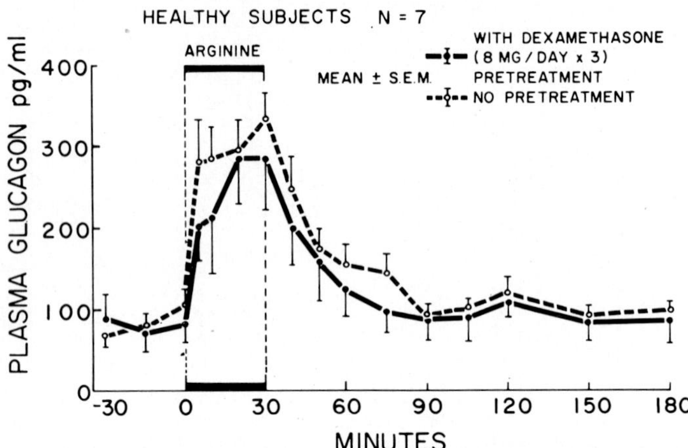

FIG. 2. Effect of pretreatment with dexamethasone (8 mg orally daily for 3 days) upon increases in plasma glucagon induced by administration of arginine (0.41 g/kg body weight; i.v. 0–30 minutes) in 7 healthy subjects. Control experiments without pretreatment were done in the same subjects.

provocative glucose tolerance tests were performed in 11 healthy subjects (Fig. 3). The fasting levels and the magnitude of the suppression of plasma glucagon were similar. In both series of experiments, the pretreatment with glucocorticoids was sufficient to induce the expected augmentation of fasting levels and of the increases in plasma insulin evoked by arginine or glucose. Further studies are needed to define the role of endogenous or exogenous glucocorticoids upon the secretion of glucagon and to establish whether hypoglucagonemia may be a factor contributing to the development of carbohydrate intolerance in patients with chronic glucocorticoid excess.

Hyperlipoproteinemia

Hyperglucagonemia has been observed in patients with Type III, IV and V hyperlipoproteinemia (Eaton and Schade, 1973). Based upon earlier observations that the administration of glucagon induces a lowering of plasma triglycerides, they have proposed that in hyperlipemic patients a resistance to endogenous glucagon could exist which in turn may result in a seemingly inappropriate increase in plasma levels of glucagon. These most interesting observations suggest that the interplay of glucagon and insulin levels may be an important factor in the pathogenesis of hyperlipoproteinemias.

Hepatic cirrhosis

A recent report by Marco et al. (1973b) indicates that hyperglucagonemia is a common finding in patients with hepatic cirrhosis. Elevated plasma levels of glucagon may be the result of reduced hepatic removal of glucagon. The contribution of hyperglucagonemia to the carbohydrate intolerance seen in patients with cirrhosis of the liver remains to be elucidated.

In summary, hyperglucagonemia has been demonstrated in a variety of diseases asso-

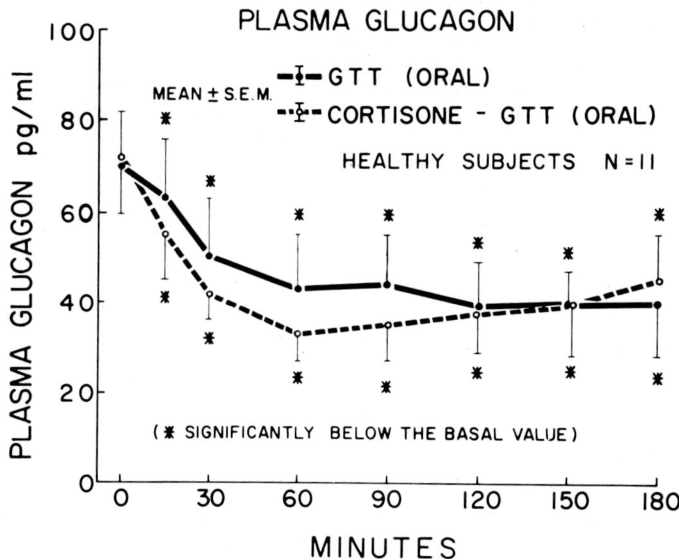

FIG. 3. Plasma levels of glucagon in 11 healthy subjects during standard oral glucose tolerance tests (glucose 1.75 g/kg ideal body weight) without and with prior administration of cortisone acetate (62.5 mg orally 8 and 2 hours preceding the test).

ciated with carbohydrate intolerance. In these clinical conditions, the mechanisms by which the production and/or disposal of glucagon may be altered are not readily apparent. Glucagon-producing islet cell tumors emerge as an entity in which a primary abnormality in glucagon secretion is present.

REFERENCES

AGUILAR-PARADA, E., EISENTRAUT, A. M. and UNGER, R. H. (1969): Pancreatic glucagon secretion in normal and diabetic subjects. *Amer. J. med. Sci., 257,* 415.

CROUGHS, R. J. M., HULSMANS, H. A. M., ISRAEL, D. E., HACKENG, W. H. L. and SCHOPMAN, W. (1972): Glucagonoma as a part of the polyglandular adenoma syndrome. *Amer. J. Med., 52,* 690.

DAY, J. L., KNIGHT, M. and CONDON, J. R. (1972): The role of pancreatic glucagon in the pathogenesis of acute pancreatitis. *Clin. Sci., 43,* 597.

DUDL, R. J., WALTER, R. and ENSINCK, J. (1972): Alpha adrenergic control of glucagon in man. *Clin. Res., 20,* 191.

EATON, R. P., CONWAY, M. and BUCKMAN, M. (1972): Role of alpha adrenergic blockade on alanine-induced hyperglucagonemia. *Clin. Res., 20,* 238.

EATON, R. P. and SCHADE, D. S. (1973): Glucagon resistance as a hormonal basis for endogenous hyperlipemia. *Lancet, 1,* 973.

GERICH, J. E., KARAM, J. H. and FORSHAM, P. H. (1972): Reciprocal adrenergic control of pancreatic alpha and beta cell function in man. *Diabetes, 21/Suppl. 1,* 332.

GERICH, J. E., LANGLOIS, M., SCHNEIDER, V., NOACCO, C. and GUSTAFSON, G. (1973a): Abnormal pancreatic alpha cell function in acromegaly. *Program, 55th Annual Meeting of the Endocrine Society, June 20–22, 1973,* p. A-173.

GERICH, J. E., LANGLOIS, M., SCHNEIDER, V., NOACCO, C. and FORSHAM, P. H. (1973b): Effect of cyclic AMP on glucagon secretion in man. *Diabetes, 22/Suppl. 1,* 301.

GOLDFINE, I. D., KIRSTEINS, L. and LAWRENCE, A. M. (1972): Excessive glucagon response to arginine in active acromegaly. *Hormone Metabol. Res., 4,* 97.

HARVEY, W., FALOONA, G. and UNGER, R. (1972): Effect of adrenergic blockade on exercise-induced hyperglucagonemia. *Clin. Res., 20,* 752.

HESS, W. (1946): Über ein endokrin-inaktives Karzinom der Langerhansschen Inseln. *Schweiz. med. Wschr., 76,* 802.

IVERSEN, J. (1971): Adrenergic receptors for the secretion of immunoreactive glucagon and insulin from the isolated perfused canine pancreas. *Diabetologia, 7,* 485.

LAWRENCE, A. M. (1966): Radioimmunoassayable glucagon levels in man: effects of starvation, hypoglycemia, and glucose administration. *Proc. nat. Acad. Sci. USA, 55,* 316.

LECLERCQ-MEYER, V., BRISSON, G. R. and MALAISSE, W. J. (1971): Effect of adrenaline and glucose on release of glucagon and insulin in vitro. *Nature New Biol., 231,* 248.

LINDSEY, C. A. and FALOONA, G. R. (1973): Adrenergic blockade in shock-induced hyperglucagonemia. *Diabetes, 22/Suppl. 1,* 301.

LUYCKX, A. S. and LEFEBVRE, P. J. (1972): Role of catecholamines in exercise-induced glucagon secretion in rats. *Diabetes, 21/Suppl. 1,* 334.

MARCO, J., CALLE, C., ROMAN, D., DIAZ-FIERROS, M., VILLANUEVA, M. L. and VALVERDE, I. (1973a): Hyperglucagonism induced by glucocorticoid treatment in man. *New Engl. J. Med., 288,* 128.

MARCO, J., DIEGO, J., VALVERDE, I. and SEGOVIA, J. M. (1973b): Hyperglucagonism in patients with cirrhosis of the liver. *Diabetes, 22/Suppl. 1,* 303.

McGAVRAN, M. H., UNGER, R. H., RECANT, L., POLK, H. C., KILO, C. and LEFIN, M. E. (1966): A glucagon-secreting alpha-cell carcinoma of the pancreas. *New Engl. J. Med., 274,* 1408.

PALOYAN, E. (1967): Recent developments in the early diagnosis of hyperparathyroidism. *Surg. Clin. N. Amer., 47,* 61.

PALOYAN, E., PALOYAN, D. and HARPER, P. V. (1967): The role of glucagon hypersecretion in the relationship of pancreatitis and hyperparathyroidism. *Surgery, 62,* 167.

PEK, S., FAJANS, S. S., FLOYD Jr., J. C., KNOPF, R. F., PRCHKOV, V. K., SHERMAN, B. M., WEISSMAN, P. N. and CONN, J. W. (1971a): Effects upon plasma glucagon of human growth hormone and of dexamethasone in man. *Clin. Res., 19,* 482.

PEK, S., FAJANS, S. S., FLOYD Jr., J. C., KNOPF, R. F., WEISSMAN, P. N. and CONN, J. W. (1971b): Augmentation of arginine-induced glucagon release by beta adrenergic receptor stimulation in man. *Clin. Res., 19,* 680.

PEK, S., FAJANS, S. S., FLOYD Jr., J. C. and KNOPF, R. F. (1973): Unpublished observations.

TYLER, J. M. and KAJINUMA, H. (1972): Influence of beta-adrenergic and -cholinergic agents in vivo on pancreatic glucagon and insulin secretion. *Diabetes, 21/Suppl. 1,* 332.

TYLER, J. M. (1973): Effects of alpha-adrenergic blockade on pancreatic glucagon secretion during administration of norepinephrine in vivo. *Program, 55th Annual Meeting of the Endocrine Society, Chicago, June 20–22, 1973,* p. A-277.

UNGER, R. H. and EISENTRAUT, A. M. (1967): Glucagon. In: *Hormones in Blood,*

Vol. 1, p. 83. Editors: C. H. Grey and A. L. Bacharach. Academic Press, London and New York.

VANCE, J. E., STOLL, R. W., KITABCHI, A. E., WILLIAMS, R. H. and WOOD, F. C. (1969): Nesidioblastosis in familial endocrine adenomatosis. *J. Amer. med. Ass., 207,* 1679.

WALTER, R. M., DUDL, R. M. and ENSINCK, J. W. (1972): Immunoreactive glucagon in islet cell tumors. *Diabetes, 21/Suppl. 1,* 333.

WALTER, R. M., PALMER, J. P. and ENSINCK, J. W. (1973): Evaluation of the role of the adrenergic nervous system in glucagon release during fasting. *Diabetes, 22/Suppl. 1,* 301.

WEIR, G. C., KNOWLTON, S. D. and MARTIN, D. B. (1973): Glucagon secretory responses to theophylline and cyclic AMP. *Diabetes, 22/Suppl. 1,* 302.

REGULATION OF METABOLIC FUELS SUPPLY

AMINO ACIDS AND GLUCONEOGENESIS: INFLUENCE OF BLOOD CELLS, OBESITY, PROLONGED EXERCISE AND GLUCOCORTICOIDS*

PHILIP FELIG** and JOHN WAHREN

Department of Internal Medicine, Yale University School of Medicine, New Haven, Connecticut 06510, U.S.A., and Department of Clinical Physiology, Karolinska Institute at the Serafimer Hospital, Stockholm, Sweden

Gluconeogenesis may be defined as the process whereby non-carbohydrate precursors are converted to glucose. The important substrates available for glucose formation in man are amino acids, lactate, pyruvate and glycerol. In recent years a variety of studies conducted in several laboratories (Ross et al., 1967; Felig et al., 1969a; Mallette et al., 1969) have directed attention to the role of amino acids in the regulation of gluconeogenesis. These studies have identified alanine as the principal endogenous aminogenic precursor (Felig et al., 1969a, 1970a) and have indicated that availability of alanine is the rate-limiting step in the regulation of gluconeogenesis in prolonged starvation (Felig et al., 1969a, 1970a) and in pregnancy (Felig et al., 1972). In addition, studies in exercising man have demonstrated that release of alanine by muscle tissue is related to glucose utilization and pyruvate availability (Felig and Wahren, 1971a). On the basis of these studies a glucose-alanine cycle analogous to the Cori cycle for lactate has been proposed (Mallette et al., 1969; Felig et al., 1970a; Felig, 1973). In this cycle, alanine is selectively extracted by the liver and converted to glucose and is subsequently reformed in muscle by transamination of glucose-derived pyruvate.

Investigation of amino acid metabolism has not only focused attention on the regulatory role of the substrate, but has also served to clarify the mechanism of insulin action. In studies in normal, intact man the inhibitory action of insulin on gluconeogenesis has been shown to involve a direct hepatic effect rather than a reduction in precursor availability (Felig and Wahren, 1971c). In contrast, in diabetes augmented gluconeogenesis has been demonstrated to occur as a result of increased hepatic extraction of amino acids in the face of a diminution in circulating levels of alanine and other glycogenic amino acids (Wahren et al., 1972; Felig et al., 1970b).

It is the purpose of the present report to review several recent studies which have further extended our understanding of amino acid metabolism in the regulation of gluconeogenesis. Specifically the role of red blood cells in inter-organ amino acid transport, the effects of obesity, prolonged exercise, and glucocorticoids on amino acid metabolism, and the influence of alanine deficiency states on gluconeogenesis will be examined.

* This work was supported by grants AM 13526 and RR 125 from the U.S. Public Health Service, and grants 19X-722 and 19X-3108 from the Swedish Medical Research Council.

** Recipient of a Research Career Development Award (AM 70219) from the U.S. Public Health Service.

P. FELIG AND J. WAHREN

ROLE OF RED BLOOD CELLS IN INTER-ORGAN AMINO ACID EXCHANGE

In previous studies demonstrating the primacy of alanine in the transfer of aminogenic substrate across the liver and peripheral tissues, amino acid concentrations were determined in plasma rather than whole blood (Felig et al., 1969a, 1970a; Felig and Wahren, 1971a, b). The use of plasma was dictated by the long-held notion that red blood cells were inert with respect to the transport of amino acids between tissues in view of their slow equilibration time across the red blood cell membrane when studied in vitro (Winter and Christensen, 1964). The demonstration by Aoki et al. (1972) that red blood cells have a dynamic role in insulin-stimulated uptake of glutamate by muscle tissue necessitated examination of the overall in vivo contribution of red blood cells to amino acid exchange. In addition, the relative importance of alanine and glutamine as hepatic gluconeogenic precursors was investigated inasmuch as studies with plasma indicated that output of glutamine by muscle tissue was comparable to that of alanine (Marliss et al., 1971).

In Figure 1 the relative contribution of red blood cells to amino acid exchange across the leg in normal postabsorptive subjects is shown. Arteriofemoral venous differences were determined using whole blood and plasma and the relative contribution of blood cells (primarily erythrocytes) was calculated (Felig et al., 1973). As shown, using whole blood, alanine output exceeded that of glutamine and all other amino acids. In the case of alanine, glutamine, leucine, isoleucine and tyrosine, significant net exchange occurred by way of blood cells. Interestingly, the net output of alanine via blood cells exceeded that of all other amino acids and accounted for 25% of total alanine release.

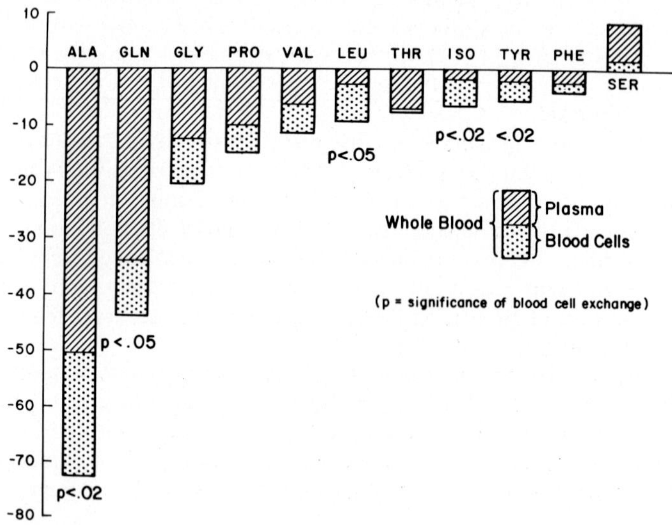

FIG. 1. Arteriofemoral venous (A-FV) differences (in μmoles/l) of individual amino acids in whole blood, plasma and blood cells. The P values indicate the significance of the exchange via blood cells. Where P values are not shown, the A-FV difference in blood cells was too small or variable to be significantly different from zero. (Based on the data of Felig et al., 1973.)

In Figure 2 arteriohepatic venous differences for individual amino acids in whole blood, plasma and blood cells are shown. The data reveal that splanchnic uptake of alanine from whole blood was greater than that of glutamine and all other amino acids, accounting for 35–40% of total net aminogenic extraction by the splanchnic bed. In the case of alanine, threonine, serine, leucine and methionine splanchnic uptake could not be accounted for solely by plasma exchange but was due in part to a significant transfer by way of blood cells. Noteworthy is the fact that splanchnic uptake of alanine from blood cells (as well as plasma) exceeded that of all other amino acids.

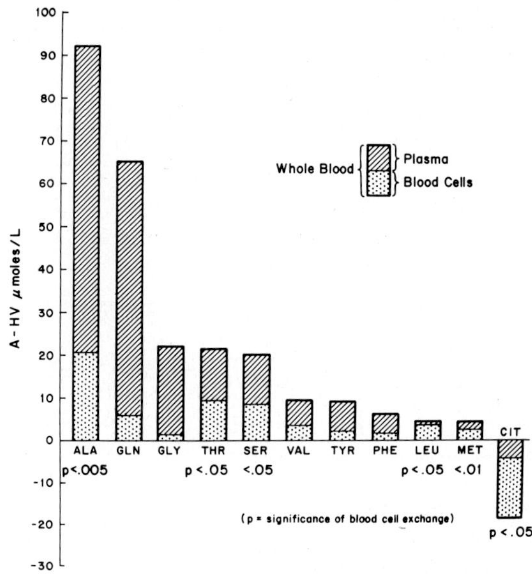

FIG. 2. Arteriohepatic venous differences (A-HV) of individual amino acids in whole blood, plasma and blood cells. P values are defined as in Figure 1. (Based on the data of Felig et al., 1973.)

The contribution of the gut to net splanchnic exchange was investigated by determining arterioportal venous differences. As shown in Figure 3, a consistent output from the gut was observed for 9 amino acids, the net release of alanine being greater than that of other amino acids. Of the total alanine released by the gut, 30% was transported via blood cells. In contrast to all other amino acids, a net uptake by gastrointestinal tissues was observed for glutamine. The transport of glutamine was also unique in that its movement on passage through the gut was in opposite directions with respect to plasma and blood cells. Thus, while glutamine was being taken up from plasma, a smaller shift was calculated to occur into blood cells.

These observations with whole blood thus indicate that blood cells contribute to inter-organ amino acid exchange. With the exception of glutamine, the tissue exchange via blood cells occurred in a direction which parallelled the net shifts occurring in plasma. With respect to alanine, 25–30% of the net release of this amino acid from muscle and gut to the liver occurs by way of blood cells. Thus previous studies employing plasma

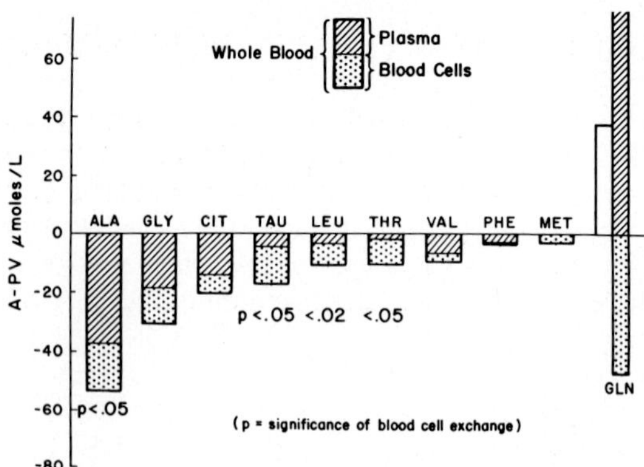

FIG. 3. Arterioportal venous (A-PV) differences of individual amino acids in whole blood, plasma and blood cells. P values are defined as in Figure 1. For glutamine (GLN) whole blood exchange is shown by the open bar, and is smaller than the value for plasma exchange (cross-hatched bar) because of the negative A-PV difference observed in blood cells (stippled bar). The A-PV difference for glutamine in blood cells was significant at the $P < 0.005$ level. (Based on the data of Felig et al., 1973.)

rather than whole blood under-estimated rather than over-estimated the actual contribution of this amino acid as a glucose precursor.

It is also of interest to compare the relative availability of alanine and glutamine as substrates for hepatic gluconeogenesis (Fig. 4). With respect to peripheral exchange, output of alanine is somewhat greater than that of glutamine but release of both amino acids occurs by way of blood cells as well as plasma. In contrast, marked differences are observed in the transfer of these amino acids across the splanchnic tissues. In the case of alanine, this amino acid is released from extrahepatic splanchnic tissues by way of plasma and blood cells and is subsequently extracted from the cells and plasma by the liver. Thus the arteriohepatic venous differences underestimate the actual hepatic uptake of alanine, since gastrointestinal tissues contribute additional alanine for hepatic extraction. In contrast, glutamine is taken up by gastrointestinal tissues and by blood cells on passage through the gut, and only a small proportion (< 50%) is available for hepatic extraction.

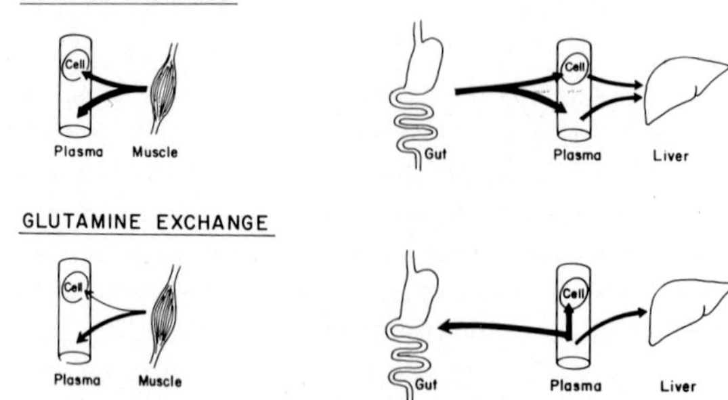

FIG. 4. Comparison of muscle and splanchnic exchange of alanine and glutamine via plasma and blood cells. Output of both amino acids from muscle is via plasma and cells. In the splanchnic bed, alanine is released from gastrointestinal tissues and is taken up by the liver from plasma and blood cells. In contrast, glutamine is taken up by the gut and by blood cells on passage of whole blood through the splanchnic bed. The residual proportion (< 50% of the total splanchnic uptake) is available for hepatic extraction.

CONDITIONS WITH INCREASED HEPATIC UPTAKE OF ALANINE

An increase in gluconeogenesis would be expected to occur in circumstances in which the availability of alanine is increased and/or the net balance of glucoregulatory hormones (insulin and glucagon) favors augmented extraction of available precursors. As shown in Table 1 a variety of conditions have now been identified in which hepatic extraction and/or availability of alanine is augmented. The increase in alanine uptake by the liver in diabetes (Wahren et al., 1972) has been commented upon above. The initial response to starvation, as indicated in patients fasted for 2–3 days, is one in which hepatic alanine uptake increases from postabsorptive levels (Felig et al., 1969a). Interestingly, this increase in gluconeogenic precursor uptake coincides with the peak increase in glucagon levels observed during the course of a prolonged fast (Marliss et al., 1970). Recently evidence has been obtained identifying 3 additional conditions in which hepatic uptake of alanine is increased: obesity, prolonged exercise and hypercorticism. In all of these circumstances it would appear that increased gluconeogenesis is a consequence of either (a) absolute insulin lack (diabetes); (b) insulin lack and hyperglucagonemia (brief starvation; prolonged exercise); or (c) resistance to insulin (obesity) which may be accompanied by hyperglucagonemia (glucocorticoid excess) (Table 1).

TABLE 1
Increased hepatic uptake of alanine: substrate availability and hormonal mechanisms

Condition	Circulating alanine levels	Insulin lack	Insulin resistance	Glucagon increase	References
Diabetes	Decreased	X		*	Wahren et al. (1972)
Brief starvation (2–3 days)	Decreased	X		X	Felig et al. (1969a) Marliss et al. (1970)
Prolonged exercise (4 hours)	Increased	X		X	Ahlborg et al. (1974)
Obesity	Increased		X		Felig et al. (1974)
Glucocorticoid excess	Increased		X	X	Wise et al. (1973)

* An absolute increase in basal glucagon levels contributes to augmented gluconeogenesis in severely decompensated (ketoacidotic) diabetics. However, increased gluconeogenesis also occurs in diabetics who are not ketoacidotic and in whom basal glucagon concentration is not increased (Wahren et al., 1972).

OBESITY

A variety of abnormalities in carbohydrate metabolism have been well documented in obesity. Hyperinsulinemia (Karam et al., 1963), decreased responsiveness of fat (Salans et al., 1968) and muscle tissue (Rabinowitz and Zierler, 1962; Felig et al., 1969b) to insulin, and an increased incidence of diabetes (Ogilvie, 1935), have all been observed in obese subjects. In view of recent studies implicating the liver as the primary site of action of endogenous insulin in normal man (Felig and Wahren, 1971c), it was of interest to determine the effects of obesity on hepatic uptake of alanine and other glucose precursors. Accordingly, the hepatic venous catheter technique was employed to examine net splanchnic balances in obese subjects with normal glucose tolerance (Felig et al., 1974).

In Figure 5 splanchnic exchange of lactate, alanine (using whole blood), and glycerol are shown for 13 obese subjects and 12 normal weight controls. In the obese group, splanchnic uptake of these glucose precursors was increased 50–75%. In the case of glycerol this augmentation in uptake was entirely a consequence of an increase in arterial concentration. However, with respect to lactate and alanine, a 50% increase in splanchnic fractional extraction was observed. It is noteworthy that in association with the augmented uptake of glucose precursors increased splanchnic consumption of free fatty acids and oxygen was observed in the obese subjects (Fig. 5).

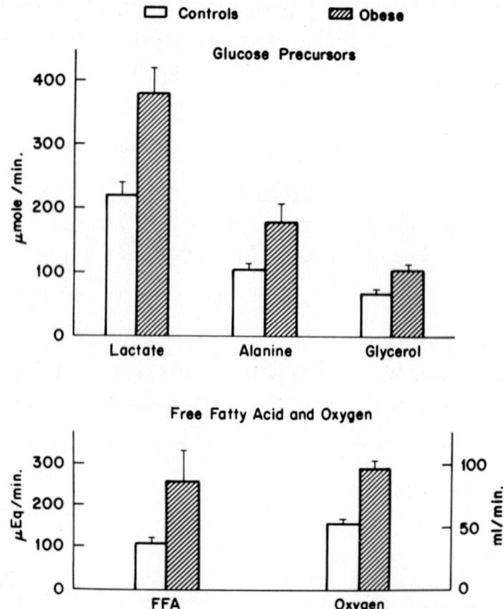

FIG. 5. Splanchnic uptake of glucose precursors, free fatty acids and oxygen in normal weight controls and in obese subjects in the basal, postabsorptive state. (Based on the data of Felig et al., 1974.)

From the observations on net precursor balance and absolute splanchnic glucose production (1.2 ± 0.1 mmoles/min. in the controls and 1.1 ± 0.1 mmoles/min. in the obese) the relative contribution of gluconeogenesis to total glucose output may be calculated (Fig. 6). As reflected in net precursor balance, it can be seen that 19% of hepatic glucose output can be accounted for by gluconeogenesis in the controls, whereas 35% was derivable from precursor substrates in the obese group. Interestingly this increase in precursor uptake in obesity corresponds closely with that previously demonstrated in diabetic subjects in whom 33% of glucose output could be attributed to utilization of gluconeogenic substrates (Wahren et al., 1972). Furthermore, in obesity as well as in diabetes the

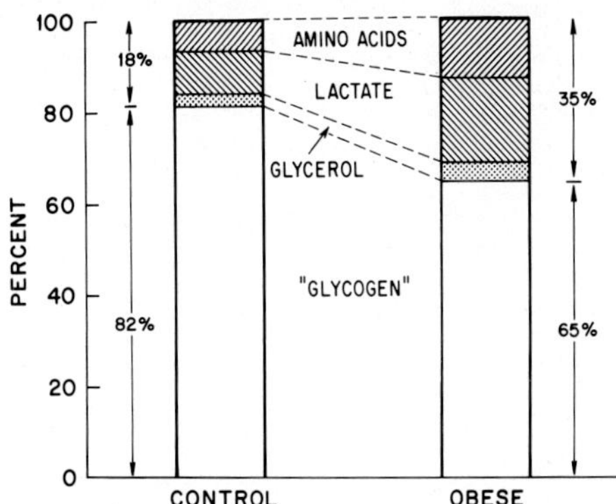

FIG. 6. Relative contributions of gluconeogenic precursors to total splanchnic glucose output in control and obese subjects as indicated by net substrate balance. That proportion of glucose output not accountable by precursor uptake is presumed to be derived from glycogen. (Based on the data of Felig et al., 1974.)

increase in precursor uptake is due in part to augmented splanchnic fractional extraction of available precursors. These similarities to diabetes with respect to hepatic uptake of gluconeogenic substrates, despite the presence of hyperinsulinemia in the obese group, suggest that the liver is resistant to insulin in obesity. It would thus appear that an accelerated rate of gluconeogenesis may occur either in the face of a diminution or lack of insulin (brief starvation, diabetes) or in circumstances in which target tissues are resistant to insulin (obesity).

PROLONGED EXERCISE

In normal man, total hepatic glycogen stores amount to 75–90 g (Hultman and Nilsson, 1971). Observations on splanchnic and peripheral exchange of glucose in subjects exercising on a bicycle ergometer for 4 hours at 30% of maximal capacity indicate a total glucose turnover during this period of approximately 75 g (Ahlborg et al., 1974). It is thus clear that hepatic glycogen stores are depleted as exercise progresses and that maintenance of glucose homeostasis in prolonged exercise requires an increasing contribution from gluconeogenesis. Indeed increased glucose production from glycerol has been observed in prolonged exercise, as indicated by isotopic technique (Young et al., 1967) as well as by substrate balances (Ahlborg et al., 1974).

With respect to amino acid metabolism, as noted above, peripheral release of alanine is increased in exercise in association with augmented glucose utilization and increased availability of pyruvate for transamination. During brief periods of exercise (up to 1 hour) splanchnic uptake of alanine remains at levels comparable to the resting state. As a consequence of this imbalance between peripheral release and splanchnic utilization rates, the arterial concentration of alanine rises (Felig and Wahren, 1971a). However, as exercise continues beyond 1 hour, an increase in splanchnic uptake of alanine and a fall in arterial levels is observed. As shown in Figure 7, splanchnic uptake of alanine after 4 hours of exercise was 50–100% higher than that observed in the resting state or after brief (40

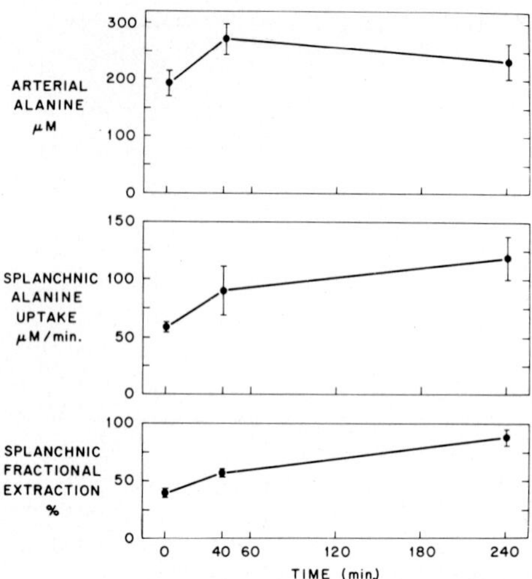

FIG. 7. Alanine metabolism in normal subjects during prolonged exercise at 30% of maximal work capacity. The values for splanchnic alanine uptake and fractional extraction at 240 minutes are significantly greater than those observed in the resting state. (Based on the data of Ahlborg et al., 1974.)

minutes) exercise. Inasmuch as arterial alanine fell between 40 and 240 minutes of exercise, the rise in alanine uptake was due to an increase in fractional extraction from 57 ± 3% at 40 minutes to 87 ± 8% at 240 minutes ($P < 0.025$). With respect to the mechanism of this increase in alanine extraction, it is noteworthy that insulin levels fell progressively during exercise while glucagon levels rose markedly as exercise was continued beyond 90 minutes (Ahlborg et al., 1974). Thus both hypoinsulinemia and hyperglucagonemia are likely to contribute to the augmented alanine uptake of prolonged exercise (Table 1).

GLUCOCORTICOID EXCESS

It has long been recognized that glucocorticoids increase glucose production by the liver. This effect has generally been ascribed to accelerated protein catabolism (Long et al., 1940), resulting in augmented availability of precursor amino acids for hepatic gluconeogenesis (Smith and Long, 1967). Despite the repeated documentation that glucocorticoids can increase the total concentration of circulating amino acids, little information is available concerning the effect of glucocorticoids on the concentrations of individual amino acids. Considering the specificity of alanine uptake in overall hepatic extraction of aminogenic glucose precursors, it is obviously of some interest to determine the pattern of amino acids in glucocorticoid-treated subjects. Consequently plasma amino acid concentrations were measured in healthy subjects before and after the short-term administration of dexamethasone (8 mg/day for 3 days) and in patients with spontaneous or iatrogenic Cushing's syndrome of at least 6 months' duration (Wise et al., 1973). In addition, the possibility that glucocorticoids may influence gluconeogenesis by altering glucagon secretion was investigated by determining plasma glucagon concentration in the basal state and following the infusion of alanine (0.15 g/kg) or the ingestion of a protein meal (boiled lean beef 3 g/kg).

In Figure 8 the effect of dexamethasone administration on the concentrations of acidic and neutral plasma amino acids is shown. As indicated, a 40% increment in plasma alanine was observed after 3 days of glucocorticoid excess. In contrast, no significant changes were observed in any of the remaining 14 amino acids which were measured. In patients with chronic hypercorticism (Cushing's syndrome) a virtually identical pattern was observed (Wise et al., 1973). Plasma alanine concentration in the Cushing's group (488 ± 31 μmoles/l) was 40% higher than that observed in normal controls (347 ± 26 μmoles/l, $P < 0.01$), while the levels of all other amino acids were uninfluenced by chronic hypercorticism. These data thus indicate a specific effect of glucocorticoids on alanine availability and further underscore the overall importance of this amino acid in gluconeogenesis. With respect to the mechanism of hyperalaninemia, it is noteworthy that glucocorticoids increase blood pyruvate levels (Hennes et al., 1957). Thus, as in the case of exercise, hyperalaninemia associated with steroid exercise may reflect greater availability of pyruvate for transamination.

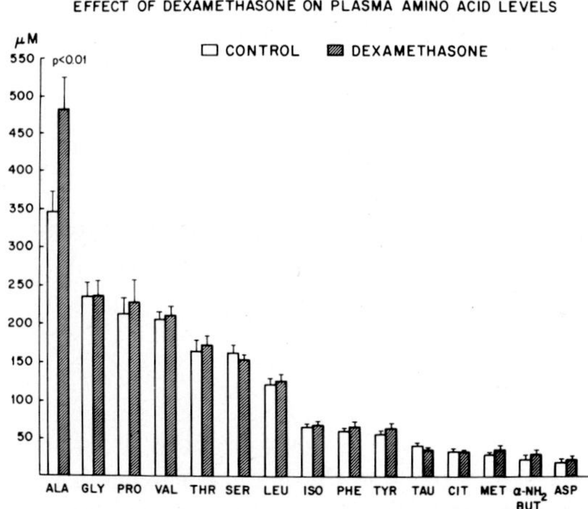

FIG. 8. Effect of dexamethasone (8 mg/day for 3 days) on basal plasma amino acid concentrations. Mean values ± S.E.M. are shown. (Based on the data of Wise et al., 1973.)

The changes in glucagon concentration induced by glucocorticoid administration were also quite striking. Dexamethasone treatment resulted in a 55% increment in basal glucagon levels and in a 60–100% increase in the maximal glucagon response to alanine infusion or protein ingestion (Wise et al., 1973). In patients with Cushing's syndrome basal glucagon levels were 100% higher and the glucagon response to alanine infusion was 170% greater than in normal controls. A similar glucocorticoid-induced increment in the glucagon response to arginine has been reported by Marco et al. (1973).

Concerning the mechanism of the hyperglucagonemia, it is noteworthy that small increases in plasma alanine have been demonstrated to increase glucagon secretion in the dog (Muller et al., 1971). Furthermore, in the dexamethasone-treated subjects a direct linear correlation was observed between the rise in alanine levels and the increase in plasma glucagon concentration (Fig. 9). In addition, a similar correlation between basal alanine and glucagon levels was observed in patients with chronic hypercorticism (Wise et al., 1973).

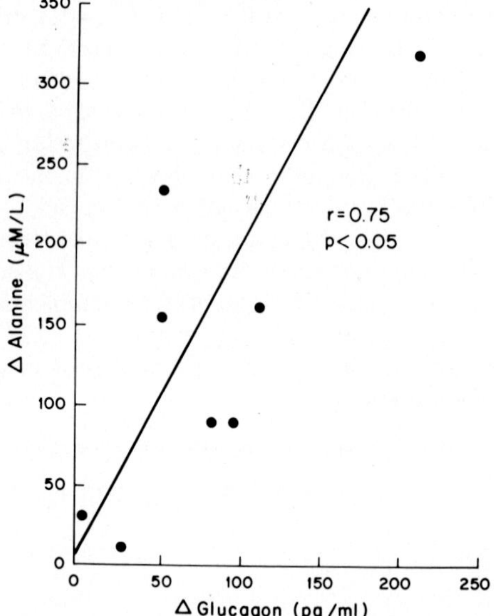

FIG. 9. Relationship between changes in plasma alanine concentration and basal glucagon levels in subjects treated with dexamethasone (8 mg/day) for 3 days. (Based on the data of Wise et al., 1973.)

On the basis of these data it is clear that the gluconeogenic effect of glucocorticoids is based on a multiplicity of actions involving hormones as well as substrate (Table 1). Increased substrate availability in the form of hyperalaninemia, augmented secretion of glucagon, and possibly direct effects of corticosteroids on the liver resulting in insulin resistance and increased activity of hepatic gluconeogenic enzymes, all contribute to the enhancement of glucose production (Fig. 10). These individual effects may in turn be interdependent and synergistic. Thus the increase in amino acids may contribute to hyperglucagonemia, while direct effects of corticoids on the liver enhance the gluconeogenic response to augmented levels of glucagon (Exton et al., 1972).

DECREASED HEPATIC GLUCONEOGENESIS FROM ALANINE

A diminution in hepatic gluconeogenesis would be anticipated in circumstances in which the hormonal milieu or other factors interfere with hepatic extraction of alanine and in those conditions in which the availability of alanine from peripheral protein reserves (muscle tissue) is diminished. Several conditions have now been identified in which substrate or hepatic factors, or a combination of the two, are responsible for decreased gluconeogenesis (Table 2).

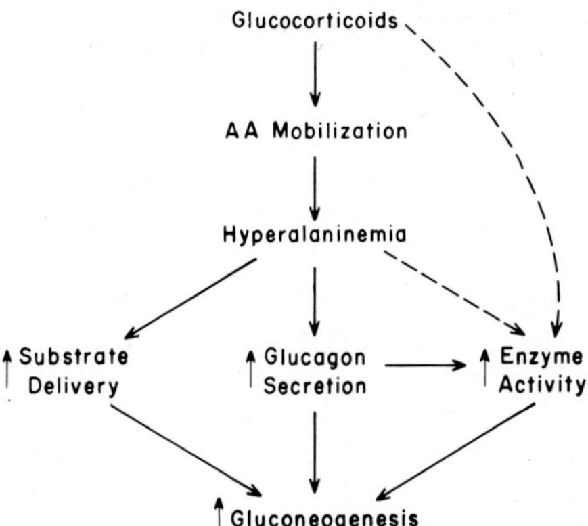

FIG. 10. Mechanisms of stimulation of gluconeogenesis by glucocorticoids. Glucocorticoid administration results in an increase in plasma alanine, which may in turn be responsible for the rise in plasma glucagon. Increases in activity of hepatic gluconeogenic enzymes may be a consequence of a direct steroid effect, hyperglucagonemia, or substrate induction.

TABLE 2
Decreased hepatic gluconeogenesis from alanine: influence of substrate availability and hepatic extraction

Condition	Circulating alanine levels	Hepatic extraction*	References
Glucose administration (hyperinsulinemia)	Unchanged	Decreased	Felig and Wahren (1971c)
Prolonged starvation (3–6 weeks)	Decreased	Unchanged	Felig et al. (1969a)
Pregnancy	Decreased	Unchanged	Felig et al. (1972) Metzger et al. (1971)
Ketotic hypoglycemia	Decreased	Unchanged	Pagliara et al. (1972)
Ethanol administration	Decreased	Decreased	Kreisberg et al. (1972) Kalkhoff and Kim (1973)

* Hepatic extraction refers to the avidity with which a given concentration of circulating alanine is taken up by the liver.

The changes shown in hepatic extraction are based on direct observations of splanchnic fractional extraction of alanine (glucose administration, prolonged starvation) or the glycemic response to infusion of alanine (pregnancy, ketotic hypoglycemia, ethanol administration).

As noted at the outset, hyperinsulinemia resulting from glucose administration in normal man is associated with a decrease in hepatic uptake of alanine (Felig and Wahren, 1971c). This effect is a consequence of a hepatic rather than peripheral action of insulin, inasmuch as arterial alanine is unchanged by the glucose infusion while splanchnic fractional extraction of alanine declines significantly (Felig and Wahren, 1971c). A reverse phenomenon is observed with respect to the diminution in gluconeogenesis accompanying prolonged (3–6 weeks) starvation. In such subjects, insulin levels are reduced and splanchnic fractional extraction of alanine is unchanged from the postabsorptive state. Nevertheless total splanchnic uptake of alanine is reduced as a consequence of diminished arterial alanine levels (Felig et al., 1969a) and decreased output of this amino acid from peripheral muscle (Felig et al., 1970a). Hypoalaninemia has also been implicated in the hypoglycemic response to starvation which occurs in pregnancy (Felig et al., 1972; Metzger et al., 1971), and in the syndrome of ketotic hypoglycemia of infancy and childhood (Pagliara et al., 1972). In these conditions direct observations of hepatic or splanchnic extraction of alanine are lacking. However, the prompt glycemic response to an infusion of alanine in these conditions suggests that hepatic extraction mechanisms are intact and that the failure to maintain normoglycemia is due to substrate lack.

The hypoglycemic effects of ethanol have received intensive interest in recent years. Studies with liver slices in the rat (Freinkel et al., 1965) and observations on incorporation of ^{14}C-alanine into blood glucose in intact man indicate that ethanol interferes with gluconeogenesis from alanine by virtue of a direct hepatic effect. Evidence of an additional mechanism has recently been reported. In normal subjects (Kreisberg et al., 1972) as well as in diabetics (Kalkhoff and Kim, 1973), ethanol administration has been demonstrated to cause a diminution in plasma alanine concentrations. Thus, in the case of alcohol hypoglycemia, interference with gluconeogenesis involves both a hepatic as well as a substrate effect (Table 2).

SUMMARY

Amino acid exchange between muscle and liver involves net transfer by way of blood cells as well as plasma. Alanine predominates in this inter-organ transfer of aminogenic glucose precursors, with 20–25% of its net release from muscle and gut and 30% of the uptake by the liver occurring via blood cells. Increased hepatic uptake of alanine has been demonstrated to occur in diabetes, brief starvation, obesity, prolonged exercise and glucocorticoid excess. The mechanisms responsible for these increases in gluconeogenesis include insulin lack (diabetes, brief starvation), insulin resistance (obesity), augmented precursor availability (exercise, glucocorticoids) and hyperglucagonemia (starvation, exercise, glucocorticoids). Stimulation of endogenous insulin secretion results in diminished hepatic alanine uptake as a consequence of a direct action of insulin on the liver. A decrease in alanine availability contributes to altered gluconeogenesis in prolonged starvation, pregnancy, ketotic hypoglycemia and following alcohol administration.

REFERENCES

AHLBORG, G., FELIG, P., HAGENFELDT, L., HENDLER, R. and WAHREN, J. (1974): *J. clin. Invest., 53,* in press.

AOKI, T. T., BRENNAN, M. F., MULLER, W. A., MOORE, F. D. and CAHILL Jr., G. F. (1972): Effect of insulin on muscle glutamate uptake. Whole blood versus plasma glutamate analysis. *J. clin. Invest., 51,* 2889.

EXTON, J. H., FRIEDMANN, N., WONG, E. H., BRINEAUX, J. A., CORBIN, J. D. and PARK, C. R. (1972): Interaction of glucocorticoids with glucagon and epinephrine in the control of gluconeogenesis and glucogenolysis in liver and of lipolysis in adipose tissue. *J. biol Chem., 247,*3579.

FELIG, P., OWEN, O. E., WAHREN, J. and CAHILL Jr., G. F. (1969a): Amino acid metabolism during prolonged starvation. *J. clin. Invest., 48,* 584.

FELIG, P., MARLISS, E. and CAHILL Jr., G. F. (1969b): Plasma amino acid levels and insulin secretion in obesity. *New Engl. J. Med., 281,* 811.

FELIG, P., POZEFSKY, T., MARLISS, E. and CAHILL Jr., G. F. (1970a): Alanine: Key role in gluconeogenesis. *Science, 167,* 1003.

FELIG, P., MARLISS, E., OHMAN, J. L. and CAHILL Jr., G. F. (1970b): Plasma amino acid levels in diabetic ketoacidosis. *Diabetes, 19,* 727.

FELIG, P. and WAHREN, J. (1971a): Amino acid metabolism in exercising man. *J. clin. Invest., 50,* 1703.

FELIG, P. and WAHREN, J. (1971b): Central role of alanine in gluconeogenesis: The glucose-alanine cycle. In: *Diabetes, Proceedings of the 7th Congress of the International Diabetes Federation,* p. 583. Editor: R. R. Rodriguez. International Congress Series No. 231, Excerpta Medica, Amsterdam.

FELIG, P. and WAHREN, J. (1971c): Influence of endogenous insulin titration on splenic glucose and amino acid metabolism in man. *J. clin. Invest., 50,* 1702

FELIG, P., KIM, H. J., LYNCH, V. and HENDLER, R. (1972): Amino acid metabolism during starvation in human pregnancy. *J. clin. Invest., 51,* 1195.

FELIG, P. (1973): The glucose-alanine cycle. *Metabolism, 22,* 179.

FELIG, P., WAHREN, J. and RAF, L. (1973): Evidence of the inter-organ amino acid transport by blood cells in humans. *Proc. nat. Acad. Sci. USA, 70,* 1775.

FELIG, P., WAHREN, J., HENDLER, R. and BRUNDIN, T. (1974): *J. clin. Invest., 53,* in press.

FREINKEL, N., COHEN, A. K., ARKY, R. A. and FOSTER, A. E. (1965): Alcohol hypoglycemia. II. A postulated mechanism of action based on experiments with rat liver slices. *J. clin. Endocr., 25,* 76.

HENNES, A. R., WAJCHENBERG, B. L., FAJANS, S. S. and CONN, J. W. (1957): *Metabolism, 6,* 339.

HULTMAN, E. and NILSSON, L. H. (1971): *Advanc. exp. Biol. Med., 11,* 143.

KALKHOFF, R. K. and KIM. H. J. (1973): Metabolic responses to fasting and ethanol infusion in obese, diabetic subjects. Relationship to insulin deficiency. *Diabetes, 22,* 372.

KARAM, J. H., GRODSKY, G. M. and FORSHAM, P. H. (1963): Excessive insulin response to glucose in obese subjects as measured by immunochemical assay. *Diabetes, 12,* 197.

KREISBERG, R. A., SIEGAL, A. M. and OWEN, W. C. (1972): Alanine and gluconeogenesis in man. Effect of ethanol. *J. clin. Endocr., 34,* 876.

LONG, C. N. H., KATZIN, B. and FRY, E. G. (1940): *Endocrinology, 26,* 309.

MARCO, J., CALLE, C., ROMAN, D., DIAZ-FIERROS, M., VILLANUEVA, M. and VALVERDE, I. (1973): Hyperglucagonism induced by glucocorticoid treatment in man. *New Engl. J. Med., 288,* 128.

MALETTE, L. E., EXTON, J. H. and PARK, C. R. (1969): Control of gluconeogenesis from amino acids in the perfused rat lever. *J. biol. Chem., 244,* 5713.

MARLISS, E.B., AOKI, T. T., UNGER, R. H., SOELDNER, J. S. and CAHILL Jr., G. F. (1970): Glucagon levels and metabolic effects in fasting man. *J. clin. Invest., 49,* 2256.

MARLISS, E. B., AOKI, T. T., POZEFSKY, T., MOST, A. S. and CAHILL Jr., G. F. (1971): Muscle and splanchnic glutamine and glutamate metabolism on postabsorptive and starved man. *J. clin. Invest., 50,* 814.

METZGER, B. E., HARE, J. W. and FREINKEL, N. (1971): Carbohydrate metabolism in pregnancy. IX. Plasma levels of gluconeogenic fuels during fasting in the rat. *J. clin. Endocr., 33,* 869.

MULLER, W. A., FALOONA, G. and UNGER, R. H. (1971): The effect of alanine on glucagon secretion. *J. clin. Invest., 50,* 2215.

OGILVIE, R. F. (1935): *Quart. J. Med., 4,* 345.

PAGLIARA, A. S., KARL, I. E., DeVIVO, D. C., FEIGIN, R. D. and KIPNIS, D. M. (1972): Hypoalaninemia: a concomitant of ketotic hypoglycemia. *J. clin. Invest., 51,* 1440.

RABINOWITZ, D. and ZIERLER, K. L. (1962): Forearm metabolism in obesity and its response to intra-arterial insulin. Characterization of insulin resistance and evidence for adaptive hyperinsulinism. *J. clin. Invest., 41,* 2173.

ROSS, B. D., HEMS, R. and KREBS, H. A. (1967): The rate of gluconeogenesis from various precursors in the perfused rat liver. *Biochem. J., 102,* 943.

SALANS, L. B., KNITTLE, J. L. and HIRSCH, J. (1968): The role of adipose cell size and adipose tissue insulin sensitivity in the carbohydrate intolerance of human obesity. *J. clin. Invest., 47,* 153.

SMITH, O. K. and LING, C. N. H. (1967): Effect of cortisol on the plasma amino nitrogen of eviscerated adrenalectomized diabetic rats. *Endocrinology, 80,* 561.

WAHREN, J., FELIG, P., CERASI, E. and LUFT, R. (1972): Splanchnic and peripheral glucose and amino acid metabolism in diabetes mellitus. *J. clin. Invest., 51,* 1870.

WISE, J. K., HENDLER, R. and FELIG, P. (1973): Influence of glucocorticoids on glucagon secretion and plasma amino acid concentrations in man. *J. clin. Invest., 52,* 2774.

WINTER, C. G. and CHRISTENSEN, H. N. (1964): Migration of amino acids across the membrane of the human erythrocyte. *J. biol. Chem., 239,* 872.

YOUNG, D. R., PELLIGRA, R., SHAPIRA, J., ADACHI, R. R. and SKRETTINGLAND, K. (1967): Glucose oxidation and replacement during prolonged exercise in man. *J. appl. Physiol., 23,* 734.

INTERACTIONS OF INSULIN, KETONE BODIES AND FREE FATTY ACIDS IN THE REGULATION OF PERIPHERAL UTILIZATION OF SUBSTRATES*

E. O. BALASSE

Laboratory of Experimental Medicine, University of Brussels, Brussels, Belgium

The rate of utilization of a metabolic substrate is essentially dependent on 3 main factors: (1) the blood concentration of the substrate, (2) the hormonal milieu, and (3) the presence of other substrates which can compete with (or sometimes enhance) the utilization of the substrate under study.

The data to be reported here summarize some of our recent personal results on the regulation of fuel consumption and the presentation will be focused on 2 main topics: (a) the role of insulin in the regulation of peripheral utilization of ketone bodies, and (b) the role of plasma FFA in glucose homeostasis. All the experiments have been performed in vivo either in dogs or in man using constant infusions of ^{14}C-labeled substrates which allow the estimation of rates of turnover and oxidation by commonly used techniques.

Part of the results have been published earlier in a more extensive form (Balasse and Havel, 1971; Balasse and Neef, 1973; Balasse and Ooms, 1973).

INFLUENCE OF INSULIN ON THE PERIPHERAL UTILIZATION OF KETONE BODIES

When present at high concentration (as in starvation or uncontrolled diabetes), ketone bodies are known to play a major role in the supply of energy to various tissues. The prominent role of insulin in the control of ketogenesis is well known, but its possible influence on the regulation of ketone utilization by peripheral tissues is still a matter of debate (Balasse and Havel, 1971). In our studies, this problem has been approached along 2 different lines.

Effect of insulin deprivation on peripheral ketone utilization

Ketotic depancreatized dogs deprived of insulin for 48–72 hours were infused at a constant rate with 3-^{14}C-acetoacetate to determine the turnover rate of ketone bodies. Comparable studies were performed in control animals. This group consisted of normal

* This work was supported in part by U.S. Public Health Service Grant HE-06285, by the Fonds de la Recherche Scientifique Médicale (Grant 20193) and by the Ministère Belge de la Politique Scientifique, within the framework of the association Euratom – University of Brussels – University of Pisa.

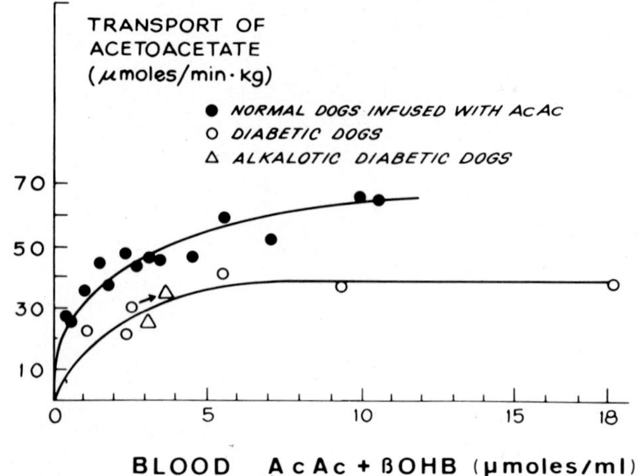

FIG. 1. Relationship between the rates of transport of acetoacetate and ketone concentration in normal and diabetic dogs. Two ketotic diabetic dogs rendered alkalotic with bicarbonate infusions showed no improvement in ketone utilization (from Balasse and Havel, 1971, by courtesy).

dogs rendered artificially ketotic by a constant infusion of unlabeled acetoacetate in variable amounts to obtain a range of ketonemia comparable to that observed in the diabetic dogs. Figure 1 shows the exponential relationship between the turnover rate of acetoacetate and corresponding ketone concentrations in the 2 groups.

Comparison of the 2 groups provides the following information: (1) maximal capacity to utilize ketones amounts to about 70 μmoles/kg/min. in normal dogs whereas it does not exceed 40 μmoles/kg/min. in diabetic animals; (2) for any turnover rate lower than 30 μmoles/kg/min., the ketone concentration in the diabetic dog is about 3 times that in the normal dog; (3) the highest rate of ketogenesis observed in diabetic dogs amounts to about 40 μmoles/kg/min. At this turnover rate, the ketone concentration in normal dogs would not exceed 2 μmoles/ml whereas actual values in diabetic animals vary between 6 and 18 μmoles/ml. These results indicate that the uptake of ketones by extrahepatic tissues is considerably impaired in insulin-deficient animals.

Effect of insulin administration on peripheral utilization of ketones

It would be interesting to know whether the ketone removal defect observed in uncontrolled diabetes can be corrected by administration of insulin. However, this possibility is difficult to test because the injection of insulin to a diabetic dog would decrease the ketone concentration by virtue of its antiketogenic action and make it difficult to detect a direct effect of this hormone on peripheral removal of ketones. Therefore, the effect of insulin on ketone utilization was tested in normal postabsorptive animals infused at a constant rate with amounts of acetoacetate greatly exceeding the expected endogenous production. Under these conditions, the rate of inflow of ketone bodies into the blood compartment is only minimally influenced by the injection of insulin, and the effects of this hormone on ketone uptake can be easily evaluated. Using this experimental approach, we were able to show (Balasse and Havel, 1971) that the infusion of large amounts of insulin (plus glucose in order to prevent hypoglycemia) induced a 35% increase in the fractional removal rate of ketone bodies and a 40% increase in their fractional oxidation.

The 2 groups of data presented above strongly suggest that peripheral utilization of ketones is, at least partly, controlled by insulin. However, they do not provide information on its mechanism of action. Experiments were designed in order to test whether the effect of insulin on peripheral ketone utilization could be mediated by the action of this hormone on the metabolism of FFA which might compete with ketones as a fuel. For this purpose, we tested the effects of an increase in plasma FFA on the uptake and the oxidation of infused acetoacetate (Fig. 2). Six normal animals were infused – at a constant rate and for 300 minutes – with acetoacetate (30.7–62.5 μmoles/kg/min.) containing 3-^{14}C-acetoacetate. After a basal period of 200 minutes, a triglyceride emulsion was infused in combination with heparin, so that plasma FFA rose to concentrations as high as 1.5 μmoles/ml. This was accompanied by a very slow rise in ketone concentration

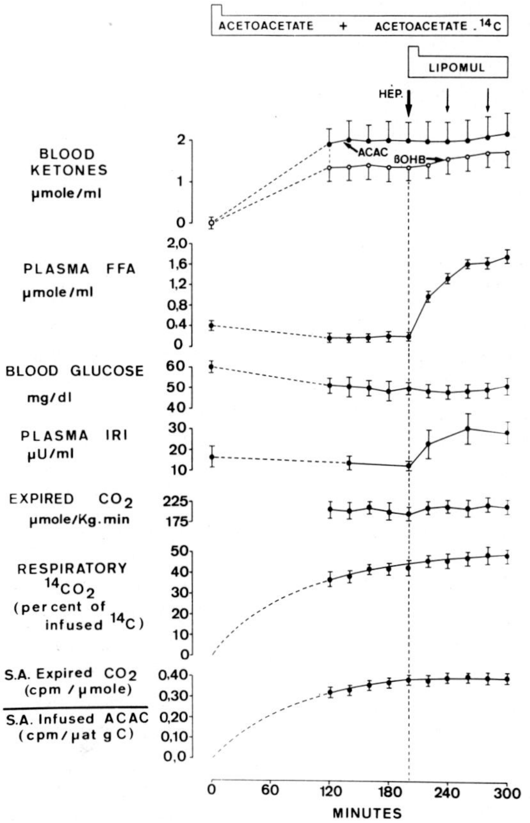

FIG. 2. Influence of an experimental increase in plasma FFA levels (obtained by administration of Lipomul and heparin) on the uptake and the oxidation of infused ketones in normal dogs. Average results ± S.E.M. (n = 6).

probably related to a slight increase in ketogenesis from circulating FFA. A small elevation in IRI concentration was also noticed but glycemia remained unchanged. The efflux of $^{14}CO_2$ and the specific activity of expired CO_2 rose slowly with time and was unaffected by the sudden increase in plasma FFA concentration. These data indicate that under our experimental conditions plasma FFA do not successfully compete with ketones as a substrate for oxidation. It is therefore unlikely that the effects of insulin on ketone utilization are mediated through changes in FFA availability to tissues.

Our results on the role of insulin in the control of ketone utilization clearly indicate that severe diabetic ketoacidosis cannot be explained only on the basis of an overproduction of this substrate. Severe hyperketonemia can only occur because the overproduction is associated with a reduced capacity of diabetic tissues to remove ketones from blood. This concept is further substantiated by the observation that in normal dogs the fractional removal rate and the oxidation of exogenous ketone bodies can be stimulated by the administration of insulin.

When the present data are integrated with other known effects of insulin on ketone metabolism, it can be concluded that this hormone regulates ketonemia by acting at 3 different levels: (1) insulin regulates adipose tissue lipolysis, thereby controlling the availability to the liver of FFA which are the primary ketogenic substrate; (2) insulin influences the intrahepatic fate of FFA in such a way that it reduces their fractional conversion to ketones (Bieberdorf et al., 1970; McGarry and Foster, 1972); (3) insulin enhances the uptake and the oxidation of ketone bodies by extrahepatic tissues. The mechanism of this latter effect is presently unknown. Some of our data suggest that it is not related to a competitive effect of FFA on ketone utilization at the peripheral level.

PARTICIPATION OF PLASMA FFA IN THE CONTROL OF INSULIN SECRETION AND GLUCOSE UTILIZATION

Two aspects of this regulation in man will be discussed: (1) the insulinotropic effects of FFA; and (2) the operation of the glucose-fatty acid cycle in vivo.

Role of plasma FFA in the control of insulin secretion in man

Long chain fatty acids are undoubtedly capable of stimulating insulin secretion in various animal species. The most remarkable demonstration of this effect has been made in dogs by Crespin et al. (1969) who showed that the infusion of oleate in dogs elicits a marked rise in insulin concentration accompanied by hypoglycemia. Several reports indicate that in man the basal insulin concentration is little affected by experimental changes in FFA levels, but there is some evidence that the insulinic response to glucose is enhanced in the presence of elevated FFA concentration (Schalch and Kipnis, 1965; Balasse and Ooms, 1968). The following data recently published by our laboratory (Balasse and Ooms, 1973) further emphasize the modulating role of plasma FFA on beta cell reactivity.

Figure 3 shows that the plasma insulin response to i.v. administration of glucose, tolbutamide or glucagon is significantly reduced when plasma FFA levels have been depressed by the injection of nicotinic acid, while basal IRI levels are minimally affected. In these experiments, each subject was tested both under basal conditions and during the administration of nicotinic acid (100 mg i.v. every 15 min., starting 2 hr before the injection of the insulinotropic agent).

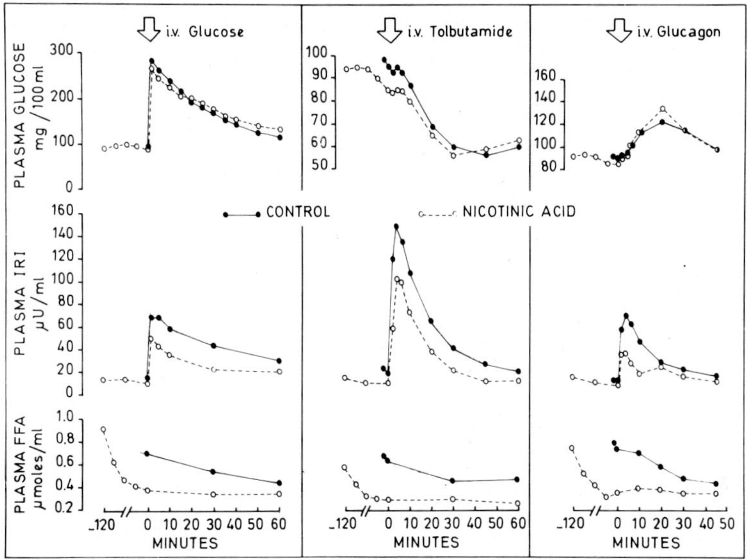

FIG. 3. Average concentration of plasma glucose, IRI and FFA after i.v. glucose (n = 13), i.v. tolbutamide (n,= 6) or i.v. glucagon (n = 7) in the basal state(●———●) and during administration of nicotinic acid (○– – – –○). The nicotinic acid-induced inhibition of IRI response averaged (± S.E.M.) 31 ± 7% ($P < 0.001$) for the glucose test, 32 ± 9% ($P < 0.02$) for the tolbutamide test and 33 ± 9% ($P < 0.02$) for the glucagon test (from Balasse and Ooms, 1973, by courtesy).

A similar experimental protocol was used to demonstrate that an increase in FFA levels amplifies the beta cell response to i.v. glucose, tolbutamide and glucagon while the basal insulin concentration remains unchanged (Fig. 4). The rise in FFA levels was obtained by the combined administration of a fat meal (100 g of triglycerides given as milk cream 4 hr before the pancreatic stimulation) and i.v. heparin (80 mg in divided doses started 2 hr after the oral fat).

Effects of changes in FFA levels on the rates of turnover and oxidation of plasma glucose in man

The effects of modifications of FFA levels on the rates of turnover and oxidation of plasma glucose have been studied using a constant infusion of $1\text{-}^{14}C$-glucose. In a first group of 6 overnight fasted obese patients, glucose kinetics has been measured both in the basal state and during the administration of nicotinic acid, each subject serving as its own control. Average results (Table 1) indicate that antilipolysis induced by nicotinic acid increases the fractional disappearance rate of plasma glucose by an average of 25% despite a small but significant fall in IRI concentration, suggesting that a decrease in FFA levels enhances the sensitivity to insulin. The increased fractional removal rate is entirely compensated by a stimulation of the hepatic glucose output (turnover rate) so that glycemia remains unchanged. The oxidation of glucose was also stimulated: the fraction of total CO_2 production deriving from plasma glucose increased by 32%, this effect resulting from

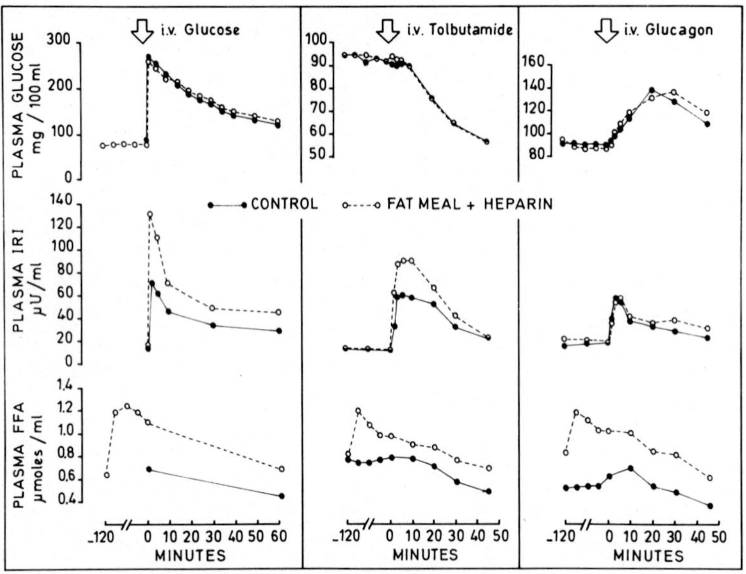

FIG. 4. Average concentration of plasma glucose, IRI, and FFA after i.v. glucose (n = 12), i.v. tolbutamide (n = 7) or i.v. glucagon (n = 8) in the basal state (●———●) and after administration of a fat meal and heparin (○– – – –○). The fat meal heparin-induced increase in IRI response averaged (± S.E.M.) 178 ± 79% ($P < 0.05$) for the glucose test, 58 ± 17% ($P < 0.02$) for the tolbutamide test and 14 ± 5% ($P < 0.05$) for the glucagon test (from Balasse and Ooms, 1973).

TABLE 1

Effect of the administration of nicotinic acid or of a fat meal and heparin on plasma FFA, plasma IRI and glucose metabolism in man

	Nicotinic acid (n = 6)	Fat meal + heparin (n = 8)
	Average percent change from control	
Plasma FFA	– 64 ± 5	+ 117 ± 22
Plasma IRI	– 37 ± 6	+ 125 ± 69
Plasma glucose		
concentration	– 3 ± 2	+ 1 ± 2
fractional removal rate	+ 25 ± 6	– 9 ± 3
hepatic output	+ 20 ± 3	– 9 ± 3
fraction oxidized	+ 20 ± 4	– 13 ± 5
% CO_2 from glucose	+ 32 ± 6	– 22 ± 3

the combination of an increase in turnover rate and in the fractional oxidation of glucose.

When nicotinic acid is used to lower FFA levels in starved (8 days) obese subjects, results obtained are qualitatively similar to those observed in overnight fasted subjects. Objections have been raised regarding the validity of conclusions drawn from studies using nicotinic acid since a direct effect of the drug on glucose metabolism cannot be excluded. However, this criticism does not seem to hold in view of our observation that glucose metabolism remains unaffected in patients who fail to respond to nicotinic acid by a significant decrease in FFA concentration (Balasse and Neef, 1973).

Studies with labeled glucose have also been undertaken in 8 normal overnight fasted subjects in order to evaluate the influence of an increase in FFA concentration on glucose metabolism; the average results are reported in Table 1. The rise in plasma FFA levels induced by the combined administration of a fat meal and heparin is accompanied by a 9% reduction in the fractional removal rate of glucose despite the occurrence of a slight although not significant hyperinsulinemia. These results are best interpreted as indicating a reduced sensitivity of tissues to insulin in the presence of elevated FFA levels. The reduced fractional disappearance rate is compensated by an inhibition of the hepatic glucose output of comparable amplitude, so that glycemia remains unaffected. The high FFA levels induced a 22% reduction in the contribution of plasma glucose to total CO_2 production, this effect resulting from a decrease in both the turnover rate and the fractional oxidation of glucose.

When all the data pertaining to the influence of FFA on glucose utilization are taken into account, it appears (Fig. 5) that a significant correlation exists between the experimentally-induced changes in FFA concentration (in plus or minus) and the corresponding modifications in glucose metabolism, whatever the parameter taken into consideration (changes in turnover rate, in fractional oxidation or in the contribution of glucose to CO_2 production). The FFA-glucose interrelationships are also clearly apparent when absolute values of parameters of glucose metabolism are plotted against corresponding absolute FFA levels (Fig. 6). These data, obtained under a variety of experimental conditions, indicate that the amplitude of glucose utilization is inversely correlated with plasma FFA over a wide range of concentrations.

Overall significance of plasma FFA in the control of glucose metabolism in man

Taken as a whole, the above results indicate that the availability of FFA to tissues is an important determinant of overall glucose metabolism. The influence of FFA can be observed at at least 2 different levels. Firstly the response of the pancreatic beta cells to a variety of stimuli seems to be modulated by the plasma FFA concentration in such a way that high FFA tend to enhance beta cell reactivity whereas low FFA levels tend to reduce it. Secondly, the sensitivity of tissues to insulin is also dependent on FFA levels, hyperlipacidemia reducing insulin sensitivity and glucose utilization and hypolipacidemia producing the opposite effect.

This dual action of FFA might account – at least partly – for the frequently observed association between high FFA levels, hyperinsulinism and insulin resistance. It is well known that this metabolic syndrome occurs in a variety of conditions such as obesity, acromegaly and pregnancy, which might represent examples of clinical situations in which the 'glucose-fatty acid cycle' plays an important pathophysiological role.

As suggested by Randle et al. (1963), the competitive effect of FFA on glucose utilization seems to be primarily located at the muscular level. Since cardiac and skeletal

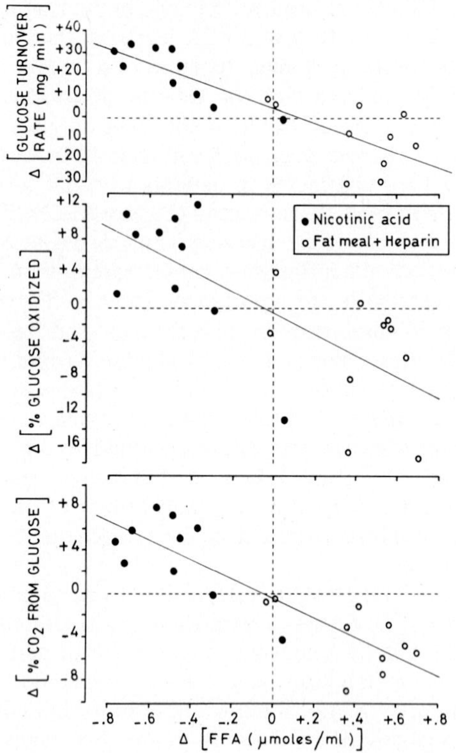

FIG. 5. Correlation between experimentally-induced changes in plasma FFA concentrations and corresponding modifications in the rates of turnover and oxidation of plasma glucose in man.

muscles account for only a small part of total glucose uptake in overnight fasted patients (30 g for a total glucose turnover of about 180 g per day), it can be calculated that the 20% rise in glucose turnover rate occurring after nicotinic acid represents a more than 100% increase in muscle glucose uptake. This figure emphasizes the considerable quantitative importance of FFA in muscle glucose utilization in vivo.

The changes in hepatic glucose output observed in our experiments cannot be directly ascribed to the changes in FFA availability to the liver. Indeed in vitro experiments on the perfused liver have shown that FFA stimulate gluconeogenesis and glucose production (Struck et al., 1966) whereas opposite effects were observed in the present experiments carried out in vivo. This discrepancy can probably be accounted for by the hormonal changes associated with the induced variations in FFA levels. The modifications in insulin concentration observed in these studies are one possible explanation of the observed changes in hepatic glucose output; the known inhibitory effect of FFA on glucagon secretion (Luyckx and Lefebvre, 1970) might represent an additional factor.

It is tempting to speculate on the fact that the operation of the glucose-fatty acid cycle is easily demonstrable under normoglycemic conditions (using a glucose tracer) whereas it has never been convincingly established from studies using glucose tolerance

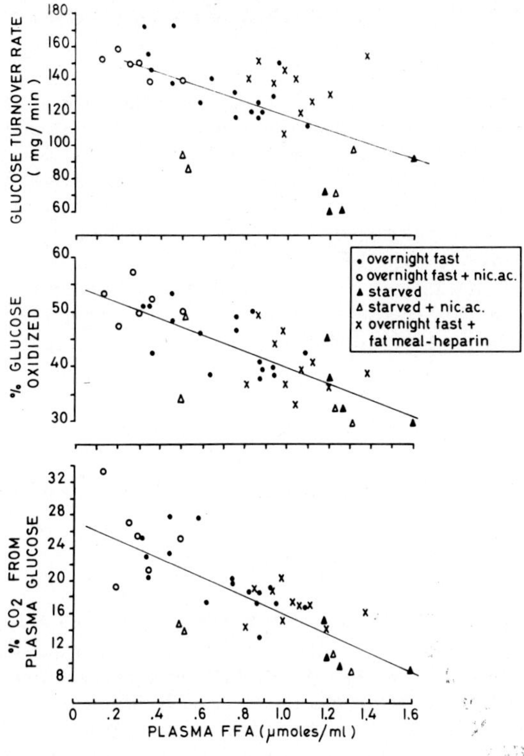

FIG. 6. Relationship between plasma FFA levels and parameters of glucose utilization under various experimental conditions in man.

tests as an index of glucose utilization. One likely explanation is that the potentiating effect of FFA on IRI response to a glucose load tends to mask their inhibitory action on glucose utilization, the overall effect of FFA on glucose tolerance being therefore highly variable.

SUMMARY

Role of insulin in the peripheral utilization of ketone bodies in dogs

a. Insulin deprivation is associated with an impairment of mechanisms for utilizing ketones. This defect contributes to ketosis and is probably essential in the development of severe ketoacidosis.

b. The administration of insulin and glucose to normal dogs increases the fractional removal rate and the oxidation of infused ketones.

c. Experimentally-induced elevations of FFA levels do not significantly reduce the uptake nor the oxidation of infused ketone bodies. It is thus unlikely that the regulatory role of insulin on ketone utilization is mediated through changes in availability of FFA to tissues.

Participation of plasma FFA in the regulation of insulin secretion and glucose utilization in man

a. The insulinic response to glucose, tolbutamide and glucagon is inhibited after experimental antilipolysis induced by nicotinic acid, whereas it is enhanced when plasma FFA levels are raised by means of a fat meal and heparin.
b. Studies with ^{14}C-glucose indicate that the experimental lowering of plasma FFA increases the fractional removal rate of plasma glucose, the hepatic glucose production, the glucose oxidation and the sensitivity to insulin. Opposite effects are observed after experimental elevations of plasma FFA.

These data suggest that plasma FFA play an important role in the regulation of insulin secretion and in the control of glucose utilization in man. They strongly support the idea that the glucose-fatty acid cycle is operative in man.

ACKNOWLEDGEMENTS

The technical assistance of M. A. Neef and D. Calay is gratefully acknowledged.

REFERENCES

BALASSE, E. O. and HAVEL, R. J. (1971): Evidence for an effect of insulin on the peripheral utilization of ketone bodies in dogs. *J. clin. Invest., 50,* 801.

BALASSE, E. O. and NEEF, M. A. (1973): Influence of nicotinic acid on the rates of turnover and oxidation of plasma glucose in man. *Metabolism, 22,* 1193.

BALASSE, E. O. and OOMS, H. A. (1968): Effet d'une élévation aiguë du taux des acides gras libres (NEFA) sur la tolérance glucidique et la réponse insulinique à l'hyperglycémie chez l'homme normal. *Rev. Franç. étud. clin. biol., 13,* 62.

BALASSE, E. O. and OOMS, H. A. (1973): Role of plasma free fatty acids in the control of insulin secretion in man. *Diabetologia, 9,* 145.

BIEBERDORF, F. A., CHERNICK, S. S. and SCOW, R. O. (1970): Effect of insulin and acute diabetes on plasma FFA and ketone bodies in the fasting rat. *J. clin. Invest., 49,* 1685.

CRESPIN, S. R., GREENOUGH III, W. B. and STEINBERG, D. (1969): Stimulation of insulin secretion by infusion of free fatty acids. *J. clin. Invest., 48,* 1934.

LUYCKX, A. S. and LEFEBVRE, P. J. (1970): Arguments for a regulation of pancreatic glucagon secretion by circulating plasma free fatty acids. *Proc. Soc. exp. Biol. Med. (N.Y.)., 133,* 524.

McGARRY, J. D. and FOSTER, D. W. (1972): Regulation of ketogenesis and clinical aspects of the ketosis. *Metabolism, 21,* 471.

RANDLE, P. J., GARLAND, P. B., HALES, C. N. and NEWSHOLME, E. A. (1963): The glucose-fatty acid cycle. Its role in insulin sensitivity and the metabolic disturbances of diabetes mellitus. *Lancet, 1,* 785.

SCHALCH, D. S. and KIPNIS, D. M. (1965): Abnormalities in carbohydrate tolerance associated with elevated plasma nonesterified fatty acids. *J. clin. Invest., 44,* 2010.

STRUCK, E., ASHMORE, J. and WIELAND, O. (1966): Effects of glucagon and long chain fatty acids on glucose production by isolated perfused rat liver. *Advanc. Enzyme Regulat., 4,* 219.

GLUCAGON REGULATION OF METABOLIC FUEL SUPPLY

E. B. MARLISS and J. R. GIRARD

Department of Medicine, University of Toronto, Toronto, Ontario, Canada
and Laboratoire de Physiologie Comparée, Université de Paris, Paris, France

Instead of entering directly into the controversy revolving around whether glucagon is an essential gluconeogenic hormone in man and other species, this review will take a rather unorthodox chronological glance at the potential roles of this hormone in a number of the physiologic and pathologic vicissitudes that befall the organism from birth through to the serious illness which usually heralds its demise. In keeping with the claim to unorthodoxy, this review will stress one aspect of the effects of glucagon which once aroused interest, then was definitively laid to rest, and is now being resurrected: the possibility of important physiologic effects on muscle metabolism. With respect to the classical hepatic glycogenolytic effect of this hormone, there is little dubiety as to its physiologic importance in situations of acute glucose need. A role for glucagon in the regulation of fatty acid mobilization from triglycerides has been proposed. This is a concept strongly supported by the Belgian investigators and has been reviewed in detail recently (Lefebvre, 1972). Therefore, this presentation will seek to correlate secretory responses and effects of glucagon to some events related to protein and amino acid metabolism.

The background requisite to the understanding of hormonal influences on amino acid fluxes bears upon the direction and magnitude of movements of individual amino acids in the intact organism. These have been reviewed by Felig (this Volume, pp. 217–230) and may be found detailed in a number of original articles (Felig et al., 1969, 1970; Felig and Wahren, 1971) and recent reviews (Marliss and Aoki, 1972; Felig, 1972; Ruderman and Lund, 1972). The effects of glucagon on amino acid metabolism have likewise been the subject of a recent review (Marliss et al., 1972). As a first approximation: in the state beginning after the last meal has been totally metabolized there is net movement of most free plasma amino acids from the muscle beds to the splanchnic circulation. This is most apparent for those amino acids destined largely for conversion by the liver into glucose: alanine, glycine, threonine, and serine; the large peripheral glutamine output appears to be dealt with by the kidney (Owen and Robinson, 1963) and the intestinal portion of the splanchnic circulation rather than the liver (Felig, this Volume pp. 217–230). Other potentially important body stores of protein, such as connective tissue and epithelia, are more difficult to study in vivo. Hence, few data are available on the contribution of such tissues to fuel fluxes, though they may well be important. Such periphery to liver (and kidney) transport serves to convey carbon skeletons which may be converted to glucose, and potentially harmful amino groups which are removed from the organism by the liver as urea and by the kidney as ammonia. This general outline has been moderately complicated by the recent demonstration of differing contributions of blood cell versus plasma compartments to the flux across specific circulatory beds (Aoki et al., 1973; Wise et al., 1973). However, the changes in interpretation are mainly quantitative, and the direction of fluxes previously demonstrated by plasma studies remains generally valid for the fasted state.

In mammals, life begins in a diametrically opposite state, namely, a continuous, unremitting, maternal amino acid supply to the fetus across the placenta. This may be considered to be the only 'continuously fed' state that the organism experiences in a physiologic context. Oxidative fuels are supplied by the maternal circulation in the form of glucose and ketone bodies, and the amino acid substrate for maximal anabolism of protein in the fetus similarly arrives via the placenta. Indeed, the studies of metabolic fuels in the pregnant rat (Metzger et al., 1971) and woman (Felig and Lynch, 1970) suggest that they are in an accelerated catabolic state to provide for the fetus. Protein mobilization is increased, and levels of glucogenic amino acids are decreased (Freinkel et al., 1972).

Such an adaptation in the rat could be attributable to the altered hormone levels shown in Table 1. In the pregnant rat, elevated glucagon level, alone responsible for the decreased insulin/glucagon ratio, is such as to convert the latter to a relationship favoring catabolism (Unger, 1971). Whereas increased glucagon levels would be expected to induce the observed maternal amino acid changes (Bromer and Chance, 1969) and protein catabolism (Marliss et al., 1970), a contributory role for the hormones of gestation is possible (Landau and Lugibihl, 1967). In addition, since other steroid hormones have been shown

TABLE 1

Plasma hormones in virgin and pregnant rats and their fetuses (21.5 days)§

	Virgin	Pregnant	Fetus
Immunoreactive insulin ng/ml	0.85 ± 0.06 (6)	0.92 ± 0.11 (9)	8.0 ± 0.8+ (12)
Immunoreactive glucagon pg/ml	200 ± 20 (6)	560 ± 40* (10)	270 ± 29+ (18)
Insulin/glucagon molar ratio	2.4	0.92	16.4
Growth hormone ng/ml	28 ± 4 (8)	103 ± 19* (12)	147 ± 8+ (29)

§ Data from Girard et al. (1973a).

* Indicates that pregnant rat values differ significantly from virgin rat values ($P < 0.05$, Student unpaired t test).

\+ Indicates that fetal values differ significantly from maternal values ($P < 0.05$, Student unpaired t test).

Data are presented as mean ± S.E.M. of number of observations indicated in parentheses.

to increase glucagon levels and responsiveness to aminogenic secretion (Marco et al., 1973; Felig and Wahren, 1973), it is conceivable that the altered hormonal milieu of pregnancy could influence the maternal alpha cell, in addition to the effects of fasting hypoglycemia (Freinkel et al., 1972; Felig and Lynch, 1970). In the present study, virgin and pregnant rats were in the fed state and glycemia was comparable. The elevation of growth hormone levels in the pregnant rat (Table 1) would appear to be appropriate to observed state (which is more akin to the fasted than the fed) in light of its adipokinetic and glucoregulatory effects.

The comparison of maternal with fetal hormone levels (Table 1) and fuels (Table 2) in the rat at term demonstrates dramatic differences. The role of glucagon as inferred by its circulating levels is opposite on the 2 sides of the placenta: on the maternal side, high levels are found, as described.

By contrast, the fetus prior to and at term has extremely high insulin levels, and lower glucagon levels, producing an insulin/glucagon ratio considered to be maximally anabolic (Unger, 1971). This would be highly appropriate to a metabolic set for which no endogenous glucose is required (hence neither significant glycogenolysis nor gluconeogenesis) and in which available amino acids are channeled into protein synthesis – and which thus relegates glucagon to a role of little importance in amino acid flux. Whether the presence of glucagon is required to assure the appearance of the appropriate enzymes for glyco-

TABLE 2

*Metabolic fuels and substrates in maternal and fetal circulations at term (21.5 days)**

	Maternal (10)	Fetal (10)	P<+
Blood glucose, mM	5.0 ± 0.4	3.7 ± 0.2	0.01
Blood lactate, mM	2.0 ± 0.1	7.8 ± 0.3	0.01
Blood pyruvate, mM	0.16 ± 0.02	0.10 ± 0.01	0.01
Lactate/pyruvate ratio	12.5	78.0	
Plasma α-amino nitrogen, mM	3.0 ± 0.2	9.2 ± 0.6	0.01
Plasma alanine, μM	210 ± 16	560 ± 40	0.01
Plasma glutamine, μM	350 ± 25	610 ± 50	0.01
Plasma free fatty acids, μM	230 ± 20	160 ± 20	0.05
Blood glycerol, μM	90 ± 10	38 ± 5	0.01
Blood β-hydroxybutyrate, μM	70 ± 8	81 ± 7	NS
Blood acetoacetate, μM	19 ± 2	18 ± 2	NS
β-hydroxybutyrate/acetoacetate ratio	3.69	4.50	

* Data from Girard et al. (1973a), presented as mean ± S.E.M.

\+ P value represents the significance of the difference between maternal and fetal values, by the Student unpaired t test.

genolysis and gluconeogenesis – though their activities are low – remains unanswered, pending a model of intrauterine alpha cell deficiency. A human newborn with probable congenital absence of pancreatic islets (i.e. both insulin and glucagon deficiency) was totally unable to withstand fasting due to hypoglycemia (without ketosis), was grossly glucose-intolerant, and was small-for-date (Sherwood et al., 1973)

It is of interest that amino acids are transported against a concentration gradient by the placenta to the fetus (Szabo and Grimaldi, 1970), so as to provide extremely high total alpha amino nitrogen levels as compared with the maternal side (Table 2). Levels of other substrates shown are equally appropriate to the metabolic state as defined: very low free fatty acids, glycerol and ketone bodies, and high levels of the gluconeogenic substrates alanine, glutamine, lactate and pyruvate.

At birth, a totally different metabolic set is imposed upon the organism: that of providing oxidative fuel from body stores on an urgent and continuing basis, until the first 'meal' arrives. Data from the rat allow for the interpretation that the glucagon secretory response is central to survival during this period. The newborn rat, in terms of body composition, is quite different from the human newborn and from the adult of its species. It has no appreciable white adipose tissue, and its only triglycerides are hepatic and in a small amount of brown adipose tissue. Hence, it must immediately produce glucose from either glycogen – of which it has large stores – or by gluconeogenesis, and it would appear to have very adequate amounts of circulating precursor (Table 2).

The hepatic conversion from a glycolytic to a glucose-producing organ occurs after a lag period. This period, lasting 1–2 hours, is associated with a rapid and profound hypoglycemia (Fig. 1). Recovery occurs over the succeeding 2 hours, in association with a

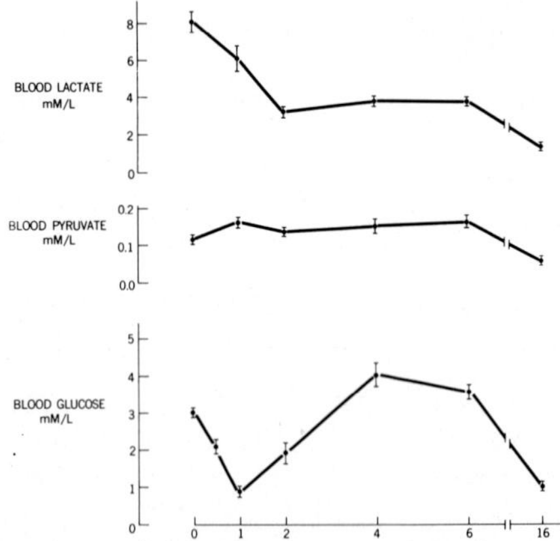

FIG. 1. Blood glucose, lactate and pyruvate in newborn rats fasted 16 hours after delivery by caesarean section at 21.5 days gestation. Animals were maintained isothermic (37°C) and 70% relative humidity. Mean ± S.E.M. From Girard et al. (1973a), by courtesy.

demonstrable increase in hepatic phosphorylase activity and a decrease in hepatic glycogen (Table 3; Cake and Oliver, 1969; Girard et al., 1972; Dawkins, 1963). However, a second phase of more gradual decline in blood glucose, but to the same marked degree, supervenes from 6 to 16 hours. The latter parallels the depletion of hepatic glycogen, essentially complete at 16 hours. It has been calculated that the glucose utilization rate of the newborn rat is 10–15 μmoles/hr (Ballard, 1971; Snell and Walker, 1973). It is apparent that at this rate of oxidation inadequate glycogen is available to maintain euglycemia after 10 hours (Table 3).

A stimulation of gluconeogenesis might be inferred based upon the fall in known glucose precursor levels (Figs 1 and 2), and the increase in assayable activity of glucose-6-phosphatase (Dawkins, 1963), and phosphoenolpyruvate carboxykinase (PEPCK, Table 3; Ballard, 1971; Yeung and Oliver, 1967), both of which occur concurrent with the restoration of normoglycemia. The K_m's and substrate levels are such as to be compatible with a significant increase in flux at these steps. However, any increment in gluconeogenesis which occurs is clearly insufficient to maintain blood glucose levels. Indeed, despite these changes in gluconeogenic enzymes, levels of amino acid substrates rise at 16 hours (Fig. 2). The implication of these findings is that gluconeogenesis is not sufficient during

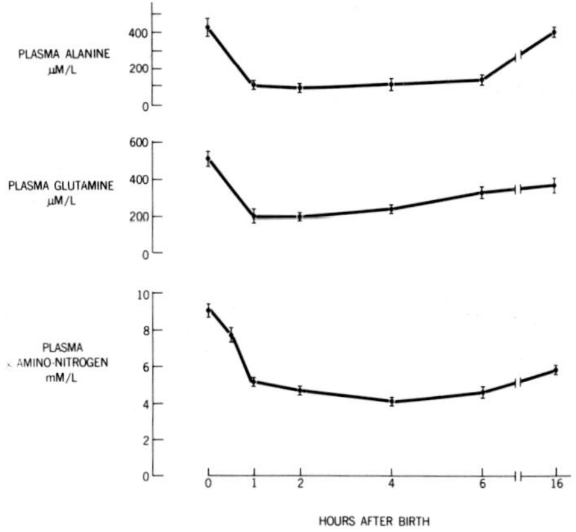

FIG. 2. Plasma α-amino nitrogen, alanine and glutamine in newborn rats fasted 16 hours. From Girard et al. (1973a), by courtesy.

this early phase of life to maintain euglycemia (in accord with previous observations (Ballard, 1971)). Data on conversion of exogenous substrates to glucose favor lactate and glycerol as precursors with relatively poor conversion of amino acids, including alanine (Vernon et al., 1968). It has been inferred previously that the sudden fall in circulating amino acid concentrations as shown in Figure 2 is due to hepatic uptake, perhaps with continued peripheral uptake. Data on the distribution ratios of infused ^{14}C-labelled aminoisobutyric acid (AIB) and cycloleucine suggest a doubling of muscle uptake and tripling of hepatic uptake between the fetus at term and the 4-hour-old newborn (Girard, unpublished results). However, after the administration of alanine-^{14}C, and following its incorporation into glucose-^{14}C, it is clear that even at the stage of restoration of blood glucose a maximum of 10–13% of the radioactivity administered appears in glucose (Table 4). Though this represents a 10-fold increase over the rate of conversion at birth, it falls short of the 23% observed on the second day of life in suckling rats. The earlier in vitro data and those presently reported suggest that transamination may in part be limiting for gluconeogenesis, since the hepatocyte appears capable of inward transport of amino acids (Christensen and Clifford, 1963) and of more efficient conversion of lactate

TABLE 3

*Blood and hepatic carbohydrate metabolism in fasted newborn rats**

	Hours after birth								
	0	1	2	4	6	8	10	12	16
Blood glucose, mM	3.0 ± 0.1	1.0 ± 0.2	1.9 ± 0.3	4.0 ± 0.3	3.5 ± 0.2	2.2 ± 0.1	1.6 ± 0.2	1.1 ± 0.1	1.0 ± 0.1
n	45	39	36	43	42	15	8	6	31
P<		0.01	0.02	0.01	NS	0.02	0.01	0.01	0.01
Phosphorylase μM P_i/hr/mg/prot.	5.30 ± 0.19	5.87 ± 0.21	6.87 ± 0.29	7.11 ± 0.34	6.54 ± 0.32				6.44 ± 0.19
n	13	9	13	10	9				13
P<		0.05	0.01	0.01	0.02				0.02
Glucose-6-phosphatase μM P_i/hr/mg/prot.	0.75 ± 0.04	1.00 ± 0.03	1.21 ± 0.06	1.43 ± 0.04	1.61 ± 0.04				2.75 ± 0.24
n	13	11	12	15	12				13
P<		0.01	0.01	0.01	0.01				0.01
PEPCK nM CO_2/hr/mg prot.	24 ± 3	48 ± 4	240 ± 28	1140 ± 90	1440 ± 120				1800 ± 120
n	12	12	15	13	13				12
P<		0.02	0.01	0.02	0.01				0.01
Glycogen mg/animal	28 ± 2	29 ± 2	25 ± 3	18 ± 3	13 ± 1	7 ± 1	3.4 ± 0.4	2.6 ± 0.2	2.0 ± 0.1
n	45	37	36	48	42	15	8	6	20
P<		NS	NS	0.05	0.01	0.01	0.01	0.01	0.01
μmoles glucose available from glycogen/hr[+]	–	–	22.3	19.5	13.9	16.7	10.0	2.2	0.8

* Data from Girard et al. (1973a), by courtesy. Presented as mean ± S.E.M.
P values represent the significance of the difference from the 0 time value (Student unpaired t test).
\+ Calculated for the time interval preceding the column in which the value appears.

TABLE 4
*Percent conversion of alanine-^{14}C to glucose-^{14}C in newborn rats**

Time after alanine-^{14}C (min.)	Hours of life: 0	1	2	4	6	48
15	0.65 ± 0.02 (12)	0.76 ± 0.04 (12)	2.0 ± 0.1 (17)	3.7 ± 0.2 (16)	6.8 ± 0.4 (16)	10.3 ± 0.2 (5)
30	0.94 ± 0.10 (5)	1.3 ± 0.2 (6)	2.3 ± 0.2 (13)	5.0 ± 0.3 (10)	12.8 ± 1.4 (5)	23.4 ± 1.0 (6)
60	0.95 ± 0.1 (6)	1.5 ± 0.2 (6)	2.3 ± 6.3 (13)	5.6 ± 0.3 (5)	10.9 ± 0.5 (5)	22.2 ± 2.2 (6)

* Calculations based upon conversion of tracer amount of alanine-^{14}C to glucose-^{14}C, with the latter assumed to be distributed into 85% of the body weight of the animal. The rats were delivered by caesarean section at 21.5 days gestation, then were fasted the number of hours indicated, prior to injection of alanine-^{14}C, except for those studied at 48 hours, which had been allowed normal suckling.

and glycerol to glucose. Since the mobilization of fatty acids is very small in this species (Fig. 3), limited hepatic oxidative substrates for the energy-requiring gluconeogenic process may also contribute.

The response of the endocrine pancreatic hormones is demonstrated in Figure 4. The very high insulin/glucagon ratio of the fetus converts rapidly to a very low one, which persists. This is contributed to by a marked fall in insulin and a 3-fold rise in glucagon levels. Such changes occur prior to the alterations in enzyme activity. In light of the demonstrated ability of exogenous glucagon to prematurely induce these enzyme changes in the rat fetus (reviewed in Girard et al., 1973a), it is probable that the observed response was in large measure responsible, and this is favored as well by the time relationships. A role for the inevitable catecholamine release at birth in inducing glycogenolysis directly, and indirectly via stimulation of glucagon secretion (Marliss et al., 1973), remains probable. It is to be noted that non-pancreatic glucagon-like immunoreactivity also rises acutely at birth in rats (Girard et al., 1972), even prior to alimentation. Thus a role for this group of substances, acting similarly, cannot be excluded. (The antiserum K47 used for the glucagon values reported would appear to be specific, though not totally, for native hormone of pancreatic origin (Heding, 1971).)

Additional arguments in favor of the altered fuel fluxes being significantly influenced by the glucagon response include: (1) the ability of exogenous glucagon to induce hypoaminoacidemia in the fetus analogous to that observed spontaneously at birth (Girard and Marliss, unpublished results). (2) The spontaneous appearance after birth of autophago-

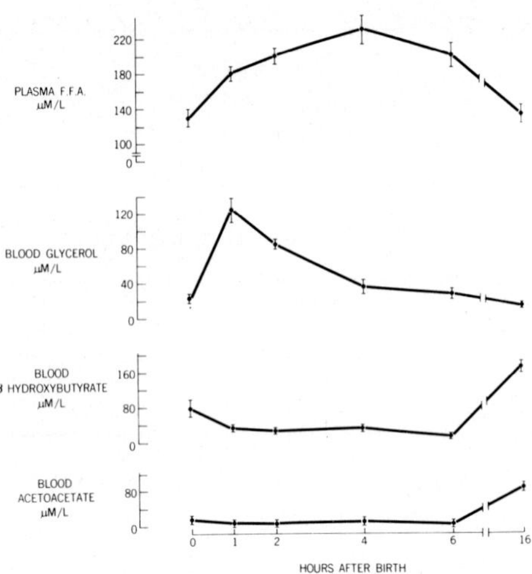

FIG. 3. Plasma free fatty acids and blood glycerol, β-hydroxybutyrate and acetoacetate in newborn rats fasted 16 hours. From Girard et al. (1973a), by courtesy.

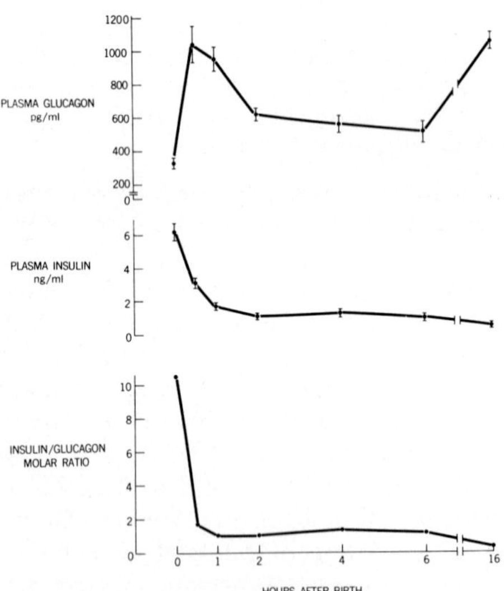

FIG. 4. Plasma immunoreactive insulin, glucagon and insulin/glucagon molar ratio in newborn rats fasted 16 hours. From Girard et al. (1973a), by courtesy.

cytosis in the hepatocyte – a phenomenon inducible by exogenous glucagon, and found in situations of increased endogenous glucagon secretion such as diabetic ketoacidosis (Amherdt et al., 1973). This increased lysosomal activity is related to catabolic processes, including glycogenolysis. (3) A marked increase in liver 3′,5′ cyclic adenosine monophosphate (cyclic AMP) has been demonstrated following birth (Novak et al., 1972), as would be expected with increased endogenous glucagon secretion, particularly if associated with a decrease in the insulin/glucagon ratio. It is probable that all of the above effects attributed in whole or in part to augmented glucagon secretion could be inhibited by insulin, and undoubtedly the concurrent fall in insulin levels contributed significantly to the changes observed.

The possibility of pathological glucagon responses at birth have already been raised in the infants of diabetic mothers (Luyckx et al., 1972; Bloom and Johnston, 1972). The high insulin and subnormal glucagon levels in such newborns could well interact at both the liver and periphery and be responsible for the frequency of neonatal hypoglycemia. Perhaps continuous glucagon infusion or long-acting glucagon preparations in such a situation, in addition to the usual glucose therapy, might accelerate recovery by stimulation of hepatic enzyme activity.

Having now considered the first absolute fast experienced by all mammals, one must begin to consider the response to feeding. The development of 'adult-type' glucagon responses, analogous to those of insulin, is not spontaneous at birth. Indeed, relative unresponsiveness to acute alterations in glycemia is the rule for the fetal and newborn alpha cell (Girard et al., 1973b, c; Edwards et al., 1972; Lernmark and Wenngren, 1972) as for the beta cell. Hence, the intermittent exposure to and absorption of potential energy substrates provided via the gastrointestinal tract must be responsible for inducing the normal adult response. Study of this phase is in its 'infancy'.

The maturing organism does not only have to respond to alternating feeding and fasting, but also to altered dietary composition and total caloric intake. The nature and magnitude of insulin responses depending upon antecedent diet have been a subject of intensive study and are well-documented. The role of glucagon in response to altered dietary composition, and hence in contributing to the distribution and metabolism of ingested foodstuffs, is less well quantified at present. In man, Unger and colleagues have shown the following changes in glucagon with isocalorically altered diet: high carbohydrate is associated with lowered basal IRG values, whereas low carbohydrate causes both increased basal levels and increased response to protein (Muller et al., 1971). Extrapolating such findings to the situation of a maximally ketogenic diet, i.e. low in both carbohydrate and protein and high in fat, one would predict high glucagon levels, and relatively low insulin. Such studies, presently in progress (Marliss, unpublished results), have shown very rapid conversion of subjects to a state in relation to fuel fluxes very akin to the prolonged-fasted state. The metabolic milieu consists of very high ketone acid levels within 3–6 days, decreased glycemia, and a rapid drop off in blood levels of alanine concurrent with a decrease in urea nitrogen excretion. Such findings suggest an adaptation such as occurs in prolonged fasting: restraint of protein mobilization, exerted at the level of the 'store', considered to be mainly skeletal muscle. Such an adaptation has not yet been explained as to the mechanism of curtailment of muscle proteolysis, though it remains possible that elevated ketone body levels themselves may be important, in an hormonal environment with low insulin and absolute or relative elevation of glucagon. Such findings have been demonstrated in the mouse fed uniquely on triglyceride and in the prolonged-fasted obese mouse (Cuendet et al., 1972).

In an earlier attempt to define the role of glucagon in prolonged fasting, IRG levels were assayed in a group of obese, non-diabetic patients undergoing prolonged therapeutic fasting, for periods of 5–6 weeks (Marliss et al., 1970). These studies confirmed the now well-documented shift toward a 'catabolic' insulin/glucagon ratio (decrease in insulin with transient or sustained increase in glucagon; Aguilar-Parada et al., 1969). Such a change early in fasting could account for early protein mobilization for stimulated gluconeogenesis, and adipokinesis with elevated free fatty acid and glycerol levels, all leading to ketosis. However, an unchanging 'bihormonal set' for the succeeding weeks, during which progressive curtailment of protein loss occurred, could hardly be attributable to the observed hormone levels. Nonetheless, after 4 weeks of fasting, glucagon was administered to such subjects by constant infusion at different dose levels for 48 hours, and produced a reversion to a catabolic state as had been previously demonstrated with even larger doses in man (Salter et al., 1960). The intermediate dose (2 mg/48 hr) gave assayable plasma glucagon concentrations equivalent to the highest levels predicted to occur physiologically in the portal vein. Though a peripheral infusion, it caused levels perfusing the liver in the range that might be found in the portal vein in physiologic settings. These subjects as well showed what could only be described in terms of a potent stimulus to gluconeogenesis: increase in urea nitrogen excretion, increase in glycemia, decrease in circulating glucogenic substrate levels, despite the presence of mild elevation in insulin concentrations. Such observations are consistent with a gluconeogenic effect of glucagon in man, at levels perfusing the liver probably consistent with portal vein levels from endogenous secretion.

However, when further analogous studies were carried out, employing an infusion rate of 0.2 mg/48 hr, peripheral IRG levels doubled, this time with no change in glycemia or insulinemia (Fig. 5). Yet a significant fall in the level of amino acids (including the

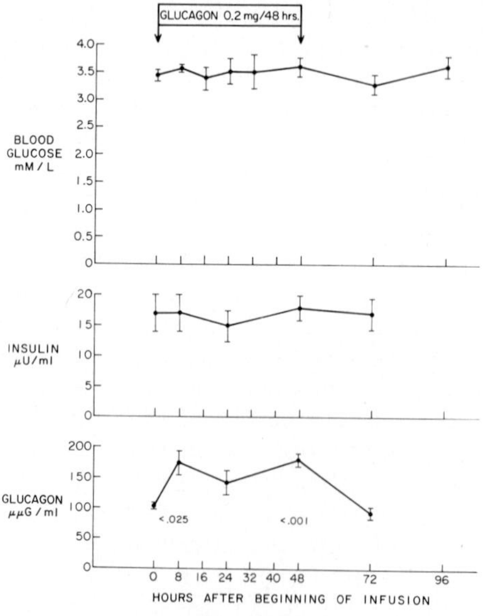

FIG. 5. Effect of glucagon infusion at 0.2 mg/48 hr into 5 prolonged-fasted (4 weeks) obese subjects upon blood glucose and plasma immunoreactive insulin and glucagon concentrations. The near doubling of glucagon levels had no influence upon glucose or insulin at the times measured. P values indicate the significance of the difference from the value observed prior to infusion (Student unpaired t test). From Marliss et al. (1970), by courtesy.

important glucogenic precursors) was observed (Fig. 6). Totally unexpected in this setting was a fall in urea excretion (Fig. 7), implying a decrease rather than an increase in hepatic gluconeogenesis. A possible interpretation of such data is that in the absence of the overriding hepatic effects observed in higher-dose studies (perhaps because doubling peripheral glucagon levels is not recognized by the liver as an increment since portal vein levels are always at least twice peripheral), a peripheral effect on amino acid metabolism was being unmasked. Such observations have been confirmed during infusions of 4 days' duration in prolonged-fasted subjects which have further shown that glutamine participates in the hypoaminoacidemia (Aoki et al., 1971). These observations were regarded as a curiosity until the recent demonstration by Liljenquist et al. (1972) that infusion of larger amounts of glucagon for shorter periods into diabetics incapable of insulin secretory responses was associated with no change in splanchnic uptake of alanine, but a decline in arterial plasma levels was observed. Again, such data might be considered to be consistent with a non-hepatic locus sensitive to glucagon. The nature and mechanism of such an effect remains unexplained, and hence its potential physiologic implications remain questionable. However, the observation again raises the possibility that fuel supplies may be subject to peripheral modulation by glucagon, a concept considered untenable since the definitive demonstration that it has no influence on insulin-mediated glucose metabolism by peripheral tissues.

The pathophysiology of glucagon secretion is considered in detail elsewhere in this Volume (pp. 137–216). Hence, suffice it to summarize by indicating that the protein catabolic effects of glucagon secreted endogenously in excess could well be primarily responsible for protein wasting in uncontrolled diabetes (Unger et al., 1970), trauma and burns (Lindsey et al., 1973), and severe infections (Rocha et al., 1973). The altered fuel fluxes in these situations may thus be a consequency of not only the altered insulin

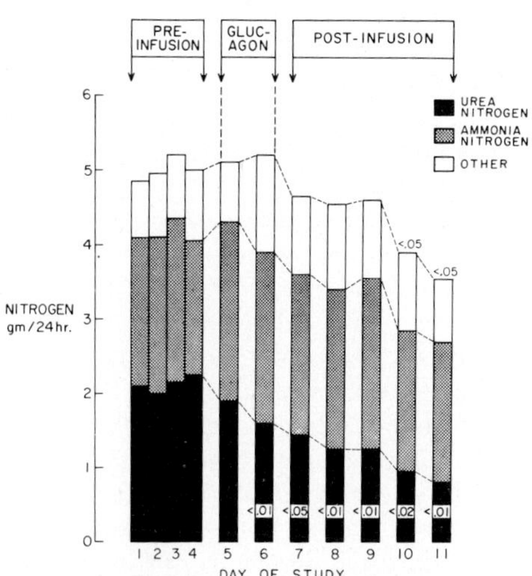

FIG. 6. Effect of glucagon infusion at 0.2 mg/48 hr on urine nitrogen components in 5 prolonged-fasted subjects. P values reflect the significance of the decrease in urea nitrogen and total nitrogen when compared with the mean of the 4-day preinfusion period. A paradoxical fall in urea nitrogen excretion occurred. From Marliss et al. (1970), by courtesy.

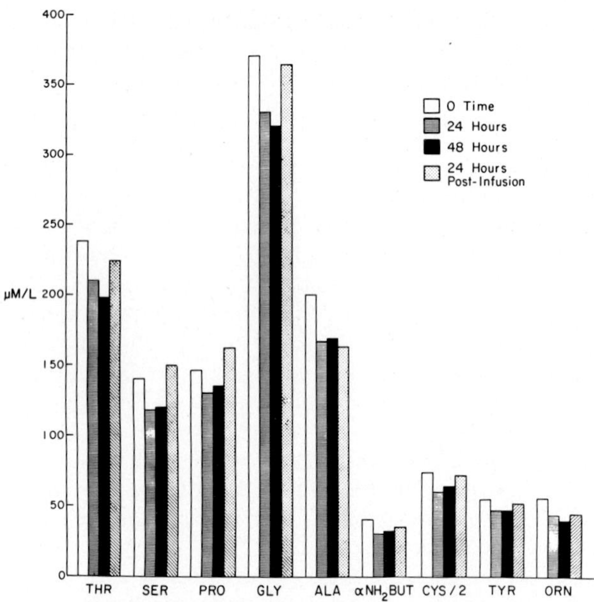

FIG. 7. Plasma amino acids showing a significant decrease during infusion of 0.2 mg/48 hr of glucagon into prolonged-fasted subjects. All but alanine returned toward preinfusion values at the termination of infusion. From Marliss et al. (1970), by courtesy.

secretion to which they have previously been attributed in large measure, but also the altered insulin-glucagon interrelationship. Similarly, a role for glucagon in fuel fluxes in exercise is now considered definitive.

To summarize, an attempt has been made to relate the effects of glucagon upon fuel fluxes to the multitude of situations in which such fluxes are altered. In following the organism chronologically from birth through life, it is presently possible to identify a number of both physiologic and pathologic states of altered fuel supply which may be attributed to altered glucagon secretion. Attention has been focused in this short review on 2 very different kinds of data relating to the role of this hormone in physiology: the first is intended to demonstrate a potentially central role for glucagon in the successful metabolic transition from intrauterine to extrauterine life. The second is presented to justify circumventing consideration of the controversial question as to whether glucagon is gluconeogenic in man (which we indeed consider it to be). The data presented and referred to raise the possibility of an equally controversial effect of this hormone: that of an effect on peripheral amino acid metabolism. No consideration of the glycogenolytic action of glucagon in the mature organism has been presented, since this is one effect of this hormone that remains unequivocal, namely its role in responding to emergency states of 'glucose need' by rapid mobilization of liver glycogen.

REFERENCES

AGUILAR-PARADA, E., EISENTRAUT, A. M. and UNGER, R. H. (1969): Effects of starvation on plasma pancreatic glucagon in normal man. *Diabetes, 18,* 717.

AMHERDT, M., HARRIS, E., RENOLD, A., ORCI, L. and UNGER, R. (1973): Hepatic autophagy and the insulin/glucagon ratio in severe diabetic ketoacidosis (abstract). *Diabetes, 22,* 302.

AOKI, T. T., MULLER, W. A., BRENNAN, M. F. and CAHILL Jr., J. F. (1973): Blood cell and plasma amino acid levels across forearm muscle during a protein meal. *Diabetes, 22,* 768.

AOKI, T. T., MULLER, W. A. and CAHILL Jr., G. F. (1972): Hormonal regulation of glutamine metabolism in fasting man. In: *Advances in Enzyme Regulation, Vol. 10,* pp. 145–151. Editor: G. Weber. Pergamon Press, Oxford.

BALLARD, F. J. (1971): Gluconeogenesis and the regulation of blood glucose in the neonate. In: *Proceedings of the VIIth Congress of the International Diabetes Federation, Buenos Aires, 1970,* pp. 592–600. Editor: R. R. Rodriguez. International Congress Series No. 231, Excerpta Medica, Amsterdam.

BLOOM, S. R. and JOHNSTON, D. I. (1972): Failure of glucagon release in infants of diabetic mothers. *Brit. med. J., 4,* 453.

BROMER, W. W. and CHANCE, R. E. (1969): Zinc glucagon depression of blood amino acids in rabbits. *Diabetes, 18,* 748.

CAKE, M. H. and OLIVER, I. T. (1969): The activation of phosphorylase in neonatal rat liver. *Europ. J. Biochem., 11,* 576.

CHRISTENSEN, H. N. and CLIFFORD, J. B. (1963): Early postnatal intensification of hepatic accumulation of amino acids. *J. biol. Chem., 238,* 1743.

CUENDET, G. S., LOTEN, E., WOLLHEIM, C. B., RABINOWITZ, A. and MARLISS, E. B. (1972): Protein conserving effect of fat-derived substrates. *Clin. Res., 20,* 942.

DAWKINS, M. J. R. (1963): Glycogen synthesis and breakdown in fetal and newborn rat liver. *Ann. N.Y. Acad. Sci., III,* 203.

EDWARDS, J. C., ASPLUND, K. and LUNDQUIST, G. (1972): Glucagon release from the pancreas of the newborn rat. *J. Endocr., 54,* 493.

FELIG, P. (1972): Interaction of insulin and amino acid metabolism in the regulation of gluconeogenesis. *Israel J. med. Sci., 8,* 262.

FELIG, P. and LYNCH, V. (1970): Starvation in human pregnancy: hypoglycemia, hypoinsulinemia and hyperketonemia. *Science, 170,* 990.

FELIG, P., OWEN, O. E., WAHREN, J. and CAHILL Jr., G. F. (1969): Amino acid metabolism during prolonged starvation. *J. clin. Invest., 48,* 584.

FELIG, P., POZEFSKY, T., MARLISS, E. and CAHILL Jr., G. F. (1970): Alanine: key role in gluconeogenesis. *Science, 167,* 1003.

FELIG, P. and WAHREN, J. (1971): Amino acid metabolism in exercising man. *J. clin. Invest., 50,* 1703.

FELIG, P. and WAHREN, J. (1973): The glucose-alanine cycle: role of red blood cells in splanchnic and peripheral alanine exchange (abstract). *Diabetes, 22,* 37.

FREINKEL, N., METZGER, B. E., NITZAN, M., HARE, J. W., SHAMBAUGH III, G. E., MARSHALL, R. T., SURMACZYNSKA, B. Z. and NAGEL, T. C. (1972): 'Accelerated starvation' and mechanisms for the conservation of maternal nitrogen during pregnancy. *Israel J. med. Sci., 8,* 426.

GIRARD, J. R., ASSAN, R. and JOST, A. (1973c): Glucagon in the rat fetus. In: *Foetal and Neonatal Physiology, Proceedings of the Sir J. Barcroft Centenary Symposium,* p. 456. Cambridge University Press, Cambridge.

GIRARD, J. R., BAL, D. and ASSAN, R. (1972): Glucagon secretion during the early postnatal period in the rat. *Hormone metabol. Res., 4,* 168.

GIRARD, J. R., CUENDET, G. S., MARLISS, E. B., KERVRAN, A., RIENTORT, M. and ASSAN, A. (1973a): Fuels, hormones and liver metabolism at term and during the early postnatal period in the rat. *J. clin. Invest., 52,* 3190.

GIRARD, J. R., KERVRAN, A., SOUFFLET, E. and ASSAN, R. (1973b): Factors affecting the secretion of insulin and glucagon by the rat fetus in utero. *Diabetes,* in press.

HEDING, L. (1971): Radioimmunological determination of pancreatic and gut glucagon in plasma. *Diabetologia, 7,* 10.

LANDAU, R. L. and LUGIBIHL, K. (1967): The effect of progesterone on the concentration of plasma amino acids in man. *Metabolism, 16,* 1114.

LEFEBVRE, P. J. (1972): Glucagon and lipid metabolism. In: *Glucagon: Molecular Physiology and Therapeutic Implications,* pp. 109–122. Editors: P. J. Lefebvre and R. H. Unger. Pergamon Press, Oxford.

LERNMARK, A. and WENNGREN, B. I. (1972): Insulin and glucagon release from the isolated pancreas of newborn mice. *J. Embryol. exp. Morphol., 28,* 607.

LILJENQUIST, J. F., BOMBOY, J. D., SINCLAIR-SMITH, B. C., LEWIS, S. B., FELTS, P. W., LACY, W. W., CROFFORD, O. B. and LIDDLE, G. W. (1972): Metabolic effects of glucagon in normal and diabetic man (abstract). *Diabetes, 21,* 332.

LINDSEY, C. A., WILMORE, D. W., MOYLAN, J. A., FALOONA, G. R. and UNGER, R. H. (1972): Glucagon and the insulin:glucagon ratio in burns and trauma (abstract). *Clin. Res., 20,* 802.

LUYCKX, A. S., MASSI-BENEDETTI, F., FALORNI, F. and LEFEBVRE, P. J. (1972): Presence of pancreatic glucagon in the portal plasma of human neonates. Differences in the insulin and glucagon responses to glucose between normal infants and infants from diabetic mothers. *Diabetologia, 8,* 296.

MARCO, J., CALLE, C., ROMAN, D., DIAZ-FIERROS, M., VILLANUEVA, M. L. and VALVERDE, I. (1973): Hyperglucagonism induced by glucocorticoid treatment in man. *New Engl. J. Med., 288,* 128.

MARLISS, E. B. and AOKI, T. T. (1972): Hormonal regulation of amino acid metabolism in man. *Acta diabet. lat., 9/Suppl. 1,* 189.

MARLISS, E. B., AOKI, T. T. and CAHILL Jr., G. F. (1972): Glucagon and amino acid metabolism. In: *Glucagon: Molecular Physiology and Therapeutic Implications, Chapter 8,* pp. 123–150. Editors: P. J. Lefebvre and R. H. Unger. Pergamon Press, Oxford.

MARLISS, E. B., AOKI, T. T., UNGER, R. H., SOELDNER, J. S. and CAHILL Jr., G. F. (1970): Glucagon levels and metabolic effects in fasting man. *J. clin. Invest., 49,* 2256.

MARLISS, E. B., GIRARDIER, L., SEYDOUX, J., KANAZAWA, Y., ORCI, L., RONALD, A. E., WOLLHEIM, C. B. and PORTE Jr., D. (1973): Glucagon release induced by pancreatic nerve stimulation in the dog. *J. clin. Invest., 52,* 1246.

METZGER, B. E., HARE, J. W. and FREINKEL, N. (1971): Carbohydrate metabolism in pregnancy. IX. Plasma levels of gluconeogenic fuels during fasting in the rat. *J. clin. Endocr., 33,* 869.

MULLER, W. A., FALOONA, G. R. and UNGER, R. H. (1971): The influence of antecedent diet upon glucagon and insulin secretion. *New Engl. J. Med., 285,* 1450.

NOVAK, E., DRUMMOND, G. I., SKALA, J. and HAHN, P. (1972): Developmental changes in cyclic AMP, protein kinase, phosphorylase kinase and phosphorylase in liver, heart, and skeletal muscle of the rat. *Arch. Biochem. Biophys., 150,* 511.

OWEN, E. and ROBINSON, R. R. (1963): Amino acid extraction and ammonia metabolism by the human kidney during the prolonged administration of ammonium chloride. *J. clin. Invest., 42,* 263.

ROCHA, D. M., SANTEUSANIO, F., FALOONA, G. R. and UNGER, R. H. (1973): Abnormal alpha cell function in bacterial infection. *New Engl. J. Med., 288,* 100.

RUDERMAN, N. B. and LUND, P. (1972): Amino acid metabolism in skeletal muscle. *Israel J. med. Sci., 8,* 295.

SALTER, J. M., EZRIN, C., LAIDLAW, J. C. and GORNALL, A. G. (1960): Metabolic effects of glucagon in human subjects. *Metabolism, 9,* 753.

SHERWOOD, W. G., CHANCE, G. W., TOEWS, C. J., MARTIN, J. M. and MARLISS, E. B. (1973): Familial pancreatic agenesis: clinical and biochemical features (abstract). *Clin. Res., 21,* 1062.

SNELL, K. and WALKER, D. G. (1973): Glucose metabolism in the newborn rat. Temporal studies in vivo. *Biochem. J., 132,* 739.

SZABO, A. J. and GRIMALDI, R. D. (1970): The metabolism of the placenta. *Advanc. metabol. Dis., 4,* 185.

UNGER, R. H. (1971): Glucagon and the insulin-glucagon ratio in diabetes and other catabolic illnesses. *Diabetes, 12,* 834.

UNGER, R. H., AGUILAR-PARADA, E., MULLER, W. A. and EISENTRAUT, A. M. (1970): Studies of pancreatic alpha cell function in normal and diabetic subjects. *J. clin. Invest., 49,* 837.

VERNON, R. G., EATON, S. W. and WALKER, D. G. (1968): Carbohydrate formation from various precursors in neonatal rat liver. *Biochem. J., 110,* 725.

WISE, J. K., HENDLER, R. and FELIG, P. (1973): Hyperglucagonemia: A new mechanism for the diabetogenic effects of glucocorticoids (abstract). *J. clin. Invest., 52,* 90A.

YEUNG, D. and OLIVER, I. T. (1967): Development of gluconeogenesis in neonatal rat liver. Effect of premature delivery. *Biochem. J., 105,* 1229.

THE REGULATION OF GLUCOSE TURNOVER (MOBILIZATION AND SUPPLY) AND FFA CONCENTRATION BY INSULIN-GLUCAGON INTERACTION IN DOGS*

MLADEN VRANIC and ALAN CHERRINGTON**

Department of Physiology, Medical Faculty, University of Toronto, Toronto, Canada

New evidence has accumulated in recent years emphasizing the importance of precise regulation of glucose in plasma. It has been suggested that in diabetic patients a chronic elevation of plasma glucose, irrespective of insulin concentration, can lead to (a) increased activity of polyol pathways in insulin-insensitive tissues resulting in lesions in peripheral nerves, aorta and development of cataracts (Winegrad et al., 1972), and (b) an increased activity of the enzyme glycosyl transferase resulting in thickening of the kidney basement membrane (Spiro, 1970). It is therefore important to discuss the role of the interplay between insulin and glucagon in the fine regulation of glucose homeostasis. An efficient glucoregulatory mechanism ensures that changes induced in blood glucose level by food ingestion or other physiological challenges will be minimal and that the fasting blood sugar levels will be re-established promptly. While it has been suggested that insulin-glucagon interactions are important under a variety of physiological and pathological conditions (diabetes, hypoglycemia, 'catabolic illness') (Unger and Lefebvre, 1972) this paper will discuss only the role of pancreatic hormones in regulating glucose turnover and free fatty acid (FFA) concentration in response to a carbohydrate or protein load and to exercise.

In order to understand the mechanisms whereby glucose homeostasis is maintained, it is necessary to measure the rates at which glucose is produced by the liver and utilized by the body. By using the tracer method, the distinct effects of insulin and/or glucagon on rates of glucose production (appearance, Ra) and utilization (disappearance, Rd) can be determined. Plasma glucose concentration does not necessarily reflect changes in the hormone levels since both production and utilization of glucose can change proportionally (for review see Vranic et al., 1971). Ra and Rd were determined using the method of primed tracer infusion (De Bodo et al., 1963) which has been recently validated experimentally for the inulin system (Radziuk et al., 1974). All the specific activities were corrected for ^{14}C recycling (Cherrington et al., 1972b).

The negative and positive feedback loops controlling the relationship between glucagon, insulin and glucose in intact animals are very complex (Vranic, 1972). In order to investigate these relationships starting from the basic feedback relationship (Fig. 1) and progressing to complex relationships operating in normal dogs, it was necessary to study

* This work was supported by Medical Research Council of Canada (Grant MT-2197).
** Recipient of a Medical Research Council of Canada Studentship.

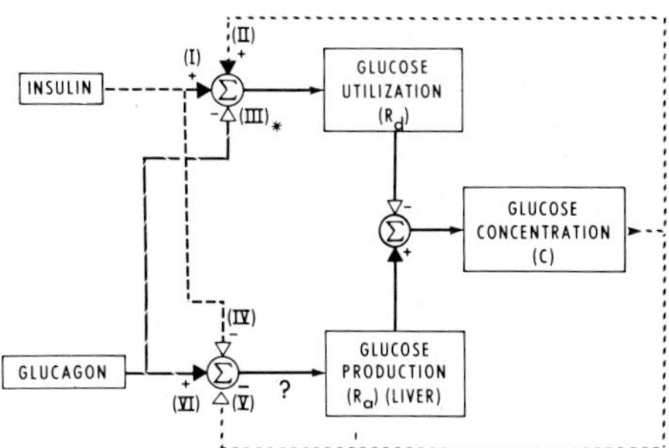

FIG. 1. Block diagram showing the feed-back loops in depancreatized dogs infused by insulin and glucagon. On each summing junction (Σ) stimulating effects are shown as +↘ and the inhibitory effects as −↘. The controlling sites are numbered with Roman numerals. The question whether glucose concentration per se inhibits Ra is discussed in the text. * Evidence is presented that glucagon does not inhibit peripheral glucose clearance, but the possibility that glucagon might interfere with glucose uptake by the liver at high glucose levels is discussed in the text.

glucose homeostasis in dogs the glucoregulatory feedback loops of which had been broken.

We have attempted to achieve an optimal experimental simulation of insulin-glucagon interaction in depancreatized dogs with respect to glucose turnover and FFA concentration. A successful simulation of an 'islet response' entails that the increments in Ra, Rd, IRI and immunoreactive glucagon (IRG) concentration approach those observed in normal dogs during glucagon or arginine infusion. It was of particular interest to find out whether or not such a simulation of a normal response could be achieved with a constant infusion of insulin, a problem related to the metabolic significance of the insulin/glucagon ratio. The approach was such that glucose turnover and FFA concentrations were measured during glucagon or arginine infusion into normal dogs and into depancreatized insulin-infused dogs concurrently given graded amounts of insulin. A '2-stage pancreatectomy (Rappaport et al., 1966) and insulin replacement' technic (Vranic and Wrenshall, 1968) was used in preparation of the depancreatized animals in order to minimize the adverse metabolic consequences which normally accompany extensive surgery and general anesthesia. In this way experiments were performed on conscious animals which had not been exposed to the stress of major surgery prior to the experiments and which had never been without constant physiological supplies of insulin. Subsequent work established that such dogs have normal turnover of glucose as well as normal plasma concentrations of glucose, FFA, and near normal immunoreactive insulin (Table 1). They cannot, however, vary their insulin supply in response to a physiological stimulus and they are devoid of pancreatic glucagon.

This experimental approach provided information about the basal rate of insulin secretion and revealed deficiencies of the homeostatic mechanisms which result from the inability of the dog to change its insulin or glucagon supply. Since the predominant effect of insulin was to increase glucose utilization and that of glucagon to increase glucose production, it seemed reasonable that simultaneous release of these 2 hormones could increase glucose turnover while maintaining normoglycemia. Such a proportional increase in Ra and Rd occurred in normal dogs given either glucagon or arginine. By attempting to

TABLE 1
The mean control period (± S.E.M.) concentrations of plasma glucose, serum immunoreactive insulin (IRI), and plasma free fatty acids (FFA), and rates of glucose production (Ra), utilization (Rd), and clearance (M) in 13 normal and 15 matched depancreatized insulin-infused dogs

	Normal dogs	Depancreatized insulin-infused dogs
Glucose (mg/100 ml)	100 ± 3	108 ± 2
IRI (μU/ml)	18.3 ± 2	15.1 ± 0.6*
FFA (mEq/l)	1.14 ± 0.12	1.00 ± 0.05
Ra (mg/kg/min.)	3.32 ± 0.29	3.47 ± 0.14
Rd (mg/kg/min.)	3.21 ± 0.29	3.67 ± 0.14
M (ml/kg/min.)	3.12 ± 0.27	3.61 ± 0.27

* Although very small this difference was significant at < 0.01 level.

reproduce in depancreatized dogs the measured profile of insulin and glucagon concentration resulting from physiological stimuli in intact dogs, and by measuring its effect on glucose turnover, we hoped to determine the secretion rates of insulin and to study the physiological significance of a given pattern of hormonal release.

THE GLUCOREGULATORY FUNCTION OF INSULIN DURING GLUCOSE INGESTION

In 1934 Soskin et al. obtained a normal glucose tolerance test in depancreatized dogs when insulin was infused at a constant rate. They concluded that excess insulin release does not play an essential role in the homeostatic mechanisms that determine glucose tolerance. Since the decay of glucose concentration in plasma after a glucose load is proportional to the difference between glucose production and utilization, this implied that hyperglycemia per se directly inhibits the endogenous release of glucose by the liver and maximally enhances glucose utilization by various tissues. The importance of a continuous steady secretion of insulin in maintaining glucose homeostasis was demonstrated by Wrenshall et al. (1965), who observed a prompt hyperglycemia following interruption of insulin supply, because glucose production increased and its utilization decreased. The diabetic changes were reversed by unclamping the pancreatic graft and allowing resumption of insulin supply. By clamping and unclamping the pedicle of the remnant pancreatic autograft it was possible to study the metabolic consequences of total but temporary diabetes in conscious dogs without stress of major surgery. In contrast to the findings of Soskin, conscious depancreatized dogs infused intraportally a basal amount of insulin (200 μU/kg/min.) had a significantly altered glucose tolerance test (Fig. 2). A lesser

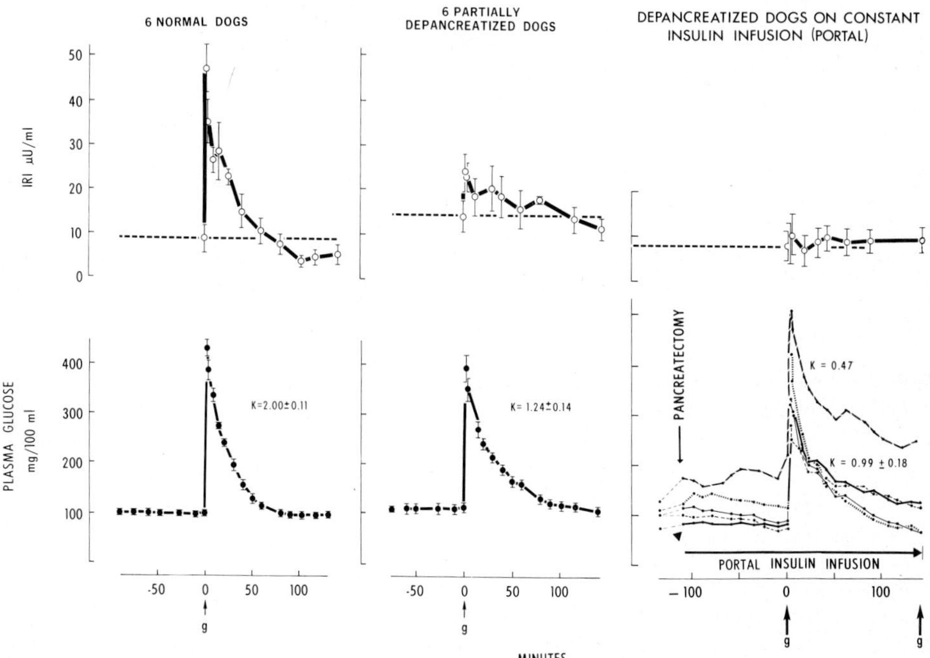

FIG. 2. Modified from Vranic et al. (1971). Mean ± S.E.M. values of immunoreactive insulin (IRI) and plasma glucose following i.v. glucose injection of 0.5 g/kg (↗g). Pancreatectomy = removal of remaining subcutaneous pancreatic autograft and start of basal constant intraportal insulin infusion (190–260 μU/kg/min.) in conscious dogs.

reduction of glucose tolerance was observed in dogs which had a pancreatic graft and were able to mobilize a reduced amount of insulin. We felt that Soskin et al. (1934) obtained different results because they infused insulin peripherally at rates up to 33 times our basal infusion rate, and because in most experiments insulin and glucose infusions were given simultaneously in order to obtain an initial steady glucose level.

Figure 3 illustrates the deficient disposal of glucose in a conscious dog which could not mobilize extra insulin. Endogenous glucose production did not decrease in response to glucose given at a rate two thirds to twice the normal rate of endogenous glucose production, even when the concentration of glucose in plasma exceeded 200 mg/100 ml. It is

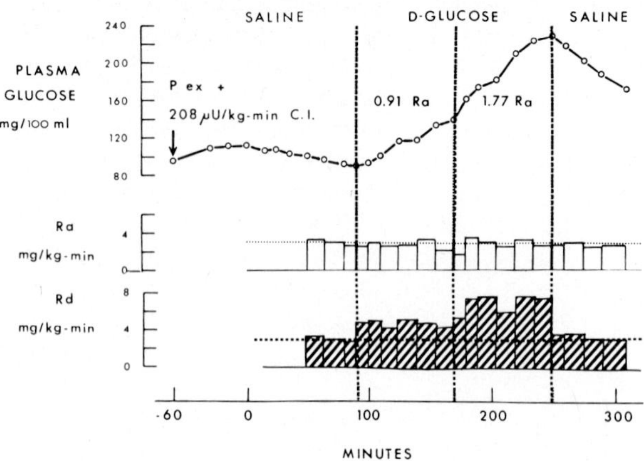

FIG. 3. Modified from Ishiwata et al. (1969). Effect of an infusion of D-glucose on the concentration and on the calculated rates of appearance (Ra) and disappearance (Rd) of glucose. Glucose was infused in the indicated intervals at 2.6 mg/kg/min. and 5.2 mg/kg/min. respectively. These rates correspond to 0.91 and 1.77 times endogenous Ra respectively. P_{ex} indicates the removal of the pancreatic autograft and the beginning of the intraportal infusion of canine insulin into the conscious dog.

known that at similar glucose concentrations in normal dogs endogenous glucose production is considerably reduced (Steele et al., 1965) or ceases (Hetenyi et al., 1973). We concluded that extra secretion of insulin, ordinarily evoked by a glucose load, plays a regulatory rather than a permissive role. It still remains to be explored whether a very rapid change of glucose concentration in plasma per se could induce some change in Ra since Herrera et al. (1966), reported that a high glucose concentration in the absence of insulin can inhibit the output of glucose in a perfused liver preparation. In normal dogs hyperglycemia depresses glucagon concentration (for review see Unger and Lefebvre, 1972) and this could also contribute to the decrease of Ra. The quantitative significance of insulin release and cessation of glucagon secretion on decreasing Ra during carbohydrate meals has, however, not been established yet. The utilization of glucose rose in proportion to its concentration in plasma in the absence of any change in the rate of insulin supply. The metabolic clearance of glucose was calculated to illustrate this relationship between the concentration and uptake of glucose. A relatively unaltered clearance indicates a linear relationship between the 2 parameters, i.e. when the concentration of glucose in plasma is doubled, Rd doubles as well. During glucose infusion the average clearance did not show marked changes. In contrast, clearance increased when insulin concentration increased in plasma (Vranic et al., 1971, 1973). Therefore the disposal of glucose in dogs unable to alter insulin supply is deficient both because the liver looses its homeostatic glucoregulatory role with respect to Ra and because the increase in Rd is deficient.

THE GLUCOREGULATORY FUNCTION OF CONCURRENT RELEASE OF INSULIN AND GLUCAGON DURING PROTEIN MEALS

The effects of glucagon without insulin release

Attempts to quantitate the metabolic effects of glucagon in vivo face the problem that glucagon stimulates insulin release, indirectly due to hyperglycemia, and directly through its effect on pancreatic beta cells (for review see Foa, 1972). It is well known that insulin increases the uptake of glucose by insulin-sensitive tissues, inhibits the production of glucose by the liver and inhibits the release of FFA from adipocytes. The metabolic effects of glucagon in normal dogs may therefore be masked by the effects of the insulin it releases. Glucagon was therefore infused into 8 depancreatized dogs maintained on constant near-basal intraportal infusions of insulin (Cherrington et al., 1972b). An infusion of glucagon, considered to produce physiological glucagon concentrations, induced in a fasting depancreatized insulin-infused dog an increase in Ra, and a marked hyperglycemia. A similar rate of glucagon infusion induced in normal dogs only a minor change in glucose concentration (Fig. 4). In depancreatized dogs Rd rose only in proportion to the

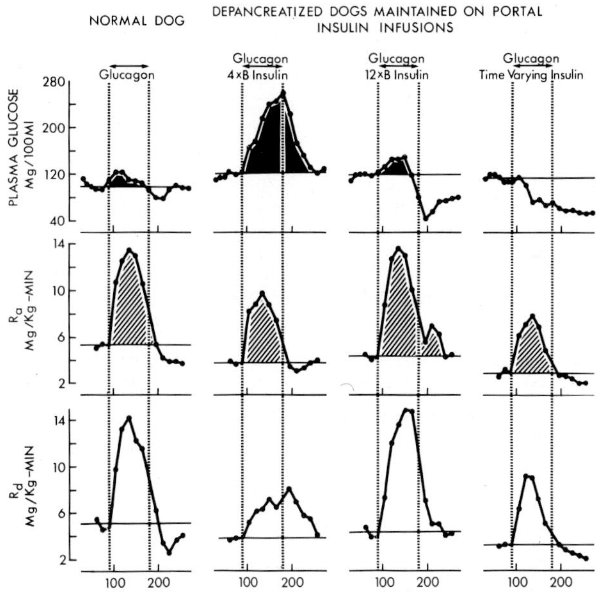

FIG. 4. Modified from Cherrington and Vranic (1971, 1974). Concentrations and rates of appearance (Ra) and disappearance (Rd) of glucose in a normal dog and 3 depancreatized insulin-infused dogs before, during, and after infusion of glucagon. Glucagon was infused for 90 minutes, starting at 13 mμg/kg/min. and reaching 29 mμg/kg/min. at 25 minutes. Concurrently, with start of infusion of glucagon into 3 depancreatized dogs, rates of insulin infusion were increased to 4 × B (960 μU/kg/min.) and 12 × B (2,880 μU/kg/min.) and in a time varying manner (16 × B for 20 min., 8 × B for 30 min., and 4 × B for 40 min.), respectively. Simultaneous with cessation of glucagon infusion, insulin infusion was returned to basal. Abscissa: time from start of tracer infusion. B: basal infusion.

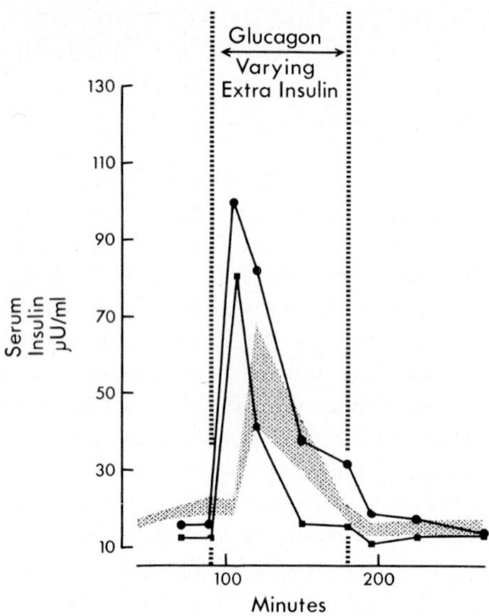

FIG. 5. Stippled area corresponds to ± 1 S.E.M. of the IRI levels observed in 6 normal dogs in response to glucagon. IRI levels of 2 depancreatized dogs given concurrently with glucagon a time-varying insulin infusion are also shown (●———●). Modified from Cherrington and Vranic (1974), by courtesy.

increased blood sugar level, so that at any given time the increase in Rd was smaller than that of Ra. The unchanged clearance of glucose illustrated the unchanged linear relationship between the concentration and uptake of glucose. In normal dogs however, glucagon induced an increase in insulin secretion (Fig. 5) and therefore the clearance of glucose increased, balance between Ra and Rd was maintained and only a small change in glucose concentration occurred (Fig. 4). The observation of unchanged glucose clearance in depancreatized dogs indicates that glucagon does not directly affect peripheral glucose uptake. The possibility that glucagon might interfere with glucose uptake in the liver at high plasma glucose concentrations has been recently discussed (Cherrington and Vranic, 1974).

Glucagon also induced an increase in the rate at which ^{14}C recycled (Cherrington and Vranic, 1974) suggesting enhanced gluconeogenesis. An enhanced rate of recirculation of the label cannot be quantitatively related to the absolute increase in gluconeogenesis in view of the crossing over of carbon which can occur when various metabolic pathways share common pools of intermediates (Krebs et al., 1966). Also recycling does not necessarily reflect the activity of the Cori cycle (glucose-lactate-glucose) because part of the glucose-derived label could be transported from the periphery to the liver via alanine (Felig, 1973).

The role of glucagon in control of lipid mobilization in different species was recently reviewed by Lefebvre (1972). Lefebvre (1966) obtained with a small dose of glucagon (0.12 μg/kg/hr, intraportal) an increase in plasma FFA in normal fasted anesthetized dogs. Larger peripheral infusions of glucagon induce in normal dogs a decrease in FFA levels, presumably because mobilized insulin inhibits the release of fatty acids. We have investigated therefore the effect of glucagon (1.00–3.00 μg/kg/hr) in conscious depancreatized insulin-infused dogs. Glucagon did not increase FFA levels in our dogs although the supply and the measured IRI concentrations were constant. A small decrease in FFA levels was noted when the rate of infusion was above 1.79 μg/kg/hr and hyperglycemia was prominent (Cherrington et al., 1972b). The difference between our approach and that of Lefebvre (1966) was in the dose applied and route of administration. In addition our dogs were conscious and could not mobilize insulin. It is difficult to ascertain which of these factors could explain the difference in the observed results.

Experimental simulation of insulin-glucagon interaction

Since ingestion of amino acids causes the plasma levels of insulin and glucagon to increase concurrently (Assan et al., 1967), we examined the effects of concomitant increase in levels of both pancreatic hormones on glucose turnover. The question arose as to whether the increased secretion of the 2 hormones maintains normoglycemia by a proportional increase of Ra and Rd or because the 2 hormones neutralize each other at their site of action. Figure 4 (left panel) shows that the glucagon infusion in a normal dog (1 experiment out of 6) induced a 100% proportional increase in Ra and Rd while glucose concentration in plasma changed only slightly. The increase in Rd was attributed to the measured increment in the serum IRI (Fig. 5).

In order to stimulate the insulin response to glucagon found in the normal dogs, graded amounts of insulin were given to the depancreatized dogs simultaneously with glucagon infusions. An experimental simulation was considered to be successful if glucose concentration, Ra, Rd and measured concentration of IRI in plasma of depancreatized dogs approximated those observed in normal dogs during glucagon infusion. Figure 4 shows experiments performed on 3 out of a series of 11 depancreatized dogs. Insulin infusion of 4 × basal infusion (B) did not prevent glucagon-induced hyperglycemia, because the initial rate of increase in Rd did not match the rate of increase in Ra. An insulin infusion of 12 × B maintained normoglycemia in a manner similar to the normal dog initially, but hypoglycemia occurred eventually since at that time the effect of insulin became predominant and Rd exceeded Ra (Cherrington and Vranic, 1971). Since normal dogs responded to glucagon infusion with a spike pattern of insulin release (Fig. 5), it was attempted to more closely simulate the insulin-glucagon interplay by applying a time-varying pattern of insulin infusion, and the spike release of insulin could be successfully approximated in the depancreatized dogs. Figure 4 shows that when the initially high rate of insulin infusion was experimentally reduced during the second half of the glucagon infusion period, Rd was increased synchronously with the waning Ra. Thus a time-varying insulin infusion did indeed correct the late imbalance between Ra and Rd, although a small imbalance between the 2 rates occurred initially. This indicates that the pattern of insulin release not only reflects a secretory characteristic of β cells but has an important glucoregulatory function. In the 11 depancreatized dogs studied, the increases in Ra induced by identical infusions of glucagon varied considerably, but these increments were not affected by increasing amounts of insulin indicating that at these physiological hormonal levels the inhibitory role of insulin is not marked. Furthermore the same average increase in Ra was induced in normal (4.34 ± 0.67) and depancreatized dogs (4.23 ± 0.70). Thus within this range of insulin and glucagon infusion rates the predominant role of the 2 pancreatic hormones is stimulatory, glucagon to increase Ra and insulin to increase Rd. The ability of glucagon to override the inhibitory effect of insulin on the liver within a range of hormonal concentrations has been recently reviewed by Exton and Park (1972).

The effect of arginine on glucose turnover

Figure 6 shows the effects of arginine in one dog out of a series of 7 (Cherrington and

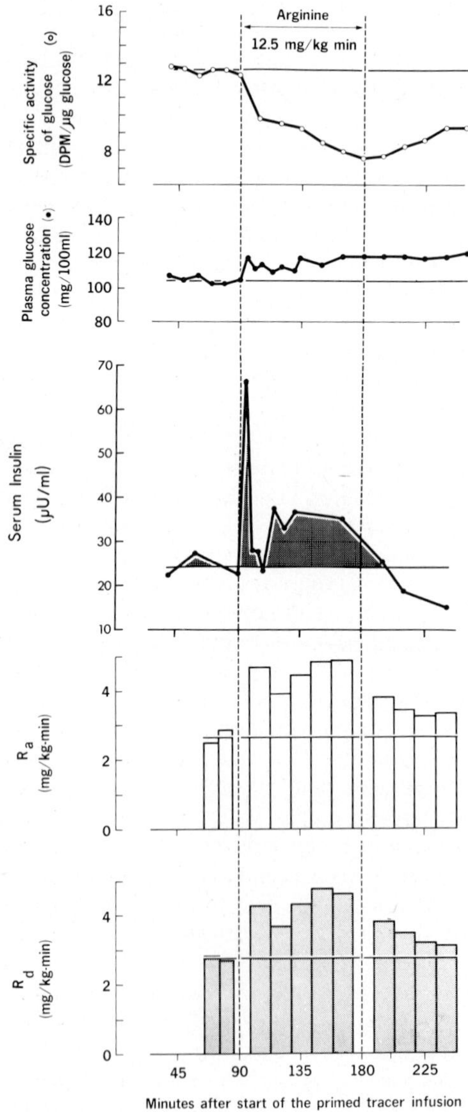

FIG. 6. Modified from Cherrington and Vranic (1973) by courtesy. The effect of arginine on IRI, specific activity and concentration and rates of production (Ra) and utilization (Rd) of glucose.

Vranic, 1973). The specific activity of plasma glucose decreased markedly during the infusion of arginine, while glucose concentration increased minimally, thus indicating that the increases in Ra and Rd were synchronous and of the same magnitude. The increase in Ra is attributed to glucagon release (for review see Unger and Lefebvre, 1972) while the increase in Rd was attributed to the release of insulin. The increase of glucose turnover fits well with the suggestion (Unger and Lefebvre, 1972) that glucose represents an important source of energy for the protein synthetic processes occurring during protein ingestion.

In order to determine whether or not the mobilized pancreatic hormones are solely responsible for the increase in glucose turnover, arginine was also infused into 6 conscious normoglycemia depancreatized insulin-infused dogs (Cherrington et al., 1972a). As Figure 7 shows (one representative experiment out of 7) there were no significant changes in Ra, Rd, glucose concentration, IRI or IRG. Thus the increased turnover of glucose observed in normal dogs was solely due to the increased secretion of glucagon and insulin and not to other metabolic or hormonal changes which arginine induces.

In order to re-establish the normal response of glucose turnover to arginine, arginine was then infused into the same depancreatized dogs simultaneously with glucagon and extra insulin. In view of the possibility that the physiological pattern of insulin release is essential in providing a glucoregulatory balance between the effects of the 2 hormones, the rates of these hormonal infusions were such as to yield plasma concentrations of IRI and IRG similar to those occurring in normal dogs in response to amino acids. A multiphasic infusion of insulin induced measured peripheral IRI concentrations (Fig. 7b) which were close to peripheral IRI concentrations in normal arginine infused dogs (Fig. 6). Glucagon was infused peripherally and the peripheral IRG concentrations were equivalent to portal concentrations induced by amino acid infusion in normal dogs (Müller et al., 1971). Since glucagon was infused peripherally it is assumed that portal and peripheral concentrations would be equal because such an infusion bypasses the liver which normally creates a gradient in concentrations of the pancreatic hormones. The infusion of the 2 hormones into depancreatized dogs increased IRI and IRG levels, which in turn increased glucose turnover in a manner equivalent to the normal dogs. Thus the main aim of these experiments was achieved, namely a simulation of metabolic response and concentrations of pancreatic hormones in depancreatized dogs.

The symptoms of glucagon deficiency in depancreatized mammals are difficult to ascertain (for review see Foa, 1972; Sokal, 1970) because they are overshadowed by more dramatic effects of insulin deprivation. When glucagon mobilization was prevented in depancreatized dogs, arginine infusion did not increase Ra. The lack of Ra response cannot be due to insulin deprivation, because excess insulin can only decrease Ra, and an increased Ra could be induced when glucagon was infused in physiological amounts. Therefore these experiments demonstrated that using the tracer method consequences of glucagon deficiency can be demonstrated in depancreatized dogs.

It is of interest that the arginine-induced decrease of FFA was of the same magnitude both in normal and depancreatized dogs, suggesting that in addition to insulin other factors such as growth hormone (Sirek et al., 1967) may play a role. In the dog arginine thus reverses the fuel utilization characteristic of fasting: the release of FFA mobilization from fat depots is inhibited, while the turnover of glucose is enhanced even though normoglycemia is maintained.

It was suggested (Unger and Lefebvre, 1972) that a given molar ratio of insulin/glucagon (I/G) determines the flux of carbohydrates: a high ratio favoring storage and a low

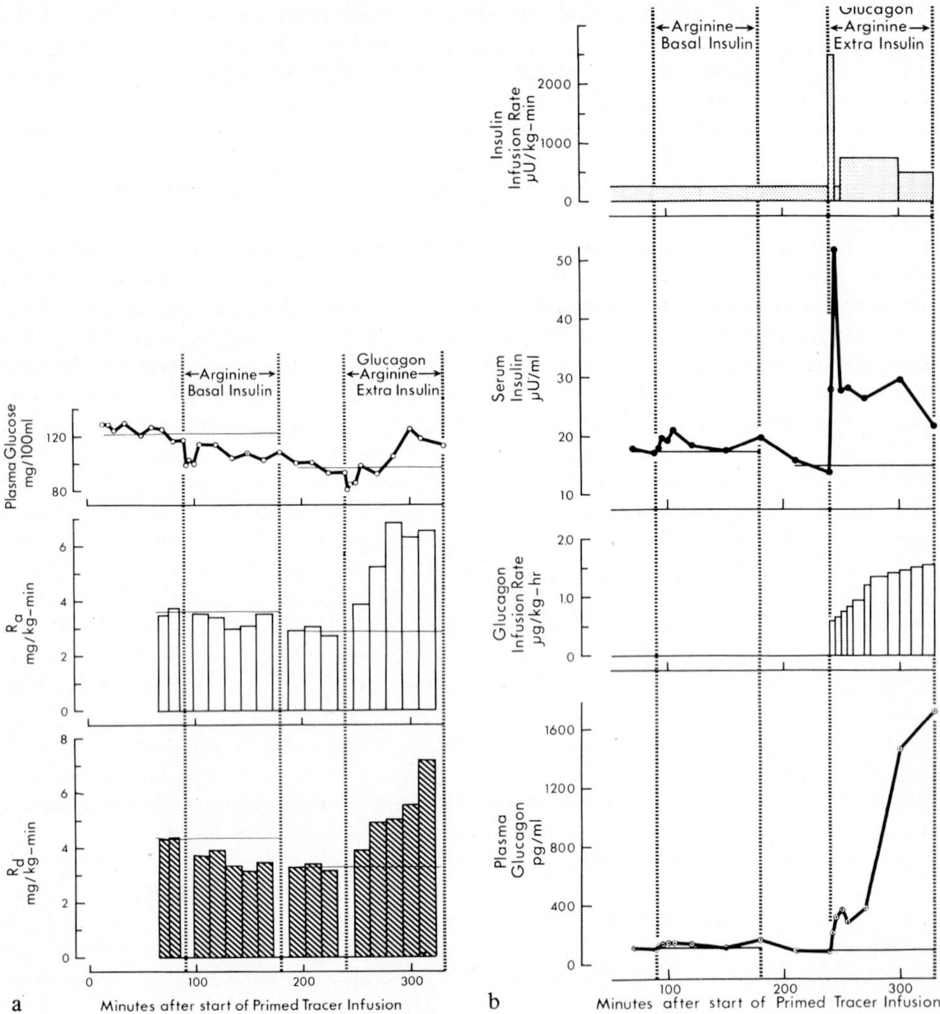

FIG. 7. From Cherrington, Vranic, Pek and Kavamori (unpublished observations). (a) The effect of arginine in a depancreatized normoglycemic insulin-infused dog with or without glucagon and extra insulin on concentration, rates of production (Ra) and utilization (Rd) of plasma glucose. Control period means are shown as horizontal solid lines. (b) The infusion rates of insulin and glucagon and the induced measured concentration of IRI and IRG.

ratio favoring gluconeogenesis. Parilla et al. (1972) have indicated that a constant I/G ratio has the same average effect on glucose output by the isolated liver regardless of absolute insulin and glucagon concentration. Our data, however, indicate that for an acute sustained increase in glucose turnover a continuously decreasing ratio of insulin to glucagon is required (Fig. 7). Furthermore glucose homeostasis depends on the balance between the effects of the 2 hormones on the liver and periphery respectively. Since glucagon presumably has no marked effect on peripheral glucose uptake this implies that only the absolute concentration of insulin is important at this site. Thus doubling of the levels of insulin and glucagon (thereby keeping I/G ratio constant) even if it does not have a major effect on glucose production will enhance peripheral glucose uptake and induce hypoglycemia. Thus we feel that in the acute regulation of glucose turnover by insulin and glucagon it is important to consider the absolute concentrations of the hormones and the duration of the challenge, rather than a given I/G ratio.

Exercise

The increased energy requirements during exercise are met partly by the circulating glucose and FFA. It was recently shown that an optimal glucose flux is essential for the muscle to exercise (Issekutz et al., 1970). It was of interest therefore that during exhaustive exercise glucagon levels increase both in dogs and human subjects (Bottger et al., 1972), an increase induced perhaps by alanine, since this amino acid is released by the exercising muscle and accumulates in plasma (Felig, 1973). The question remains, however, whether or not glucagon is an essential mediator of the increased glucose mobilization during exercise, since we have shown previously that both normal and depancreatized dogs (insulin-infused or insulin-deprived) were able to mobilize from the liver essentially the same extra amount of glucose during moderate exercise (Vranic and Wrenshall, 1969). It is of course possible that this essential amount of extra glucose is mobilized in the absence of pancreatic glucagon through metabolic and hormonal compensatory mechanisms. The metabolic significance of such compensations remains, however, to be explored.

SUMMARY

The distinct and combined effects of insulin and glucagon were studied in conscious depancreatized dogs by independent or combined graded infusions of the pancreatic hormones. The rates of glucose production (Ra), utilization (Rd), and metabolic clearance, and measured concentrations of insulin and glucagon were compared in glucose-, arginine- or glucagon-infused intact and depancreatized dogs. This permitted the precise evaluation of the individual and combined effects of these hormones in homeostatic regulations by eliminating interfering responses by the islets.

Dogs deprived of pancreatic glucagon and insulin given only a constant basal insulin supply showed an abnormal glucose tolerance. Ra did not decrease in response to a glucose load. Glucagon in these dogs increased Ra, did not affect peripheral glucose clearance, and did not stimulate FFA release. Normal plasma profiles of glucose, FFA and glucose turnover were achieved by multiphasic insulin infusions. This indicates that the physiological pattern of insulin release reflects not only an inherent secretory characteristic of beta cells, but also serves an important glucoregulatory function, counterbalancing the effect of glucagon. Arginine infusion to intact dogs increased Ra and Rd proportionally, thus maintaining normoglycemia. The increases in Ra and Rd are attributed to simultaneous mobilization of glucagon and insulin, since arginine did not affect glucose turnover in normoglycemic depancreatized insulin-infused dogs. The normal response could be fully re-established by concurrent physiological infusions of glucagon and insulin (biphasic). Thus the tracer method was able to reveal the consequences of both glucagon and insulin deficiency. Maintenance of increased glucose turnover required a continuously decreasing insulin-glucagon ratio. This suggests that the absolute concentrations rather than the relative ratio between the 2 pancreatic hormones play the important glucoregulatory function in intact dogs. The observed decrease of FFA in the arginine-stimulated depancreatized dogs suggests that in addition to insulin other humoral factors can also inhibit lipolysis during arginine infusion.

ACKNOWLEDGEMENT

We are grateful to Mrs. N. Kovacevic, P. Eng. and Mrs. J. Wilkins for their excellent assistance. The gifts of Hoechst Pharmaceuticals Ltd. (Festal tablets), Ames Co. Ltd. (dextrostix strips, reflectance meter) and Connaught Laboratories (canine insulin) are also gratefully acknowledged.

REFERENCES

ASSAN, R., ROSSELIN, G. and DOLAIS, J. (1967): Effêts sur la glucagonémie des perfusions et ingestions d'acides aminées. *J. Ann. Diabétol. Hôtel Dieu, 7,* 25.

BOTTGER, I., SCHLEIN, E. M., FALOONA, G. R., KNOCHEL, J. P. and UNGER, R. H. (1972): The effect of exercise on glucagon secretion. *J. clin. Endocr., 35,* 117.

CHERRINGTON, A., KAWAMORI, R. and VRANIC, M. (1972a): Role of insulin and glucagon in the response of glucose turnover to arginine. *Proc. Canad. Fed. biol. Soc., v. 15,* Abstract 388.

CHERRINGTON, A. and VRANIC, M. (1971): Role of glucagon and insulin in control of glucose turnover. *Metabolism, 20,* 625.

CHERRINGTON, A. D. and VRANIC, M. (1973): Effect of arginine on glucose turnover and plasma free fatty acids in normal dogs. *Diabetes, 22,* 537.

CHERRINGTON, A. D. and VRANIC, M. (1974): Effect of interaction between insulin and glucagon on glucose turnover in normal and depancreatized dogs. *Metabolism,* in press.

CHERRINGTON, A., VRANIC, M., FONO, P. and KOVACEVIC, N. (1972b): Effect of glucagon on glucose turnover and plasma free fatty acids in depancreatized dogs maintained on matched insulin infusions. *Canad. J. Physiol., 50,* 946.

DE BODO, R. C., STEELE, R., ALTSZULER, N., DUNN, A. and BISHOP, J. S. (1963): On the hormonal regulation of carbohydrate metabolism. *Rec. Progr. Hormone Res., 19,* 445.

EXTON, J. H. and PARK, C. R. (1972): Interaction of insulin and glucagon in the control of liver metabolism. In: *Handbook of Physiology, Section 7, Vol. 1,* pp. 437–455. Editors: N. Freinkel and D. F. Steiner. American Physiological Society, Washington, D.C.

FELIG, P. (1973): The glucose-alanine cycle. *Metabolism, 22,* 179.

FOA, P. O. (1972): The secretion of glucagon. In: *Handbook of Physiology, Section 7, Vol. 1,* pp. 261–277. Editors: D. F. Steiner, N. Freinkel. American Physiological Society, Washington, D.C.

HERRERA, M. G., KAMM, D., RUDERMAN, N. and CAHILL JR., G. F. (1966): Non hormonal factors in the control of gluconeogenesis. In: *Advances in Enzyme Regulation, 4,* pp. 225–235. Pergamon Press, Oxford.

HETENYI Jr., G., NORWICH, K. H. and ZELIN, S. (1973): Analysis of the glucoregulatory system in dogs. *Amer. J. Physiol., 224,* 635.

ISHIWATA, K., HETENYI Jr., G. and VRANIC, M. (1969): Effect of d-glucose or d-ribose on the turnover of glucose in pancreatectomized dogs maintained on a matched intraportal infusion of insulin. *Diabetes, 12,* 820.

ISSEKUTZ Jr., B., ISSEKUTZ, A. C. and NASH, D. (1970): Mobilization of energy sources in exercising dogs. *J. appl. Physiol., 29,* 691.

KREBS, H. S., HEMS, R. and WEIDEMANN, M. J. (1966): The fate of isotopic carbon in kidney cortex synthesizing glucose from lactate. *Biochem. J., 101,* 242.

LEFEBVRE, P. (1966): *Contribution à l'Etude du Rôle Physiologique du Glucagon.* Aiscia, Brussels.

LEFEBVRE, P. (1972): Glucagon and lipid metabolism. In: *Glucagon, Chapter 7,* pp. 109–121. Editors: P. J. Lefebvre and R. H. Unger. Pergamon Press, Oxford.

MÜLLER, W. A., FALOONA, G. R. and UNGER, R. H. (1971): The effect of alanine on glucagon secretion. *J. clin. Invest., 50,* 2215.

PARRILLA, R., TOEWS, C. J. and GOODMAN, M. N. (1972): The influence of the glucagon:insulin ratio on hepatic metabolism (abstract). *Diabetes, 21/Suppl. 1,* 341.

RADZIUK, J., NORWICH, K. H. and VRANIC, M. (1974): Measurement and validation of nonsteady turnover rates with applications to the inulin and glucose systems. Proceedings of the tracer methodology group meeting, Atlantic City, April, 1973. *Fed. Proc., 34,* in press.

RAPPAPORT, A. M., VRANIC, M. and WRENSHALL, G. A. (1966): A pedunculated subcutaneous autotransplant of an isolated pancreas remnant for the temporary deprivation of internal pancreatic secretion in the dog. *Surgery, 59,* 792.

SIREK, O. V., SIREK, A., PRZYBYLSKA, K., DOOLAN, H. and NIKI, A. (1967): Plasma free fatty acid concentrations in Houssay dogs following a single injection of growth hormone. *Endocrinology, 81,* 395.

SOKAL, J. E. (1970): Glucagon. In: *Diabetes Mellitus, Theory and Practice, Chapter 5,* pp. 112–131. Editors: M. Ellenberg and H. Rifkin. McGraw Hill, New York, N.Y.

SOSKIN, S., ALLWEISS, M. D. and COHN, D. J. (1934): Influence of pancreas and the liver upon the dextrose tolerance curve. *Amer. J. Physiol., 109,* 155.

SPIRO, R. G. (1970): Chemistry and metabolism of the basement membrane. In: *Diabetes Mellitus, Theory and Practice, Chapter 9,* p. 210. Editors: M. Ellenberg and H. Rifkin. McGraw Hill, New York, N.Y.

STEELE, R., BISHOP, J. S., DUNN, A., ALTSZULER, N., RATHGEB, I. and DE BODO, R. C. (1965): Inhibition by insulin of hepatic glucose production in the normal dog. *Amer. J. Physiol., 208,* 301.

UNGER, R. H. (1972): Circulating pancreatic glucagon and extra pancreatic glucagon like materials. In: *Handbook of Physiology, Chapter 32,* pp. 529–544. Editors: D. F. Steiner and N. Freinkel. American Physiological Society, Washington, D.C.

UNGER, R. H. and LEFEBVRE, P. J. (1972): Glucagon physiology. In: *Glucagon, Chapter 15,* pp. 213–244. Editors: P. J. Lefebvre and R. H. Unger. Pergamon Press, Oxford.

VRANIC, M. (1972): Insulin and glucagon. A dual feedback system to control glucose homeostasis. In: *Insulin Action, Chapter 21,* pp. 529–541. Editor: I. B. Fritz. Academic Press, New York, N.Y.

VRANIC, M., FONO, P., KOVACEVIC, N. and LIN, B. J. (1971): Glucose kinetics and fatty acids in dogs on matched insulin infusion after glucose load. *Metabolism, 20,* 954.

VRANIC, M., RADZIUK, J. and CHERRINGTON, A. (1973): The role of glucagon and insulin in the glucoregulatory system as assessed by tracer methods. In: *Regulation and Control, in Physiological Systems, Ch. 16,* pp. 487–490. Editors: A. Iberall and A. Guyton. Instrument Society of America Press, Pittsburgh.

VRANIC, M. and WRENSHALL, G. A. (1968): Matched rates of insulin infusion and secretion and concurrent tracer-determined rates of glucose appearance and disappearance in fasting dogs. *Canad. J. Physiol. Pharmacol., 46,* 383.

VRANIC, M. and WRENSHALL, G. A. (1969): Exercise, insulin and glucose turnover in dogs. *Endocrinology, 85,* 165.

WINEGRAD, A. I., CLEMENTS Jr., R. S. and MORRISON, A. D. (1972): Insulin independent pathways of carbohydrate metabolism. In: *Handbook of Physiology, Section 7, Chapter 29,* pp. 456–473. Editors: D. F. Steiner and N. Freinkel. American Physiological Society, Washington, D.C.

WRENSHALL, G. A., VRANIC, M., COWAN, J. S. and RAPPAPORT, A. M. (1965): Effects of sudden deprivation and restoration of insulin secretion on glucose metabolism in dogs. *Diabetes, 14,* 689.

CONTROL OF HEPATIC KETOGENESIS IN VIVO. THE PRESENT POSITION

D. H. WILLIAMSON

Medical Research Council External Staff, Metabolic Research Laboratory,
Nuffield Department of Medicine, Radcliffe Infirmary,
Oxford, United Kingdom

The clinician generally associates ketone bodies with diabetes and the need for a particular form of treatment. For the biochemist ketone bodies (acetoacetate and 3-hydroxybutyrate) represent an area of metabolism which, in spite of considerable effort and numerous publications, still contains many unsolved problems. As a biochemist interested in clinical problems my aim in this contribution is to give an outline of the factors which may control the formation of ketone bodies in the whole animal and to deal in more detail with the recent advances in this field. It is important to stress this emphasis on the whole animal because, although many elegant in vitro experiments have demonstrated control points at various steps in the conversion of fatty acids to ketone bodies, it is by no means certain how many of these apply in vivo. For recent, more comprehensive reviews of ketone body metabolism the reader is referred to Williamson and Hems (1970) and McGarry and Foster (1972).

IN VIVO METABOLISM

First a simplified view of ketone body metabolism in the whole animal (Fig. 1). The major precursors of ketone bodies are the plasma free fatty acids (FFA) released from adipose tissue stores. They are transported to the liver and are oxidized to acetyl-CoA which is then converted to acetoacetate. The latter can be reduced to 3-hydroxybutyrate

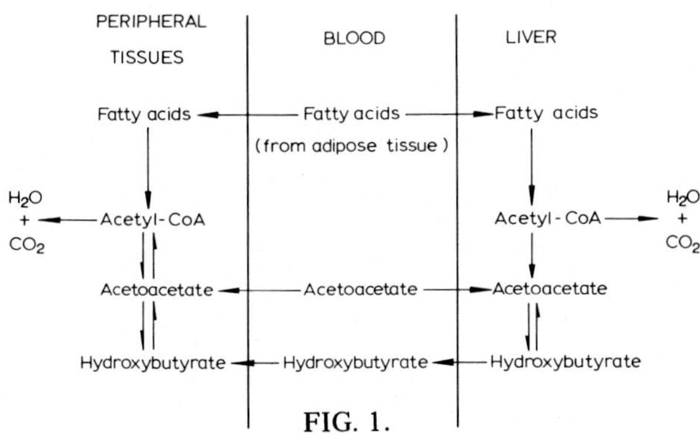

FIG. 1.

with 3-hydroxybutyrate dehydrogenase and NADH. The 2 ketone bodies leave the liver and are transported via the circulation to the peripheral tissues. In these tissues (brain, muscle, kidney) ketone bodies are reconverted to acetyl-CoA and can thus act as a metabolic fuel or, in certain circumstances, as a substrate for lipid synthesis. An essential difference between liver and peripheral tissues is that in the former the reactions leading from acetyl-CoA to acetoacetate are irreversible, while in the latter they are freely reversible.

Recent studies on the importance of ketone bodies as substrates for peripheral tissues, especially brain (Owen et al., 1967; Williamson and Buckley, 1973), support the concept that moderate hyperketonaemia is a physiological response and is beneficial to the animal (Krebs, 1961). Some of the situations in which hyperketonaemia is encountered in humans are listed in Table 1. Most of these examples are associated with increased concentrations of plasma FFA and decreased availability of carbohydrate. Therefore perhaps it is not surprising that in these situations an increase in ketone body concentrations in blood occurs to fulfil their role as alternative metabolic fuels.

TABLE 1
*Occurrence of hyperketonaemia in the human**

Situation	Ketone body concentration (mmole/l)
Normal subjects (fed)	0.1
Normal subjects (fasted 16 hr)	up to 0.3
Normal subjects (fasted 72 hr)	2 to 3
Normal subjects (postexercise)	up to 1
Obese subjects (starved 5–6 weeks)	7 to 8
Pregnancy (3rd trimester)	up to 1
Neonatal period	0.5 to 1
Idiopathic hypoglycaemia of childhood	1 to 5
Diabetic coma	up to 25

* The approximate range of total ketone bodies (acetoacetate plus 3-hydroxybutyrate) refer to whole blood and enzymatic measurements of ketone bodies.

ROLE OF FATTY ACID FLUX TO LIVER

Does this association between increased plasma fatty acids and hyperketonaemia provide the explanation for the increased rates of hepatic ketogenesis in these examples? Certainly, administration of anti-lipolytic drugs, such as nicotinic acid or insulin, will cause an immediate decrease in plasma FFA with a slightly slower fall in ketone bodies (Carlson et al., 1967; Williamson et al., 1971) as might be expected from the precursor-product relationship. It is from such evidence that the following sequence of events leading to hyperketonaemia has been formulated. A change in the hormonal balance (e.g. insulin versus glucagon) in the circulation leads to increased release of FFA from adipose tissue stores; this in turn results in increased delivery of fatty acids to the liver with a concomitant increase in ketogenesis. Although there is no question that the flux of FFA to the liver is a major factor in the control of ketogenesis, it is not the only one. A considerable amount of evidence indicates that presentation of a load of FFA to a fed liver produces considerably less ketone bodies than does the same load in a starved liver. Conversely it is possible to obtain a decrease in ketogenesis without any appreciable change in plasma FFA.

McGarry et al. (1973) have elegantly demonstrated that in the rat the time course of the changes in ketonaemia on transition from the fed state to starved and back to fed is closely correlated with the rates of ketogenesis in isolated livers perfused with a constant concentration of oleate. These findings mean that there must be intrahepatic site(s) for the regulation of ketogenesis. Most of the present research effort is being directed to discovering where this intrahepatic control is exerted because, although it is relatively easy to control the flux of FFA to the liver with insulin or anti-lipolytic drugs, direct influence on intrahepatic events is more difficult unless the regulatory site is identified.

FATE OF FATTY ACID WITHIN THE LIVER

Free fatty acid entering the liver has 2 metabolic options after its conversion to fatty acyl-CoA (Fig. 2): catabolism via the β-oxidation pathway to acetyl-CoA, or reaction with

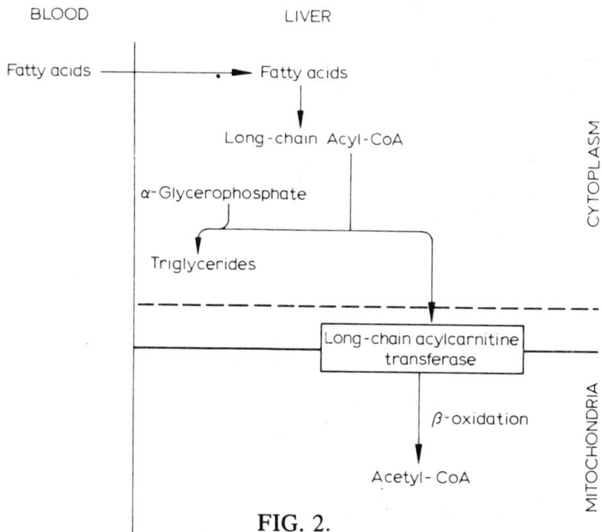

FIG. 2.

glycerol-3-phosphate to form triglycerides. Clearly, the proportion of fatty acyl-CoA diverted to triglycerides could control the amount available for the β-oxidation pathway and vice versa. One method of testing the importance of control at this branch-point in fatty acid metabolism is the use of a short-chain fatty acid such as octanoate or butyrate which is not converted to triglyceride. Such experiments indicate that the difference in ketogenesis between fed and starved livers is much less, suggesting that this branch-point is indeed an important control point.

How then is triglyceride synthesis from exogenous FFA regulated? Three possible mechanisms have been proposed: (a) availability of glycerol-3-phosphate; (b) alterations in the activities of the enzymes involved in glyceride synthesis; and (c) alterations in the rate of lipolysis of intrahepatic triglyceride. The current concept is that it is not the concentration of glycerol-3-phosphate itself which exerts control at this stage. Indeed, an often forgotten fact is that in any situation where active lipolysis occurs in adipose tissue the amount of glycerol released and made available to the liver is more than sufficient to re-esterify all of the fatty acid taken up by the liver. The activity of glycerophosphate acyl-transferase decreases in rat liver in situations associated with increased ketogenesis (Table 2; Aas and Daae, 1971) and this might direct more of the available long-chain acyl-CoA to β-oxidation. Evidence on the other mechanism (c) is lacking.

TABLE 2

*Comparison of in vitro capacities of reactions related to ketogenesis in liver of fed and starved rats**

Reaction	State of animal		Reference
	Fed	Fasted (48 hr)	
1. Palmitate → Palmityl-CoA	560	464	Aas and Daae (1971)
2. Glycerophosphate acylation	21.6	10.4	Aas and Daae (1971)
3. Palmitylcarnitine transferase	20	increased 100%	Norum (1965) Hoppel and Tomec (1972) Van Tol and Hülsmann (1969)
4. Acetyl-CoA → Acetoacetate	40	48	Williamson et al. (1968a)
5. Citrate synthase	18	18	Srere and Foster (1967)
6. Lipogenesis in vivo	4	0.2	Brunengraber et al. (1973)
7. Ketogenesis in vivo	3.4	9.4	Bates et al. (1968)

* The values are expressed as μmole C_2 units formed or removed/100 g body weight/min. at 37°C and have been taken from the cited references. Where necessary corrections have been made for temperature and liver weights. Measurements of the in vivo rates of lipogenesis and ketogenesis are included for comparison.

ROLE OF LONG-CHAIN ACYLCARNITINE TRANSFERASE

There is no evidence for a control site in the complex of enzymes concerned in β-oxidation and indeed the capacity of this system is probably high. An important potential point of regulation, however, is the entry of fatty acyl-CoA into the mitochondrial matrix, the site of β-oxidation. This process is facilitated by long-chain acylcarnitine transferase which is located on the inner mitochondrial membrane (Fig. 2). This enzyme is considered to be the rate-limiting step in the oxidation of long-chain acyl-CoA and its activity increases in situations associated with increased fatty acid oxidation (Norum, 1965; Harano et al., 1972). The apparent reciprocal changes in the in vitro activities of glycerophosphate acylation (triglyceride synthesis) and acylcarnitine transferase (fatty acid oxidation; Table 2) can be interpreted as contributing to the control of ketogenesis. The alterations in the measured activities of these enzymes appear small in relation to the manifold changes in hepatic ketone body production which can occur. However, it must be remembered that reciprocal changes in the activities of 2 enzymes competing for the same substrate can provide a sensitive form of control on the disposition of the substrate between the 2 pathways.

That acylcarnitine transferase is a potential point of control in ketogenesis is indicated by the fact that inhibition of this enzyme with (+)-decanoylcarnitine in livers perfused with oleate results in decreased ketogenesis and virtually complete esterification of the fatty acid (Williamson et al., 1968b; McGarry and Foster, 1973). This finding has been interpreted as indicating no defect in the ability of starved liver to form triglycerides. However, this type of experiment does not necessarily rule out possible control of fatty acyl-CoA disposition via changes in the activities of the 2 key enzymes, because inhibition of the transferase may increase the hepatic concentrations of long-chain acyl-CoA and thus allow glycerophosphate acylation to proceed more rapidly without the need for alteration of the concentration of the relevant enzymes.

The extension of the studies with (+)-decanoylcarnitine to the diabetic animal has shown that insulin plus (+)-decanoylcarnitine is more effective than either agent alone in decreasing the excessive ketosis (McGarry and Foster, 1973). In these experiments part of the effectiveness of (+)-decanoylcarnitine may be due to increased ketone body utilization by extra-hepatic tissues secondary to inhibition of peripheral fatty acid oxidation at the long-chain acylcarnitine step. This postulate is based on the converse findings that addition of fatty acids to kidney cortex slices can result in ketone body synthesis due to excessive production of acetyl-CoA via β-oxidation and consequent reversal of the direction of flux in the reactions involved in ketone body uptake (Weidemann and Krebs, 1969).

This recent work on long-chain acylcarnitine transferase raises 2 important questions: (1) how might the activity of this enzyme(s) be regulated so as to allow the relatively rapid changes in rates of ketogenesis which have been observed in vivo (Williamson et al., 1969; McGarry et al., 1973), and (2) is the disposition of long-chain acyl-CoA between triglyceride synthesis and the β-oxidation pathway the only intrahepatic site for the regulation of ketogenesis in vivo? At this moment there appears to be very little information on the first question, and any studies are made more complex by the fact that at least 2 long-chain acylcarnitines with different properties appear to exist on the inner mitochondrial membrane (Kopec and Fritz, 1973). The fact that short-chain fatty acids (octanoate or butyrate) produce a more pronounced hyperketonaemia in starved rats than in fed rats (McGarry and Foster, 1971; Williamson et al., 1974) means that other intrahepatic sites for the control of ketogenesis must exist. Unlike long-chain fatty acids, the short-chain acids are converted to the respective CoA derivatives within the mitochondrial matrix (Aas and Bremer, 1968; Haddock et al., 1970; Williamson et al., 1974) and consequently they are not converted to triglycerides nor do they require long-chain acylcarnitine transferase for transport to the site of β-oxidation, the mitochondrial matrix. The rate of uptake of octanoate is similar in perfused livers of fed and starved rats (McGarry and Foster, 1971) which suggests that the regulatory site is after the formation of acetyl-CoA.

FATE OF ACETYL-CoA FORMED FROM FATTY ACIDS

Like the FFA which enter the liver, the acetyl-CoA formed in β-oxidation also stands at a metabolic branch-point (Fig. 3). It can either enter the tricarboxylic acid cycle via condensation with oxaloacetate in the citrate synthase reaction, or be converted to ketone bodies via the hydroxymethylglutaryl-CoA (HMG-CoA) pathway. The hepatic activities of the enzymes of the HMG-CoA pathway in the rat liver increase in certain situations associated with hyperketonaemia, e.g., experimental diabetes, fat-feeding and the suckling period, and this may contribute to the increase in ketogenesis in these situations by directing more of the available acetyl-CoA to this pathway. There is, however, no signifi-

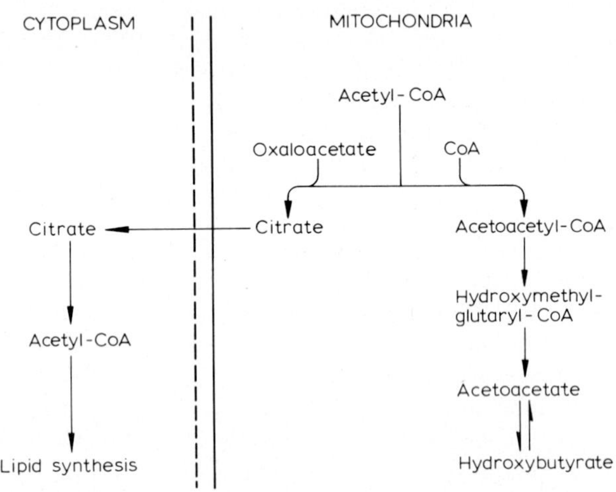

FIG. 3.

cant change in the activities of the relevant enzymes in starvation (Table 2). The in vitro measured capacity of the HMG-CoA pathway exceeds that of glycerophosphate acylation, long-chain acylcarnitine transferase or citrate synthase (Table 2), and the present evidence suggests that it is controlled by the concentrations of the substrates acetyl-CoA and acetoacetyl-CoA, though further information is required on the kinetics and other properties of the enzymes concerned. The finding that ketogenesis can be diminished without change in acetyl-CoA concentrations and in calculated values for acetoacetyl-CoA (Williamson et al., 1969; Foster 1967) means that either a regulatory step exists in the HMG-CoA pathway or the measurements of whole tissue acetyl-CoA are not meaningful in relation to the concentrations available to HMG-CoA pathway enzymes.

THE SUPPLY OF OXALOACETATE

One of the most controversial areas in the consideration of the control of hepatic ketogenesis is the role of citrate synthase and its substrate oxaloacetate, which is present in extremely low concentrations in tissues (below 10 μM). Citrate synthase is inhibited by a number of physiological effectors, such as ATP, long-chain acyl-CoA, acetoacetyl-CoA and NADH. Although a plausible theory of control can be made for each of these inhibitors, no evidence exists as yet for such a role in vivo and so this possible mechanism for the regulation of acetyl-CoA disposition will not be discussed further.

The activity of citrate synthase can also be regulated by the availability of oxaloacetate and it has been suggested by Krebs (1966) that in situations associated with increased rates of gluconeogenesis oxaloacetate is diverted from the citrate synthase reaction to the formation of phosphoenolpyruvate and ultimately glucose (Fig. 4). This is an attractive hypothesis in some ways because it would link the demand for glucose with increased production of alternative substrates, ketone bodies, which in turn can decrease the uptake of glucose by peripheral tissues.

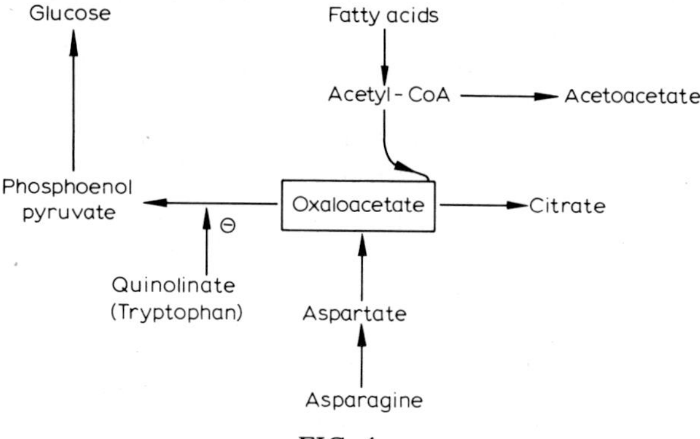

FIG. 4.

Few experiments have so far been carried out to test the 'oxaloacetate availability' hypothesis and the results obtained are conflicting. One approach is to inhibit gluconeogenesis at the stage of conversion of oxaloacetate to phosphoenolpyruvate with quinolinic acid (Veneziale et al., 1967). This results in large increases in the hepatic concentrations of oxaloacetate, aspartate, malate and citrate in starved rats, but no significant change in total ketone bodies (Table 3). Contrary to these findings, Bässler and Brinkrolf (1971)

TABLE 3

*Effects of quinolinate on the in vivo concentrations of hepatic metabolites of starved rats**

Treatment	Time after injection (min.)	Ketone bodies	Oxaloacetate	Malate	Aspartate
Saline	30	2.02	0.006	0.27	0.92
Quinolinate	30	1.98	0.015	1.91	1.64
Quinolinate	60	1.75	0.027	2.01	1.51

* Starved (48 hr) rats were injected i.p. with either saline or sodium quinolinate (500 mg/kg body weight). The rats were killed at the times indicated and the livers 'freeze-clamped'. The metabolite concentrations are expressed as μmole/g fresh weight of liver and are the mean of at least 10 observations.

reported that injection of tryptophan (which can form quinolinic acid) to starved rats caused a decrease in hyperketonaemia and suggested that this was due to the increased availability of oxaloacetate. An alternative approach is the use of the amino acid asparagine which is rapidly taken up by the liver (Woods and Handschumacher, 1971) and converted to oxaloacetate via aspartate (Fig. 4). Administration of asparagine to starved rats caused increases in aspartate and glutamate, but no significant fall in total ketone bodies (Table 4). The failure of these experiments to demonstrate any appreciable effect on ketogenesis of increasing the availability of oxaloacetate must, however, be interpreted with caution because it does not rule out the possibility of an effect in diabetic rats in which the rate of gluconeogenesis is higher than in starved rats and in which the demand for oxaloacetate is consequently greater.

TABLE 4

*Effects of L-asparagine on the in vivo concentrations of hepatic metabolites in starved rats**

Treatment	Time after injection (min.)	Ketone bodies	Aspartate	Glutamate
Saline	7	1.58	0.83	2.83
L-Asparagine	7	1.30	1.37	4.90

* Starved (48 hr) rats were anaesthetized with Nembutal and given an i.v. injection of saline or L-asparagine (2.5 mmoles/kg body weight). The rats were killed exactly 7 min. later and the livers 'freeze-clamped'. The metabolite concentrations are expressed as μmole/g fresh weight of liver and are the mean of at least 10 observations.

RELATIONSHIP BETWEEN LIPOGENESIS AND KETOGENESIS

Lipogenesis is diminished in all situations associated with increased fatty acid oxidation and concomitant increased ketogenesis. The inhibition of lipogenesis is necessary from the physiological standpoint to prevent the cycling of acetyl-CoA derived from fatty acid oxidation from being reconverted to fatty acids in an energy-wasting 'futile' cycle. It is tempting to speculate that the acetyl-CoA diverted from lipogenesis in situations where this process is inhibited might make a major contribution to ketone body synthesis. Indeed, comparison of the relative in vivo rates of hepatic lipogenesis and ketogenesis in fed and starved rats suggests that this could be so (Table 2). Short-term control of fatty acid synthesis appears to occur at the acetyl-CoA carboxylase and citrate cleavage enzyme steps and this means that any diversion of acetyl-CoA from lipogenesis to ketogenesis would have to be exerted at the level of the citrate synthase reaction (see above). Experiments in which an inhibitor of fatty acid synthesis, kynurenate, has been used in perfused livers of fed rats did not show any increase in ketogenesis (Barth et al., 1973). Thus there is no evidence for a direct link between the reciprocal rates of lipogenesis and ketogenesis which occur in vivo.

ROLE OF INSULIN

A vital question about which there is little information is: does insulin play a role in the regulation of ketogenesis other than by its effects on lipolysis in adipose tissue and the flux of FFA to the liver? Evidence that insulin may act at an intrahepatic site comes from the work of Bieberdorf et al. (1970) who were able to reverse the hyperketonaemia of starvation in rats by injection of insulin while maintaining a high concentration of plasma FFA by a constant infusion technique. The finding that insulin does not affect the hyperketonaemia of rats infused with octanoate (McGarry and Foster, 1971) or butyrate (Williamson et al., 1974) suggests that the locus of insulin action is on the disposition of long-chain acyl-CoA (Fig. 2), either by increasing esterification or by decreasing transfer into the mitochondria. Clearly, more work is required to clarify the mechanisms involved.

CONCLUSIONS

The regulation of ketogenesis is a complex subject with a multiplicity of potential control points, and it is likely that in vivo the predominant control site may vary with the physiological situation. At this stage of knowledge it is possible to provide a tentative assessment of the relative importance of the various sites for the regulation of ketogenesis in vivo. I would place them in the following order: (1) availability of plasma FFA; (2) changes in the relative rates of triglyceride synthesis and entry of long-chain acyl-CoA into the β-oxidation pathway; (3) regulation of the citrate synthase step; (4) activities of enzymes of ketone body synthesis. In severe diabetes, all 4 may play a role in the excessive hyperketonaemia.

In such a brief review much of importance has been omitted but it is hoped that the content will stimulate other biochemists to enter this 'happy hunting ground' of metabolic regulation and will convince clinicians that some progress is being made in solving the problem of pathological ketoacidosis.

REFERENCES

AAS, M. and BREMER, J. (1968): Short-chain fatty acid activation in rat liver. A new assay procedure for the enzymes and studies on their intracellular localization. *Biochim. biophys. Acta (Amst.), 164,* 157.

AAS, M. and DAAE, L. N. (1971): Fatty-acid activation and acyl transfer in organs from rats in different nutritional states. *Biochim. biophys. Acta (Amst.), 239,* 208.

BARTH, C. A., HACKENSCHMIDT, H. J., WEIS, E. E. and DECKER, K. F. A. (1973): Influence of kynurenate on cholesterol and fatty-acid synthesis in isolated perfused rat liver. *J. biol. Chem., 248,* 738.

BÄSSLER, K. H. and BRINKROLF, H. (1971): Role of oxaloacetate in increased ketogenesis and in antiketogenic action. *Z. ges. exp. Med., 156,* 52.

BATES, M. W., KREBS, H. A. and WILLIAMSON, D. H. (1968): Turnover rates of ketone bodies in normal, starved and alloxan-diabetic rats. *Biochem. J., 110,* 655.

BIEBERDORF, F. A., CHERNICK, S. S. and SCOW, R. O. (1970): Effect of insulin and acute diabetes on plasma FFA and ketone bodies in the fasting rat. *J. clin. Invest., 49,* 1685.

BRUNENGRABER, H., BOUTRY, M. and LOWENSTEIN, J. M. (1973): Fatty-acid and 3-beta-hydroxysterol synthesis in perfused rat liver including measurements on production of lactate, pyruvate, beta-hydroxybutyrate, and acetoacetate by fed liver. *J. biol. Chem., 248,* 2656.

CARLSON, L. A., FREYSCHUSS, U., KJELLBERG, J. and ÖSTMAN, J. (1967): Suppression of splanchnic ketone body production in man by nicotinic acid. *Diabetologia, 3,* 494.

FOSTER, D. W. (1967): Studies in ketosis of fasting. *J. clin. Invest., 46,* 1283.

HADDOCK, B. A., YATES, D. W. and GARLAND, P. B. (1970): The localization of some coenzyme A-dependent enzymes in rat liver mitochondria. *Biochem. J., 119,* 565.

HARANO, Y., KOWAL, J., YAMAZAKI, R., LAVINE, L. and MILLER, M. (1972): Carnitine palmitoyltransferase activities (1 and 2) and rate of palmitate oxidation in liver-mitochondria from diabetic rats. *Arch. Biochem. Biophys., 153,* 426.

HOPPEL, C. L. and TOMEC, R. J. (1972): Carnitine palmityltransferase. Location of two enzymatic activities in rat liver mitochondria. *J. biol. Chem., 247,* 832.

KOPEC, B. and FRITZ, I. B. (1973): Comparison of the properties of carnitine palmitoyltransferase I with those of carnitine palmitoyltransferase II, and preparation of antibodies to carnitine palmitoyltransferases. *J. biol. Chem., 248,* 4069.

KREBS, H. A. (1961): The physiological role of the ketone bodies. *Biochem. J., 80,* 225.

KREBS, H. A. (1966): The regulation of the release of ketone bodies by the liver. *Advanc. Enzyme Reg., 4,* 339.

McGARRY, J. D. and FOSTER, D. W. (1971): The regulation of ketogenesis from octanoic acid. *J. biol. Chem., 246,* 1149.

McGARRY, J. D. and FOSTER, D. W. (1972): Regulation of ketogenesis and clinical aspects of the ketotic state. *Metabolism, 21,* 471.

McGARRY, J. D. and FOSTER, D. W. (1973): Acute reversal of experimental diabetic ketoacidosis in rat with (+)-decanoylcarnitine. *J. clin. Invest., 52,* 877.

McGARRY, J. D., MEIER, J. M. and FOSTER, D. W. (1973): Effects of starvation and refeeding on carbohydrate and lipid metabolism in vivo and in perfused rat liver – relationship between fatty acid oxidation and esterification in regulation of ketogenesis. *J. biol. Chem., 248,* 270.

NORUM, K. R. (1965): Activation of palmityl-CoA:carnitine palmityl-transferase in livers from fasted, fat-fed, or diabetic rats. *Biochim. biophys. Acta (Amst.), 98,* 652.

OWEN, O. E., MORGAN, A. P., KEMP, H. G., SULLIVAN, J. M., HERRERA, M. G. and CAHILL, G. F. (1967): Brain metabolism during fasting. *J. clin. Invest., 46,* 1589.

SRERE, P. A. and FOSTER, D. W. (1967): On proposed relation of citrate enzymes to fatty acid synthesis and ketosis in starvation. *Biochem. biophys. Res. Commun., 26,* 556.

VAN TOL, A. and HÜLSMANN, W. C. (1969): The localization of palmitoyl-CoA:carnitine palmitoyltransferase in rat liver. *Biochim. biophys. Acta (Amst.), 189,* 342.

VENEZIALE, C. M., WALTER, P., KNEER, N. and LARDY, H. A. (1967): Influence of L-tryptophan and its metabolites on gluconeogenesis in isolated perfused liver. *Biochemistry, 6,* 2129.

WEIDEMANN, M. J. and KREBS, H. A. (1969): The fuel of respiration of rat kidney cortex. *Biochem. J., 112,* 149.

WILLIAMSON, D. H., BATES, M. W. and KREBS, H. A. (1968a): Activity and intracellular distribution of enzymes of ketone-body metabolism in rat liver. *Biochem. J., 108,* 353.

WILLIAMSON, J. R., BROWNING, E. T., SCHOLZ, R., KREISBERG, R. A. and FRITZ, I. B. (1968b): Inhibition of fatty acid stimulation of gluconeogenesis by (+)-decanoylcarnitine in perfused rat liver. *Diabetes, 17,* 194.

WILLIAMSON, D. H., VELOSO, D., ELLINGTON, E. V. and KREBS, H. A. (1969): Changes in the concentrations of hepatic metabolites on administration of dihydroxyacetone or glycerol to starved rats and their relationship to the control of ketogenesis. *Biochem. J., 114,* 575.

WILLIAMSON, D. H. and HEMS, R. (1970): Metabolism and function of ketone bodies. In: *Essays in Cell Metabolism,* p. 257. Editors: W. Bartley, H. L. Kornberg and J. R. Quayle. Wiley-Interscience, London, New York.

WILLIAMSON, D. H., MAYOR, F., VELOSO, D. and PAGE, M. A. (1971): Effects of nicotinic acid and related compounds on ketone body metabolism. In: *Metabolic Effects of Nicotinic Acid and its Derivatives,* p. 227. Editors: K. F. Gey and L. A. Carlson. Hans Huber, Berne.

WILLIAMSON, D. H. and BUCKLEY, B. M. (1973): The role of ketone bodies in brain development. In: *Inborn Errors of Metabolism,* p. 80. Editors: F. A. Hommes and C. J. Van Den Berg. Academic Press, London, New York.

WILLIAMSON, D. H., ILIC, V., ELLINGTON, E. V. and SAAL, J. (1974): Hepatic effects of saturated and unsaturated short-chain fatty acids and the control of ketogenesis in vivo. In: *Liver Metabolism,* 5th Alfred Benson Symposium, in press.

WOODS, J. S. and HANDSCHUMACHER, R. E. (1971): Hepatic homeostasis of plasma L-asparagine. *Amer. J. Physiol., 221,* 1785.

INSULITIS AND VIRUS

INSULITIS AND VIRUSES. INTRODUCTORY REMARKS

WILLY GEPTS

Department of Pathology, Brugmann University Hospital, Brussels, Belgium

The relationship between infection and diabetes has been looked upon mainly from one side. All students of diabetes readily agree that, at least in uncontrolled diabetics, infections are more common than in non-diabetics. This increased frequency has been attributed to a lower resistance, but the intimate nature of the latter remains unknown.

The task here is not to discuss why infections occur more frequently in diabetics, but to debate whether diabetes can be caused by an infection. From the beginning of this century, the hypothesis of an infectious origin of diabetes has been proposed time and again, but it has always met with discouraging scepticism. However, new facts have been discovered in recent years, which provide the infection theory with somewhat more solid foundations. The present arguments in favour of an infectious etiology of some cases of diabetes can be grouped under 4 headings:

1. Many diabetologists have been impressed by the frequency of acute infections prior to or shortly after the onset of diabetes in young individuals. Mumps has particularly been held in suspicion, and there have been several reports of cases of diabetes appearing within a relatively short time after an epidemic of viral parotitis (Gundersen, 1927; Cole, 1934a, b; Kremer, 1947; Hinden, 1962).

2. Inflammatory infiltration, mainly lymphocytic, is present in the islets of many juvenile diabetics of recent onset (LeCompte, 1958; Gepts, 1965). This lesion, for which von Meyenburg (1940) coined the name insulitis, has been described well before insulin was discovered. Classically it is considered of rare occurrence, but we found it in 68% of a group of young diabetics, who had died within a few years of the onset of the disease (Gepts, 1965). On the other hand Doniach (1973) could not find one example of insulitis in 12 cases of recent onset juvenile diabetes. In late onset diabetics insulitis had never been observed, until recently LeCompte and Legg (1972) reported 2 cases in elderly patients.

3. Epidemiological studies, carried out in Great Britain (Gamble et al., 1969; Gamble and Taylor, 1969), disclosed elevated levels of anitbodies against a strain of Coxsackie viruses in young diabetics with a disease of short duration. Such an increase was not found in other diabetics, nor did it occur for antibodies against other viruses.

4. Craighead et al. (1968, 1971), later on confirmed by others (Müntefering et al., 1971; Burch et al., 1972; Taylor, 1973), reported that diabetes can be induced in mice, by inoculating them with selected virus strains. In some of these mice, insulitis was present in the islets.

These 4 headings represent the landmarks around which the contributions to this panel will be oriented. The pathological and epidemiological evidence for a possible infectious etiology in some cases of diabetes will first be reviewed and evaluated critically by Craighead and Taylor. All the participants to the panel will report on their personal experience with experimental viral insulitis. Its ultramicroscopic appearance will be described by Müntefering. Freytag will compare viral and immune insulitis and discuss a possible relationship between these two. Grodsky will present new data on viral infection in a species with a mild form of, or predisposed to diabetes.

Each member of this panel has made important contributions to the problem of insulitis, and therefore introductions will not be necessary. I feel confident that their presentations and discussions will greatly help the audience to have a clear view of a subject which is becoming increasingly interesting. Although it is much too early to raise unwarranted hopes, it is clear that the decisive demonstration of an infectious origin in some cases of diabetes, particularly juvenile diabetes, would open new possibilities for the prevention of one of the most grievous diseases of mankind.

REFERENCES

BURCH, G. E., TSUI, C. J. and HARB, J. M. (1972): Pancreatic islet damage in mice produced by Cocksackie B_1 and encephalomyocarditis viruses. *Experientia (Basel), 28/3,* 310.

COLE, L. (1934a): Diabetes mellitus in children. *Lancet, i,* 947.

COLE, L. (1934b): Diabetes mellitus in children. *Lancet, i,* 998.

CRAIGHEAD, J. E. (1965): Necrosis of the pancreas, lacrimal and parotid glands associated with encephalomyocarditis virus infection. *Nature (Lond.), 207,* 1268.

CRAIGHEAD, J. E. (1966): Pathogenicity of the M. and E. variants of the encephalomyocarditis (EMC) virus. II. Lesions of the pancreas, parotid and lacrimal glands. *Amer. J. Path., 48,* 375.

CRAIGHEAD, J. E. and McLANE, M. F. (1968): Diabetes mellitus: induction in mice by encephalomyocarditis virus. *Science, 162,* 913.

CRAIGHEAD, J. E. and STEINKE, J. (1971): Diabetes mellitus-like syndrome in mice infected with EMC virus. *Amer. J. Path., 116,* 119.

DONIACH, I. (1973): In: *Immunology in Diabetes,* Francqui Foundation Colloquium, Brussels, May 1973. Excerpta Medica, in press.

GAMBLE, D. R., KINSLEY, M. L., FITZGERALD, M. G., BOLTON, R. and TAYLOR, K. W. (1969): Viral antibodies in diabetes mellitus. *Brit. med. J., 3,* 627.

GAMBLE, D. R. and TAYLOR, K. W. (1969): Seasonal incidence of diabetes mellitus. *Brit. med. J., 3,* 631.

GEPTS, W. (1965): Pathologic anatomy of the pancreas in juvenile diabetes mellitus. *Diabetes, 14,* 619.

GUNDERSON, E. (1927): Is diabetes of infectious origin? *J. infect. Dis., 41,* 197.

HINDEN, E. (1962): Mumps followed by diabetes. *Lancet, i,* 138.

KREMER, H. U. (1947): Juvenile diabetes as sequel of paratitis. *Amer. J. Med., 3,* 257.

LeCOMPTE, P. M. (1958): 'Insulitis' in early juvenile diabetes. *Arch. Path., 66,* 450.

LeCOMPTE, P. M. and LEGG, A. (1972): Insulitis (lymphocytic infiltration of pancreatic islets) in late-onset diabetes. *Diabetes, 21,* 762.

MÜNTEFERING, H., SCHMIDT, W. A. K. and KÖRBER, W. (1971): Zur Virusgenese des Diabetes mellitus bei der weiszen Maus. *Dtsch. med. Wschr., 96,* 693.

TAYLOR, K. W. (1973): In: *Immunology in Diabetes,* Francqui Foundation Colloquium, Brussels, May 1973. Excerpta Medica, in press.

VON MEYENBURG, H. (1940): Über 'Insulitis' bei Diabetes. *Schweiz. med. Wschr., 21,* 554.

VIRAL LESIONS OF THE PANCREATIC ISLETS OF LANGERHANS*

JOHN E. CRAIGHEAD

Department of Pathology, University of Vermont, Burlington, Vt., U.S.A.

A variety of viruses multiply in the pancreatic tissue of man and animals. Experimental and epidemiological observations suggest that these agents may play an etiologic role in some cases of human diabetes mellitus. This paper is concerned with the viral pathogenesis of pancreatic insular lesions and their possible importance in the causation of diabetes mellitus.

INSULAR LESIONS IN HUMAN VIRAL INFECTIONS

Although mumps virus is well recognized as a cause of pancreatitis in man, the pathogenesis of the lesion is poorly understood. Epidemiological studies and anecdotal case reports suggest that diabetes mellitus occasionally occurs in the wake of mumps virus involvement of the pancreas. If, indeed, the islets of Langerhans are affected during the course of this disease, the pathologic features of the insular lesion remain to be defined. The available information is confined to autopsy observations on a few individuals who succumbed inadvertently during the course of clinical mumps. Clearly, critically-designed epidemiological and experimental studies must be undertaken before an association between mumps virus infection and diabetes mellitus can be established.

An unusual prevalence of diabetes mellitus in children and young adults with the congenital rubella syndrome is suggested by the recent reports of several groups of investigators (Forrest et al., 1971). Although the pancreas appears to support the replication of rubella virus in the infant with a disseminated infection, lesions of the parenchyma of the organ are rarely observed. Since rubella virus affects the multiplication rate and growth of a variety of tissues in the congenitally-infected individual, it seems plausible to surmise that at least under some circumstances the beta cell mass may be compromised. Bunnell and Monif (1972) reported a case of congenitally-acquired disease in which interstitial pancreatitis was found at autopsy. Although the islets of Langerhans in this child were said to be shrunken and degranulated (Monif, personal communication), evidence of pancreatic endocrine insufficiency was not detected. It seems likely that the role of rubella virus in the pathogenesis of diabetes mellitus could be clarified by epidemiological investigations.

* Work of the author cited in this paper was supported by U.S. Public Health Service Grant No. AI 09118 from the National Institute of Allergy and Infectious Diseases.

Pathologists long have recognized the characteristic lesions of cytomegalic inclusion disease in human pancreatic tissue. Interestingly enough, the cells of the islets of Langerhans commonly exhibit typical inclusions, both in infants and adults with generalized cytomegalovirus infection. Indeed, insular cells often are affected even when inclusion-bearing cells infrequently are found in the acinar pancreas. Gepts et al. (1973) studied an infant dying of an obscure disease in which virions consistent with cytomegalovirus were present in alpha cells of the islets of Langerhans. At present, one can only speculate regarding the significance of these findings. Increasing clinical and pathologic evidence suggests that non-fatal disseminated cytomegalovirus infections occur commonly in members of the general population, and in individuals with abnormalities of immunologic responsiveness. It seems plausible to suggest that covert lesions of the pancreatic insular tissue could occur as a consequence of these subtle infections.

Pancreatic lesions have been observed in infants with congenitally-acquired group B Coxsackie virus infections. In addition to a fatal myocarditis and meningoencephalitis, these patients occasionally exhibit interstitial inflammation of the pancreatic parenchyma. Sussman et al. (1959) described a unique necrotizing lesion of the islets of Langerhans in an infant succumbing with congenitally-acquired group B, type 3, Coxsackie virus infection. In this case, interstitial inflammatory disease of the exocrine pancreas was not prominent. On the other hand, Drs. Lotte Strauss (New York) and William J. Newton, Jr. (Columbus, Ohio) have brought to our attention additional cases of congenitally-acquired group B Coxsackie virus infection, in which interstitial pancreatitis was prominent. In the pancreases of these cases, mononuclear cells frequently had accumulated around the islets of Langerhans and occasionally were found in and around the cords of beta cells in the islets. Moreover, aldehyde fuchsin stains of this tissue showed that the beta cells were degranulated. Thus, the evidence suggests that, on occasion, lesions of the pancreatic parenchyma and of the islets of Langerhans develop in the course of Coxsackie virus infections. Although the metabolic consequences of these changes have yet to be defined, the recent epidemiological studies of Gamble et al. (1969) and Gamble and Taylor (1973) suggest an association between abrupt-onset diabetes in man and infection with group B Coxsackie virus.

The occurrence of pancreatic disease in the course of systemic virus infections is recognized but incompletely studied. The possible role of viruses in the causation of metabolically-significant lesions of the islets of Langerhans in man remains to be elucidated.

INSULAR LESIONS IN ENCEPHALOMYOCARDITIS (EMC) VIRUS-INFECTED MICE

The encephalomyocarditis (EMC) virus is a member of the picornavirus group. Thus, it is a small RNA-containing agent which has biological properties similar to many of the common enteroviruses of man, i.e. the polio-, Coxsackie and echoviruses. As with the group B Coxsackie viruses, EMC multiplies in the myocardium and central nervous system of experimental animals. It also replicates in zymogen organs, specifically the lacrimal and the parotid glands, and the pancreas (Craighead, 1965). Some strains of this virus appear to grow in the exocrine tissue of the pancreas, where they cause necrosis of acinar cells (Craighead, 1966b). On the other hand, a virus selected in our laboratory, the M variant, multiplies in the pancreas, but causes lesions exclusively of the islets of Langerhans (Craighead and McLane, 1968; Craighead and Steinke, 1971). The reasons for this tropism for insular tissue are unclear. No other recognized virus possesses this unique property.

The M variant of EMC virus can be recovered from the pancreatic tissue of adult mice for as long as 18 days after inoculation by the subcutaneous route. The amounts of virus in the pancreas during the first week of the infection are substantial, and exceed the quantities in the blood serum. Fluorescence microscopy shows that viral antigens are located exclusively in beta cells of the islets of Langerhans (Boucher et al., 1973).

Characteristic histopathologic alterations appear in the insular tissue approximately 4 to 6 days after virus inoculation (Craighead and Steinke, 1971; Wellmann et al., 1972; Müntefering et al., 1971). The uniform architecture and arrangement of cells in the islets is distorted. The tissue is edematous and mononuclear cells are located around small blood vessels and at the periphery of the islets. Aldehyde fuchsin stains of the insular tissue at this time show that the beta cells are degranulated, and electron micrographs confirm this observation. Despite the multiplication of virus in the islets, necrosis of individual beta cells occurs uncommonly. This is of considerable interest, since EMC virus is cytolytic for many types of cultured cells.

Early in the course of the infection, macrophages appear in the islets of Langerhans, where they phagocytize degenerate beta cells (Wellmann et al., 1972). Lymphocytes are observed somewhat later. These cells often are intimately associated with beta cells, and frequently are found at sites of tissue necrosis. Interestingly enough, lymphocytes rarely are located in the islets of infected mice by the 14th day after inoculation.

As might be expected, degranulation of islets is associated with a prompt decrease in the total pancreatic content of immunologically-reactive insulin. Initially, a transient hypoglycemia is observed. This event is followed promptly by the appearance of increased concentrations of glucose in the blood. During the acute stages of infection, the biochemical and pathologic alterations differ in inidividual animals. Some exhibit severe hyperglycemia and prominent lesions of the islets, whereas in a few there is little or no evidence of abnormal carbohydrate metabolism. As will be discussed below, the severity of the lesion appears to be influenced by genetic and metabolic factors which are defined incompletely at present.

Hyperglycemia persists in individual mice for variable periods of time. The quantitative aspects of these experiments are complicated by the death of some animals, primarily due to the severe myocardial necrosis which accompanies the infection (Craighead, 1966a). Approximately 60% of mice of the CD-1 strain survive for 3 weeks or longer. At this time, some are normoglycemic and have a normal response to a carbohydrate challenge, whereas others persistently have elevated concentrations of glucose in the blood. A few additional mice with normal or slightly elevated amounts of blood glucose exhibit evidence of beta cell insufficiency when challenged in a glucose tolerance test.

Approximately 40% of convalescent animals exhibit chronic hyperglycemia. A few of these mice lose weight and become ketotic (Boucher and Notkins, 1973). Eventually they die. If members of this group are studied biochemically before death, the amounts of immunologically-reactive insulin in the pancreas and blood are reduced. A variety of morphologic changes are observed in the insular tissue of these animals. The cells of the islets of Langerhans are degranulated and substantially reduced in number. Often, there are ultrastructural features of hyperactivity in the residual beta cells as evidenced by a hyperplasia of the cytoplasmic organelles and changes in the nuclei. In addition, regeneration of beta cells in the form of mitoses and metaplasia of acinar cells at the periphery of the islets is found (Craighead and Kessler, 1974).

Animals with less severe degrees of hyperglycemia survive indefinitely. A variety of morphological changes are observed in the insular tissue of these mice, although the total beta cell mass appears sufficient to maintain a degree of metabolic compensation. With the passage of time, some animals appear to recover, for they exhibit a normal response to a carbohydrate challenge months after the original infection.

A number of factors influences the severity of the lesion in the islets of Langerhans of virus-infected animals. Metabolic influences have an important effect. When experimental animals are administered pharmacological dosages of corticosteroid hormone, the islets undergo severe necrosis (Craighead, 1966b). Similarly, the severity of the insular lesion and the consequent hyperglycemia is accentuated when animals are made obese by the administration of gold-thioglucose* (Craighead and Steinke, 1974).

Genetic factors also influence the extent of the damage to the beta cells in the islets of Langerhans. For example, infected inbred mice of the DBA/2 strain regularly develop necrosis of beta cells and inflammation of the islets, whereas animals of several other inbred strains (C3H, C57BL) show only minor insular lesions during the acute stages of virus infection. The relative severity of these lesions is reflected by the degree of carbohydrate intolerance exhibited by the animal (Craighead, 1974).

It is apparent that many features of human diabetes mellitus are simulated by the mouse model. The metabolic abnormalities and pathologic lesions in the severely affected, acute and convalescent animals strikingly resemble the picture observed in juvenile-type human diabetes. On the other hand, it is clear that many virus-infected animals sustain damage to insular tissue which results in a condition comparable to chemical prediabetes, and possibly the maturity-onset form of the disease. In man, genetic and metabolic factors strikingly affect the expression and severity of diabetes mellitus. Similarly, in the animal model, these influences play an important role.

Classical concepts of infection relate the micro-organism and disease in a cause and effect association. This view may be simplistic, for it ignores environmental factors and genetic susceptibility or resistance. If a uniquely susceptible group of individuals exists in the population, a common infectious organism could cause an unusual disease syndrome. Indeed, the agent may not be as important as the host response to the agent. In this context, we might address ourselves to the question 'Could diabetes mellitus in man have an infectious etiology?'

REFERENCES

BOUCHER, D. W., HAYASHI, K. and NOTKINS, A. L. (1974): Virus-induced diabetes mellitus in mice. *Amer. J. Pathol.*, in press.

BOUCHER, D. W. and NOTKINS, A. L. (1973): Virus-induced diabetes mellitus. I. Hyperglycemia and hypoinsulinemia in mice infected with encephalomyocarditis virus. *J. exp. Med., 137/5,* 1226.

BUNNELL, C. E. and MONIF, G. R. G. (1972): Interstitial pancreatitis in the congenital rubella syndrome. *J. Pediat., 80/3,* 465.

CRAIGHEAD, J. E. (1965): Necrosis of the pancreas, parotid and lachrymal glands associated with encephalomyocarditis virus infection. *Nature (Lond.), 207/5003,* 1268.

* Gold-thioglucose appears to act on the satiety center of the hypothalamus when administered intravenously. This results in hyperphagia and obesity (Marshall et al., 1955).

CRAIGHEAD, J. E. (1966a): Pathogenicity of the M and E variants of the encephalomyocarditis (EMC) virus. I. Myocardiotropic and neurotropic properties. *Amer. J. Pathol., 48/2,* 333.

CRAIGHEAD, J. E. (1966b): Pathogenicity of the M and E variants of the encephalomyocarditis (EMC) virus. II. Lesions of the pancreas, parotid and lacrimal glands. *Amer. J. Pathol., 48/3,* 375.

CRAIGHEAD, J. E. and HIGGINS, D. A. (1974): Genetic influences affecting the occurrence of a diabetes mellitus-like disease in mice infected with the encephalomvocarditis virus. *J. exp. Med.,* in press.

CRAIGHEAD, J. E. and KESSLER, J. B. (1974): Lesions of islets of Langerhans in mice with EMC virus induced diabetes mellitus: late changes. Submitted for publication.

CRAIGHEAD, J. E. and McLANE, M. F. (1968): Diabetes mellitus: induction in mice by encephalomyocarditis virus. *Science, 162,* 913.

CRAIGHEAD, J. E. and STEINKE, J. (1971): Diabetes mellitus-like syndrome in mice infected with encephalomyocarditis virus. *Amer. J. Pathol., 63/1,* 119.

CRAIGHEAD, J. E. and STEINKE, J. (1974): The effect of gold-thioglucose induced obesity on the diabetes-like disease in encephalomyocarditis virus infected mice. In preparation.

FORREST, J. M., MENSER, M. A. and BURGESS, J. A. (1971): High frequency of diabetes mellitus in young adults with congenital rubella. *Lancet, 1,* 332.

GAMBLE, D. R., KINSLEY, M. L., FITZGERALD, M. G., BOLTON, R. and TAYLOR, K. W. (1969): Viral antibodies in diabetes mellitus. *Brit. med. J., 3,* 627.

GAMBLE, D. R. and TAYLOR, K. W. (1973): Coxsackie B virus and diabetes. *Brit. med. J., 1,* 289.

MARSHALL, N. B., BARRNETT, R. J. and MAYER, J. (1955): Hypothalamic lesions in gold-thioglucose injected mice. *Proc. Soc. exp. Biol. Med., 90/1,* 240.

MÜNTEFERING, H., SCHMIDT, W. A. K. and KORBER, W. (1971): Zur Virusgenese des Diabetes Mellitus bei der Weissen Maus. *Dtsch. med. Wschr., 16/16,* 693.

SUSSMAN, M. L., STRAUSS, L. and HODES, H. L. (1959): Fatal Coxsackie group B virus infection in the newborn. *J. Dis. Child., 97,* 483.

WELLMANN, K. F., AMSTERDAM, D., BRANCATO, P. and VOLK, B. W. (1972): Fine structure of pancreatic islets of mice infected with the M variant of the encephalomyocarditis virus. *Diabetologia, 8/5,* 349.

Detailed reference lists are published in 'Inflammatory lesions of the islets of Langerhans', *Handbook of Physiology, Section 7: Endocrinology* (American Physiological Society, 1972) and 'Role of viruses in diabetes mellitus', in *Progress in Medical Virology, Vol. 16* (S. Karger, 1974).

IMMUNE INSULITIS, COMPARISON WITH VIRAL INSULITIS*

G. FREYTAG and G. KLÖPPEL

Department of Pathology, University of Hamburg, Federal Republic of Germany

Similar or almost identical pathohistological changes as described by Drs. Craighead and Müntefering (see this Volume, pp. 287–291 and 316–320) in the pancreas of mice infected with encephalomyocarditis (EMC) virus, can be observed in animals injected repeatedly or over prolonged periods with anti-insulin serum (Lacy and Wright, 1965; Logothetopoulos and Bell, 1966; Klöppel et al., 1971; Freytag, 1972) or immunized with crystalline insulin (Toreson et al., 1964; Renold et al., 1964; Klöppel et al., 1972; for further literature see Freytag and Klöppel, 1973). These 2 types of immune insulitis depend on the immunogenicity of insulin extracted from the mammalian pancreas:

Experimental immune response to insulin

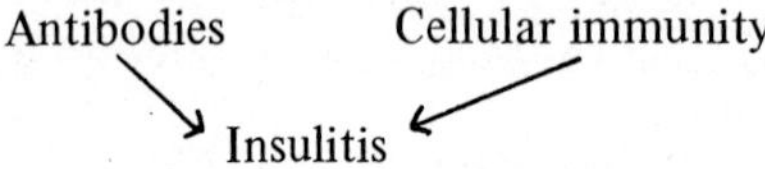

ACTIVE IMMUNIZATION

Active immunization of rabbits with bovine insulin and Freund's adjuvant resulted in insulitis in 40–60% of the animals. In general a great number of islets are infiltrated. The extent of the inflammation as well as the destructive character of the insulitis vary in the individual animals.

Insulitis starts with a peri-insular infiltration. In a few cases the inflammatory process extends and leads to a destructive infiltration of the whole islet (Fig. 1). Following Gomori's aldehyde-fuchsin staining the beta cells are often degranulated to some extent and show hyperactive alterations. The nuclei of those cells are markedly enlarged, the cytoplasm is swollen and the granules are frequently displaced to the cell surface, indicating a temporarily increased insulin release. The alpha and delta cells are intact and show no changes in size or staining reaction.

* Supported by the Deutsche Forschungsgemeinschaft, Sonderforschungsbereich 34, 'Endokrinologie'.

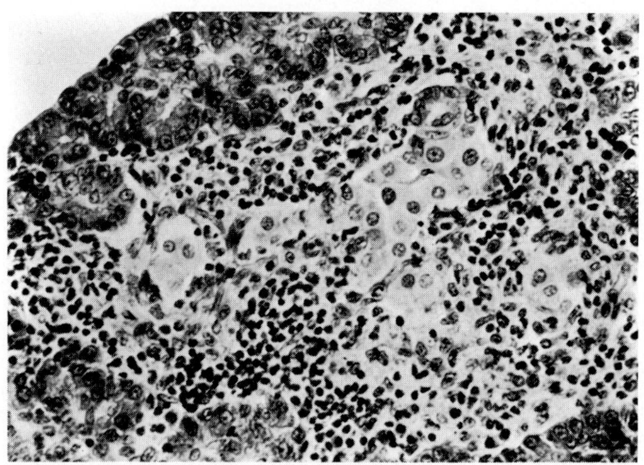

FIG. 1. Islet of rabbit after weekly immunization with crystalline bovine insulin, predominantly in Freund's adjuvant incomplete (4th week): extensive insulitis with extensive peri-insular and intra-insular infiltrates of lymphoid cell. PAS, × 197.

By electron microscopy, lymphocytes and immunoblasts are found to be the main cell types of the infiltrate. These cells are characterized by their nuclei and their cytoplasmic structures. Furthermore macrophages are observed. As a rule plasma cells are very rare.

The lymphocytes are generally in very close contact with the beta cells. Pseudopod-like structures of immune cells are the main characteristics of these contact areas (Fig. 2).

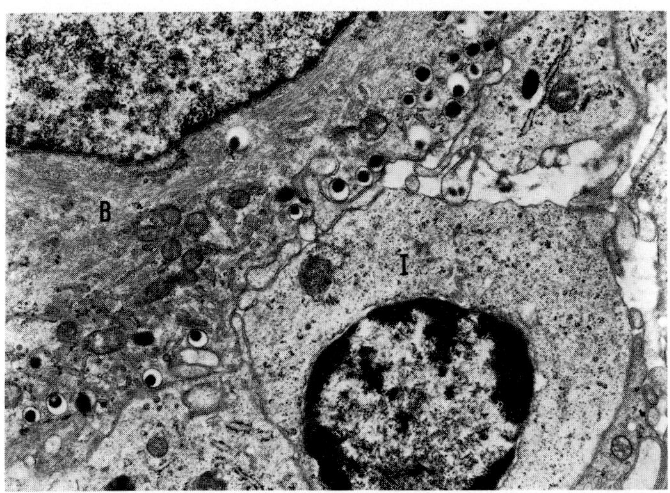

FIG. 2. Islet of rabbit after weekly immunization with crystalline bovine insulin (4th week): immunoblast (I) in close contact to a beta cell (B); pseudopod-like structures of the immunoblast invading the beta cell cytoplasm. × 9,750.

In cases with permanent diabetes the beta cells are severely degenerated. The nucleus is shrunken, the perinuclear space is enlarged, and the rough endoplasmic reticulum undergoes cystic dilatation. The necrotic beta cells are obviously phagocytized by macrophages. Despite the close contact with some immune cells the alpha cells show no degenerative changes. Thus the alpha cell is well granulated, and its nucleus is preserved (Fig. 3).

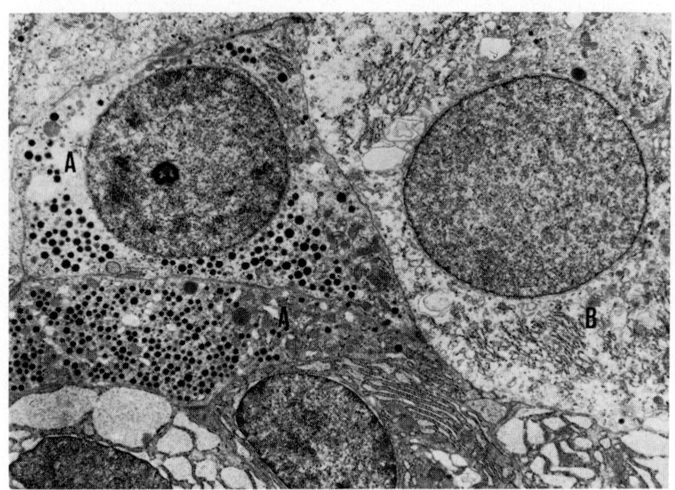

FIG. 3. Islet of rabbit with overt diabetes following insulin immunization. Note the severely degranulated beta cell (B) with degenerative changes of the cytoplasmic matrix. In contrast, alpha cells (A) are well preserved. X 6,560.

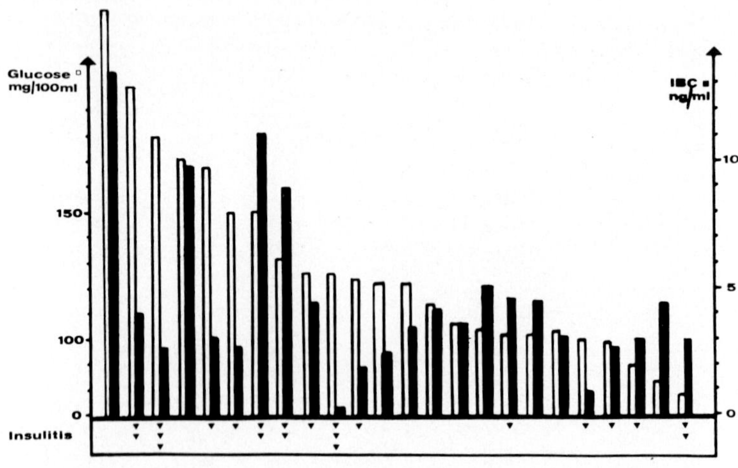

FIG. 4. Intensity and incidence of insulitis, fasting blood glucose levels and insulin-binding capacity (IBC) after immunization with crystalline bovine insulin in predominantly Freund's adjuvant incomplete. IBC is calculated on that dilution of serum with 30% binding 0.1 ng of porcine ^{127}I insulin/ml.

In our series about 10% of the animals temporarily showed hyperglycemic episodes, but only one rabbit out of 22 developed frank diabetes. Animals with transient hyperglycemia in general seem to show a poor relation between antibody titre and blood glucose levels, whereas there was no correlation at all between antibody titre and insulitis. In contrast, manifest diabetes appears to be associated with most severe insulitis (Fig. 4). The glucose tolerance of the diabetic animal was clearly decreased, whereas the glucose tolerance of those rabbits which showed a temporary elevation of fasting blood sugar had normal curves following glucose injection.

PASSIVE TRANSFER OF INSULIN ANTIBODIES

The injection of insulin antibodies leads to another type of insulitis. The single injection of high titre guinea pig anti-insulin serum into rats or mice results in degranulation of beta cells and, 3 hours following the injection, in an acute but reversible type of islet inflammation (Fig. 5a). Polymorphonuclear cells, especially eosinophil *granulocytes* migrate into the intra- and peri-insular spaces. This inflammatory reaction depends on the presence of precipitated immune complexes produced by the injected insulin antibodies and insulin. They develop in the area of highest insulin concentration, the specific antigen, i.e. in the islet area. Insulitis is therefore thought to be an immune reaction of the immediate type. A cytotoxic effect of the injected antibodies on the beta cells has not been observed. Electron microscopically the beta cell is well separated from the infiltrate. Precipitated protein-like material can be observed between beta cells and capillaries, or phagocytized in the cytoplasm of granulocytes (Fig. 5b).

Repeated injections of antibodies are parallelled by marked increases in blood sugar. A permanent diabetic lesion is not observed in these early stages of the study. Using low titre anti-insulin serum the type of insulitis changes. Now the first infiltrates are noted about the third day of the study. The infiltrate is mainly localized between small veins and adjacent islets (Fig. 6a). During the following days the infiltrate may increase and extend into the islet area. Sometimes a typical halfmoon-like shape can be observed (Fig. 6b).

Cytologically large round cells with a pyroninophilic nucleus are most noticeable within the infiltrate, whereas leukocytes are less obvious (Fig. 7a). The proliferating character of these mononucleated cells can be demonstrated by the tritiated thymidine technique. After injection of tritiated thymidine most of the mononuclear cells have been found to incorporate the radioactive substance. This indicates high mitotic activity in these cells (Fig. 7b).

Electron microscopically the late infiltrate mainly consists of large macrophages, filled out with phagocytized cloudy material, probably precipitated immune complexes. Furthermore, lymphoid cells, probably *immunoblasts*, as well as plasma cells and single eosinophil cells can be demonstrated. Immunofluorescence with labelled anti-guinea pig gamma globulin serum suggests the phagocytosis of proteins from guinea pigs. Fluorescent material can be demonstrated within infiltrate cells.

In long-term studies throughout a period of 4 6 weeks extensive infiltration of the peri-insular and insular areas becomes evident. The normal islet architecture is greatly altered, and in some cases almost completely destroyed (Figs 6c and d). Finally this destruction results in islet fibrosis.

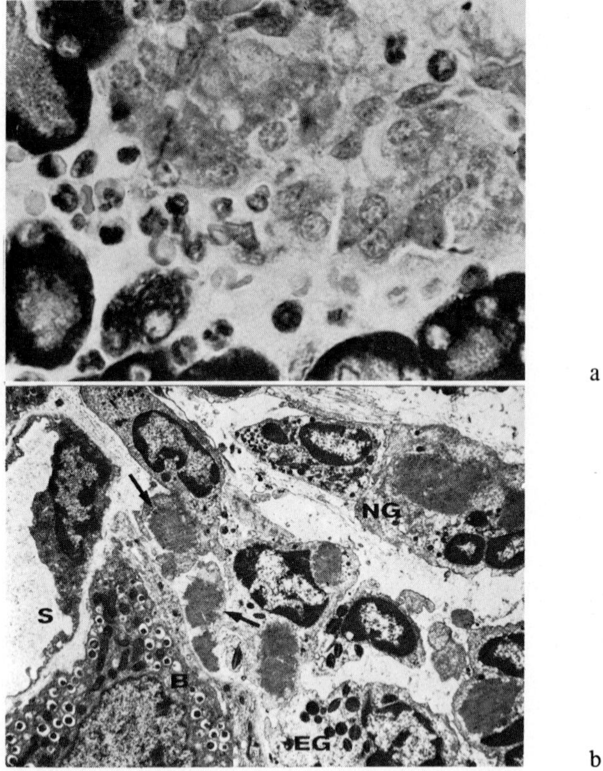

FIG. 5. Islet of mice 180 minutes after injection of 0.5 ml of high titer anti-insulin serum. (a) Acute polymorphocellular peri-insulitis. Giemsa, × 700. (b) Acute peri-insulitis with interstitial infiltration by eosinophil (EG) and neutrophil granulocytes (NG). Cloudy electron-dense material (precipitated insulin antibody complex?) in close contact to a beta cell (B), being phagocytized by neutrophils (↗). Sinusoid (S). × 5,660. (from Klöppel et al., 1971, by courtesy).

COMPARISON WITH VIRAL INSULITIS

When the histopathological characteristics of immune insulitis, mentioned above, are compared with those of virus insulitis, one can find some parallels, but also some differences. These differences between insulitis produced by virus infection and insulitis induced immunologically probably depend on the different pathogenetic mechanisms of aggression to the insular system (Table 1). The virus multiplication damages the beta and alpha as well as the delta cells, and leads to their necrosis. In some animals this in turn results in cellular infiltration. Thus islet cell necrosis plays the main role at the beginning of the pathogenesis of virus-induced insulitis. Immune insulitis, however, is the result of certain immune mechanisms to insulin, which in consequence exclusively involve the beta cells, the source of insulin.

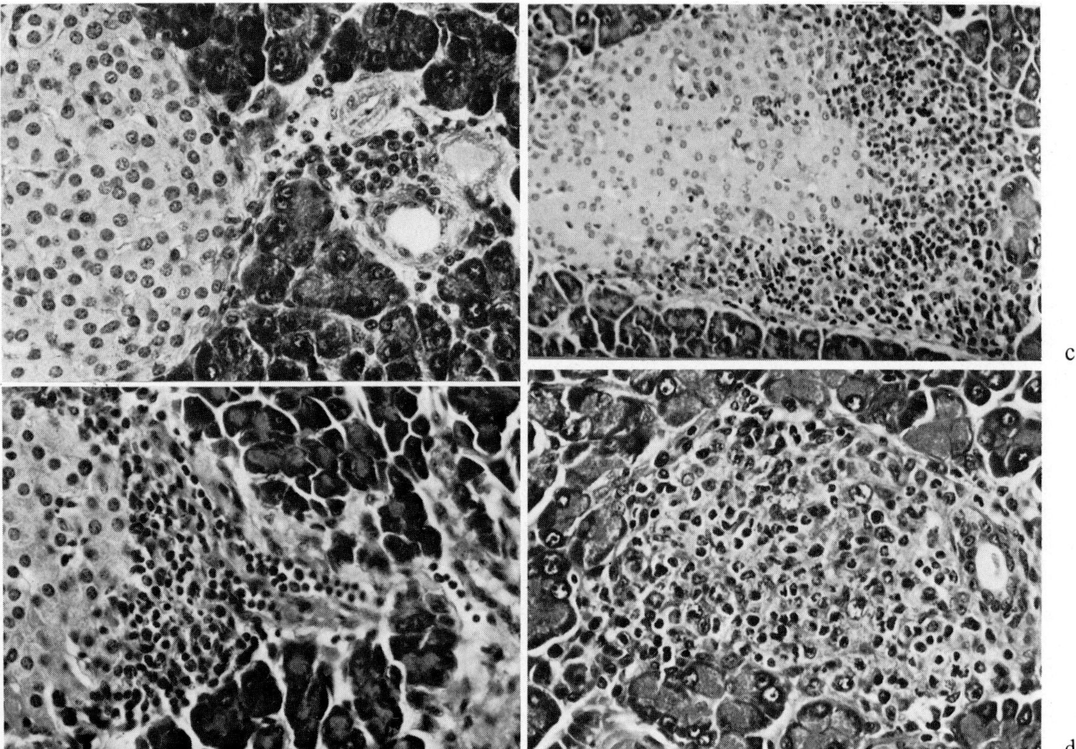

FIG. 6. Islet of mice repeatedly injected with medium titer anti-insulin serum: (a) Small round cells infiltrate at the vascular pool of the islet (first week). PAS, X 292. (b) Small half moon-like infiltrate in the peri-insular area (2nd week). PAS, X 292. (c) Marked half moon-like islet infiltrate of predominantly round cells (4th week). H & E, X 183. (d) Inflammatory islet destruction (6th week). PAS, X 305.

Virus insulitis is characterized by mononucleated cells, mainly macrophages and lymphoid cells, but also by some polymorphonuclear cells (Table 2). In addition to its temporary appearance these findings suggest that virus insulitis represents a resorptive mechanism to damaged cell material. Immune insulitis in animals injected with anti-insulin serum or immunized with insulin is, in contrast, thought to be a pure immune reaction of the immediate or delayed type. Pure eosinophilic or lymphocytic infiltrates of the islets are therefore its characteristics, associated with selective beta cell alterations.

If one compares virus-induced insulitis and immune insulitis with insulitis in man, parallels can be drawn as follows: the fact that lymphocytic insulitis is a rare finding in young diabetics may be explained by a short and only temporary duration of this islet lesion. This would be supported by a similar course and incidence of insulitis in mice infected with viruses, according to the reports of Drs. Craighead and Müntefering (this Volume, pp. 287–291 and 316–320). However, necrosis and phagocytosis of islet cells as

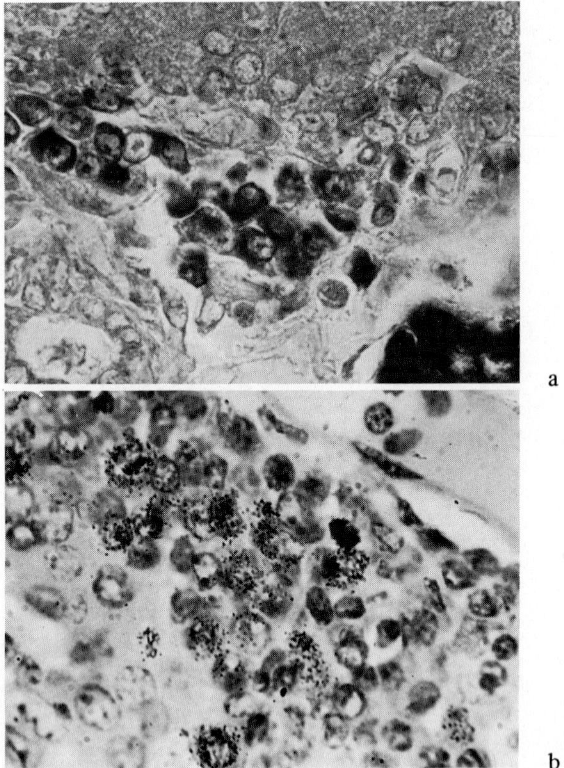

FIG. 7. Insulitis following repeated injections of anti-insulin serum: (a) Part of the infiltrate consisting of large mononuclear cells. (Giemsa, X 720). (b) Marked incorporation of ^{3}H-thymidine in infiltrate cells indicating high mitotic activity. X 720.

well as the occurrence of leukocytes, as they are found in virus insulitis, were in general not described in lymphocytic insulitis of diabetics (Gepts, 1965; for further literature see Freytag and Klöppel, 1973). Insulitis in animals immunized with insulin, however, closely imitates the pure lymphocytic character of insulitis in man (Table 3). Our studies on immune insulitis indicate that the antigenicity of insulin-like components, probably produced by the chemical procedures during extraction, may account for the induction of the insular lesion. In this connection it is of some interest to point to the results of Nerup et al. (1973) who found cellular hypersensitivity to pancreatic extracts in diabetics and immunized animals. Finally it should be mentioned that eosinophilic insulitis induced by means of anti-insulin serum has its possible parallels in the eosinophilic infiltrates of newborns of diabetic mothers.

Since some of the experimental data of the 2 models of insulitis induced by viruses or by immunization seem to have parallels in clinical and pathohistological findings in diabetics, the question arises whether there might be some relations between virus infection and immune mechanisms at the level of the pancreatic islets. The theoretical basis for this hypothetical concept will be shortly explained in the following.

TABLE 1
Alterations of islet cells in insulitis

	Man	Virus infection	Insulin immunization Active	Insulin immunization Passive
Islet necrosis	–	++	–	–
B cell necrosis	?	++	–	–
A cell necrosis	–	++	–	–
B cell degeneration	+	+	+	++
B cell hyperactivity	+	+	+	+
Islet hyperplasia	+	+	–	+

TABLE 2
Cytological composition of insulitis

	Man	Virus infection	Insulin immunization Active	Insulin immunization Passive
Leukocytes	(+)	+	–	++–(+)
Lymphocytes	++	+	++	+
Monocytes	+	+	++	++
Macrophages	?	++	+	++
Plasma cells	–	(+)	(+)	+
Fibrosis	+	+	(+)	+

TRIGGERING OF AUTOIMMUNE MECHANISMS BY VIRUSES

Various possibilities of the interaction of virus and host cell inducing autoimmune mechanisms can be discussed.

1. The most simple way by which viruses are thought to evoke an immune response against cell components, is damage of the host cell. The chemical alteration of certain proteins may result in sufficiently different structures from 'self' so that antibodies are produced, which may cross-react with the intact proteins. This seems to occur, for example, in the chronic aggressive type of hepatitis which tends to progress into cirrhosis (Fig. 8 I).

TABLE 3
Course of insulitis

	Frequency	Time until occurrence	Duration	Manifest diabetes
Man (1)	?	3–150 d	?	Constantly
Virus infection (2)	50–100%	3–7 d	7 d	Frequently
Insulin immunization active (3)	30–60%	14–21 d	Chronic	Very rare
Insulin immunization passive (4)	100%	3 h–4 d	Dependent on injection	Rare

(1): Gepts (1965).
(2): see Craighead and Müntefering (this Volume, pp. 297–291 and 316–320).
(3): Toreson et al. (1964); Renold et al. (1964); Klöppel et al. (1972).
(4): Lacy and Wright (1965); Logothetopoulos and Bell (1966); Freytag (1972).

2. A second pathogenetic mechanism seems to be of greater importance: the formation of antibodies to viruses. Hotchin (1962) has shown that the infection of mice with viruses of lymphocytic choriomeningitis leads to a special disease which only starts when specific virus antibodies have been produced. This probably also proves to be right for the groups of 'slow viruses' (Johnson, 1967). Immune complexes seem to lead to an autonomous immune disease by localizing on the surface of capillary membranes in some organs. A similar effect is well known in poststreptococcus glomerulonephritis due to streptococcus-antistreptococcus globulin complexes (Fig. 8 I).

3. A more differentiated pathogenic mechanism that may lead to a pathologic immune response is suggested for some RNA viruses which contain a lipid envelope in their structure (Drzeniek and Rott, 1969). Virus particles of the lipid-containing RNA viruses appear during multiplication which, after cell damage, carry on their surface host-specific antigens in addition to virus-specific antigens. The antibody formation is stimulated because these lipid-containing viruses work as an ideal adjuvant for material which is by itself only weakly antigenic. Virus- and host-specific antigenic sites are in very close vicinity at the virus surface (Fig. 8 I).

4. The fourth possibility that viruses induce an immune disease depends upon the close relation between lipid-containing RNA virus and the lipids in the cell membranes (Drzeniek and Rott, 1969). In these cases of virus host cell interaction without cytolysis, the intracellular virus replication leads to an incorporation of virus-specific substances into the cell membrane of the host cell. It is well known that virus-specific antibodies react with antigenic sites of virus protein on the surface of the cell membrane (Fig. 8 II).

5. Membrane alterations of the infected cell may take place because viral incorporation results in exposing of pre-existing but masked antigens. Herpes simplex virus is an example. As shown by Brooke and Karnovsky (1961) the membrane of the host cell is altered by these viruses. In consequence new antigenic sites appear on the surface of the

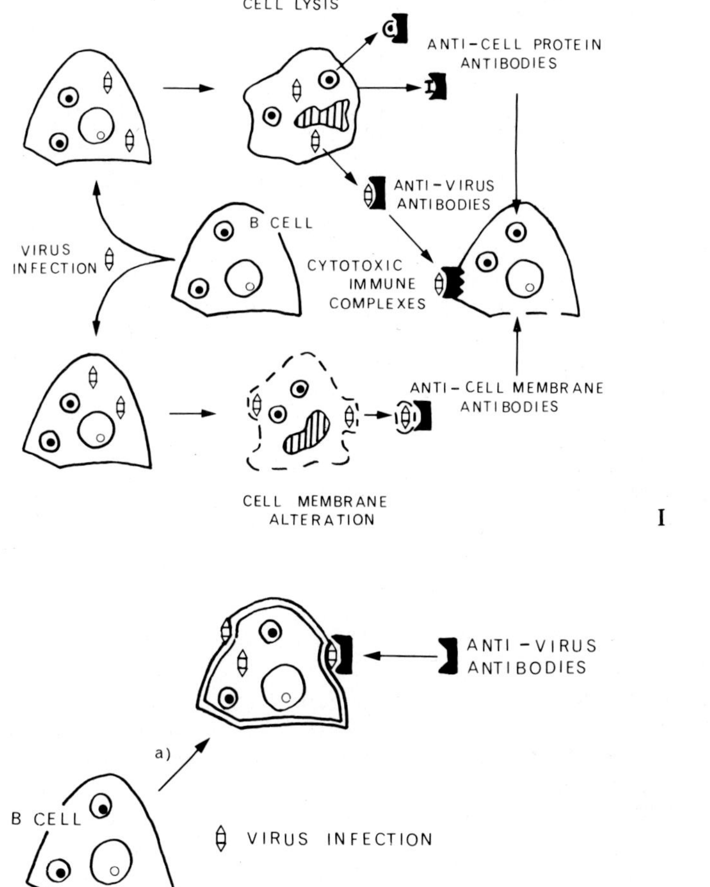

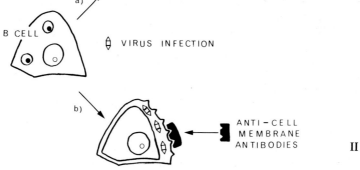

FIG. 8. Theoretical induction of immune mechanisms by virus infections of the beta cell possibly resulting in insulitis. The survey schemes are based on conceptions considered to play a role in triggering immune mechanisms due to viral infections. (I) Immune mechanisms due to acute cytolytic beta cell virus interaction. (II) Immune mechanisms due to chronic beta cell virus interaction at the level of the cell membrane. (a) Incorporation of virus particles into the cell membrane resulting in antigenic sites. (b) Incorporation of viruses in the cell membrane resulting in structural alteration of the whole membrane matrix. (III) Immune mechanisms due to chronic host cell-virus interactions at the level of the DNA-RNA system.

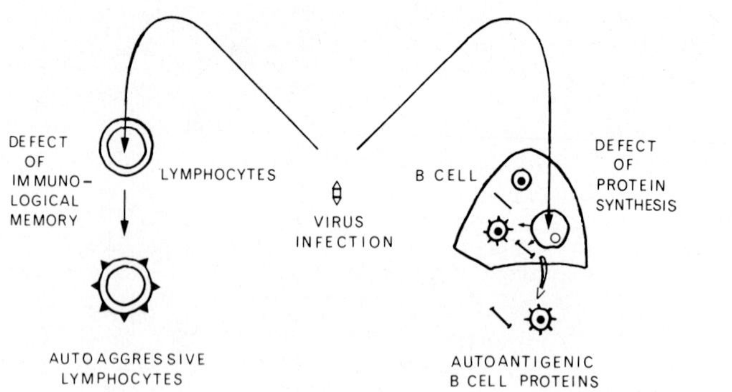

FIG. 8

cell membrane. This interaction may lead to a damage of the infected cell and to a production of specific immunopathological changes in certain organs (Fig. 8 II).

6. In DNA virus infections, the viral DNA or a part of it becomes intergrated into the chromosomal DNA of the host cell. The incorporation of virus DNA into the DNA structure of the host cell leads to essential changes in cell metabolism. The transformation of the cell metabolism may then result in the production of altered proteins inducing autoimmunological reactions (Fig. 8 III).

7. Hypothetically viruses might also interact with immune competent cells. A loss of 'immunological memory' may be the result of the incorporation of virus DNA into the DNA of lymphocytes. This in turn would account for a breakdown of immunological tolerance (Fig. 8 III).

In summarizing one can state that there is evidence from virus research suggesting a mediator role of viruses in cytotoxic immunologic mechanisms. However, concerning the beta cell system, this assumption has still to be proved.

ACKNOWLEDGEMENT

The authors are very grateful to Dr. F. K. Jansen (Diabetes Research Institute, Düsseldorf) for radioimmunological determination of the insulin-binding capacity of the sera, and to Dr. E. Altenähr for his cooperation at the electron microscope.

REFERENCES

BROOKE, M. S. and KARNOVSKY, M. J. (1961): Immunological paralysis and adoptive immunity. *J. Immunol., 87,* 205.

DRZENIEK, R. and ROTT, R. (1969): The possible role of lipid-containing RNA viruses for the etiology of autoimmune diseases. In: *Bayer-Symposium I. Current Problems in Immunology,* pp. 245–250. Springer Verlag, Berlin – Heidelberg – NewYork.

FREYTAG, G. (1972): *Immunpathologie des Diabetes mellitus. Veröffentlichungen aus der Morphologischen Pathologie, Vol. 88.* Editors: W. Giese, W. Büngler, G. Seifert and G. Peters. Gustav Fischer, Stuttgart.

FREYTAG, G. and KLÖPPEL, G. (1973): Insulitis – a morphological review. *Current Topics in Pathology, Vol. 58,* pp. 49–90. Springer, Berlin, Heidelberg, New York.

GEPTS, W. (1965): Pathologic anatomy of the pancreas in juvenile diabetes mellitus. *Diabetes, 14,* 619.

HOTCHIN, J. E. (1962): The biology of lymphocytic choriomeningitis infection: virus-induced immune disease. *Cold Spr. Harb. Symp. quant. Biol., 27,* 479.

JOHNSON, R. T. (1967): Pathways of invasion and spread. Symposium on chronic infectious agent ('slow virus' infections). *Curr. Top. Microbiol. Immunol., 40,* 3.

KLÖPPEL, G., ALTENÄHR, E. and FREYTAG, G. (1971): Elektronenmikroskopische Untersuchungen zur experimentellen Insulitis nach Injektion von Anti-Insulin-Serum. *Virchows Arch. path. Anat. Abt. A, 354,* 324.

KLÖPPEL, G., ALTENÄHR, E. and FREYTAG, G. (1972): Studies on ultrastructure and immunology of the insulitis in rabbits immunized with insulin. *Virchows Arch. path. Anat. Abt. A, 356,* 1.

NERUP, J., ANDERSEN, O. O., BENDIXEN, G., EGEBERG, J., KROMANN, H. and POULSEN, J. E. (1973): Spontaneous and experimental antipancreatic cellular hypersensitivity in man and rodents. In: *Abstracts, VIII Congress of the International Diabetes Federation, Brussels, 1973,* p. 134. Editors: J. J. Hoet and P. Lefebvre. International Congress Series No. 280, Excerpta Medica, Amsterdam.

LACY, P. E. and WRIGHT, P. H. (1965): Allergic interstitial pancreatitis in rats injected with guinea pig anti-insulin serum. *Diabetes, 14,* 634.

LOGOTHETOPOULOS, J. and BELL, E. G. (1966): Histological and autoradiographic studies of the islets of mice injected with insulin antibody. *Diabetes, 15,* 205.

RENOLD, A. E., SOELDNER, J. S. and STEINKE, J. (1964): Immunological studies with homologous and heterologous pancreatic insulin in the cow. *Ciba Foundation Colloquia Endocrinol., 15,* 122.

TORESON, W. E., FELDMAN, R., LEE, J. C. and GRODSKY, G. M. (1964): Pathology of diabetes mellitus produced in rabbits by means of immunization with beef insulin. *Amer. J. clin. Path., 42,* 531.

CHARACTERISTICS OF M-VARIANT ENCEPHALOMYOCARDITIS VIRUS (EMC) IN THE CHEMICALLY DIABETIC NON-OBESE CHINESE HAMSTER*

G. M. GRODSKY, B. FRANKEL, A. RUDNICK, J. SCHACHTER, J. LEE, R. FANSKA and L. WEST

Metabolic Research Unit, Hooper Foundation and Departments of Medicine, Biochemistry and Pathology, University of California Medical Center, San Francisco, Calif., U.S.A.

It is well established that human diabetes has a strong genetic component although the exact mode of inheritance is unknown. Recent studies indicate that environmental factors such as an insulin-induced autoimmune response (Grodsky et al., 1966; Renold et al., 1966), or a pancreatic-directed viral infection can precipitate overt diabetes in normal animals (Craighead and Steinke, 1971; Müntefering, 1972; Wellman et al., 1972; Burch et al., 1971). Possibly a combination of these factors may be important in many forms of human diabetes (Monif, 1973; Gepts, 1965; Le Compte, 1958).

Heretofore, the effect of viral infection on an experimental animal model with a genetic tendency to diabetes has not been studied. Using the perfused pancreatic preparation the investigations presented here indicate that the overt diabetic Chinese hamster is a good model for non-obese diabetes in man. Furthermore, a small percentage of the offspring from these animals have normal fasting blood sugar but carry the diabetic trait and resemble the human *chemical* diabetic.

The M strain of EMC virus has been shown (Craighead and Steinke, 1971) to cause specific islet cell lesions and hyperglycemia in Swiss mice. As part of a proposed prolonged study, the acute effects of this virus on the intact *chemical* diabetic Chinese hamster is reported. Data indicate this virus causes pancreatic lesions in this species which are not islet cell-specific.

MATERIAL AND METHODS

Animals

Adult Chinese hamsters (*Cricetulus griseus*), aged 7–17 months and weighing 17–30 g were studied. *Overt* diabetic hamsters all had fasting hyperglycemia and glucosuria but only occasional ketonuria. Table 1 (Gerritsen and Dulin, personal communication) shows that approximately 20% of the offspring of some sublines of diabetic hamsters have normal fasting blood sugars. These animals, once categorized at 5 months of age, do not

* This work was supported in part by Grant AM-01401 from the National Institutes of Arthritis and Metabolic Diseases, U.S. Public Health Service, a grant from the Hoechst Pharmaceutical Company, Somerville, N.H., a grant from the Upjohn Company, Kalamazoo, Mich., and by a grant from the Levi J. and Mary Skaggs Foundation and the Kroc Foundation.

TABLE 1
Results of brother-sister mating of non-ketotic diabetics in the subline, XA

	XA^{++++}	X	XA^{++++}	
	Normal	Trace	$Diabetic^{++++}$	Ketotic
%	20	10	50	20

progress to the overt diabetic category, but remain euglycemic and apparently normal (Gerritsen and Dulin, 1967). However, our experiments to be reported here show that this type of animal has elevated blood glucose during surgical stress and that its pancreas secretes abnormally low insulin when perfused with glucose. These animals are referred to subsequently as *chemical* diabetics and were selected for the viral studies. Non-diabetic, age- and sex-matched hamsters from 5 normal inbred sublines of the same colony served as controls; these animals had no demonstrable glucosuria for at least 5 generations.

Experimental techniques

The apparatus and dissection procedure for the in vitro perfusion of a Chinese hamster pancreas were adapted from that for the perfused rat pancreas previously described (Grodsky et al., 1967; Grodsky and Fanska, 1973; Curry et al., 1968). Surgical procedures, apparatus and tubing were modified to accommodate the 0.2 g hamster pancreases instead of the 1.2 g rat pancreases. Flow rates of the unrecycled perfusate were 1.5 ml/min., and mean oxygen tension was 500–600 mM Hg. Oxygen uptake per gram tissue was similar to that previously observed with the perfused rat pancreas (Grodsky et al., 1967).

Insulin was assayed in the perfusion experiments using a solid-phase modification of a single antibody radioimmunoassay incorporating the Automated Pipetting Station (Micromedia System Incorporated, Philadelphia, Penn.). Experiments where serial dilutions of pancreatic extracts from the Chinese hamster were compared with rat, beef, and pork insulin standards showed there was proportional cross-reaction with pork or beef but not rat insulin. All samples from the perfusion experiments, therefore, were assayed against pork insulin standards. Glucagon was measured against beef-glucagon standards with a single antibody radioimmunoassay (Unger and Eisentraut, 1967). The glucagon levels reported here are comparable to those reported from this laboratory from normal rat pancreases (Gerich et al., 1972).

Animals were subjected to mild anesthesia with methoxyflurane (Pitman-Moore Inc., Metofane) and blood was collected from the retro-orbital sinus using a heparinized capillary tube. Blood glucose levels were determined with Dextrostix evaluated by the Ames Reflectance Meter. This method gave a reproducibility of ± 10% and was used to minimize viral contamination of other laboratory equipment.

Viral experiments

A sample of the M strain of EMC virus was obtained from Dr. John Craighead, Department of Pathology, College of Medicine, University of Vermont. The virus was passed 2 times in 3-week-old weanling mice as a 10% heart suspension in albumin-Hanks solution. Diluted suspensions (0.1 ml) were injected i.p. into both normal and *chemical* diabetic non-fasting animals. The dilution used as the approximate LD_{50} was $10^{-5.5}$.

Tissues were examined by light microscopy after fixation in 10% Zenker-formal solution followed by H and E stain. Circulating antibody to EMC virus was determined by the plaque reduction neutralization test of Russell et al. (1967).

RESULTS

Overt diabetics

Figure 1 is taken from studies by Frankel et al. (1973a, b) and shows the results when pancreas from normal or non-ketotic but overtly diabetic Chinese hamsters are continuously perfused with glucose (300 mg/100 ml). Basal (unstimulated) secretion of *insulin* was similar from all pancreas. From the normal pancreas, glucose elicited the characteristic diphasic insulin response previously described for the perfused rat pancreas (Grodsky et al., 1969; Curry et al., 1968) and in man (Porte and Pupo, 1969; Cerasi et al., 1972). With the diabetic pancreas, the first and second phases of insulin release were significantly reduced to a similar extent (54 ± 15% and 50 ± 13% of normal, respectively). Insulin secretion from the individual diabetic pancreas varied. However, there was no

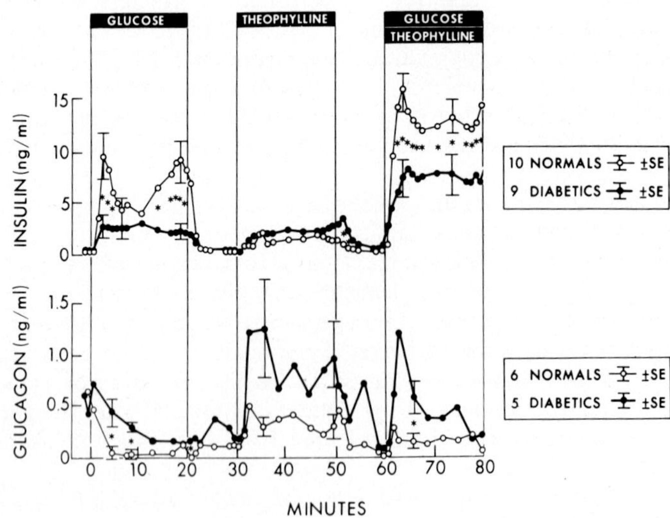

FIG. 1. Insulin and glucagon secretion from the perfused pancreases of *overt* diabetic Chinese hamsters. Glucose, 300 mg/100 ml, theophylline, 10 mM. Figure taken from Frankel et al. (1973b), by courtesy.

linear correlation of secretion with duration or severity of diabetes in the donor animals.

As with insulin, basal *glucagon* secretion was similar from both diabetic and normal pancreas (Fig. 1). From the normals, glucose promptly suppressed glucagon release, a maximum suppression to less than 10% of basal values occurring by 10 minutes. However, from the diabetic pancreas, glucose-induced suppression was both delayed and impaired.

The results of a sequence of different stimulation patterns is also shown in Figure 1. Theophylline caused similar non-phasic *insulin* secretion from both normal and diabetic pancreas. Theophylline also stimulated non-phasic *glucagon* secretion in both groups. Although the mean glucagon secretion of diabetic pancreas exceeded that of the normals, the difference was not significant. In additional experiments reported elsewhere, an initial stimulus with theophylline caused identical glucagon release from diabetic and normal pancreas (Frankel et al., 1973b).

When theophylline and glucose were combined, the normal pancreatic *insulin* release was biphasic and greater than when either stimulus was perfused alone (Fig. 1). Similarly, the response of the diabetic pancreas to the combined stimulus was also greater than either stimulus alone. However, although insulin release was 'normalized', the diabetic's response was still less than that of the normal pancreas. A distinct first phase was not apparent in the diabetic's response, suggesting theophylline action was most pronounced in the second phase. The addition of glucose to theophylline reduced the *glucagon* response in normal pancreas but had less suppressive effect in the diabetics.

Chemical diabetics

Although the non-ketotic, non-obese Chinese hamsters parallel human diabetes (Unger, 1971) in that both their beta and alpha cells are insensitive to glucose, they were inappropriate for the proposed viral studies since they are already diabetic with marked fasting hyperglycemia.

Approximately 20% of the offspring of the non-ketotic, non-obese Chinese hamsters have approximately normal fasting blood sugar levels and normal glucose tolerance (Table 1; Gerritsen and Dulin, personal communication). However, when blood sugar was measured in our laboratory during the surgical-anesthetic stress prior to pancreatic excision, we found most animals studied had elevated levels compared to similarly operated normals (Fig. 2). When pancreases from these animals were perfused (Fig. 3), glucose-stimulated insulin secretion was impaired in those animals with elevated glucose and was normal in the normoglycemic animal. Glucose tolerance tests in a large series of these animals showed a small but significant elevation in basal and poststimulatory glucose levels compared to normals (Fig. 4). The large overlap of individual data in each group, however, emphasized the mildness of the abnormality and the general inability of a glucose tolerance test to distinguish the *chemical* diabetics from normal. Thus, these animals seemed uniquely suited for viral studies since (1) they have a strong genetic component for diabetes, both siblings and parents being overt diabetics; (2) they do not spontaneously become overt diabetics; (3) they have impaired insulin secretion; and (4) their glucose tolerance tests are essentially normal.

Effect of M-strain EMC virus in the chemically diabetic Chinese hamster

The LD_{50} for EMC virus was estimated in a necessarily limited number of normal Chinese hamsters. Results shown in Figure 5 illustrate the extreme sensitivity of the Chinese

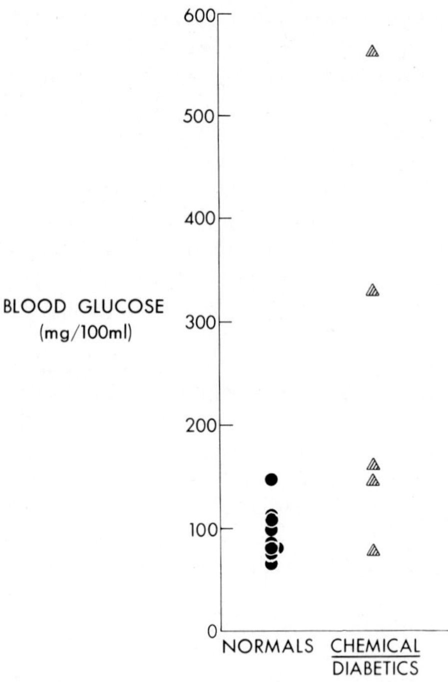

FIG. 2. Blood glucose (vena cava) in normal and *chemical* diabetic hamsters during surgical-anesthetic stress.

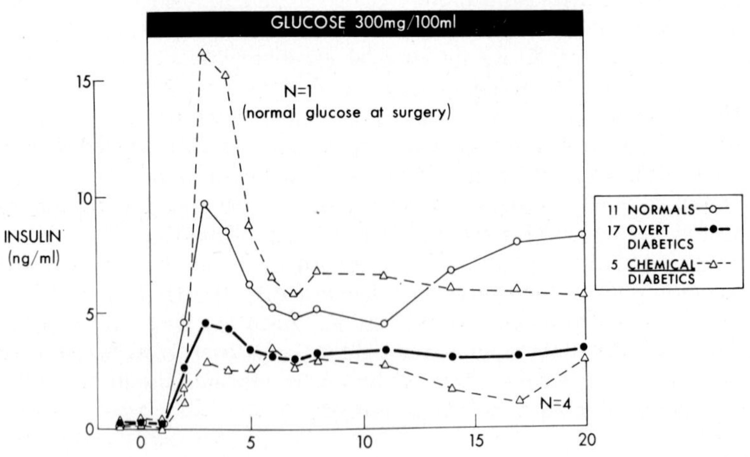

FIG. 3. Insulin secretion from the perfused pancreas of *chemical* diabetic Chinese hamsters. N = 1 refers to the *chemical* diabetic animal with normal blood glucose at surgery (85 mg/100 ml, see Fig. 2); N = 4 refers to *chemical* diabetics with high glucose.

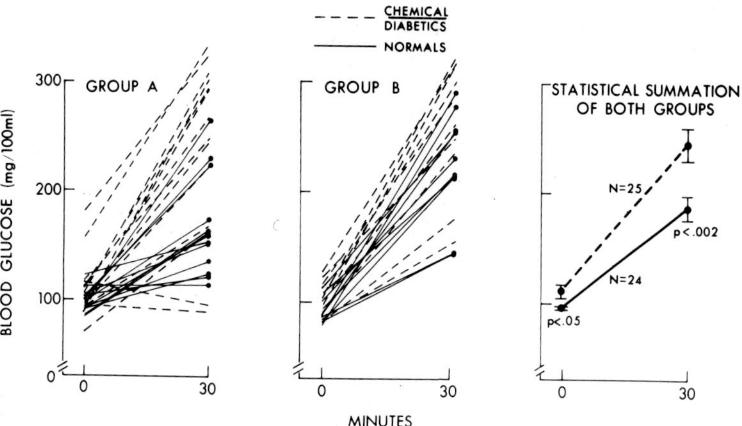

FIG. 4. Glucose tolerance tests in normal and *chemical* diabetic hamsters. Groups A and B refer to similar shipments of animals studied on 2 different occasions.

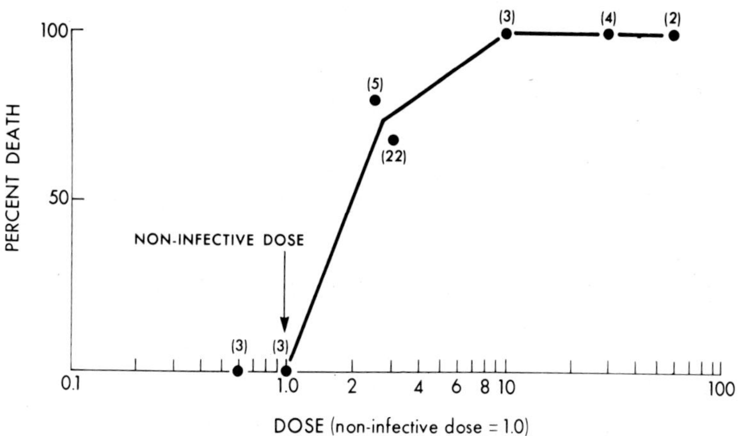

FIG. 5. Lethality of M-EMC virus in the normal Chinese hamster. LD_{50} was approximately 2 times the non-infective dose.

hamster to the EMC virus. The viral non-infective dose (characterized by no deaths, undetectable heart lesions and no circulating antibody to EMC virus) was taken as 1.0. The approximate LD_{50} was estimated at only 2 times this dose. All survivors at the LD_{50} dose or above had circulating viral antibody and, when sacrificed, massive heart lesions. In these preliminary studies, diffuse pancreatic lesions (described below), were observed in 3 of 18 normal animals.

Weight- and sex-matched normal and *chemically* diabetic animals were injected with EMC virus at doses corresponding to 1.0 or 1.25 LD_{50}. The incidence of lesions in all normal and diabetic animals examined by light microscopy is shown in Table 2. Massive

TABLE 2
Incidence of lesions in Chinese hamsters infected with EMC virus

Dose (LD_{50} units)	Heart	Pancreas*	
0	0/4	0/4	
⩽0.5	0/6	0/6	
1.0	22/22	4/22	
1.25	28/28	4/28	18%
> 1.5	12/12	3/12	

* Pancreatic lesions – diffuse lymphocytes.

heart lesions consisting of necrosis and predominantly round cell infiltrates were found in all animals who had received doses of LD_{50} or above.

Pancreatic lesions were discernible by light microscopy in 18% of the total animals. Lesions consisted of a mild scattering of round cells (mostly lymphocytes) in interstitial tissue, generally randomized between islets and acinar tissue. Brain tissue was normal with no detectable involvement of the CNS; there was no difference noted between normals and *chemical* diabetics.

The survival rate of the animals injected with 1 and 1.25 LD_{50} is shown in Table 3. Most animals died at days 3–5 with only occasional deaths occurring thereafter. There was no difference in the time of death or survival rate between the normal and *chemically* diabetic animals; death rate was over 75% at both dose levels in the 2 groups.

Fasting blood glucose in both normal and *chemically* diabetic animals was not altered

TABLE 3
Incidence of death in normal and chemically *diabetic hamsters after a single infection with M-EMC virus*

Animals	Dose (LD_{50})	Survival after viral infection										
		Days										
		1	2	3	4	5	6	7	8	9	> 14	
Normals (10)	1.0			II	𝍸		I				II	(5)
Normals (14)	1.5			II	𝍸	IIII					III	
Diabetics (10)	1.0				𝍸	II					III	(4)
Diabetics (15)	1.5			IIII	IIII	IIII		I		I	I	

up to 4 weeks after infection (Fig. 6). As shown in Figure 7, glucose tolerance tests at 2 weeks post infection were characteristic of those seen prior to infection in both groups. One normal animal, however, had an elevated glucose curve which was significantly abnormal when compared to either the normal or *chemically* diabetic groups (See Fig. 4).

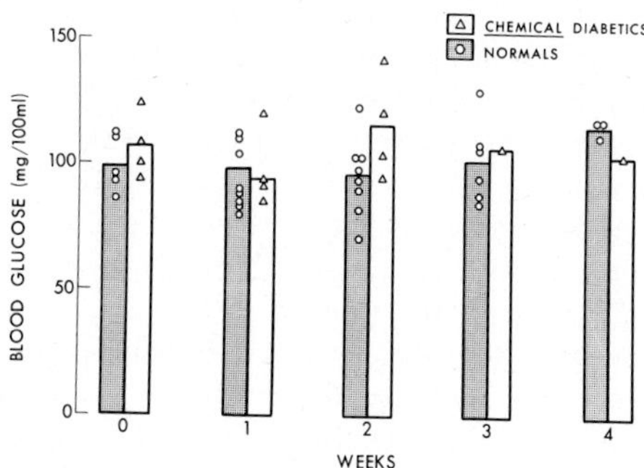

FIG. 6. Influence of M-EMC virus on fasting blood sugars of normal and *chemical* diabetic hamsters. Data refer to time after infection. Included are some normal animals who had received infective doses in the preliminary studies (Fig. 5).

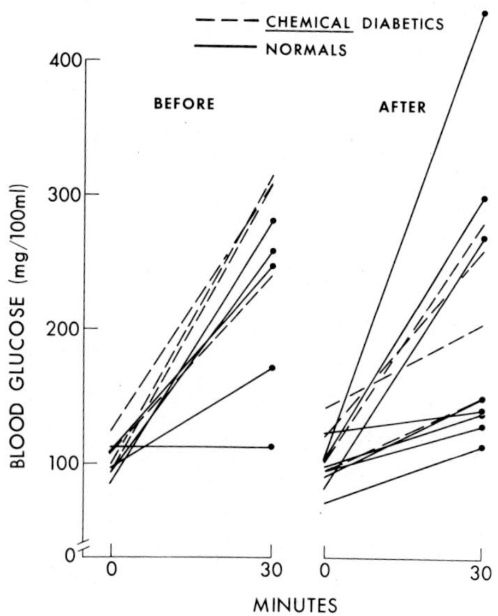

FIG. 7. I.p. glucose tolerance tests in normal and *chemical* diabetic hamsters before and 2 weeks after infection with M-EMC virus.

DISCUSSION

The non-obese, non-ketotic diabetic Chinese hamster may be a particularly good model for lean human diabetes of both maturity-onset and juvenile-onset types. This animal was previously shown to have hyperglycemia and impaired insulin responses to glucose, diminished pancreatic insulin content (Gerritsen and Dulin, 1967; Malaisse et al., 1967) and abnormal islet morphology (Dulin and Gerritsen, 1967). Our studies with the perfused pancreases of these animals (Frankel et al., 1973b) show that both the first and second phases of insulin release during glucose stimulation are impaired similarly to man (Cerasi et al., 1972). The identical impairment of both phases of insulin release in the diabetic hamster and man suggests the occurrence in diabetes of a defect early in glucose action, possibly involving a glucoreceptor rather than a preferential defect in some mechanism underlying one of the phases (Grodsky, 1972; Cerasi et al., 1972).

There was impaired suppression of glucagon release by glucose suggesting the inability to recognize glucose occurs in both alpha and beta cells. A similar inability for alpha cell recognition of glucose may occur in man (Unger, 1971).

Finally, our data show that the diabetic hamster pancreas, as in the human diabetic (Cerasi and Luft, 1969), secretes additional insulin if the glucose signal is augmented with theophylline. However, the diabetic pancreas still does not secrete as well as normal pancreas subjected to the same combined stimulus. Theophylline alone also increases glucagon secretion in normal and diabetic pancreas; however, suppression by glucose was not as great in the diabetic hamsters.

These results thus indicate that the genetic diabetic hamster's beta and alpha cells do not respond normally to glucose, that theophylline can compensate for but not restore to normal the diabetic's defective glucose action in either cell, and that the mechanism by which theophylline acts (presumably by cAMP elevation) is relatively normal in the diabetic pancreas.

Since these animals are already overt diabetics, they are not ideal for studying the diabetogenic characteristics of viral infection. Surprisingly, despite their high genetic purity (6 to 22 generations of brother-sister matings), 20% of their offspring have normal fasting blood sugar and negative urine sugar. Although these offspring were originally considered 'normals', we found their fasting blood sugar was elevated during surgical stress compared to normals, indicating they more closely resemble the human *chemical* diabetic. These *chemically* diabetic Chinese hamsters are a particularly good model for studying the role of virus superimposed on genetic diabetes since (1) they have a strong genetic component for diabetes (diabetic parents and siblings); (2) insulin secretion during glucose stimulation in vitro is impaired; (3) they have only mild glucose intolerance and normal fasting blood sugar; and (4) there is no natural progression to overt diabetes with time (Gerritsen and Dulin, personal communication). As in human *chemical* diabetes, there may be a mean increase in fasting blood sugar and a decreased glucose tolerance in these animals but the changes are small; the glucose tolerance test therefore is not sufficient to distinguish individual *chemical* diabetics from normals.

The M-variant of the EMC virus was chosen for these studies since in certain strains of mice it produces a specific islet cell lesion, a high incidence of acute diabetes, and a comparatively low mortality (Craighead and Steinke, 1971). It is recognized, however, that the characteristics of this virus in other strains of mice and the Golden Hamster differ in both ability to specifically attack the islets and in production of acute diabetes (Craighead, 1972). Heretofore, no studies in the Chinese hamster were available.

This virus caused massive heart lesions and proved extremely lethal in the Chinese hamster, the approximate LD_{50} being only twice the non-infective dose. Despite this narrow margin, the survivors of the LD_{50} dose were definitely infected as indicated by cardiac lesions (in those sacrificed), or circulating EMC antibodies. However, the number of survivors of these comparatively rare animals was disappointingly low. Although an increased sensitivity to infection is a characteristic of human diabetes, there was no difference in survival rate or time of death (3–5 days) between the *chemical* diabetics and the normals. Pancreatic lesions were seen in only 18% of the animals studied. Since the pancreases were examined only by light microscopy, this should be considered a minimum estimate of lesions in this tissue and strongly suggests the pancreas of the Chinese hamster is a target for EMC virus. The lesions, consisting of mild diffuse lymphocytic infiltration, were not restricted to the islets but were generalized throughout the pancreatic tissue. The lesion in the Chinese hamster, therefore, is not specific to the islet and may more closely resemble that produced by other picornaviruses such as the E variant of EMC or Coxsackie B_4 virus (Craighead, 1966; Burch et al., 1971). Although a greater incidence of islet lesions would have been desirable, the primary purpose of the study was to evaluate whether animals bearing a genetic diabetic trait show increased sensitivity of the islets to the virus or an inability to repair. Too dramatic impairment of islet function in the normal animals could complicate interpretation of long term studies.

In contrast to certain mice (Craighead and Steinke, 1971), elevated fasting blood sugar was not observed in any normal or *chemically* diabetic hamsters during the 4 weeks following infection. Glucose tolerance tests in normals and diabetics at 2 weeks were not consistently different from those before infection. However, the abnormal glucose tolerance test in one of the normal animals at this period suggests that significant pancreatic lesions can be produced which may or may not be exacerbated with time.

CONCLUSION

The *chemically* diabetic Chinese hamster appears a particularly useful animal model for studying the role of virus on genetic diabetes since it has a strong genetic component for diabetes and only mild glucose intolerance and normal fasting blood sugar. The choice of the M-EMC virus may be less ideal because of its high lethality and relatively non-specific islet cell infectivity in these animals. Acutely, no consistent change in fasting glucose or glucose tolerance in either normal or *chemically* diabetic animals was demonstrable. However, these studies can now be extended to evaluate the long-term effect of a single mild viral attack on an animal with genetic diabetic tendencies but, normally, with no progression to diabetes.

ACKNOWLEDGEMENTS

We wish to thank Drs. George C. Gerritsen and W. E. Dulin of the Upjohn Company, Kalamazoo, Mich., for generously supplying the hamsters and technical information regarding their characteristics. We also thank Dr. John Craighead, University of Vermont, both for supplying the M-EMC virus and his invaluable advice. Albumin required in the perfusion experiments was obtained from Drs. M. Mozen and A. Pappenhagen of Cutter Labs., Berkeley, Calif., and James B. Lesh of the Armour Pharmaceutical Co., Kankakee, Ill.

REFERENCES

BURCH, G. E., TSUI, C., HARB, J. M. and COLCOLOUGH, H. H. (1971): Pathologic findings in the pancreas of mice infected with Coxsackie virus B_4. *Arch. intern. Med., 128,* 40.

CERASI, E. and LUFT, R. E. (1969): The effect of an adenosine-3′,5′-monophosphate diesterase inhibitor (aminophylline) on the insulin response to glucose infusion in prediabetic and diabetic subjects. *Hormone metabol. Res., 1,* 162.

CERASI, E., LUFT, R. and EFENDIC, S. (1972): Decreased sensitivity of the pancreatic beta cells to glucose in prediabetic and diabetic subjects. A dose-response study. *Diabetes, 21,* 224.

CRAIGHEAD, J. E. (1966): Pathogenicity of the M and E variants of the encephalomyocarditis (EMC) Virus. II. Lesions of the pancreas, parotid, and lacrimal glands. *Amer. J. Pathol., 48,* 375.

CRAIGHEAD, J. E. (1972): Workshop on viral infection and diabetes mellitus in man. *J. infect. Dis., 125,* 568.

CRAIGHEAD, J. E. and STEINKE, J. (1971): Diabetes mellitus-like syndrome in mice infected with Encephalomyocarditis virus. *Amer. J. Pathol., 63,* 119.

CURRY, D. L., BENNETT, L. L. and GRODSKY, G. M. (1968): Dynamics of insulin secretion by the perfused rat pancreas. *Endocrinology, 83,* 572.

DULIN, W. E. and GERRITSEN, G. C. (1967): Summary of biochemical, physiological and morphological changes associated with diabetes in the Chinese hamster. In: *Proceedings of the VIth Congress of the International Diabetes Federation,* pp. 806–812. Editor: J. Östman. International Congress Series No. 172, Excerpta Medica, Amsterdam.

FRANKEL, B. J., GERICH, J. E., FANSKA, R. E. and GRODSKY, G. M. (1973a): Subnormal insulin and excessive glucagon release from *in vitro* perfused pancreases of nonobese, genetically diabetic Chinese hamsters. *Diabetes, 22/Suppl. 1,* 307.

FRANKEL, B. J., GERICH, J. E., HAGURA, R., GERRITSEN, G. C. and GRODSKY, G. M. (1973b): Abnormal secretion of insulin and glucagon by the *in vitro* perfused pancreas of the genetically diabetic Chinese hamster. *J. clin. Invest.,* in press.

GEPTS, W. (1965): Pathological anatomy of the pancreas in Juvenile diabetes mellitus. *Diabetes, 14,* 619.

GERICH, J. E., CHARLES, M. A., LEVIN, S. R., FORSHAM, P. H. and GRODSKY, G. M. (1972): *In vitro* inhibition of pancreatic glucagon secretion by diphenylhydantoin. *J. clin. Endocr., 35,* 823.

GERRITSEN, G. C. and DULIN, W. E. (1967): Characterization of diabetes in the Chinese hamster. *Diabetologia, 3,* 74.

GRODSKY, G. M. (1972): A threshold distribution hypothesis for packet storage of insulin and its mathematical modeling. *J. clin. Invest., 51,* 2047.

GRODSKY, G. M., BENNETT, L. L., SMITH, D. F. and SCHMID, F. G. (1967): Effect of pulse administration of glucose or glucagon on insulin secretion *in vitro. Metabolism, 16,* 222.

GRODSKY, G. M., CURRY, D., LANDAHL, H. and BENNETT, L. (1969): Further studies on the dynamic aspects of insulin release *in vitro* with evidence for a two-compartmental storage system. *Acta diabet. lat., 6/Suppl. 1,* 554.

GRODSKY, G. M. and FANSKA, R. (1973): *Methods in Enzymology,* in press.

GRODSKY, G. M., TORESON, W. E., FELDMAN, R. and LEE, J. C. (1966): Diabetes mellitus in rabbits immunized with insulin. *Diabetes, 15,* 579.

LE COMPTE, P. M. (1958): Insulitis in early Juvenile diabetes. *Arch. Pathol., 66,* 450.

MALAISSE, W., MALAISSE-LAGAE, F., GERRITSEN, G. C., DULIN, W. E. and WRIGHT, P. H. (1967): Insulin secretion *in vitro* by the pancreas of the Chinese hamster. *Diabetologia, 3,* 109.

MONIF, G. R. G. (1973): Can diabetes mellitus result from an infectious disease? *Hosp. Pract., March,* 124.

MÜNTEFERING, H. (1972): Pathology of diabetes mellitus in the white mouse infected with EMC virus. Histological, electron microscopical and quantitative morphological findings in the islets of Langerhans. *Virchow's Arch. path. Anat., 356,* 207.

PORTE, D. and PUPO, A. A. (1969): Insulin responses to glucose: evidence for a two pool system in man. *J. clin. Invest., 48,* 2309.

RENOLD, A. E., STEINKE, J., SOELDNER, J. S., ANTONIADES, H. N. and SMITH, R. E. (1966): Immunological response to the prolonged administration of heterologous and homologous insulin in cattle. *J. clin. Invest., 45,* 702.

RUSSELL, P. K., NISALAK, A., SUKHAVACHANA, P. and VIVONA, S. (1967): A plague reduction test for dengue virus neutralizing antibodies. *J. Immunol., 99,* 285.

UNGER, R. H. (1971): Glucagon physiology and pathophysiology. *New Engl. J. Med., 285,* 443.

UNGER, R. H. and EISENTRAUT, A. M. (1967): Glucagon. In: *Hormones in Blood, 2nd Edition,* pp. 83–128. Editors: C. H. Gray and A. L. Bacharach. Academic Press, New York.

WELLMAN, K. F., AMSTERDAM, D., BRANCATO, P. and VOLK, B. W. (1972): Fine structure of pancreatic islets of mice infected with the M variant of the encephalomyocarditis virus. *Diabetologia, 8,* 349.

ULTRASTRUCTURE OF VIRAL INSULITIS*

H. MÜNTEFERING

Pathologisches Institut, Universität Düsseldorf, Federal Republic of Germany

Up to now no case of human insulitis of certified viral origin could be examined electron microscopically. For that reason we have chosen an animal model using the M variant of the encephalomyocarditis (EMC) virus, which exclusively causes lesions of the islets of Langerhans (accompanied by a diabetes-like syndrome) whereas nearly all the exocrine pancreas tissue is spared (Craighead and McLane, 1968).

We were able to demonstrate, by extensive series of systematic preliminary experiments, that an insulitis could be produced. It occurs regularly but is transitory in nature, being observed from the seventh to the twelfth day as a rule and in extreme cases from the third to the sixteenth day (Müntefering et al., 1971; Müntefering, 1972). Alterations of the mitochondria in the form of edematous disaggregation as well as destruction and wasting of the cristae were already observed on the first day. From the second day many, but not all islets show single and grouped A and B cells with lesions extending even to necrosis (Fig. 1) and an interstitial edema (Fig. 2).

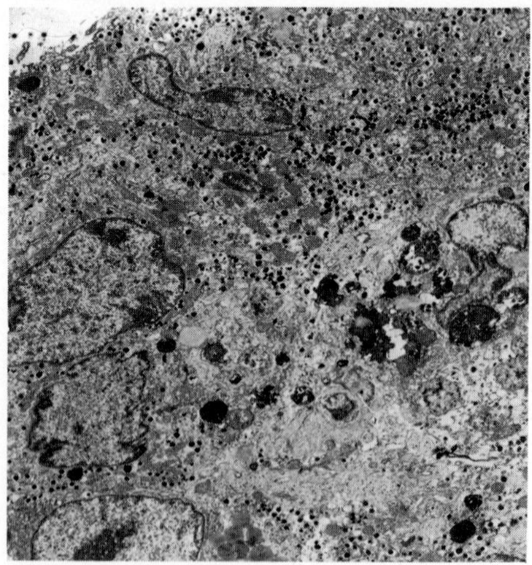

FIG. 1. Necrosis of several cells in the center of an islet of Langerhans 4 days after inoculation of the M variant of the EMC virus. X 2,245.

* This investigation was supported in part by Sonderforschungsbereich 113 (Diabetologie) of the Deutsche Forschungsgemeinschaft.

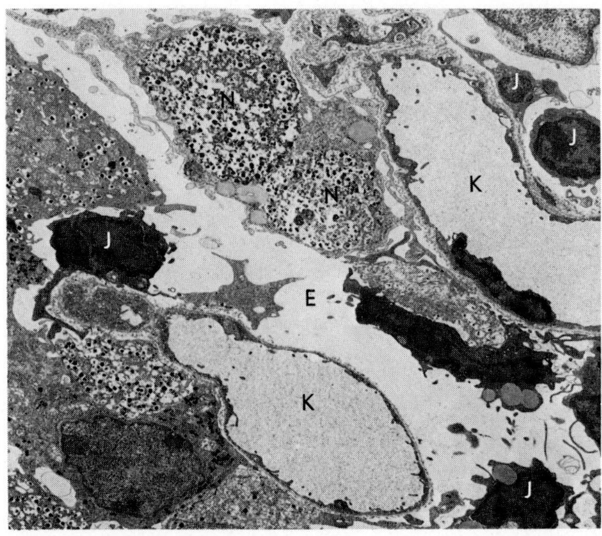

FIG. 2. Necrosis of the islet cells (N), intense interstitial edema (E), inflammatory infiltrates (I) and dilatated blood capillaries (K) in an islet of Langererhans 3 days after inoculation of the EMC virus. X 2,350. (From Müntefering, 1972, by courtesy.)

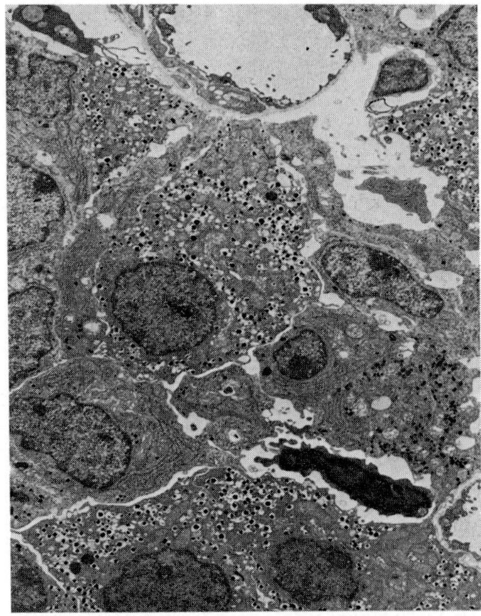

FIG. 3. Phagocytes between largely degranulated B cells 3 days after inoculation of the M variant of the EMC virus. X 1,812.

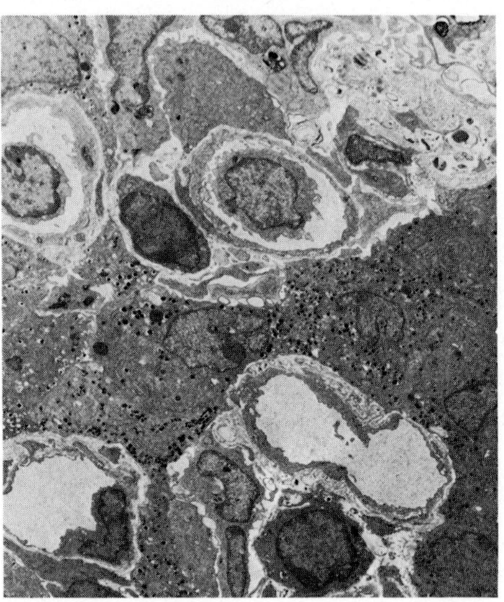

FIG. 4. Inflammatory infiltrates between necrotic cells, widened capillaries and very few, partly degranulated B cells but normally granulated A cells, being the residues of an islet of Langerhans 5 days after inoculation of the EMC virus. X 2,620.

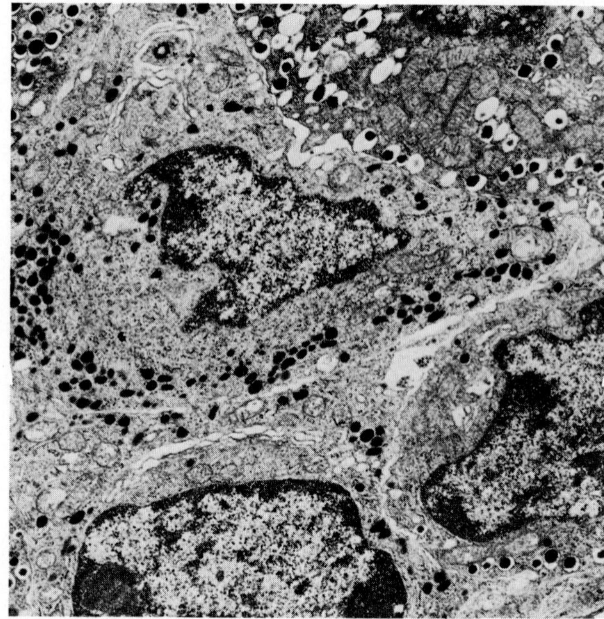

FIG. 5. B cells of an islet of Langerhans with diabetes mellitus 7 days after the inoculation of the M variant of the EMC virus. Far-reaching degranulation partly with shifting of the remaining granules to the periphery of the cell. Increase of the endoplasmic reticulum and of the mitochondria. × 8,350.

Mostly cytoplasm shows organelles with blurred contours and a focal decay of the cell membranes. At that time dilated blood and lymph capillaries can be seen more often, so that the islet cells appear to be bordered by such vessels.

Beginning on the third day after the inoculation we also found, near to damaged or necrotic islet cells, infiltrated ones with phagocytic properties (Fig. 3). These were polymorphs and lymphocytes as well as monocytic cells with cytosomal inclusions. The disappearance of the cell necrosis coincides with the decrease in the infiltrates, so that on the seventeenth day after inoculation we could not observe any insulitis.

In contrast to the A cells the still intact B cells also show alteration. They are remarkably degranulated and show an increase in endoplasmic reticulum and mitochondria (Fig. 4). Also in islets without necrosis the B cells show a depletion of secretory granules. The few remaining granules are shifted to the cell periphery (Fig. 5). The endoplasmic reticulum and the mitochondria are increased. Nearly always the Golgi apparatus is widened. In animals with severe diabetes tiny tubular structures, vesicles, and vacuoles of all sizes are seen after weeks or even one month (Fig. 6).

The A cells on the contrary, do not show corresponding alterations after the acute infection phase. Up to now we also could not observe new formations of islet cells, mitosis or definite transformations.

The EMC virus has a diameter of 20 μ and so corresponds to ribosomes in size and shape. Therefore it can only be proved electron microscopically in cells if present in the form of so-called cristals. As shown in other studies the viral strain used here never

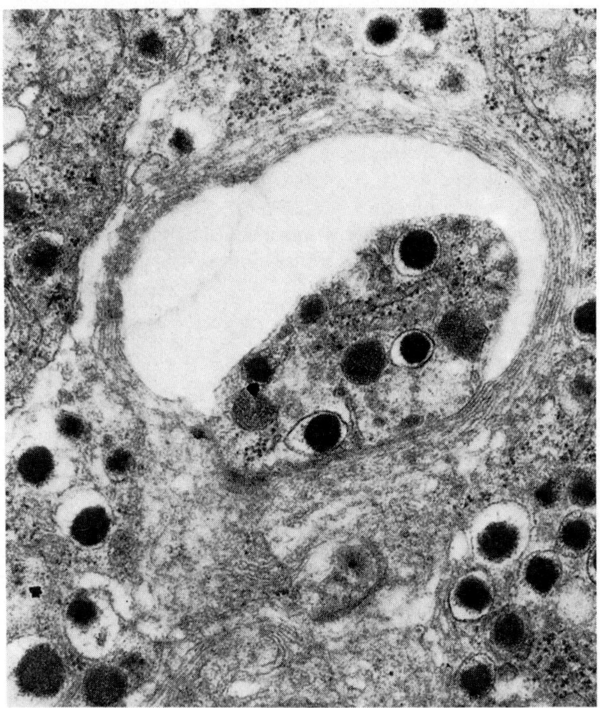

FIG. 6. Giant formation of a vacuole, focal degranulation, increased and parallelled endoplasmic membranes and multiplication of free ribosomes in a still existing B cell 16 days after inoculating the M variant of the EMC virus. X 51,700.

formed crystals in tissue cells so the presence of the virus cannot be definitely proved by electron microscopy.

We, however, were able to prove virus multiplication by immunofluorescence. Thus there is no doubt that the findings described are caused by viruses.

CONCLUSIONS

1. Viruses damage the islet cells directly.
2. This is followed by a transitory inflammation with infiltrates of phagocytes, polymorphs and finally lymphocytes.
3. The localization of infiltrating cells depends on the localization of the damaged secretory cells in the islets, so infiltrates would surround islet cells only by chance.
4. The secondary alteration with remaining B cells depends on the severity of the viral lesions.

REFERENCES

CRAIGHEAD, J. E. and McLANE, M. F. (1968): Diabetes mellitus: Induction in mice by encephalomyocarditis virus. *Science, 162,* 913.

MÜNTEFERING, H. (1972): Zur Pathologie des Diabetes mellitus der weissen Maus bei der EMC-Virusinfektion. Histologische, elektronenmikroskopische und quantitativ morphologische Befunde an den Langerhansschen Inseln. *Virchows Arch. path. Anat. Abt. A, 356,* 207.

MÜNTEFERING, H., SCHMIDT, W. A. K. and KÖRBER, W. (1970): Experimenteller Beitrag zur Virusgenese des Diabetes mellitus bei der weissen Maus. *Verh. Dtsch. Ges. Path., 54,* 669.

MÜNTEFERING, H., SCHMIDT, W. A. K. and KÖRBER, W. (1971): Zur Virusgenese des Diabetes mellitus bei der weissen Maus. *Dtsch. med. Wschr., 96,* 693.

EPIDEMIOLOGICAL AND EXPERIMENTAL STUDIES IN RELATION TO COXSACKIE VIRUSES AS AN AETIOLOGICAL FACTOR IN DIABETES

D. R. GAMBLE, T. J. COLEMAN and K. W. TAYLOR

Public Health Laboratories, West Park Hospital, Epsom, and Biochemistry Group, University of Sussex, Brighton, United Kingdom

SOME OBSERVATIONS ON THE POSSIBLE VIRAL AETIOLOGY OF DIABETES IN MAN

This paper will mainly be about diabetes of the juvenile kind as it is seen developing in Britain. Most of the conclusions are based on work carried out at the Public Health Laboratories, Epsom, Surrey. Every year there may be at least as many as 2,000 diabetics who are newly diagnosed under the age of 15. Such figures are beginning to emerge from the survey done under the auspices of the British Diabetic Association which is now being carried out on juvenile diabetics in Britain. By contrast, the larger group of patients are mainly a middle-aged group with diabetes which is of much milder type and which is often associated with obesity.

The clinical features of the juvenile patients are so well known that they need not be mentioned here, except for the briefest of summaries. Such patients exhibit diabetes of an acute onset, that is a child will develop diabetes suddenly, after being in apparently normal health for many years. The duration of symptoms may frequently be only 2 or 3 weeks and the progression of the disease is rapid, leading to ketosis, extreme hyperglycaemia and wasting. Many of these patients, though of course not all, lack a family history of the disease. Their diabetes is typically insulin-deficient and bears close resemblances to what can be produced in animals by destructive lesions of the islets of Langerhans from any cause. The suddenness of onset in this group suggests a dramatic event which precipitates the disease rather than the operation of a genetic factor the full expression of which may take some years to become evident. We do not of course wish to imply that genetic factors may not sometimes play an important role in the genesis of this kind of diabetes. We would rather wish to emphasize that the clinical pattern more closely suggests the operation of an environmental factor which may be superimposed, sometimes on an already pre-existing genetic defect.

Some recent work conducted mainly by Dr. D. A. Pyke and his associates in London (Tattersall and Pyke, 1972) on the identical twins of diabetics has tended to support this conclusion. Such twins, say of an insulin-taking type, may frequently have a normal or near normal glucose tolerance which does not deteriorate over a period of years. Moreover, there are many normal twins of diabetics who have remained free from the disease for many years, even though their identical sib has had the disease in an overt form. Such considerations do not suggest a genetic factor as the primarily operative one in inducing the acute type of the disease.

Seasonal incidence data

Because there had been no detailed studies on the seasonal incidence of diabetes, apart from those of Adams in 1926 and Danowski in 1957 we decided to examine how acute diabetes might vary by month in newly diagnosed diabetics. This data, which we know will be familiar to some of the readers, shows that in diabetics under the age of 20 there is a peak in the latter part of the year with a fall off in notifications of the disease in the summer months. In some much more recent data analyzed by us the same broad pattern obtains. This data represents the month of onset of the disease in a further group of patients, this time taken from 9 Centres in England and Wales between May, 1970 and April, 1973. The patients in this particular survey were of course a selected group and it is always possible that they do not conform to a more general pattern. However, this data reinforces our earlier conclusions that there is a low incidence of diabetes in the summer months with peaks in October and in January (Gamble and Taylor, 1969). Such data seemed to us compatible with the suggestion that there might be a viral etiology for this type of diabetes though we are sure we do not have to remind the reader that there are many other possible reasons for such a pattern of seasonal distribution.

At about this time we were becoming aware of a number of reports of experimental diabetes in animals being produced by enteroviruses. These included of course the well-known outbreak of foot and mouth disease in cattle in Italy, 1962 and the elegant and important studies of Craighead and McLane (1968) on EMC virus. There has also been a large body of evidence which incriminated various enteroviruses in the production of pancreatitis in man and in animals. Such work suggested in addition that those forms of diabetes in man which are associated with pancreatitis might also be viral in origin.

It was because of these observations that we began systematic surveys of the presence of antibody for various types of virus in the sera of recently diagnosed juvenile diabetics. These results, derived from patients mainly in the south-east area of England when compared to controls from the same geographical locality, showed that 65% of the diabetics were positive for the presence of Coxsackie B4 virus as opposed to only 40% of the controls (Gamble et al., 1969). An excess of antibodies to other common viruses was not found among the diabetic population. In addition an excessive titre of antibodies to other Coxsackie viruses was not evident. Such results by themselves, while they are interesting, were in no sense finally conclusive. They suggested some association between Coxsackie B4 virus and diabetes among a considerable proportion of juvenile diabetics but a large number of such patients did not give evidence of recent Coxsackie infection. These earlier studies have therefore been repeated on a wider scale. Serum specimens were collected in 9 Centres in England and Wales from 162 patients with diabetes onset between May, 1970 and April, 1973. Control serum specimens were also obtained, using 2 control specimens for each patient matched for age within 5 years and for date of collection within 28 days.

In some observations there appears to be an excess of diabetics with antibody to type B4 virus, although this is only so with patients over the age of 10 years. Thus, in the 10- to 19-year age group 87% of diabetics were positive compared with 65% of controls, and 63% of patients over the age of 20 years were positive compared with 55% of controls. When all the patients are studied 70% had Coxsackie B4 virus against only 58% of the controls. Antibodies to other Coxsackie virus types did not differ significantly in patients or controls but diabetics of 20 or more years of age had antibody to Coxsackie B2 virus slightly more frequently than the controls.

Discussion

The present paper is concerned with speculating about a possible viral aetiology in some cases of juvenile diabetics. The general characteristics of the disease itself are all compatible with this idea. Moreover, as we have indicated within the last 10 years, there has been evidence of a type of diabetes closely resembling that seen in juveniles which may be produced in animals by a number of enteroviruses including, as we shall see later, members of the Coxsackie group.

The data derived from work on viruses and antibodies has shown an association between Coxsackie B4 virus and juvenile diabetes but the association is not evident in more than a proportion of juvenile diabetics. Moreover, surprisingly there was absence of evidence for an excessive infection with Coxsackie B4 virus in diabetics under the age of 10. It may be that susceptibility to virus-induced diabetes is relatively low at birth and increases with age – or alternatively diabetes may result from repeated viral infection. It is also possible that in very young children diabetes may be induced by infection with viruses other than of the Coxsackie group; mumps virus is a possible candidate, although we would not wish to exclude some other viruses.

Supposing that Coxsackie B4 virus may sometimes be involved in the genesis of juvenile diabetes in the 10 to 19 age group, how might this process take place? If it does so, it seems more likely that the virus can induce pancreatic damage from infection late in the year which may not, however, manifest itself in a full diabetic syndrome for a period of some months. A delay in the induction of diabetes due to Coxsackie B4 virus has been noted in mice. There are many possible explanations for a delay of this kind which might for example be due to a hypersensitivity phenomenon.

We have tried in this survey to indicate the present position with regard to virally induced diabetes in man. You will see that the picture is a complicated and difficult one from which it is at present impossible to formulate a completely unifying hypothesis. However, present experiments strongly indicate the possibility of a viral etiology of some kind for many cases of juvenile diabetics and it is essential that further work with larger groups of patients and more complex analyses should be carried out to explore the possibility in further detail.

INSULITIS IN COXSACKIE-INFECTED MICE

It has already been mentioned that a number of viruses may cause islet damage and diabetes and in what follows I am going to discuss some recent work carried out mainly by Dr. T. Coleman in Dr. Gamble's laboratory and in our own laboratory at Sussex, using Coxsackie B viruses.

That Coxsackie viruses can cause a generalized pancreatitis in animals has been known for some time. Recently Burch et al. (1971) have in addition suggested that both Coxsackie B4 and Coxsackie B1 viruses may cause islet damage which was evident on histological examination and electron microscopy. There has not, however, been a detailed study so far published of the effects of viruses on blood sugar, blood insulin, or the metabolic characteristics of the islets of Langerhans. Because of this we have attempted a comprehensive assessment of various parameters of islet cell function in mice infected with a number of strains of Coxsackie B3 and B4 viruses.

Infection with Coxsackie B3 virus

Coxsackie B3 virus, as others have found, can easily produce a generalized pancreatitis in some strains of mice. This was true for unadapted strains, pancreas-adapted strains, as well as a heart-adapted strain of Coxsackie B3 virus injected either into Porton mice or DBA mice. The islets of such animals appeared normal by light microscopy as did serum insulins and blood sugar levels. However, using a different strain of mouse (CD_1) in some instances it was possible to produce some deterioration in carbohydrate tolerance and some evidence of beta cell degranulation. In these animals the acinar tissue was largely unaffected. In such animals the diabetes was mild and blood sugar did not exceed 200 mg/100 ml.

An interesting feature of this work was that in some animals a depressed blood sugar was noted 3 to 4 days following infection with a raised serum insulin level. A change of this type suggested an initial disintegration of the islet with release of preformed insulin. However, on account of the generalized pancreatitis it was not possible to be certain that islet damage was due only to changes in beta cells. It seemed equally probable that some damage to islets might accompany the more generalized acinar cell disorganization produced by the B3 virus. Clearly the strain of mouse is of great importance in determining the nature of the diabetogenic effect.

Effects of Coxsackie B4 virus

Work with Coxsackie B4 virus was carried out with a prototype strain, propagated in tissue culture. The virus was inoculated into CD_1 mice at 8 or 9 weeks. Blood glucose and serum insulin levels were measured at intervals of time following inoculation and for histology the pancreases were examined by conventional stains and rhodenile blue. Again a fall in blood sugar is evident 5 days after inoculation, but by day 12 the blood sugar was rising, and between day 17 and 21 marked hyperglycaemia was present in some mice with blood glucose values of 400 mg/100 ml. Approximately 30% of such mice show levels of blood glucose greater than 160 mg/100 ml. These changes in blood sugar were accompanied by inappropriately low serum insulin levels. These results have been shown in greater detail elsewhere (Coleman et al., 1973). Once again a small rise in serum, 5 days after inoculation of the virus, was noted.

Glucose tolerance tests

Glucose tolerance tests were carried out at various intervals of time following Coxsackie B4 inoculation. In these tests, glucose was injected intraperitoneally into 12 hour fasted mice at a dose of 1 mg/g body weight, and blood samples were taken from the tail vein at half-hour intervals for 2 hours. Such tests showed abnormalities of tolerance on the 2nd, 7th and 16th days and at 10 weeks following inoculation. With this virus there is therefore a marked disturbance of tolerance which has persisted in some animals for 10 weeks.

Work on islets and pancreatic slices

Studies on insulin release from pancreatic slices isolated from mice inoculated with B3 virus were also attempted. Such studies showed an increased basal release rate of insulin, accompanied by a diminished response to increased concentration of glucose. In the case of mice inoculated with Coxsackie B4 virus, however, it was possible to isolate individual islets. Studies with such islets showed a normal rate of insulin release in the basal state, but once again a markedly diminished response to raised glucose concentrations.

Histology on microscopy

While the pancreas from Coxsackie B4-treated animals shows little evidence of pancreatitis, the islets show degranulation and a lymphocytic type of infiltration. This type of picture is not dissimilar to that obtained after EMC virus infection.

GENERAL DISCUSSION

The results we have shown confirm those of others in indicating that picorna viruses may be diabetogenic agents. It is of interest that 2 types of pancreatic damage may be produced. In the first place, there may be predominantly a generalized pancreatitis with little change in blood sugar or in the islets themselves, as is the case in most of our experiments with Coxsackie B3. On the other hand, the islets may be more specifically affected with considerable changes in the characteristics of insulin release. Under these last circumstances the acinar tissue has been largely spared.

The strain of mice involved also appears to be of considerable significance, as was found by Craighead (1966) in his studies on EMC virus. This suggests that genetic susceptibility is of great importance in producing the disease picture in animals. Secondly, a rather constant feature in this work has been the lowering of blood glucose with a corresponding rise in blood insulin 3–4 days following inoculation of a virus. This effect, as we have emphasized elsewhere, is rather reminiscent of the phase of islet disintegration seen after alloxan or streptozotocin treatment of islets. Thirdly, we have also noted in our experiments that there is a prolonged time interval between inoculation and the development of a frankly diabetic state. A similar time gap has been observed by Nerup (personal communication) in his experiments on EMC diabetes in mice. The timing of this event would appear to indicate that it is secondary to the phase of viral multiplication in tissues, rather than the result of some primary damage to islet cells. The nature of this delay is of great interest.

Finally, though the induction of diabetes by Coxsackie B4 virus in mice might seem important in linking the onset of human diabetes with a particular agent, it could be dangerous to draw analogies with the human disease at this stage. We would prefer to regard Coxsackie B4 diabetes as a useful experimental model until further very extensive epidemiological investigations have been carried out in man.

REFERENCES

ADAMS, S. F. (1926): The seasonal variation in the onset of acute diabetes. *Arch. int. Med., 37,* 861.

BURCH, G. E., TSUI, C. Y., HARB, J. M. and COLOCLOUGH, H. L. (1971): Pathologic findings in the pancreas of mice infected with Coxsackievirus B4. *Arch. int. Med. 128,* 40.

BURCH, G. E., TSUI, C. Y. and HARB, J. M. (1972): Pancreatic islet cell damage in mice produced by Coxsackie B1 or encephalomyocarditis viruses. *Experientia (Basel), 28/3,* 310.

COLEMAN, T. J., GAMBLE, D. R. and TAYLOR, K. W. (1973): Diabetes in mice after Coxsackie B4 virus infection. *Brit. med. J., 3,* 25.
CRAIGHEAD, J. E. (1966): Pathogenicity of the M and E variants of the encephalomyocarditis virus. *Amer. J. Path., 48,* 325.
CRAIGHEAD, J. E. and McLANE, F. M. (1968): Diabetes mellitus induction in mice by encephalomyocarditis virus. *Science, 162,* 913.
DANOWSKI, T. S. (1957): *Diabetes Mellitus with Emphasis on Children and Young Adults,* p. 129. Williams and Wilkins, Baltimore, Md.
GAMBLE, D. R., KINSLEY, M. L., FITZGERALD, M. G., BOLTON, R. and TAYLOR, K. W. (1969): Viral antibodies in diabetes mellitus. *Brit. med. J., 3,* 627.
GAMBLE, D. R. and TAYLOR, K. W. (1969): Seasonal incidence of diabetes mellitus. *Brit. med. J., 3,* 631.
KROMANN, H., FABER-WESTERGAARD, B., EGEBERG, J. and NERUP, J. (1973): Low and high dose encephalomyocarditis-virus infection in mice. In: *Abstracts, VIII Congress of the International Diabetes Federation, Brussels, 1973,* p. 138. Editors: J. J. Hoet and P. Lefebvre. International Congress Series No. 280, Excerpta Medica, Amsterdam.
TATTERSALL, R. B. and PYKE, D. A. (1972): Diabetes in identical twins. *Lancet, II,* 1120.

NATURAL HISTORY AND PREVENTION OF DIABETES

SOME ASPECTS OF THE NATURAL HISTORY OF DIABETES MELLITUS*

STEFAN S. FAJANS, CHARLES I. TAYLOR, JOHN C. FLOYD, Jr. and JEROME W. CONN

Department of Internal Medicine, Division of Endocrinology and Metabolism and the Metabolism Research Unit, The University of Michigan, Ann Arbor, Mich., U.S.A.

In this introduction and contribution to the panel discussion on the 'Natural History and Prevention of Diabetes' we wish to (1) review some concepts of the natural history of diabetes mellitus and (2) to review and to bring up to date a study dealing with the natural history of asymptomatic or latent diabetes with emphasis on findings obtained in young people. The course of diabetes in such individuals can be ascertained only by the use of prospective studies in groups of such patients.

Various definitions of the stages in the natural history of genetic diabetes mellitus are based on the absence or presence and on the degree of abnormalities of glucose metabolism. Table 1 presents a scheme depicting the natural history of diabetes divided into 4 stages. The terminology employed in this table includes only the definitions used by our group (Fajans and Conn, 1965) and that employed by the British Diabetic Association and the World Health Organization (W.H.O.). In Tables 2 and 3 only our terminology is given.

Overt (or clinical) diabetes is the most advanced of these stages. Classical symptoms may be present; there is gross fasting hyperglycemia and glucosuria; a glucose tolerance test is not necessary for diagnosis. This stage can be divided into the ketotic and non-ketotic forms of the disease.

The preceding stage is latent (or asymptomatic, chemical) but clinically detectable diabetes. A latent diabetic is an individual who has no symptoms, signs or complications referable to the disease (except for reactive hypoglycemia in some patients) but in whom a diagnosis of diabetes can be established by presently accepted laboratory procedures. This stage may also be characterized by an elevated fasting blood glucose level but of lesser severity than in overt diabetes. When the fasting level of blood glucose is below diagnostic levels this stage can be recognized by a definitely abnormal standard glucose tolerance test.

An earlier stage is subclinical diabetes (Conn and Fajans, 1961) or latent diabetes by the W.H.O. definition. In this stage, not only the fasting blood sugar level but also the glucose tolerance test is normal under usual circumstances. However, diabetes may be suspected because of evidence of insufficient functional reserve of the islet cells under

* Supported in part by U.S. Public Health Service Grants AM-00888, AM-02244, and T1-AM05001, National Institute of Arthritis and Metabolic Diseases, and by Grants from the Upjohn Company, Kalamazoo, Michigan, and Chas. Pfizer & Co., Inc., New York, N.Y.

TABLE 1

Stages in the natural history of diabetes mellitus

Terminology by:				
University of Michigan	Prediabetes ⇄	Subclinical diabetes ⇄	Latent diabetes ⇄	Overt diabetes
World Health Organization	Potential diabetes	Latent diabetes	Asymptomatic diabetes (subclinical or chemical)	Clinical diabetes
Fasting blood sugar	Normal	Normal	Normal or ↑	↑
Glucose tolerance test (GTT)	Normal	Normal Abnormal during pregnancy, stress	Abnormal	Not necessary for diagnosis
Cortisone-GTT	Normal	Abnormal	Not necessary	----
Delayed and/or decreased insulin response to glucose	+	++	+++	++++
Vascular changes	? +	++	+++	++++

stress. An example would be a woman who has a normal glucose tolerance test but who has a history of abnormality of standard glucose tolerance during pregnancy. The latter has been termed pregnancy or gestational diabetes. A high proportion of such women develop latent or overt diabetes in the years which follow. Another example of subclinical diabetes may be an individual with a normal standard glucose tolerance test but an abnormal cortisone glucose tolerance test in the non-pregnant state.

The earliest stage is prediabetes (Conn and Fajans, 1961) or potential diabetes (W.H.O.). This stage exists prior to the onset of identifiable diabetes mellitus whether it be overt, latent or subclinical. It identifies the interval of time from conception until the demonstration of impaired glucose tolerance in an individual predisposed to diabetes on genetic grounds. This period can be identified with certainty only retrospectively. Prediabetes or potential diabetes can be suspected to be present in the individual who has an increased probability of developing diabetes on genetic grounds such as the non-diabetic identical twin of a diabetic patient or the offspring of 2 diabetic parents. During the prediabetic period, glucose tolerance and cortisone-glucose tolerance tests are normal. A number of findings suggest that groups of prediabetic subjects can be differentiated from groups of normal control subjects, although reliable diagnostic tests are not available for detection of prediabetes in the individual. A delayed and/or decreased increase in plasma insulin in response to the stimulus of glucose has been demonstrated in groups of genetic prediabetic individuals (Cerasi and Luft, 1967; Pyke and Taylor, 1967; Colwell and Lein, 1967; Rojas et al., 1969) and in other non-diabetic relatives of diabetic patients (Floyd et al., 1968; Fajans et al., 1969a; Rull et al., 1970) by a number of investigators. This defect is similar to that demonstrated in the majority of patients with overt, latent and subclinical diabetes. Vascular changes, reflected by thickening of the capillary basement membrane of muscle obtained by biopsy, have been found by Siperstein et al. (1968) in 52% of a group of 'prediabetic' individuals; however, cortisone-glucose tolerance tests were not performed in these subjects.

In the natural history of diabetes progression or regression from one stage to the next stage (a) may never occur, (b) may occur very slowly over many years, or (c) may be rapid or even explosive (Fajans and Conn, 1965). The concept, supported by appropriate findings (Fajans, 1971, 1973), that there may be fluctuations in the expression of the carbohydrate aspects of the disease in either direction is an important one. Such fluctuations are particularly common when carbohydrate intolerance is mild (O'Sullivan and Hurwitz, 1966; Kahn et al., 1969). However, even the overt stage of the disease may regress. Extreme examples such as regression from overt ketotic diabetes to prediabetes have been reported in individuals who have been in diabetic coma and who subsequently exhibited normal standard and normal cortisone-glucose tolerance tests (Peck et al., 1958). Remission of overt (clinical) diabetes with ketoacidosis to latent (chemical, asymptomatic) diabetes after a period of therapy with insulin has been documented more frequently. More recently this has been shown to be associated with improvement of beta cell secretory activity (Block et al., 1973; this report contains references to previous relevant reports; see also the review of Pirart and Lauvaux (1971) on the problem of remission). On the other hand rapid progression from prediabetes to overt or asymptomatic diabetes without recognition of the intermediary stage of latent diabetes can be documented (Fajans, 1973).

It is well recognized that the carbohydrate intolerance of latent or asymptomatic diabetes in middle age may show little or no progression in severity over many years. On the other hand, until recently it has generally been assumed that diabetes in children and adolescents can rarely be recognized at an early stage, since the first symptoms of overt diabetes are frequently of sudden and explosive onset (White, 1956). It has also been assumed by some that the course of diabetes in the young is characterized by a rapid and progressive decrease in insulin reserves (Murthy et al., 1968). Since 1960, we have reported that latent, asymptomatic or chemical diabetes can be recognized in children, adolescents and young adults by the finding of abnormal carbohydrate tolerance and that such patients may exhibit the non-progressive course of the carbohydrate intolerance of 'maturity-onset type' of diabetes (Fajans and Conn, 1960, 1962, 1965; Fajans et al., 1969b, 1970, 1971, 1973a). Since 1966 other reports have appeared which also indicate that asymptomatic diabetes can be discovered in young people by the use of the glucose tolerance test (Lister, 1966; Burkeholder et al., 1967; Johansen and Lundbaek, 1967; Paulsen et al., 1968; Sisk, 1968; Chiumello et al., 1969; Kahn et al., 1969; Rosenbloom, 1970; Workshop on Chemical Diabetes in Childhood, 1973).

We wish to report our latest follow-up observations on levels of blood glucose and plasma insulin obtained during glucose tolerance tests on 87 children, adolescents and young and older adults in whom a diagnosis of latent diabetes was made. Follow-up observations over periods of up to 19.6 years have been made in 80 of these individuals. These results extend observations reported previously (Fajans et al., 1969b, 1970, 1971, 1973a).

Some characteristics of the whole group of patients studied are given in Table 2. The majority had a strong family history of diabetes. Twenty-four patients were between the ages of 9 and 17 years at diagnosis (Group I), and 33 between the ages of 18 and 25 years (Group II). Twelve patients in each of the 2 groups had fasting hyperglycemia. This is defined as fasting blood glucose levels greater than 120 mg/100 ml at some time during their period of observation. Another 9 and 8 in the 2 groups had had fasting blood glucose levels between 100–120 mg/100 ml. For Groups I and II the mean sum of increments ± S.E.M. in blood glucose above fasting levels for all 6 intervals of the initial diagnostic glucose tolerance tests were 613 ± 57 and 505 ± 32 mg/100 ml, respectively. For 67 healthy control subjects without a family history of diabetes, aged 18 to 25 years, the corresponding value was 119 ± 19 mg/100 ml which is significantly less ($P < 0.001$) than those of the 2 groups of patients. As mentioned previously, considerable fluctuation in glucose tolerance in the direction of improvement or worsening may occur in some patients when the test is repeated at intervals of months or years, whether such patients are untreated or treated with diet or diet and hypoglycemic agents.

In these 2 groups of patients the mean sums of increments of their most abnormal glucose tolerance tests recorded during their periods of observation were 835 ± 88 and 689 ± 61 mg/100 ml, respectively (prior to the development of insulin-dependent diabetes in 4 and 3 patients in Groups I and II, respectively). In the non-obese patients (percent ideal body weight < 116%, Metropolitan Life Insurance tables) the mean of increments of plasma insulin above fasting levels at half an hour of the initial diagnostic glucose tolerance test (or the first test after 1962; see Fajans et al., 1969b, 1970) was 27.5 ± 6.5 μU/ml for 17 of the younger patients and 30.1 ± 5.2 μU/ml for 26 of the older patients. These values were significantly less ($P < 0.001$) than the 89.7 ± 7.7 μU/ml for the control subjects. Obesity was present in 4 patients of each of the 2 groups.

Among the 16 patients aged 26–35 years at diagnosis (Group III), 12 have had fasting blood glucose levels above 100 mg/100 ml. Of the 14 patients aged 36–47 years at diagnosis (Group IV), 11 have had fasting blood glucose levels above 100 mg/100 ml. The mean sums of increments in blood glucose above fasting levels for all 6 intervals of the glucose tolerance tests for these 2 groups were 485 ± 79 and 435 ± 36 mg/100 ml, respectively. These values were significantly greater ($P < 0.001$) than those for the healthy control subjects. Corresponding figures for the most abnormal tests were 629 ± 74 and 627 ± 75 mg/100 ml, respectively. In the non-obese patients the means of increments in plasma insulin above fasting levels at half an hour were 67.3 ± 33 for 8 of the patients of Group III and 40.3 ± 8.4 μU/ml for 8 of the patients of Group IV. When compared with the control subjects, only the patients of Group IV had increments in plasma insulin which were significantly less (< 0.01).

Table 2 gives the sum of increments in plasma insulin over control levels for all 6 intervals of the glucose tolerance tests, in addition to the increments at half an hour of the test. For Groups II, III and IV the insulin values are further subdivided. The means of tests of individuals in which the sum of increments exceeded the mean sum of increases plus 1 S.D. of the control subjects are given separately. Four tests in Group II and 2 tests in each of Group III and IV fell into this category. For Group II 2 of 4 of the higher tests exceeded the mean plus 2 S.D. of the sum of increases of the control subjects (1108 μU/ml).

TABLE 2

Characterization of patients with latent diabetes and of control subjects

	Patients Age 9–17 (Group I)	Patients Age 18–25 (Group II)	Control subjects Age 19–25	Patients Age 26–35 (Group III)	Patients Age 36–47 (Group IV)
Number of subjects	24	33	67	16	14
Mean age, years	13.2	21.7	21.9	30.8	39.8
FBS (highest)					
< 100 mg/100 ml	3	13	67	4	3
100–120 mg/100 ml	9	8	0	8	8
> 120 mg/100 ml	12	12	0	4	3
GTT – Sum of increments above FBS, mg/100 ml					
Initial diagnostic	613 ± 57	505 ± 32	119 ± 8	485 ± 79	435 ± 36
Highest (before insulin-dependent diabetes)	835 ± 88	689 ± 61		629 ± 74	627 ± 75
Diagnostic GTT Plasma insulin, μU/ml Increments at 1/2 hr	27.5 ± 6.5 (17)	30.1 ± 5.2 (26) 24.1 ± 4.4 (22) 66.3 ± 12.3 (4)	89.7 ± 7.7	67.3 ± 33 (8) 36.3 ± 23 (6) 160.5 ± 60 (2)	40.3 ± 8.4 (8) 32.8 ± 11.5 (6) 62.5 ± 5 (2)
Sum of increments	205 ± 37 (17)	357 ± 67 (26) 229 ± 33 (22) 1059 ± 91 (4)	464 ± 39	516 ± 182 (8) 251 ± 41 (6) 1312 ± 167 (2)	670 ± 276 (8) 288 ± 45 (6) 1625 ± 388 (2)
Obese	4	4	0	7	6
Progression to insulin-dependent diabetes	4	3		1	1
Age at diagnosis, years	11, 14, 11, 17	21, 22, 22		33	39
Initial FBS, mg/100 ml	125, 99, 106, 77	92, 81, 111		123	134
Time interval from initial diagnosis, years	0.3, 0.3, 2, 2	9, 7, 1.5		18.1	15.2
Years of follow-up	3.9–19.4 (19)	1–15.7 (27)		9.0–19.6 (13)	1.4–14.7 (12)
Mean	9.2	6.8		14.7	10.8

Of the 2 higher tests of Groups III and IV, one test exceeded, while one test approached (1076 and 1078 μU/ml, respectively) the mean plus 2 S.D. of the sum of increases of the control subjects. The mean sums of increments of the remainder of the tests were considerably lower. This demonstrates that in non-obese patients with latent diabetes a variety of insulin responses to glucose may be observed: (a) those with delayed and subnormal insulin responses, (b) those with delayed and 'supernormal' insulin responses and (c) those with 'supernormal' insulin responses to glucose without an initial delay in rise in plasma insulin (Table 2). Thus there is a heterogeneity of insulin responses to glucose in what we call 'genetic diabetes mellitus'.

Four patients in Group I have progressed to insulin-dependent diabetes within 2 years after diagnosis, while 3 patients in Group II progressed to insulin-requiring diabetes within 1.5–9 years. In each of Groups III and IV one patient has progressed to insulin-requiring diabetes after periods of 18.1 and 15.2 years. Follow-up observations have been performed in patients in each of the 4 groups over periods of up to 19.4, 15.7, 19.6 and 14.7 years, respectively.

In the diabetic patients aged 9–17 years at diagnosis (Group I), the initial fasting and the postglucose blood glucose levels were significantly higher than in the control subjects aged 18–25 years (Fig. 1). Also shown are the results of the highest glucose tolerance

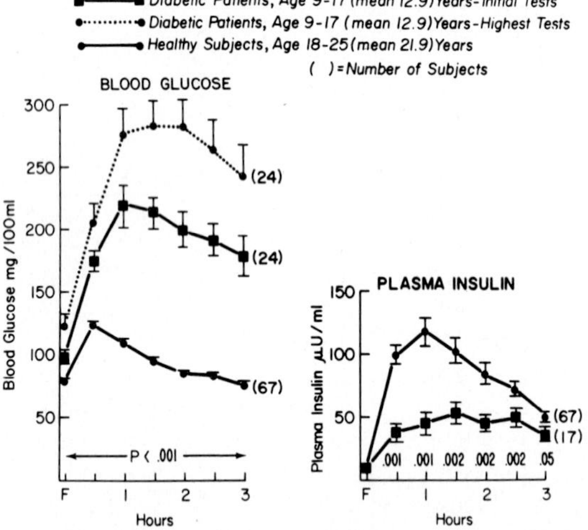

FIG. 1. Initial diagnostic standard glucose tolerance tests (1.75 g glucose/kg ideal body weight) and highest glucose tolerance tests in patients with latent diabetes (Group I, ages 9–17 years at diagnosis) and glucose tolerance tests in healthy control subjects.

tests obtained in these subjects (prior to the development of insulin-dependent diabetes in 4 of them) (Fig. 1). Plasma levels of insulin for 17 of these patients who were non-obese are shown also. After the administration of glucose the diabetic group exhibited a significantly delayed and subnormal increase in plasma insulin (Fig. 1). The mean sum of increments of plasma insulin above fasting levels for all 6 intervals of the test was significantly less than for the control subjects (205 ± 37 and 464 ± 39 μU/ml, respectively; $P<0.001$; Table 1).

The mean results of the initial diagnostic and highest glucose tolerance tests performed on the patients aged 18–25 years at diagnosis (Group II) are shown in Figure 2. The

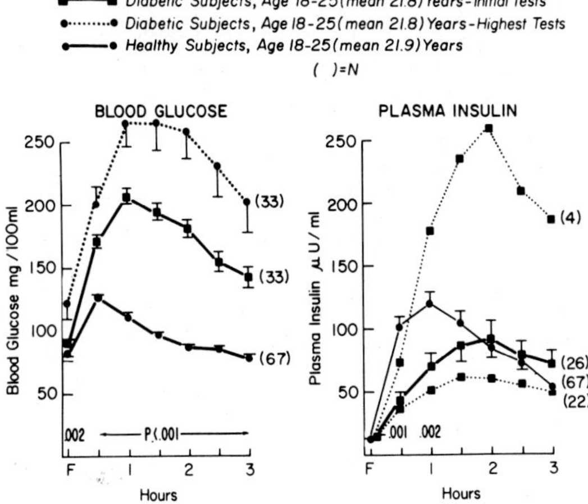

FIG. 2. Initial diagnostic standard glucose tolerance tests (1.75 g glucose/kg ideal body weight) and highest glucose tolerance tests in patients with latent diabetes (Group II, ages 18–25 years at diagnosis) and glucose tolerance tests in healthy control subjects. (P values in right-hand panel apply to comparison of 26 non-obese diabetic patients and 67 control subjects.)

mean sum of increments in plasma insulin after ingestion of glucose was significantly delayed in 26 of these patients who were non-obese. Twenty-two of these 26 patients had subnormal levels similar to those of the younger patients, while 4 showed responses which were greater than the mean plus S.D. of the sum of increases of the control subjects (Fig. 2; Table 1).

In 4 of the 24 patients aged 9–17 years at diagnosis (Group I), carbohydrate tolerance deteriorated to insulin-dependent diabetes. Nineteen of the other 20 patients have had follow-up tests for periods of 3.9–19.4 (mean 9.2) years. Although the abnormality in glucose tolerance has definitely progressed in 2 of these patients, the mean glucose tolerance of this group shows no evidence of decompensation (Fig. 3). The mean plasma insulin responses during glucose tolerance tests performed 2.6–10.8 (mean 6.3) years after the one on which the initial insulin determinations were made have shown no evidence of deterioration (Fig. 3).

Three patients of Group II have progressed to insulin-requiring diabetes. Twenty-seven of the other patients of this group have been retested at intervals of 1–15.7 (mean 6.8) years. The mean results of glucose tolerance tests obtained in these patients (including 3 of the 4 that had an excessive insulin response initially) indicate that some improvement in mean glucose tolerance has occurred at this time period of follow-up. In the patients who had a subnormal insulin response initially, there is no evidence of a significant change in the insulin response to glucose after intervals of up to 11.1 years (Fig. 4). In 3 of the 4 patients who had an excessive insulin response to glucose initially and who have been followed for more than one year, there has been a decrease in insulin levels subsequently, associated with improvement in glucose tolerance (Fig. 4).

In Groups III and IV initial glucose tolerance tests, highest glucose tolerance tests

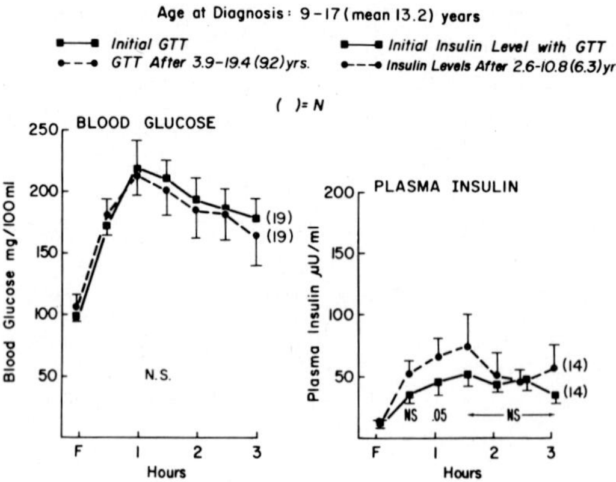

FIG. 3. Initial and last follow-up glucose tolerance tests in latent diabetic patients, ages 9–17 years at diagnosis (Group I).

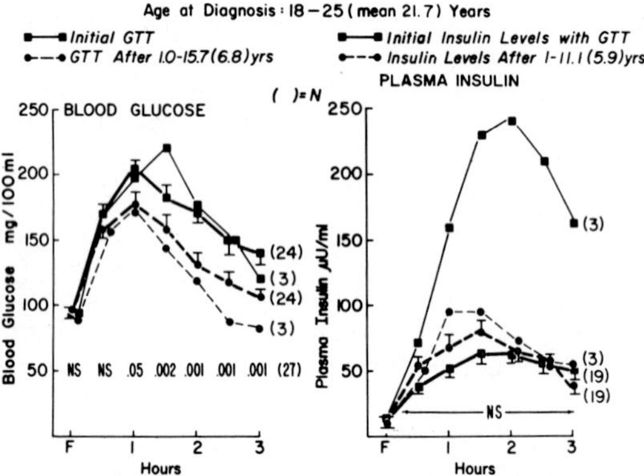

FIG. 4. Initial and last follow-up glucose tolerance tests in latent diabetic patients, ages 18–25 years at diagnosis (Group II).

(Table 2) and results of glucose tolerance tests after follow-up periods of up to 19.6 and 14.7 years, respectively, were similar to those of Group 2.

As stated above considerable fluctuation in glucose tolerance may occur in some patients when the test is repeated at intervals of days, months or years. Similar fluctuations may occur in the insulin response to glucose. On repetitive tests in an individual patient there may be no consistent relationship between glucose tolerance and the accompanying plasma insulin response as measured by levels of insulin in peripheral blood by conventional radioimmunoassay (Fajans et al., 1969b, 1970, 1971, 1973a). On repeated tests there may be (1) the expected inverse relationship between changes in glucose tolerance and the associated insulin response, (2) glucose tolerance may vary while the insulin response is unchanged, or (3) the insulin response may vary while glucose tolerance remains constant. Some representative examples of these findings have been reported previously (Fajans et al., 1969b, 1970, 1971, 1973a).

Studies were undertaken to ascertain whether evidence of microangiopathy could be detected in patients with latent diabetes. These studies have been reported in greater detail (Fajans et al., 1973b).

Muscle biopsies for determination of the width of basement membrane of muscle capillaries were performed in 71 patients who had been followed prospectively for periods of up to 18.1 years with a mean of 8.4 years. (One of these 71 patients had a grossly abnormal cortisone-glucose tolerance test at the time of biopsy but had his first of 3 definitely abnormal glucose tolerance tests when tested 8 months later.) When latent diabetes was diagnosed, 20 of the 71 patients were between the ages of 9 and 17 years, 24 between the ages of 18 and 25 years, 15 were between the ages of 26 and 35 and 12 were between the ages of 36 and 47 years. The latter 2 groups had a prevalence of basement membrane thickening (25.9%) which was similar to that of the younger 2 groups (22.8%). Estimation of capillary basement membrane width was made by Dr. Williamson by the method of Williamson et al. (1969).

Mean widths of basement membrane for the 71 patients with latent diabetes and for 71 control subjects (matched according to age and sex) are given in Table 3. The mean

TABLE 3

Basement membrane width (BMW) in patients with latent diabetes** and in age- and sex-matched control subjects***

	Latent diabetics BMW (Å) Mean ± S.E.M.	P	Control subjects (N = 71) BMW (Å) Mean ± S.E.M.
Patients (N)			
All (71)	1019 ± 25	< 0.001	916 ± 15
Without BMT+ (54)	938 ± 13		916 ± 15
	< 0.001		
With BMT (17)	1279 ± 60	< 0.001	916 ± 15

* BMW – Age and sex adjusted to 40-year-old male equivalent
** Diabetic patients (71) – Mean age 32.6 years
Control subjects (71) – Mean age 32.7 years
+ BMT – Basement membrane thickening

age of the diabetic patients at time of biopsy was 32.6 years, while the mean age of the control subjects was 32.7 years. Mean basement membrane width in the 71 latent diabetic patients, adjusted for age and sex differences to 40-year-old males, was 1019 ± 25 Å, as compared to 916 ± 15 A for the control subjects. Although mean basement membrane width in the latent diabetics is only 11.2% greater than that in the control subjects, the difference is highly significant statistically.

The 71 patients were then divided into 2 groups: those judged individually to be without basement membrane thickening (54 patients), and those with basement membrane thickening (17 patients). Patients were placed in these 2 categories according to their mean basement membrane width, or its standard deviation, employing slightly revised 95% confidence limits from those previously published by Kilo et al. (1972) and based on a larger number of control subjects in the younger age groups. The 17 patients with basement membrane thickening had a mean width much greater than that of the control subjects (Table 3). It is of interest that among the 17 patients with basement membrane thickening there was a significant correlation between basement membrane width and duration of known carbohydrate intolerance ($P < 0.05$). Among the 71 age- and sex-matched control subjects 3 individuals had basement membrane thickening giving a prevalence of 4.2%. However, among the diabetic patients, 17 of the 71 (24%) had basement membrane thickening, a prevalence that is significantly greater ($P < 0.001$) than that seen in the control subjects.

It is of considerable interest to note that of the 17 patients with basement membrane thickening, 8 have had occasional or intermittently normal glucose tolerance tests among the many performed during their respective follow-up periods ranging from 4.0–19.6 years. (Three of the 8 patients had normal and one a non-diagnostic glucose tolerance test at the time of biopsy. Four patients had their first of many abnormal glucose tolerance tests 5–17 years before biopsy but had normal tests 4 months to 3 years before or after biopsy.) If the normal tests would have been the only ones available at the time of the muscle biopsy it would have been tempting to conclude that basement membrane thickening precedes carbohydrate intolerance.

SUMMARY

The studies presented have led us to the following conclusions: (1) Although asymptomatic diabetes may progress to overt diabetes in some children, adolescents and adults, in the majority of such individuals studied, glucose intolerance does not necessarily increase in severity over periods of up to 19 years. (2) In the majority of these patients the mean insulin responses to glucose are delayed and subnormal, but the insulin response may not deteriorate further over periods of up to 11 years. (3) In individual patients there may be no consistent relationship between glucose tolerance and the insulin response to glucose as measured by plasma levels of insulin in peripheral blood by conventional radioimmunoassay. Our findings suggest that factors in addition to the abnormal pancreatic insulin response to glucose may determine normality or abnormality of glucose tolerance. (4) The slow progression of latent diabetes in many children, adolescents and young adults suggests that, with early detection, there may be time for the institution of prophylactic procedures which have the potentiality of being effective in preventing progression or in reversing abnormalities of insulin secretion and glucose intolerance. (5) A significant increase in basement membrane width and in prevalence of basement membrane thickening was found in patients with latent diabetes. Among the 17 patients with basement membrane thickening there was a significant correlation between basement membrane width and duration of known carbohydrate intolerance, a finding which parallels that of Kilo et al. (1972), who observed a correlation between basement membrane width and known duration of diabetes in insulin-requiring diabetic patients. (6) Many individual subjects with asymptomatic diabetes of long duration showed no statistically significant basement membrane thickening. This suggests: (a) that in young people with latent diabetes who have slow progression of insulin insufficiency and carbohydrate intolerance, there may also be slow progression of basement membrane changes; and (b) that if basement membrane thickening is a forerunner of clinically significant microvascular disease in later life in such patients, its early detection as demonstrated here might permit prophylactic procedures that have the potentiality of preventing serious vascular disease.

REFERENCES

BLOCK, N. B., ROSENFIELD, R. L., MAKO, M. E., STEINER, D. F. and RUBENSTEIN, A. H. (1973): Sequential changes in beta-cell function in insulin-treated diabetic patients assessed by C-peptide immunoreactivity. *New Engl. J. Med., 288,* 1144.

BURKEHOLDER, J. M., PICKENS, J. C. and WOMACK, W. N. (1967): Oral glucose tolerance test in siblings of children with diabetes mellitus. *Diabetes, 16,* 156.

CERASI, E. and LUFT, R. (1967): Insulin response to glucose infusion in diabetic and non-diabetic monozygotic twin pairs. Genetic control of insulin response? *Acta endocr. (Kbh.), 55,* 330.

CHIUMELLO, G., DEL GUERCIO, M. J., CARNELUTTI, M. and BIDONE, G. (1969): Relationship between obesity, chemical diabetes and beta pancreatic function in children. *Diabetes, 18,* 238.

COLWELL, J. A. and LEIN, A. (1967): Diminished insulin responses to hyperglycemia in prediabetes and diabetes. *Diabetes, 16,* 560.

CONN, J. W. and FAJANS, S. S. (1961): The prediabetic state. A concept of dynamic resistance to a genetic diabetogenic influence. *Amer. J. Med., 31,* 839.

FAJANS, S. S. (1971): What is diabetes? Definition, diagnosis and course. *Med. Clin. N. Amer., 55,* 794.

FAJANS, S. S. (1973): The definition of chemical diabetes. *Metabolism, 22,* 211.

FAJANS, S. S. and CONN, J. W. (1960): Tolbutamide-induced improvement in carbohydrate tolerance of young people with mild diabetes mellitus. *Diabetes, 9,* 83.

FAJANS, S. S. and CONN, J. W. (1962): The use of tolbutamide in the treatment of young people with mild diabetes mellitus – a progress report. *Diabetes, 11/Suppl.,* 123.

FAJANS, S. S. and CONN, J. W. (1965): Prediabetes, subclinical diabetes and latent clinical diabetes: interpretation, diagnosis and treatment. In: *On the Nature and Treatment of Diabetes,* pp. 641–656. Editors: B. S. Leibel and G. S. Wrenshall. International Congress Series No. 84, Excerpta Medica, Amsterdam.

FAJANS, S. S., FLOYD Jr., J. C., CONN, J. W., PEK, S., RULL, J. and KNOPF, R. F. (1969a): Plasma insulin responses to ingested glucose and to infused amino acids in subclinical diabetes and prediabetes. In: *Diabetes, Proceedings VI Congress of the International Diabetes Federation, Stockholm 1969,* pp. 515–521. Editor: J. Ostman. International Congress Series No. 172, Excerpta Medica, Amsterdam.

FAJANS, S. S., FLOYD Jr., J. C., PEK, S. and CONN, J. W. (1969b): The course of asymptomatic diabetes in young people, as determined by levels of blood glucose and plasma insulin. *Trans. Ass. Amer. Physcns, 82,* 211.

FAJANS, S. S., FLOYD Jr., J. C., CONN, J. W. and PEK, S. (1970): The course of asymptomatic diabetes of children, adolescents, and young adults. In: *Early Diabetes,* p. 377. Editors: R. A. Camerini-Davalos and H. S. Cole. Advances in Metabolic Disorders, Suppl. 1., Academic Press, New York.

FAJANS, S. S., FLOYD Jr., J. C., PEK, S. and CONN, J. W. (1971): Studies on the natural history of asymptomatic diabetes in young people. In: *Recent Advances in Endocrinology, Proceedings Seventh Pan-American Congress of Endocrinology, São Paulo, Brazil, 1970,* pp. 456–464. Editors: E. Mattar and G. B. Mattar. International Congress Series No. 238, Excerpta Medica, Amsterdam.

FAJANS, S. S., WEISSMAN, P. N., FLOYD Jr., J. C., WILLIAMSON, J. R., VOGLER, N. J., KILO, C. and CONN, J. W. (1973a): Studies on the natural history of asymptomatic diabetes in young people. In: *Modern Problems in Pediatrics, Proceedings 2nd International Beilinson Symposium on the Various Faces of Diabetes in Juveniles, Israel, 1972.* Jerusalem Academic Press and Karger, Basel, in press.

FAJANS, S. S., WILLIAMSON, J. R., WEISSMAN, P. N., VOGLER, N. J., KILO, C. and CONN, J. W. (1973b): Basement membrane thickening in latent diabetes. In: *Advances in Metabolic Disorders, Suppl. 2 – Vascular and Neurological Changes in Early Diabetes. Proceedings 2nd International Symposium on Early Diabetes, Curaçao, W. I., 1971*, pp. 393–399. Editors: R. A. Camerini-Dávalos and H. S. Cole. Academic Press, New York.

FLOYD Jr., J. C., FAJANS, S. S., CONN, J. W., THIFFAULT, C., KNOPF, R. F. and GUNTSCHE, E. (1968): Secretion of insulin induced by amino acids and glucose in diabetes mellitus. *J. clin. Endocr., 28,* 266.

JOHANSEN, K. and LUNDBAEK, K. (1967): Plasma-insulin in mild juvenile diabetes. *Lancet, 1,* 1257.

KAHN, C. B., SOELDNER, J. S., GLEASON, R. E., ROJAS, L., CAMERINI-DAVALOS, R. A. and MARBLE, A. (1969): Clinical and chemical diabetes in offspring of diabetic couples. *New Engl. J. Med., 281,* 343.

KILO, C., VOGLER, N. and WILLIAMSON, J. R. (1972): Muscle capillary basement membrane changes related to aging and diabetes mellitus. *Diabetes, 21,* 881.

LISTER, J. (1966): The clinical spectrum of juvenile diabetes. *Lancet, 1,* 386.

MURTHY, D. Y. N., GUTHRIE, R. A. and WOMACK, W. N. (1968): Progressive decrease in insulin reserve in children with chemical diabetes. *J. Pediat., 72,* 567.

O'SULLIVAN, J. B. and HURWITZ, D. (1966): Spontaneous remissions in early diabetes mellitus. *Arch. intern. Med., 117,* 769.

PAULSEN, E. P., RICHENDERFER, L. and GINSBERG-FELLNER, F. (1968): Plasma glucose, free fatty acids, and immunoreactive insulin in 66 obese children. *Diabetes, 17,* 261.

PECK Jr., F. B., KIRTLEY, W. R. and PECK Sr., F. B. (1958): Complete remission of severe diabetes. *Diabetes. 7,* 93.

PIRART, J. and LAUVAUX, J. P. (1971): Remission in diabetes. In: *Handbook of Diabetes, Vol. II,* p. 443. Editor: E. Pfeiffer. Lehmanns, Munich.

PYKE, D. A. and TAYLOR, K. W. (1967): Glucose tolerance and serum insulin in unaffected identical twins of diabetics. *Brit. med. J., 4,* 21.

ROJAS, L., SOELDNER, J. S., GLEASON, R. E., KAHN, C. B. and MARBLE, S. (1969): Offspring of two diabetic parents: differential serum insulin responses to intravenous glucose and tolbutamide. *J. clin. Endocr., 29,* 1569.

ROSENBLOOM, A. L. (1970): Insulin responses of children with chemical diabetes mellitus. *New Engl. J. Med., 282,* 1228.

RULL, J. A., CONN, J. W., FLOYD Jr., J. C. and FAJANS, S. S. (1970): Levels of plasma insulin during cortisone glucose tolerance tests in 'nondiabetic' relatives of diabetic patients. Implications of diminished insulin secretory reserve in subclinical diabetes. *Diabetes, 19,* 1.

SIPERSTEIN, M. D., UNGER, R. H. and MADISON, L. L. (1968): Studies of muscle capillary basement membranes in normal subjects, diabetic and prediabetic patients. *J. clin. Invest., 47,* 1973.

SISK, C. W. (1968): Application of a one-hour glucose tolerance test to genetic studies of diabetes in children. *Lancet, 1,* 262.

WHITE, P. (1956): Natural course and prognosis of juvenile diabetes. *Diabetes, 5,* 445.

WILLIAMSON, J. R., VOGLER, N. J. and KILO, C. (1969): Estimation of vascular basement membrane thickness. Theoretical and practical considerations. *Diabetes, 18,* 567.

WORKSHOP ON CHEMICAL DIABETES IN CHILDHOOD (1973): *Metabolism, Vol. 22,* No. 2, pp. 211–419. Guest editors: A. L. Rosenbloom, A. Drash and R. A. Guthrie.

METABOLIC CONSEQUENCES OF LOW INSULIN RESPONSE IN NON-DIABETIC SUBJECTS

EROL CERASI

Department of Endocrinology and Metabolism, Karolinska Hospital, Stockholm, Sweden

The old concept of insulin deficiency as the basic mechanism in the development of diabetes in man has, in recent years, seen a revival. It has been amply demonstrated that not only the ketosis-prone juvenile but also the mild mature-onset diabetics and even latent diabetics (with decreased glucose tolerance only) respond to glucose with a subnormal elevation of plasma insulin (Yalow and Berson, 1960; Cerasi and Luft, 1967a; Seltzer et al., 1967; Parker et al., 1968).

For this reason we presented some years ago the working hypothesis that a diminished insulin response to glucose is the basic pathogenic factor on which foundation the different stages of the diabetic syndrome develop (Cerasi and Luft, 1967b). The presence of low insulin response in healthy monozygotic twins of diabetic patients indicates that this insulin deficiency is inherited and precedes the appearance of decreased glucose tolerance (Cerasi and Luft, 1967c; Pyke et al., 1970). We therefore concluded that the combination of normal glucose tolerance and decreased insulin response to glucose characterizes the so-called prediabetic state. With this definition, the frequency of prediabetes in normal adults (Cerasi and Luft, 1967a) and children (Cerasi and Luft, 1970) was found to be about 20%. Since the frequency of manifest diabetes is much lower, it is obvious that not all prediabetics will eventually develop diabetes. The term is used in order to designate the group of subjects in which diabetes mellitus *may* develop. 'Low insulin responder' might be a more appropriate term in this connection.

FOLLOW-UP OF LOW INSULIN RESPONDERS

The important question is whether a low insulin response does indeed represent a prediabetic state, i.e., a disturbed hormonal situation, or simply reflects the left tail of a Gaussian distribution of normal pancreatic function. If, as we have postulated, the first alternative is the correct one, the majority of subjects with genetic diabetes should originate from the population of low insulin responders. One must remember, however, that in that case not more than 10% of the prediabetics can eventually develop overt diabetes (assuming an incidence of manifest diabetes of 2%) and about 30% will have decreased glucose tolerance (incidence 6%) sometimes during their adult life. Thus, substantial groups of controls and low insulin responders have to be followed for decades before a definite answer to the above question can be obtained.

By definition and by selection low insulin responders have a normal glucose tolerance.

However, the high insulin responders demonstrate a significantly higher k-value in the intravenous glucose tolerance test (IVGTT) than the lower responders (1.90 ± 0.69 versus 1.56 ± 0.40, $P < 0.01$), indicating a tighter control of the glucose tolerance. Furthermore, the rate of peripheral utilization of glucose, calculated from studies with liver vein catheterization (see below), was significantly lower than normal in low insulin responders (Cerasi et al., 1973a) and monozygotic healthy twins of diabetic subjects (Wahren et al., 1973). These facts probably make the low insulin responder more vulnerable to factors which tend to lower the glucose tolerance. In such subjects the diabetic range would thus be reached more easily.

So far, 97 high insulin responders and 39 prediabetics have been followed with repeated IVGTTs for ½–10 years. Of 356 tests performed in the controls, 4 showed k-values below 1.0, at one instance in one subject, and at 3 instances in another subject. None had fasting hyperglycemia. In low insulin responders, 151 tests were performed. Of these, 20 had k-values below 1.0 (occurring in 10 subjects). Thus, in 25.6% of the low responders a decreased glucose tolerance was noted at least at one occasion. The corresponding number in the control material was only 2.1%. One low insulin responder has repeatedly shown slight fasting hyperglycemia.

REGULATION OF LIPOLYSIS IN LOW INSULIN RESPONDERS

Lipolysis is accelerated to a greater extent in diabetic patients than in controls during submaximal work loads, resulting in a more marked elevation of the plasma levels of glycerol and free fatty acids (FFA) (Nordlander et al., 1973). A similar trend was found in low insulin responders in whom muscular work induced a significantly greater lipolytic response than in the normal group (Nordlander et al., 1973). In some of the subjects, the response was within the diabetic range. Thus, these subjects could be regarded as normal from the point of view of glucose tolerance, but as diabetic at the adipose tissue level. The cause of the exaggerated lipolytic response in low insulin responders is not known, but from an analogy with the situation in overt diabetics it may be presumed that insulin deficiency at the peripheral tissue level, and hence decreased anti-lipolysis, is a main factor.

PREGNANCY IN LOW INSULIN RESPONDERS

Pregnancy is a well-known diabetogenic situation. Many studies during recent years have demonstrated that there exists a certain degree of insulin resistance in pregnancy and that, as a compensatory factor, insulin secretion is enhanced as pregnancy progresses.

In a prospective study, glucose tolerance and the insulin response to glucose infusion were followed in 14 women with normal and 13 with low insulin response, before and during pregnancy (Edström et al., 1974). The k-value of IVGTT increased during the first 2 trimesters, but decreased to below the control level at the last trimester of pregnancy both in normals and in low insulin responders, the latter group reaching the lowest values. However, none of the subjects developed glucose intolerance. Insulin response to glucose increased with the duration of pregnancy in both groups, but the low insulin responders showed a significantly reduced response throughout pregnancy. Sensitivity to endogenous insulin (as calculated by computer analysis of the glucose infusion tests) decreased continuously during pregnancy in both groups, but more so in low insulin responders. It is therefore suggested that low insulin responders who either do not sufficiently enhance their insulin response, or demonstrate a more marked decrease in insulin sensitivity, or both, may develop gestagenic diabetes.

It is well-known that diabetic mothers often give birth to children with higher than normal glucose tolerance and a tendency to develop hypoglycemia. Although none of the pregnant low insulin responders developed glucose intolerance, preliminary data show that, during the first 24 hours of life, many children of prediabetic mothers behave like those of diabetic subjects regarding glucose tolerance. Thus, while 8 out of 14 newborns of healthy mothers had k-values below 1.0 and only 2 demonstrated a value above 1.30, in the children of prediabetic women only 2 out of 11 had a k-value less than 1.0, while in 5 a value above 1.30 was found. In other words, a substantial percentage of newborns of low insulin responders may behave like children of diabetic mothers. The factor(s) responsible for the early maturation of the islet apparatus in the offspring of prediabetic women is completely obscure.

It can be seen from the above data that low insulin responders, in addition to deranged insulin response to glucose, may share other characteristic abnormalities with diabetic subjects. Our findings give rise to a number of questions that remain to be answered: are there any basic differences between low insulin responders with and without the above metabolic abnormalities? In other words, of the total group of low insulin responders, are the real prediabetics only those who demonstrate such metabolic derangements? Or do these derangements come as late consequences of an inherited insulin deficiency? Can the metabolic abnormalities we have demonstrated so far occur successively in one and the same subject? If so, does the abnormal metabolic state of the diabetic result from the successive addition of 'partial abnormalities' already present during the prediabetic stage? Finally, what are the long-term consequences of these 'partial abnormalities' in subjects who remain prediabetics throughout life?

REGULATION OF GLUCOSE HOMEOSTASIS IN LOW INSULIN RESPONDERS

Although low insulin responders may demonstrate a decrease in insulin output of similar magnitude as that of patients with overt diabetes, and they may share a number of metabolic changes with diabetics (see above), they retain a normal glucose tolerance. We postulated earlier, therefore, the presence of some mechanisms that might be operating in the prediabetics in order to compensate for the insulin deficiency (Cerasi and Luft, 1967b). Our demonstration, in the prediabetic subjects, of decreased insulin response also to orally administered glucose (Cerasi et al., 1973b) excludes the possibility of the presence of intestinal factors which might stimulate the beta cells and thereby correct the glucose insensitivity as demonstrated on i.v. glucose.

We have earlier demonstrated that prediabetics are more sensitive to exogenous insulin (Cerasi and Luft, 1969). The site of this increased insulin sensitivity, on the basis of studies on the conversion of ^{14}C-pyruvate to ^{14}C-glucose and $^{14}CO_2$, was earlier suggested to be the liver (Cerasi and Luft, 1967b; Shreeve et al., 1970). We recently demonstrated that the splanchnic glucose production in the basal state in prediabetics was 25–45% lower than in the controls (Wahren et al., 1973; Cerasi et al., 1973a). Since both groups had normal fasting blood glucose levels, this finding indicates that the prediabetic subject had a decreased turnover rate of glucose. When blood glucose was slightly increased by the infusion of small amounts of glucose, the splanchnic glucose production fell more rapidly and to a significantly greater extent in the prediabetics, declining to less than 5% of the basal output as compared to 30% in the controls. In contrast, diabetic subjects did not diminish hepatic glucose output during glucose infusion (Wahren et al., 1972).

These findings suggest that the prediabetic subject may keep the glucose tolerance normal by shutting off the production of glucose in the liver at an earlier stage of glucose intake. The mechanisms responsible for this adaptation are not clear to us. Anyway, failure of such a mechanism might be responsible for the appearance of glucose intolerance. We have no data available at present which would permit us to conclude that there is a transition from supranormal regulation of hepatic output of glucose over a normal one to the hepatic hyporesponsiveness demonstrated in diabetes.

CONCLUSIONS

The prediabetic state is characterized by normal glucose tolerance and decreased insulin secretion on glucose stimulation. In spite of earlier belief, this state is not always devoid of metabolic consequences. Thus, the disappearance rate of intravenously administered glucose (k-value), although within the normal range, is significantly lower than in the control group. In some prediabetics, the lipolytic response to physical exercise is increased to the extent found in manifest diabetes. Furthermore, prediabetic mothers may give birth to children with diabetic fetopathy. Many of the newborns of these women show high k-values, as do children of diabetic women.

The transition from prediabetes to diabetes may be induced by several factors such as progressive deterioration of insulin output, or addition of diabetogenic factors like obesity and HGH-overproduction. Hepatic glucose output in the prediabetic is regulated with a higher than normal efficiency, thus compensating for the deficient insulin secretion. The failure of this important mechanism may be a major precipitating factor for diabetes.

REFERENCES

CERASI, E. and LUFT, R. (1967a): The plasma insulin response to glucose infusion in healthy subjects and in diabetes mellitus. *Acta endocr. (Kbh.), 55,* 278.

CERASI, E. and LUFT, R. (1967b): 'What is inherited – what is added' hypothesis for the pathogenesis of diabetes mellitus. *Diabetes, 16,* 615.

CERASI, E. and LUFT, R. (1967c): Insulin response to glucose infusion in diabetic and non-diabetic monozygotic twin pairs. Genetic control of insulin response? *Acta endocr. (Kbh.), 55,* 330.

CERASI, E. and LUFT, R. (1969): Disappearance rate of exogenous insulin, insulin sensitivity, responses of plasma growth hormone and cortisol and urinary epinephrine to hypoglycemia in prediabetic subjects. *Hormone metabol. Res., 1,* 221.

CERASI, E. and LUFT, R. (1970): The occurrence of low insulin response to glucose infusion in children. *Diabetologia, 6,* 85.

CERASI, E., WAHREN, J., LUFT, R., FELIG, P. and HENDLER, R. (1973a): The regulation of splanchnic glucose production in subjects with low insulin response – a compensatory mechanism in prediabetes? *Europ. J. clin. Invest., 3,* 193.

CERASI, E., EFENDIĆ, S. and LUFT, R. (1973b): Dose-response relationship of plasma insulin and blood glucose levels during oral glucose loads in prediabetic and diabetic subjects. *Lancet, i,* 794.

EDSTRÖM, K., CERASI, E. and LUFT, R. (1974): Insulin response to glucose infusion during pregnancy. A prospective study of high and low insulin responders with normal carbohydrate tolerance. *Acta endocr. (Kbh.),* in press.

NORDLANDER, S., ÖSTMAN, J., CERASI, E., LUFT, R. and EKELUND, L. G. (1973): Occurrence of diabetic type of plasma FFA and glycerol responses to physical exercise in prediabetic subjects. *Acta med. scand., 193,* 9.

PARKER, M. L., PILDES, R. S., KUEN-LAN, C., CORNBLATH, M. and KIPNIS, D. M. (1968): Juvenile diabetes mellitus, a deficiency in insulin. *Diabetes, 17,* 27.

PYKE, D. A., CASSAR, J., TODD, J. and TAYLOR, K. W. (1970): Glucose tolerance and serum insulin in identical twins of diabetics. *Brit. med. J., 4,* 649.

SELTZER, H. S., ALLEN, E. W., HERRON, A. L. and BRENNAN, M. T. (1967): Insulin secretion in response to glycemic stimulus: relation of delayed initial release to carbohydrate intolerance in mild diabetes mellitus. *J. clin. Invest., 46,* 323.

SHREEVE, W. W., CERASI, E. and LUFT, R. (1970): Metabolism of (2-^{14}C)pyruvate in normal, acromegalic and HGH-treated human subjects. *Acta endocr. (Kbh.), 65,* 155.

WAHREN, J., FELIG, P., CERASI, E. and LUFT, R. (1972): Splanchnic and peripheral glucose and amino acid metabolism in diabetes mellitus. *J. clin. Invest., 51,* 1870.

WAHREN, J., FELIG, P., CERASI, E., LUFT, R. and HENDLER, R. (1973): Splanchnic glucose production and its regulation in healthy monozygotic twins of diabetics. *Clin. Sci., 44,* 493.

YALOW, R. S. and BERSON, S. A. (1960): Plasma insulin concentrations in non-diabetic and early diabetic subjects. *Diabetes, 9,* 254.

GENETICS OF DIABETES MELLITUS

DAVID L. RIMOIN

Departments of Pediatrics and Medicine, Harbor General Hospital, UCLA School of Medicine, Torrance, Calif., U.S.A.

Hereditary factors are generally accepted to be of great importance in the etiology of diabetes, but there is little agreement as to the nature of the genetic mechanisms involved (Rimoin, 1971; Rimoin and Schimke, 1971; Simpson, 1971). Evidence in favor of a large genetic component in the etiology of diabetes is based primarily on studies of the familial aggregation of the disease, twin studies and population studies using markers such as clinical diabetes, glucose tolerance testing, insulin secretion and basement membrane thickening (Burkeholder et al., 1967; Cerasi and Luft, 1967; Conn and Fajans, 1961; Gottlieb and Root, 1968; Harvald and Hauge, 1963; Neel, 1970; Pincus and White, 1933; Pyke and Taylor, 1967; Rimoin and Schimke, 1971; Simpson, 1964). Irregardless of the marker used, be it clinical diabetes or abnormal glucose tolerance, there is a significantly greater prevalence of abnormality among the relatives of diabetics than among similar relatives of non-diabetics. In almost none of these studies, however, were individual family units examined, nor was there any attempt to define different genetic forms of diabetes. Although the evidence derived from studies of familial aggregation and twins leaves no doubt as to the importance of genetic factors in the etiology of diabetes, the mode of inheritance of the diabetic trait(s) is unknown (Rimoin, 1971; Rimoin and Schimke, 1971). During the past several decades, every possible mode of genetic transmission has been proposed, objections to all of them have been raised, and yet even today there are proponents of each of these hypotheses. This disagreement is due in part to a number of obstacles to which the geneticist is confronted in his attempts to unravel this problem. These include vast differences in the definition; in some an affected individual must have significant clinical symptoms of the disease, while in others only a mildly abnormal glucose tolerance test is accepted. The clinical variability, variability in the age of onset of the disease, and susceptibility to environmental factors present further difficulties in the delineation of an affected individual. Furthermore, the high prevalence of the disease in the population raises questions of relative genetic fitness. The most important impediment to genetic analysis, however, is the lack of knowledge concerning the basic defect in diabetes. Because of this, there is no certain method for detecting prediabetics, i.e., individuals with the mutant genotype who have, as yet, no signs of carbohydrate intolerance.

Although the mode of transmission of the diabetic genotype is obviously in question, many investigators have accepted the autosomal recessive hypothesis as fact and have based their definition of 'prediabetics' on this assumption. If such were the case, all offspring of 2 diabetics must possess the diabetic genotype. However, only about 50% of such individuals have been found to be affected, irrespective of the marker used to define diabetes (Kahn et al., 1969; Navarrete and Torres, 1967; Siperstein et al., 1968; Taton et al., 1964). These observations may be the result of several factors, including lack of penetrance, since accurate markers of the diabetic genotype are not available. Secondly, these data would be expected if diabetes was not inherited as a simple, autosomal recessive trait, but as a dominant or polygenic trait. Multiple factors are certainly involved in the variability of normal blood sugar levels but polygenic inheritance as a cause of clinical diabetes mellitus has not been adequately proven. Indeed, recent studies by Steinberg et al. (1970) have demonstrated bimodality in blood sugar concentrations in populations with a high prevalence of the disease. Thirdly, diabetes mellitus may be a heterogeneous group of disorders, i.e., a number of distinct disorders caused by different gene mutations at different loci, each of which results in carbohydrate intolerance (Rimoin, 1971; Rimoin and Schimke, 1971).

Evidence in favor of the heterogeneity hypothesis includes: (a) clinical variability in the disease, as exemplified by the differences between juvenile-onset and maturity-onset diabetes; (b) ethnic variability in the clinical and metabolic features of diabetes apparently not directly related to environmental factors; (c) biochemical heterogeneity as exemplified by both insulinopenic and hyperinsulinemic forms of diabetes; and (d) the occurrence of abnormal glucose tolerance in over 30 distinct genetic syndromes due to mutations at many different loci, as well as to several chromosomal aberrations (Table 1) (Rimoin and Schimke, 1971). Furthermore, genetic heterogeneity has been well documented in the mouse, being associated with at least 4 simply inherited disorders due to mutations at different loci, as well as being present in high frequency in a number of distinct strains which have been developed by selection and inbreeding (Bray and York,

TABLE 1

Genetic syndromes associated with glucose intolerance

Alstrom syndrome	Ocular hypertension induced by dexamethasone
Ataxia telangiectasia	Optic atrophy and diabetes
Cockayne syndrome	Optic atrophy, diabetes insipidus, and diabetes mellitus
Cystic fibrosis	Hereditary relapsing pancreatitis
Friedreich's ataxia	Photomyoclonus, diabetes, deafness, nephropathy, and cerebral dysfunction
Glucose-6-phosphate dehydrogenase deficiency	Pineal hyperplasia and diabetes
Type I glycogen storage disease	Acute intermittent porphyria
Hemochromatosis	Pheochromocytoma
Huntington's chorea	Prader-Willi syndrome
Hyperlipemia, diabetes, hypogonadism, and short stature	Retinitis pigmentosa, neuropathy, ataxia and diabetes
Hyperlipoproteinemia III	Schmidt syndrome
Hyperlipoproteinemia IV	Werner syndrome
Hyperlipoproteinemia V	Turner syndrome
Isolated growth hormone deficiency	Klinefelter syndrome
Laurence-Moon-Biedl syndrome	Down's syndrome
Lipoatrophic diabetes	
Muscular dystrophy	
Myotonic dystrophy	

1971; Dickie, 1970). Thus, all of this evidence points toward the possibility that diabetes represents a heterogeneous group of disorders and that hyperglycemia is a non-specific manifestation of a variety of different mechanisms. Indeed, hyperglycemia may be no more specific than anemia and the use of diet, oral hypoglycemic agents or insulin may be as non-specific as a blood transfusion.

Theoretically, there are a number of ways in which a gene mutation could affect insulin synthesis, secretion, transport or action so as to produce carbohydrate intolerance. Some of these possibilities include a structural mutation in the insulin molecule, a defect in the enzyme which cleaves insulin from proinsulin, decreased synthesis or secretion of a normal insulin molecule, glandular hypoplasia or degeneration, peripheral unresponsiveness to the actions of insulin, or circulating antagonists to insulin action. It is likely that many, if not all, of these mechanisms do produce abnormal glucose tolerance, and future research into this symptom-complex must provide a means of identifying the specific pathogenetic mechanism operative in each diabetic patient before accurate genetic counseling can be given.

Since the mode of inheritance of diabetes is still in question, accurate genetic counseling is impossible. Various tables listing the risk of an individual inheriting the diabetic genotype have been published, based on the assumption that diabetes is inherited as a simple autosomal recessive trait (Grunnet, 1957) or on the basis of a statistical analysis of morbid risk figures, calculated from a limited clinical experience (Simpson, 1968). Simpson (1968, 1971) has constructed relative risk figures for developing clinical diabetes among first degree relatives of diabetics, based on data obtained from questionnaires on a large population (Table 2). The risk of a given relative developing diabetes varies with the age of onset of diabetes in the proband. If the proband developed diabetes under the age

TABLE 2

Risk of developing diabetes with a parent, sibling or child who is a diabetic (Simpson, 1971)

Age of non-diabetic (years)	Risk of developing diabetes
0–19	> 1%
20–39	1%
40–59	3%
60+	10%

of 20 years, the risk figures should be approximately doubled, except for the over 60-year-old category. If there is more than one parent, sibling or child who is diabetic, the risks are also approximately doubled. These relative risk figures are, of course, approximations and must be related to the age-specific risk for diabetes in the specific population from which the counselee is derived. Although these risk figures allow one the satisfaction of quoting a number to the counselee, he should be made aware of its inexactness.

There has recently been some controversy on whether or not diabetics should be allowed to marry one another and have children. The World Health Organization (1965) advises that diabetics should be counseled not to marry each other, or if they do, they should not have children. They base this advice on the presumption that 'conjugal diabetics may increase the number of diabetic offspring and perhaps determine the appearance of diabetics at earlier ages'. Edwards (1969) has pointed out the fallacy of this advice and claimed that these recommendations would probably not increase the number of subsequent diabetics, but simply influence their allocation. It is apparent that with our limited knowledge concerning the genetics of diabetes, it is difficult to offer informative genetic counseling to an individual couple, and foolhardy to attempt eugenic measures.

REFERENCES

BRAY, G. A. and YORK, D. A. (1971): Genetically-transmitted obesity in rodents. *Physiol. Rev., 51,* 3.

BURKEHOLDER, J. N., PICKENS, J. M. and WOMACK, W. N. (1967): Oral glucose tolerance tests in siblings of children with diabetes mellitus. *Diabetes, 16,* 156.

CERASI, E. and LUFT, R. (1967): Insulin response to glucose infusion in diabetic and non-diabetic monozygotic twin pairs. Genetic control of insulin response. *Acta Endocr. (Kbh.), 55,* 330.

CONN, J. W. and FAJANS, S. S. (1961): The prediabetic state. *Amer. J. Med., 31,* 839.

DICKIE, M. M. (1970): Genetics of animals with spontaneous diabetes. *Advanc. metabol. Dis., Suppl. 1,* 23.

EDWARDS, J. H. (1969): Should diabetics marry? *Lancet, 1,* 1045.

GOTTLIEB, M. S. and ROOT, H. F. (1968): Diabetes mellitus in twins. *Diabetes, 17,* 693.

GRUNNET, J. (1957): *Heredity in Diabetes Mellitus, a Proband Study. Opera ex Domo Biologiae Hereditariae, Humanae Universitatis Hafniensis.* Munksgaard, Copenhagen.

HARVALD, B. and HAUGE, M. (1963): Selection in diabetes in modern society. *Acta med. scand., 173,* 459.

KAHN, C. B., SOELDNER, J. S., GLEASON, R. E., ROJAS, L., CAMERINI-DAVALOS, R. A. and MARBLE, A. (1969): Clinical and chemical diabetes in offspring of diabetic couples. *New Engl. J. Med., 281,* 343.

NAVARRETE, V. N. and TORRES, I. H. (1967): Triamcinolone provocative test in offspring of two diabetic parents. *Diabetes, 16,* 57.

NEEL, J. V. (1970): The genetics of diabetes mellitus. *Advanc. metabol. Dis., Suppl. 1,* 3.

PINCUS, G. and WHITE, P. (1933): On the inheritance of diabetes mellitus. I. An analysis of 675 family histories. *Amer. J. med. Scis, 186,* 1.

PYKE, D. A. and TAYLOR, K. W. (1967): Glucose tolerance and serum insulin in unaffected identical twins of diabetics. *Brit. med. J., 2,* 21.

RIMOIN, D. L. (1971): Inheritance in diabetes mellitus. *Med. Clin. N. Amer., 55,* 807.

RIMOIN, D. L. and SCHIMKE, R. N. (1971): *Genetic Disorders of the Endocrine Glands.* C.V. Mosby Company, St. Louis, Mo.

SIMPSON, N. E. (1964): Multifactorial inheritance. A possible hypothesis for diabetes. *Diabetes, 13,* 462.

SIMPSON, N. E. (1968): Diabetes in the families of diabetics. *Canad. med. Ass. J., 98,* 427.

SIMPSON, N. E. (1971): *Genetic Considerations in Diabetes Mellitus; Diagnosis and Treatment, Vol. III,* p. 71. Editors: S. S. Fajans and K. E. Sussman. American Diabetes Association, New York, N.Y.

SIPERSTEIN, M. D., UNGER, R. H. and MADISON, L. L. (1968): Studies of muscle capillary basement membranes in normal subjects, diabetic, and pre-diabetic patients. *J. clin. Invest., 47,* 1973.

STEINBERG, A. G., RUSHFORTH, N. B., BENNETT, P. H., BURCH, T. A. and MILLER, M. (1970): Preliminary report on the genetics of diabetes among the Pima Indians. *Advanc. metabol. Dis., Suppl. 1,* 11.

TATON, J., POMETTA, D., CAMERINI-DAVALOS, R. A. and MARBLE, A. (1964): Genetic determinism to diabetes and tolerance to glucose. *Lancet, 2,* 1360.

WORLD HEALTH ORGANIZATION (1965): *Techn. Rep. Ser. Wld Health Org., 310,* 15.

LIPID DISORDERS AND DIABETES

LIPID TRANSPORT AND INSULIN RESISTANCE*

RICHARD J. HAVEL

Cardiovascular Research Institute and Department of Medicine, University of California, San Francisco, Calif., U.S.A.

The intimate, generally reciprocal relationship between the transport and metabolism of fat and carbohydrate is evident in a variety of physiological states and pathological conditions in man (Havel, 1972a). The influence of diabetes on these relationships has been reviewed by several of the participants in this Panel. A systematic alteration in lipid transport leading to fatty liver and hyperlipemia also occurs in a group of different disorders characterized by varying degrees of glucose intolerance, in which impedance to the action of insulin appears to be fundamental. This syndrome is observed in many obese individuals, in some women taking contraceptive steroids and in chronic renal failure.

These antecedents of endogenous and mixed forms of hyperlipemia, like increased intake of calories (particularly in the form of carbohydrate or ethanol), bring out the hyperlipemic 'constitution' or 'phenotype'. Varying degrees of fatty liver and hyperlipemia are also the rule in the various forms of partial and total lipodystrophy – again, states regularly accompanied by ineffective action of insulin.

It is the purpose of this brief survey to review what is known about the manifestations of insulin resistance in these conditions and to indicate the likely mechanisms that lead to the disordered metabolism of fat.

DIRECT MANIFESTATIONS OF INSULIN RESISTANCE

Impedance to the hypoglycemic effect of insulin is a reliable, but insensitive index of resistance in euglycemic individuals. The test devised by Himsworth (Himsworth and Kerr, 1939) is probably equally reliable and more sensitive. The increase in peripheral venous insulin level after glucose challenge is usually augmented, but the reliability of tests utilizing this measure is open to question, in part because of problems relating increments in glucose and insulin levels. This is not surprising in view of the imprecise relationship between secretion of insulin and glucose tolerance (Reaven et al., 1971). Other more complex tests have been devised (Shen et al., 1970) but they have not been widely used.

Key questions about the mechanism by which insulin resistance leads to disordered

* This work was supported in part by a grant (HL 06285) from the U.S. Public Health Service.

lipid metabolism are first, which organs and tissues are the site of impedance (i.e., is the impedance local or global), and second, which actions of insulin are impeded?

Important evidence on these questions was first provided by the study of Rabinowitz and Zierler (1962) on the influence of obesity on the glucose-permease and antilipolytic actions of insulin in the human forearm. Their observations led them to conclude that both muscle and adipose tissue are insensitive to the former action and that the inhibitory effect of insulin on mobilization of fat from adipose tissue is also impeded. Quite recently, studies of Felig et al. (1973) have shown that the effect of insulin on net splanchnic glucose production is also diminished in obese individuals. Thus, the abnormality in obesity evidently is global, extending to 3 of the major tissues in which insulin affects glucose transport or metabolism and also to the rapid antilipolytic action of insulin in adipose tissue. Equivalent information is not available for other conditions characterized by insulin resistance.

MANIFESTATIONS OF INSULIN RESISTANCE IN LIPOATROPHIC DIABETES

Glucose intolerance, often accompanied by hyperinsulinism, together with fatty liver and hyperlipemia are the rule in both partial and complete forms of lipodystrophy (Piscatelli et al., 1970). Studies performed several years ago in a woman with the late-onset form of total lipodystrophy (lipoatrophic diabetes) are consistent with severe global impedance to the direct actions of insulin, similar to that observed to a lesser degree in obesity (Havel et al., 1967). Since the results of this study have not been reported previously in detail, certain aspects will be summarized here.

When the patient was first seen in 1966 at the age of 40, she had had diabetes for 5 years and was poorly controlled on 125 U of insulin daily. Loss of subcutaneous fat was evident from photographs taken during adolescence. In addition, she had muscular dystrophy involving the upper part of her body of the type known as 'ophthalmoplegia plus', accompanied by nerve deafness. Subcutaneous fat was evident only in the face. Her liver was grossly enlarged; microscopic examination of a sample obtained at biopsy showed severe fatty infiltration without fibrosis. Upon withdrawal of insulin, fasting blood glucose rose from about 200 to 350 mg/dl and she excreted 100–125 g glucose in her urine daily. However, urine tests for ketone bodies remained negative to 'trace'. Plasma triglyceride level rose from 1500 mg/dl on admission to 6,000 mg/dl on the eighth day after insulin was stopped and the level of free fatty acids (FFA) rose to about 1.5 mM. Insulin was withheld for a total of 4 weeks. During this period, a single insulin tolerance test (1 U/kg i.v.) showed poor response of glucose and FFA levels (Fig. 1). Large amounts of sodium nicotinate i.v. similarly produced a limited fall in concentration of FFA (Fig. 2). Intravenous infusion of norepinephrine (0.2 μg per kg $\times$ min. for 30 min.) increased the concentration of FFA from 1.7 to 2.1 μmoles/ml. Lipoprotein lipase activity in plasma 10 min. after intravenous injection of 0.1 mg heparin per kg body weight (Boberg and Carlson, 1964) was 0.11 μmoles FFA/ml $\times$ min. (inhibited 82% by 0.5 M NaCl). Subsequent treatment with 350–400 U insulin daily reduced glucosuria to about 25 g daily and levels of FFA fell to about 0.6 mM. Plasma triglyceride concentration fell to 1200 mg/dl after 4 days of treatment with insulin but the activity of lipoprotein lipase in postheparin plasma changed little (0.13 μmoles FFA/ml $\times$ min.).

After 4 months of treatment with 380 U insulin daily, triglyceride levels were about 500 mg/dl and lipoprotein lipase activity was essentially unchanged (0.11 μmoles

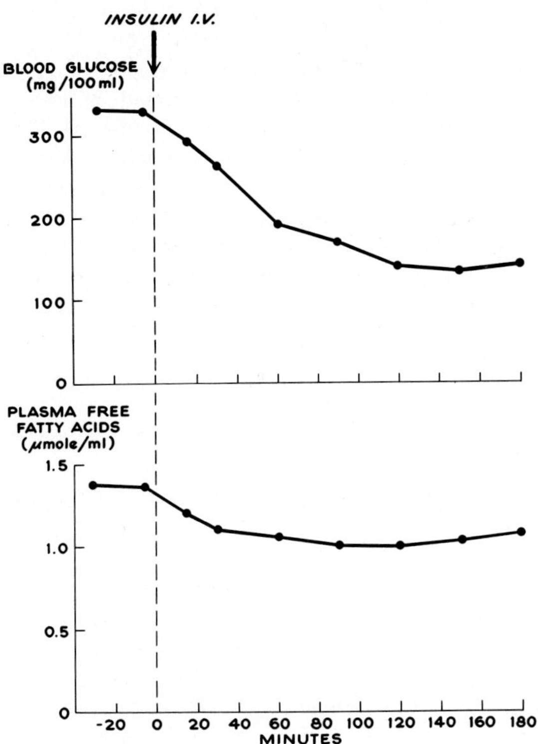

FIG. 1. Response of blood glucose and plasma FFA to 36 U insulin (1 U/kg body weight) intravenously in patient C. K. with lipoatrophic diabetes. At this time, no insulin had been given for 12 days, the patient had no ketonuria and she was utilizing approximately 210 g of dietary glucose daily.

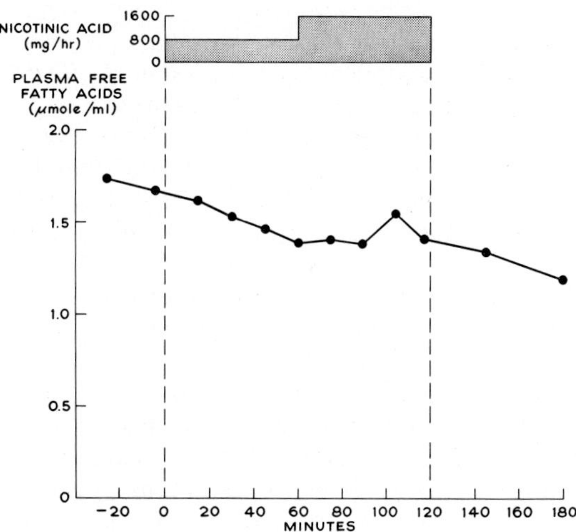

FIG. 2. Response of plasma FFA to intravenous administration of a large amount of sodium nicotinate in patient C. K. This study was performed 2 days before the one shown in Figure 1.

FFA/ml × min.). Ingestion of a meal containing 1.5 g fat/kg body weight increased plasma triglyceride level to 1200 mg/dl after 6 hours, with reduction to 650 mg/dl after 12 hours. Fasting triglyceride level increased to about 700 mg/dl 4 days after she was placed on a diet containing 5 g fat, 475 g carbohydrate and 100 g protein. At this time, she was given a pulse injection of palmitate-1-^{14}C intravenously and ^{14}C was measured in triglyceride fatty acids of very low density lipoproteins (VLDL-TGFA) for 2 days (Fig. 3). The rate of disappearance of ^{14}C was markedly delayed. Inflow transport of FFA was found to be within normal limits, but that of VLDL-TGFA was reduced (Table 1) and a maximum of only 3.3% of injected ^{14}C appeared in VLDL-TGFA.

TABLE 1

Transport of FFA and TGFA in blood plasma of patient C. K. with lipoatrophic diabetes

	FFA	VLDL-TGFA
Concentration (μmoles/ml)	0.55	15.5
Turnover rate (min^{-1})	0.33	0.00055
Net inflow transport (μmoles/min·m^2)	185	9.5

In 1968, while she was maintained on 360 U insulin daily, response to sodium nicotinate was again found to be subnormal (concentration of FFA fell from 0.61 to 0.48 μmoles/ml after injection of 800 mg nicotinic acid in one hour). No evidence of gross hypersecretion of anti-insulin hormones was obtained. Basal levels of growth hormone were normal (3 ng/ml) 6 days after insulin was stopped in 1966 and responded normally to intravenous infusion of 30 g arginine (31 ng/ml after 2 hours). Basal levels of growth hormone were similar in 1973 and fell to $<$ 1 ng/ml 2 hours after 50 g of oral glucose, 70 U insulin subcutaneously and 0.5 U/kg insulin intravenously. In the same test, basal glucagon level was 185 pg/ml and fell to 20 pg/ml after one hour. However, the level of glucagon changed little when the same amount of glucose was ingested without insulin. Circulating insulin antibody titer (Feldman et al., 1963) was in the range usually seen in insulin-dependent diabetics treated with insulin.

At present, she has no evidence of diabetic microangiopathy. No thickening of the basement membrane of capillaries in the vastus lateralis was evident in 1966 (935 Å) (Siperstein et al., 1968). A few fat cells were seen on microscopic examination of subcutaneous tissue and skeletal muscle in 1966. Masses in the left breast and axilla obtained at operation in 1968 proved to be dysplastic breast tissue and lymph nodes; the latter were largely replaced by fat. Small amounts of subcutaneous and mammary fat were also evident. The adipose tissue was unremarkable histologically.

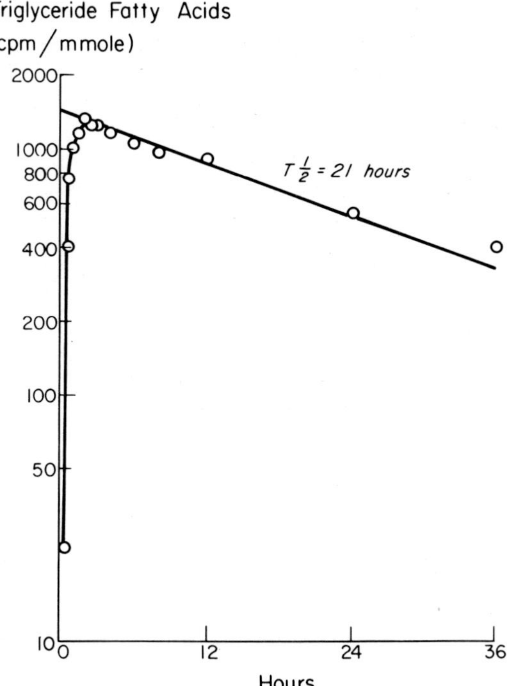

FIG. 3. Specific activity of VLDL-TGFA in blood plasma of C. K. following pulse-injection of palmitate-1-^{14}C. At this time, the patient was maintained on an isocaloric diet containing 5 g fat and was receiving 380 U insulin in 2 doses daily. The rates of turnover and transport of FFA and VLDL-TGFA determined in this study are shown in Table 1. This method of estimating the turnover rate of VLDL-TGFA is considered to be valid in patients with levels of VLDL-TGFA in the range present here, but not in normotriglyceridemic individuals (Havel et al., 1970).

The greatly impaired hypoglycemic effect of insulin in this patient cannot be explained by circulating antibodies and it must reflect severe impedance to its action in liver and extrahepatic tissues. The antilipolytic effect of insulin in her remaining adipose tissue is also greatly reduced. It is of interest that this abnormality extends to another potent antilipolytic agent, nicotinic acid. Substantial amounts of insulin in the presence of hyperglycemia likewise fail to promote secretion of VLDL-TGFA; rather the secretion rate is reduced and fat accumulates in her liver as it does in uncontrolled diabetes mellitus. Her hyperlipemia thus clearly results from impaired utilization of plasma triglycerides. Activity of lipoprotein lipase in postheparin plasma is moderately reduced and unaffected by insulin. Her failure to develop ketosis upon withdrawal of insulin cannot be ascribed simply to lack of adipose tissue, since the levels of FFA rose substantially and remained high for a period of 2 weeks. Most probably, she continues to secrete sufficient insulin to prevent gross proteolysis and to promote utilization of ketone bodies (Balasse and Havel, 1971).[1]

[1] This is supported by the observation that the level of insulin increased from 93 to 133 μU/ml plasma 60 minutes after intravenous injection of arginine in 1966.

Thus, it appears that severe global resistance to insulin accounts for the observed metabolic abnormalities in this patient with lipoatrophic diabetes. The failure of large amounts of insulin to normalize metabolism in her liver and skeletal muscle when the rate of fat mobilization was reduced to normal values is consistent with the hypothesis that the basic defect is present in all insulin-sensitive tissues.

INSULIN RESISTANCE IN OTHER HYPERLIPEMIC STATES

The results obtained in obesity and lipoatrophic diabetes raise the question whether global insulin resistance characterizes other similar metabolic states, such as uremia (Bagdade et al., 1968) and administration of contraceptive steroids (Beck, 1973). Impaired glucose tolerance associated with increased insulinogenic response characterizes these 2 states (Horton et al., 1968; Beck, 1973). Given its importance in the disposal of administered glucose, it is reasonable to postulate that the liver participates in the impeded response to insulin.

The importance of insulin resistance in the pathogenesis of primary endogenous hyperlipemia remains uncertain (Kane et al., 1965; Bagdade et al., 1971; Havel, 1972b), although there is no reason to doubt that aggravation of these states by obesity reflects impedance to insulin's effects in extrahepatic tissues. However, the maintenance of normal splanchnic metabolism of FFA (Havel et al., 1970) provides no support for the suggestion that increased availability of insulin promotes hepatic triglyceride synthesis and secretion in this syndrome. In fact, there is little to support the concept (Reaven et al., 1967; Bagdade et al., 1968) that insulin antagonism in hyperlipemic states is confined to 'peripheral' tissues, whereas the liver increases its rate of secretion of triglycerides in response to increased insulinogenic stimulation. Rather, available evidence suggests that insulin resistant states are generally global and that these states lead to hyperlipemia primarily by impeding normal mechanisms for removal of triglycerides from the blood.

ACKNOWLEDGEMENTS

I wish to express my appreciation to L. V. Basso and J. P. Kane for their contributions to the original work reported here and to J. H. Karam for the assays of growth hormone, insulin and glucagon and of antibodies to insulin in blood plasma.

REFERENCES

BAGDADE, J. D., BIERMAN, E. L. and PORTE, D. (1971): Influence of obesity on the relationship between insulin and triglyceride levels in endogenous hypertriglyceridemia. *J. Amer. Diabetes Ass., 20,* 664.

BAGDADE, J. D., PORTE, D. and BIERMAN, E. L. (1968): Hypertriglyceridemia: a metabolic consequence of chronic renal failure. *New Engl. J. Med., 279,* 181.

BALASSE, E. O. and HAVEL, R. J. (1971): Evidence for an effect of insulin on the peripheral utilization of ketone bodies in dogs. *J. clin. Invest., 50,* 801.

BECK, P. (1973): Contraceptive steroids: Modifications of carbohydrate and lipid metabolism. *Metabolism, 22,* 84.

BOBERG, J. and CARLSON, L. A. (1964): Determination of heparin-induced lipoprotein lipase activity in human plasma. *Clin. chim. Acta, 10,* 420.

FELDMAN, R., GRODSKY, G. M., KOHOUT, F. W. and WILLIAMS, N. B. (1963): Immunologic studies in a diabetic subject resistant to bovine insulin but sensitive to porcine insulin. *Amer. J. Med., 73,* 411.

FELIG, P., WAHREN, J., HENDLER, R. and BRUNDIN, T. (1973): Obesity: evidence of hepatic resistance to insulin. *J. clin. Invest., 41,* 2173.

HAVEL, R. J. (1972a): Caloric homeostasis and disorders of fuel transport. *New Engl. J. Med., 287,* 1186.

HAVEL, R. J. (1972b): Mechanisms of hyperlipoproteinemia. In: *Pharmacological Control of Lipid Metabolism, Advances in Experimental Medicine and Biology, Vol. 26,* pp. 57–70. Editors: W. L. Holmes, R. Paoletti and D. Kritchevsky. Plenum Press, New York, N.Y.

HAVEL, R. J., BASSO, L. V. and KANE, J. P. (1967): Mobilization and storage of fat in congenital and late-onset forms of 'total' lipodystrophy. *J. clin. Invest., 73,* 963.

HAVEL, R. J., KANE, J. P., BALASSE, E. O., SEGEL, N. and BASSO, L. V. (1970): Splanchnic metabolism of free fatty acids and production of triglycerides of very low density lipoproteins in normotriglyceridemic and hypertriglyceridemic humans. *J. clin. Invest., 49,* 2017.

HIMSWORTH, H. P. and KERR, R. B. (1939): Insulin-sensitive and insulin-insensitive types of diabetes mellitus. *Clin. Sci., 4,* 119.

HORTON, E. S., JOHNSON, C. and LEBOVITZ, H. E. (1968): Carbohydrate metabolism in uremia. *Ann. intern. Med., 68,* 63.

KANE, J. P., LONGCOPE, C., PAVLATOS, F. C. and GRODSKY, G. M. (1965): Studies of carbohydrate metabolism in idiopathic hypertriglyceridemia. *Metabolism, 14,* 471.

PISCATELLI, R. L., VIEWEG, W. V. R. and HAVEL, R. J. (1970): Partial lipodystrophy: metabolic studies in three patients. *Ann. intern. Med., 73,* 963.

RABINOWITZ, D. and ZIERLER, K. L. (1962): Forearm metabolism in obesity and its response to intra-arterial insulin. Characterization of insulin resistance and evidence for adaptive hyperinsulinism. *J. clin. Invest., 41,* 2173.

REAVEN, G. M., LERNER, R. L., STERN, M. P. and FARQUHAR, J. W. (1967): Role of insulin in endogenous hypertriglyceridemia. *J. clin. Invest., 46,* 1756.

REAVEN, G. M., SHEN, S.-W., SILVERS, A. and FARQUHAR, J. W. (1971): Is there a delay in the plasma insulin response of patients with chemical diabetes mellitus? *J. Amer. Diabetes Ass., 20,* 416.

SHEN, S.-W., REAVEN, G. M. and FARQUHAR, J. W. (1970): Comparison of impedance to insulin-mediated glucose uptake in normal subjects and in subjects with latent diabetes. *J. clin. Invest., 49,* 2151.

SIPERSTEIN, M. D., UNGER, R. H. and MADISON, L. L. (1968): Studies of muscle capillary basement membranes in normal subjects, diabetic and prediabetic patients. *J. clin. Invest., 47,* 1973.

INSULIN LEVELS AND PLASMA TRIGLYCERIDE REMOVAL IN DIABETES*

EDWIN L. BIERMAN

Department of Medicine, University of Washington School of Medicine and VA Hospital, Seattle, Wash., U.S.A.

There is a spectrum of insulin insufficiency in diabetic individuals associated with a variety of recognizable alterations in plasma triglyceride removal related to lipoprotein lipase. Gross deficiency of insulin secretion in severe diabetes is associated with markedly reduced activity of lipoprotein lipase (indirectly assessed as plasma post heparin lipolytic activity or PHLA) (Bagdade et al., 1967). In this situation impaired removal of triglyceride from plasma is reflected by the progressive accumulation of chylomicrons in the circulation on normal fat containing diets ('diabetic lipemia'). Diabetics with this syndrome have fasting hyperglycemia, symptomatic glucosuria, and no insulin response to a glucose load. This pathophysiological sequence can be mimicked acutely by brief periods of insulin withdrawal from insulin-dependent diabetics which results in lower PHLA and a reciprocal increase in plasma triglyceride levels (Bagdade et al., 1968). These abnormalities are promptly reversed by insulin treatment. In such patients impaired maximal removal of intravenously administered exogenous particulate fat has been demonstrated (Lewis et al., 1972). Accumulation of endogenous triglyceride-rich lipoproteins in PHLA deficiency associated with insulin lack probably results from impaired removal as well, since endogenous triglyceride-rich lipoproteins and chylomicrons are presumed to be removed from plasma by a common lipoprotein lipase-related mechanism (Brunzell et al., 1973a). This conclusion is supported by studies of others in animals, which indicate that hepatic endogenous triglyceride production is not increased in experimental chronic insulin deficiency (Heimberg et al., 1967; Basso and Havel, 1970), perhaps a result of impaired synthesis of apolipoproteins (Wilcox et al., 1968).

In less severe diabetics with fasting hyperglycemia associated with less marked deficiency of insulin secretion, triglyceride-rich lipoprotein levels in plasma may become elevated due to a removal defect despite normal PHLA (standard assay). Often chylomicronemia is present. This removal defect appears to be related to a more subtle abnormality of lipoprotein lipase in which enzyme levels cannot be normally sustained in the circulation during several hours of a high dose constant heparin infusion (Fig. 1) (Brunzell et al., 1972a). This 'PHLA depletion' (average 30% fall after 2 hours) may reflect impaired synthetic capacity of new enzyme related to insulin insufficiency when the system is stressed. In contrast, enzyme is normally available from readily releasable storage sites.

* This research was supported in part by grant AM 06670 from the National Institutes of Health and by the Veterans Administration.

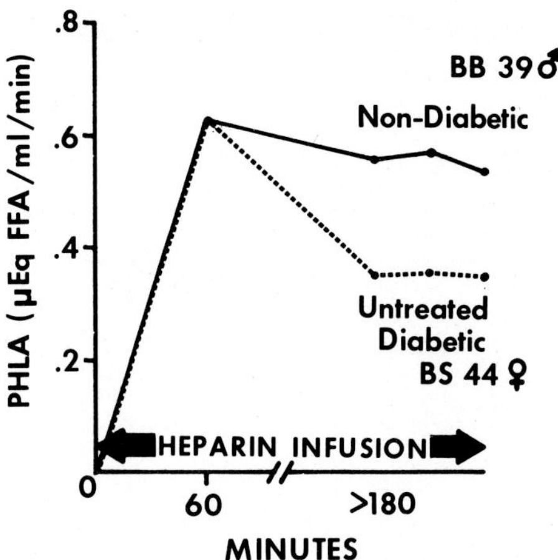

FIG. 1. Example of PHLA depletion during prolonged constant high-dose heparin infusion in an untreated diabetic subject with fasting hyperglycemia compared to normally sustained PHLA levels in a non-diabetic with comparable PHLA, both in the standard assay and after 60 minutes of infusion.

The degree of PHLA depletion is directly related to the severity of hyperglycemia ($r = 0.7$, $P < 0.01$) and hence to the severity of insulin insufficiency. Chronic insulin or sulfonylurea treatment is associated with reversal of the abnormality in PHLA and reduction of hypertriglyceridemia. PHLA depletion during prolonged heparin infusion can be mimicked by administration to dogs of the protein synthesis inhibitor cycloheximide, which selectively decreases PHLA release after two hours (Brunzell et al., 1972a). These results suggest that PHLA release is multiphasic, with early prompt release after heparin derived from readily accessible storage sites and late release from a synthesis-related tissue pool which is sensitive to insulin availability (Fig. 2) (Brunzell et al., 1972b). These results are also supported by observations in perfused hearts from alloxan-diabetic rats (Atkin and Meng, 1972). Lipoprotein lipase release was normal after brief perfusion with heparin, but considerably decreased during prolonged heparin exposure. Furthermore, the time for repletion of tissue enzyme was slower in diabetic rats. Pretreatment with insulin restored both tissue and releasable enzyme activity to normal levels.

These abnormalities of PHLA in diabetic states are apparent with the variety of substrates acted on by the enzyme (triglycerides, monoglycerides, phospholipid, and chylomicrons). Although PHLA in the circulation may be derived from lipoprotein lipase in multiple tissue sites, it is adipose tissue lipoprotein lipase that appears to be critically sensitive to circulating insulin levels (Borensztajn et al., 1972). The enzyme abnormality appears to be related to the production of hypertriglyceridemia in these diabetics since endogenous triglyceride lipolysis during prolonged heparin infusion is low (Brunzell et al., unpublished observations).

In contrast, individuals with only mild impairment of glucose tolerance without fasting hyperglycemia whose only abnormality in insulin secretion is a reduction of early insulin release after an intravenous glucose pulse do not appear to generate hypertriglyceridemia through any detectable abnormality of PHLA or plasma triglyceride removal. In such

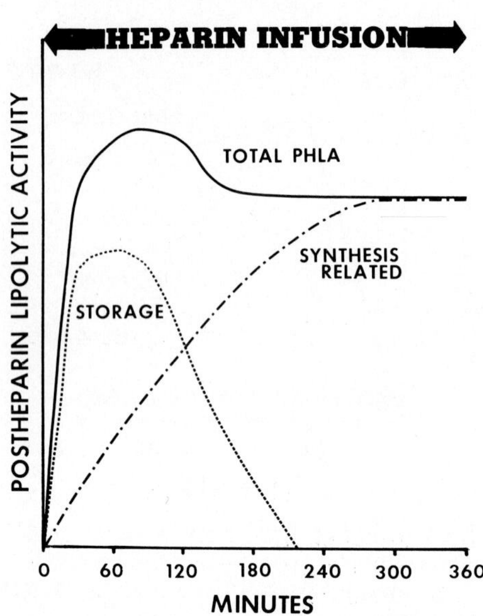

FIG. 2. A model for multiphasic PHLA release during prolonged constant heparin infusion. An immediate release phase is postulated to be derived from readily accessible storage sites and a late release phase from synthesis-related tissue pools. Early insulin insufficiency may lead to selective impairment of PHLA release during the later, synthesis-related phase.

mild diabetics who are hypertriglyceridemic, basal and stimulated insulin levels may be elevated, but remain directly proportional to their degree of adiposity (Bagdade et al., 1971). Since serum insulin levels appear to be significantly correlated with plasma triglyceride levels in a variety of unselected normal and hypertriglyceridemic individuals (Bierman et al., 1970; Bierman, 1972) and insulin promotes secretion of endogenous triglyceride-rich lipoproteins by the liver (Topping and Mayes, 1972), it is possible that increased endogenous triglyceride production, superimposed on a readily saturable removal system related to lipoprotein lipase (Brunzell et al., 1973a) plays a major pathogenetic role for hypertriglyceridemia in the typical mild obese diabetic.

In any type of diabetic with hypertriglyceridemia, both the degree of hypertriglyceridemia and its mechanism may vary with the genetic history (Brunzell et al., 1973b). For example, although both PHLA deficiency and PHLA depletion are secondary (to diabetes) and reversible disorders, triglyceride levels post insulin treatment are closely related to levels in affected relatives in those families with one of the two monogenic autosomal dominant varieties of hypertriglyceridemia (familial hypertriglyceridemia; familial combined hyperlipidemia) (Goldstein et al., 1973) and thus may remain elevated. In such families, diabetes and hypertriglyceridemia appear to segregate independently (Brunzell et al., 1973b). The effect of superimposed adiposity, with its acceleration of endogenous triglyceride production rates, presumably via enhanced insulin secretion (Robertson et al., 1973) may also vary with the genetic type of hypertriglyceridemia and lead to dual mechanisms for hypertriglyceridemia in some diabetic hypertriglyceridemic individuals (impaired removal secondary to the diabetic state coupled with enhanced production of

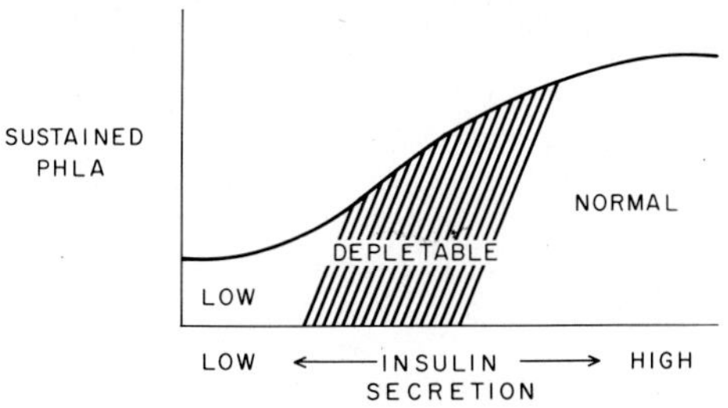

FIG. 3. A hypothetical representation of the relation between insulin secretion and the maintenance of PHLA in plasma during prolonged high dose heparin infusion. (From Bierman, 1972, by courtesy.)

triglyceride associated with an underlying genetic disorder unrelated to diabetes). Such dual mechanisms have been postulated on the basis of kinetic studies of triglyceride transport in a wide variety of diabetics (Nikkilä and Kekki, 1973).

In summary, triglyceride removal ability appears to be very sensitive to variations in insulin secretion since the hormone appears to be critical for the maintenance of normal enzyme activity and availability. Therefore progressive impairment of early insulin responses to a rapid glucose stimulus, which is closely associated with the degree of glucose intolerance, appears to result in a progressive defect in lipoprotein lipase-related triglyceride removal, first manifest as PHLA depletion (inability to sustain normal circulating levels during prolonged heparin infusion) (Fig. 3) and ultimately as overt PHLA deficiency.

REFERENCES

ATKIN, E. and MENG, J. C. (1972): Release of clearing factor lipase (lipoprotein lipase) in vivo and from isolated perfused hearts of alloxan diabetic rats. *Diabetes, 21,* 149.

BAGDADE, J. D., BIERMAN, E. L. and PORTE Jr., D. (1967): Diabetic lipemia – a form of acquired fat-induced lipemia. *New Engl. J. Med., 276,* 427.

BAGDADE, J. D., PORTE Jr., D. and BIERMAN, E. L. (1968): Acute insulin withdrawal and the regulation of plasma triglyceride removal in diabetic subjects. *Diabetics, 17,* 127.

BAGDADE, J. D., BIERMAN, E. L. and PORTE Jr., D. (1971): The influence of obesity on the relationship between insulin and triglyceride levels in endogenous hypertriglyceridemia. *Diabetes, 20,* 664.

BASSO, L. V. and HAVEL, R. J. (1970): Hepatic metabolism of free fatty acids in normal and diabetic dogs. *J. clin. Invest., 49,* 537.

BIERMAN, E. L. (1972): Insulin and hypertriglyceridemia. *Israel J. med. Sci., 8,* 303.

BIERMAN, E. L., PORTE Jr., D. and BAGDADE, J. D. (1970): Hypertriglyceridemia and glucose intolerance in man. In: *Adipose Tissue Regulation and Metabolic Functions,* pp. 209–212. Editors: B. Jeanrenaud and D. Hepp. Academic Press, New York, N.Y.

BORENSZTAJN, J., SAMOLS, D. R. and RUBINSTEIN, A. H. (1972): Effect of insulin on lipoprotein lipase activity in the rat heart and adipose tissue. *Amer. J. Physiol., 223,* 1271.

BRUNZELL, J. D., PORTE Jr., D. and BIERMAN, E. L. (1972a): PHLA depletion: a defect in plasma triglyceride removal related to hyperglycemia. *Diabetes, 21,* 342.

BRUNZELL, J. D., SMITH, N. D., PORTE Jr., D. and BIERMAN, E. L. (1972b): Evidence for multiphasic release of postheparin lipolytic activity (PHLA). *J. clin. Invest., 51,* 16a.

BRUNZELL, J. D., HAZZARD, W. R., PORTE Jr., D. and BIERMAN, E. L. (1973a): Evidence for a common saturable, triglyceride removal mechanism for chylomicrons and very low density lipoproteins in man. *J. clin. Invest., 52,* 1578.

BRUNZELL, J. D., SCHROTT, H. G., GOLDSTEIN, J. L., BIERMAN, E. L. and MOTULSKY, A. G. (1973b): Family studies in hypertriglyceridemia. *Clin. Res., 21,* 618.

GOLDSTEIN, J. H., HAZZARD, W. R., SCHROTT, H. G., BIERMAN, E. L. and MOTULSKY, A. G. (1973): Hyperlipidemia in coronary heart disease. II. Genetic analysis of lipid levels in 176 families and delineation of a new inherited disorder: combined hyperlipidemia. *J. clin Invest., 52,* 1544.

HEIMBERG, M., VanHARKEN, D. R. and BROWN, T. O. (1967): Hepatic lipid metabolism in experimental diabetes. II. Incorporation of (1-C-14) palmitate into lipids of the liver and of the $d < 1.020$ perfusate lipoproteins. *Biochim. biophys. Acta (Amst.), 137,* 435.

LEWIS, B., MANCINI, M., MATTOCK, M., CHAIT, A. and FRASER, T. R. (1972): Plasma triglyceride and fatty acid metabolism in diabetes mellitus. *Europ. J. clin. Invest., 2,* 445.

NIKKILÄ, E. A. and KEKKI, M. (1973): Plasma triglyceride transport kinetics in diabetes mellitus. *Metabolism, 22,* 1.

ROBERTSON, R. P., GAVARESKI, D. J., HENDERSON, J. D., PORTE Jr., D. and BIERMAN, E. L. (1973): Accelerated triglyceride secretion: a metabolic consequence of obesity. *J. clin. Invest., 52,* 1620.

TOPPING, D. L. and MAYES, P. A. (1972): The immediate effects of insulin and fructose on the metabolism of the perfused liver. *Biochem. J., 126,* 295.

WILCOX, H. G., DISHMAN, G. and HEIMBERG, M. (1968): Hepatic lipid metabolism in experimental diabetes. IV. Incorporation of amino acid ^{14}C into lipoprotein-protein and triglyceride. *J. biol. Chem., 243,* 665.

INDICES OF LIPID TRANSPORT AND SERUM INSULIN IN PATIENTS WITH ASYMPTOMATIC GLUCOSE INTOLERANCE

J. BOBERG, B. FURBERG and H. HEDSTRAND

Departments of Geriatrics, Medicine and Clinical Physiology,
University of Uppsala, Uppsala, Sweden

Glucose intolerance in man has been characterized in several ways. During recent years the interest has been focussed on release of insulin after glucose administration, which has been shown to be decreased in patients with diabetes mellitus. The acute, early insulin response to an intravenous glucose stimulation seems to be of special interest in this context (Lerner and Porte, 1972).

Long ago serum lipid elevations were described in diabetes mellitus (Berzelius, 1806). This rise primarily involves the triglyceride (TG) rich serum lipoproteins and is thought to be due either to a defect in removal (Bagdade et al., 1967) or to increased production of serum TG from increased lipogenesis in the liver (Reaven et al., 1967) or from an increased flux to the liver of the main precursor of serum TG, the plasma free fatty acids (FFA) (Carlson et al., 1965; Boberg, 1971).

In the present study some indices of impaired lipid transport and its relationship to serum insulin have been studied not only in patients with diabetes mellitus but also in subjects with asymptomatic intravenous glucose intolerance found at a health screening survey of 50-year-old men.

MATERIALS AND METHODS

In about 1,000 men an intravenous glucose tolerance test (IVGTT) was performed in connection with a health screening survey, where an examination was offered to 50-year-old men in Uppsala, a town of 150,000 inhabitants.

The subjects reported fasting over night at 7.30 in the morning. After 10 minutes rest in supine position 0.5 g glucose per kg body weight was given as a 50% solution into a cubital vein during 2 minutes. Blood samples were then taken for blood glucose determinations at 6, 20, 30, 40, 50, and 60 minutes and at 0, 4, 6, 8 and 60 minutes after beginning of the glucose injection for determinations of serum insulin concentrations (Phadebas insulin test Pharmacia). The fractional removal of glucose from the blood was calculated and expressed as the k-value (Ikkos and Luft, 1957). The early insulin response was calculated from the serum insulin concentrations found in 0, 4, 6 and 8 minutes samples according to the method described by Thorell et al. (1973). This method calculates the 'early response', to be the increase in serum insulin concentration from zero time to 8 minutes after start of injection plus the amount that has been eliminated (following first order kinetics) during this time. The removal rate constant for serum insulin is approximately fixed at 0.1.

The subjects, who had a k-value of the IVGTT less than 1.1 and who had no chronic treatment for diabetes mellitus or for any other metabolic disease, were referred for further investigation and treatment. The further investigation included a second identical IVGTT, serum lipid concentrations (Rush et al., 1970), an intravenous fat tolerance test (IVFTT) according to Rössner and Carlson (1972), and in a limited number of patients turnover rates of plasma FFA at rest and during exercise.

RESULTS AND COMMENTS

The subjects have been divided into 4 groups according to glucose tolerance: (1) a diabetic group with fasting blood glucose above 120 mg/100 ml and k-value < 1.1 on the IVGTT; (2) a group of latent diabetics with fasting blood glucose below 120 mg/100 ml and the IVGTT k-value < 1.1 on 2 occasions; (3) subclinical diabetics who had fasting blood glucose below 120 mg/100 ml, $k < 1.1$ on screening but $k > 1.1$ on the second IVGTT; (4) a randomly selected group of controls with normal glucose tolerance.

Serum concentrations of insulin and lipids related to glucose intolerance

The patients in the diabetic group had hyperinsulinemia with a fasting serum insulin concentration of 28.5 ± 4.3 μU per ml (Table 1). This value was significantly higher ($p < 0.001$) than the mean value for any of the other groups. This hyperinsulinemia is probably best explained by the obesity also found in this group illustrated by a weight index 1.24 ± 0.06 (Table 1).

TABLE 1
Fasting serum insulin concentration, early response of serum insulin and weight index in patients with asymptomatic glucose intolerance

	Diabetics n = 12	Latent diabetics n = 28	Subclinical diabetics n = 38	Controls n = 47
Fasting serum insulin concentration μU/ml	28.5 ± 4.3	11.5 ± 1.1	11.5 ± 0.8	13.4 ± 0.9
Early response of serum insulin μU/ml	2.1 ± 7.6	26.4 ± 3.6	45.6 ± 5.2	101.1 ± 13.8
Weight index*	1.24 ± 0.06	1.13 ± 0.03	1.06 ± 0.02	1.10 ± 0.02

Mean value ± S.E.M.
n = number of subjects
* Weight index = Actual/ideal weight (Lindberg et al., 1956)

The acute insulin response caused by the stimulus of an i.v. glucose bolus injection has been shown to be very low in diabetic patients (Robertson and Porte, 1973). Similarly we found very low values for early insulin response in the diabetic group, as shown in Table 1. This early serum insulin response to glucose is also significantly lower compared with the controls both in the latent diabetic and in the subclinical diabetic group ($P < 0.001$ for both groups).

Table 2 gives the serum lipid values for the 4 groups. There were significantly higher serum TG values in the diabetic and in the latent diabetic groups ($P < 0.01$ and $P < 0.05$ respectively) compared with the subclinical diabetics who were not significantly different from the controls. The concentration of serum cholesterol was similar in all groups.

TABLE 2
Serum lipid concentrations in patients with asymptomatic glucose intolerance

	Diabetics n = 12	Latent diabetics n = 28	Subclinical diabetics n = 38	Controls n = 47
Serum triglyceride concentrations mMoles/l	3.60 (0.557 ± −1.889) [0.557 ± (−1.889)]	2.14 (0.331 ± −1.965)	1.71 (0.234 ± −1.967)	1.77 (0.248 ± −1.976)
Serum cholesterol concentration mg/100 ml	260 ± 11	258 ± 10	243 ± 8	245 ± 6

Mean value ± S.E.M. Logarithmic values within brackets.
n = number of subjects.

Serum TG removal

The removal of the serum TG was studied by IVFTT in a limited number of patients with glucose intolerance and is shown in Figure 1. The results show a decreased removal capacity (k_2-value) in patients with elevated serum TG concentrations. However, in the patients with a k_2-value between 3 and 4% per minute, the serum TG concentration varies between 1 and 3 mmoles per litre. This finding indicates that not only impaired removal but also individual variations in production of serum TG occur in the patients with various degrees of glucose intolerance.

Serum FFA at rest and during exercise

Serum FFA has been shown to be the most important precursor for synthesis of serum TG (Boberg, 1971). Thus it was of interest to study FFA turnover rates in some of these patients with glucose intolerance, particularly since higher serum FFA levels have been

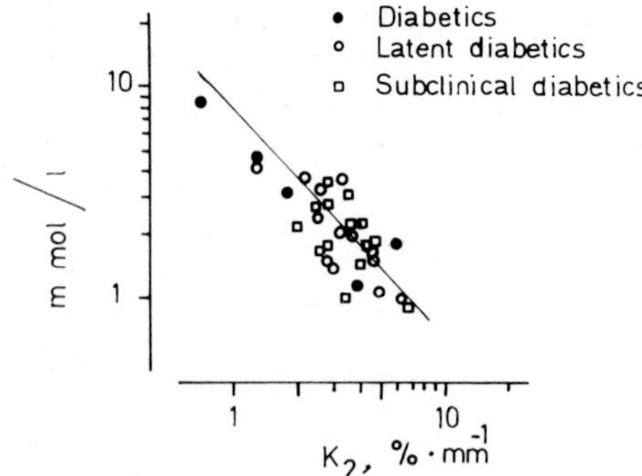

FIG. 1. Relationship between fractional removal rate of exogenous triglycerides, tested by intravenous fat tolerance (IVFTT), and serum triglyceride concentration in patients with asymptomatic glucose intolerance. The regression line represents previously described healthy controls and patients with hypertriglyceridemia, whose endogenous triglyceride turnover was also determined (Rössner et al., 1973, by courtesy).

found in fasting diabetic patients compared with controls, both at rest and during exercise (Carlström, 1967; Nordlander et al., 1973).

Figure 2 shows that higher mean values for serum FFA were found at rest, during exercise and at rest after exercise in the diabetic group compared with controls, but not so in the latent diabetic group. Similar differences were found in serum glycerol concentration during exercise and at rest after exercise. However, none of the differences were significant.

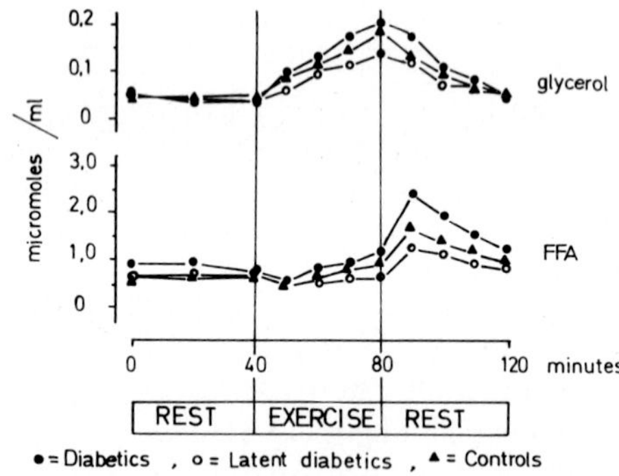

FIG. 2. Serum concentrations of free fatty acids and glycerol at rest and during exercise at a work load equal to 50% of $^{W}170$ in patients with asymptomatic glucose intolerance. Each symbol is the mean value from 5 subjects.

Whether these elevated concentrations of serum FFA are due to decreased removal of serum FFA or increased mobilization of FFA from adipose tissue has already been discussed. The latter is the more probable explanation and has also been suggested by earlier authors. Figure 3 shows that the specific radioactivity did reach the lowest mean values at rest after exercise in the diabetic subjects, which indicates more pronounced FFA mobilization in these subjects. However, in all 3 groups removal of FFA at rest after exercise seemed to be slightly impaired. This is indicated by the slightly higher concentration of labelled FFA during the period at rest after exercise compared with the resting period before exercise. This might be explained by the decreased splanchnic blood flow which occurs during exercise and which may persist for some time after the exercise period.

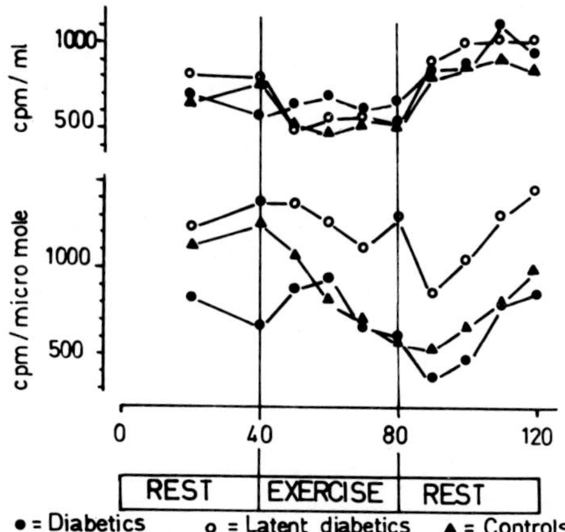

FIG. 3. Serum free fatty acid radioactivity and specific radioactivity at rest and during exercise at a work load level equal to 50% of $^{W}170$ in patients with asymptomatic glucose intolerance. A constant infusion of ^{3}H-labeled palmitate (10^5 cpm/min.) was given during the study. Each symbol is the mean value from 5 subjects.

At rest before exercise when steady state levels of serum FFA concentration were achieved the average total turnover rate of serum FFA was 715 μM per minute for the diabetics and 432 and 435 μM per minute for the latent diabetics and controls.

These results would only indicate increased serum TG production from serum FFA in the diabetic patients but not in the group of latent diabetics. However, in another presentation given at this congress, Dr. Hagenfelt showed an increased fractional splanchnic uptake of serum oleic acid in diabetic patients compared with controls. More studies including splanchnic turnover of serum FFA and TG are necessary to determine how serum TG production varies in the subjects with glucose intolerance.

CONCLUSION

In most subjects studied there is a correlation between serum FFA and serum TG total turnover (Boberg et al., 1972). However, an increase of serum TG total turnover (due to increased flux of serum FFA to the liver) does not give rise to hypertriglyceridemia unless serum TG removal is impaired, which probably is the case in insulin-deficient situations. A definite answer as to why hypertriglyceridemia is a common feature in patients with glucose intolerance must await detailed studies of serum TG and FFA splanchnic turnover in these patients and studies of the removal mechanisms of serum TG at the tissue level.

REFERENCES

BAGDADE, J. D., PORTE JR., D. and BIERMAN, E. L. (1967): Diabetic lipemia. A form of acquired fat-induced lipemia. *New Engl. J. Med., 276,* 427.

BERZELIUS, J. J. (1806): *Lehrbuch der Thier-Chemie.*

BOBERG, J. (1971): *Mechanisms of Hypertriglyceridaemia in Man.* Thesis. Acta Universitas Uppsaliensis. Abstracts of Uppsala Dissertations from the Faculty of Medicine, 105. Editor: The dean of the Faculty of Medicine. Almqvist and Wiksell, Stockholm.

BOBERG, J., CARLSON, L. A., FREYSCHUSS, U., LASSERS, B. W. and WAHLQVIST, M. L. (1972): Splanchnic secretion rates of plasma triglycerides and splanchnic turnover of plasma free fatty acids in men with normo- and hypertriglyceridaemia. *Europ. J. clin. Invest., 2,* 454.

CARLSON, L. A., BOBERG, J. and HÖGSTEDT, B. (1965): Some physiological and clinical implications of lipid mobilization from adipose tissue. In: *Handbook of Physiology. Adipose Tissue, Vol. V, chapter 63,* pp. 625–644. Editors: A. E. Renold and G. F. Cahill Jr. American Physiological Society, Washington D.C.

CARLSON, L. A. and RÖSSNER, S. (1972): A methodological study of an intravenous fat tolerance test with intralipid emulsion. *Scand. J. clin. lab. Invest., 29,* 271.

CARLSTRÖM, S. (1967): Studies on fatty acid metabolism in diabetics during exercise. *Acta med. scand., 181,* 609.

IKKOS, D. and LUFT, R. (1957): On the intravenous glucose tolerance test. *Acta Endocr. (Kbh.), 25,* 312.

LERNER, R. L. and PORTE Jr., D. (1972): Acute and steady-state insulin responses to glucose in nonobese diabetic subjects. *J. clin. Invest., 51,* 1624.

LINDBERG, W., NATWIG, H., RYGH, A. and SVENDSEN, K. T. (1956): *T. Norske Laegeforen., 76,* 351.

NORDLANDER, S., ÖSTMAN, J., CERASI, E., LUFT, R. and EKLUND, L. G. (1973): Occurrence of diabetic type of plasma FFA and glycerol response to physical exercise in prediabetic subjects. *Acta med. scand., 193,* 9.

REAVEN, G. M., LERNER, R. L., STERN, M. P. and FARQUHAR, J. W. (1967): Role of insulin in endogenous hypertriglyceridaemia. *J. clin. Invest., 46,* 1756.

ROBERTSON, R. P. and PORTE Jr., D. (1973): The glucose receptor. A defective mechanism in diabetes mellitus distinct from the beta adrenergic receptor. *J. clin. Invest., 52,* 870.

RUSH, R. L., LEON, L. and TURRELL, J. (1970): Automated simultaneous cholesterol and triglyceride determination of the autoanalyzer II instrument. In: *Advances in automated analysis, Vol. I,* p. 503. Thurman Association Suite, Miami, Fla.

RÖSSNER, S., BOBERG, J., CARLSON, L. A., FREYSCHUSS, U. and LASSERS, B. W. (1973): Comparison between fractional turnover rate of endogenous plasma triglycerides and of Intralipid (intravenous fat tolerance test) in man. *Europ. J. clin. Invest.,* in press.

THORELL, J. I., NOSSLIN, B. and STERKY, G. (1973): Estimation of the early insulin response to intravenous glucose injection. *J. lab. clin. Med., 82,* 101.

PLASMA TRIGLYCERIDE METABOLISM IN RELATION TO INSULIN SECRETION IN MAN*

ESKO A. NIKKILÄ

Third Department of Medicine, University Central Hospital,
Helsinki, Finland

A mild or moderate hypertriglyceridemia is common in patients with clinical diabetes but the degree of the abnormality is highly variable and poorly correlated with the severity of diabetes. Thus, completely normal serum lipid levels may occur in a patient with insulin-deficient uncontrolled juvenile diabetes while a gross hyperlipemia can develop in conjunction with a mild adult-onset type disease. Indeed, there seems to be no sharp delineation between primary familial Type III, IV or V hypertriglyceridemia with decreased glucose tolerance on the one hand and a diabetes-associated gross hyperlipemia on the other. However, cases with more severe forms of hyperlipemia are exceptional among diabetics as they are also in a non-diabetic population (Nikkilä and Kekki, 1973). These extreme cases arouse special interest, however, and therefore they are studied and published more frequently than the milder forms of diabetic lipid disorders and they may erroneously be taken as representative examples of the mode of disturbance of lipid metabolism in diabetes.

The mechanism by which diabetes induces an elevation of plasma triglycerides is still unsettled (for review see Nikkilä, 1973). Opinions differ on whether the major defect resides in the production or removal of triglyceride of the very low density lipoproteins (VLDL) of plasma and it is not clear which biochemical abnormality of diabetes is mainly responsible for the disturbance of lipid metabolism. It is likely that more than one cause and mechanism will be revealed for the hypertriglyceridemia of diabetes. At present some *indirect* evidence favors the view that removal of VLDL and chylomicron triglycerides from the blood is impaired in diabetes and that this accounts for the increase of plasma triglycerides. This view is based on observations in chronically insulin-deficient animals, in which the hepatic production of VLDL triglycerides is inhibited (Heimberg et al., 1966; Basso and Havel, 1970) and the fractional removal of exogenous fat is decreased (Kessler, 1962). In contrast to these results an overproduction of plasma triglycerides has been demonstrated in acute experimental insulin deficiency (Balasse et al., 1972) and in many diabetic patients (Nikkilä and Kekki, 1973). It should be emphasized that results obtained in chronically diabetic animals cannot be extrapolated to human diabetes with its protean nature. The hypertriglyceridemia which is associated with clinical diabetes is usually caused by a combination of enhanced produc-

* This study has been supported by a grant from National Research Council for Medical Sciences, Finnish Academy.

tion and relative inefficiency of removal of plasma triglycerides. A marked hyperlipemia cannot develop without a more severe defect in the tissue uptake of triglycerides.

Since it is clearly evident that the degree of diabetic control is poorly correlated with the plasma triglyceride level there is need for search of other hormonal and metabolic parameters which could show a better association with the severity of the lipid disorder. The most plausible factor in this respect is circulating insulin which is known to vary from almost zero to clearly increased levels in human diabetes. Moreover, insulin is known to exert major regulatory effects on both production and removal of plasma VLDL-triglycerides and the influences of insulin lack and insulin excess are not exactly opposite in these respects. Insulin has been shown to increase the production of VLDL triglycerides by a perfused rat liver (Topping and Mayes, 1972) and high plasma insulin response to glucose is significantly associated with fasting hypertriglyceridemia in man (Reaven et al., 1967). In the absence of insulin the lipoprotein lipase activity of adipose tissue vanishes (Robinson, 1970) and this may influence the overall efficiency of removal of circulating triglycerides.

We have examined the correlation between insulin secretion and plasma triglyceride kinetics in man under those clinical and experimental conditons where insulin output is known to vary from one extreme to another. Production and removal of endogenous triglycerides has been measured by ^{3}H-glycerol label-decay method and the elimination of exogenous lipids from the circulation is determined with intravenous Intralipid.

PLASMA ENDOGENOUS TRIGLYCERIDE TURNOVER IN DIABETES

Simultaneous assays of plasma insulin and plasma endogenous triglyceride turnover have been carried out in 47 patients with different types of uncomplicated and untreated diabetes and free of other major diseases. It is not claimed that the material is representative of a diabetic population in general but there was no selection on the basis of plasma triglyceride levels. The cases are divided into 2 groups by the fasting plasma insulin level of 20 μU/ml. This cut-off point also gave a rather good prediction of the later response to treatment so that most of the subjects having insulin values less than 20 μU/ml in the presence of hyperglycemia had an insulin-dependent diabetes. None of the subjects had severe ketoacidosis.

The turnover (production) rate and concentration of plasma triglycerides are shown in Figure 1. The concentration was within the normal range in 15 cases (32%), moderately elevated (less than 300 mg/100 ml) in another 15 patients while the remaining 17 diabetics (36%) had a marked elevation of plasma triglycerides. Eight of the 32 hypertriglyceridemic subjects (25%) had a normal plasma triglyceride production rate and they thus must have some difficulties in the elimination of triglycerides from the circulation. Only one of these patients with a removal defect had a gross hypertriglyceridemia. Six additional patients were located in the plot below the regression line extrapolated from a normal material and they thus had a higher plasma triglyceride concentration than predicted on the basis of production rate. In other words, their hypertriglyceridemia was caused by a combination of overproduction and impaired removal efficiency. In 18 cases (57%) the hypertriglyceridemia was caused by an increased rate of production of plasma triglycerides.

The amount of insulin secretion did not show any correlation with plasma triglyceride concentration or production rate in the diabetic subjects. Only a few of the insulin-defi-

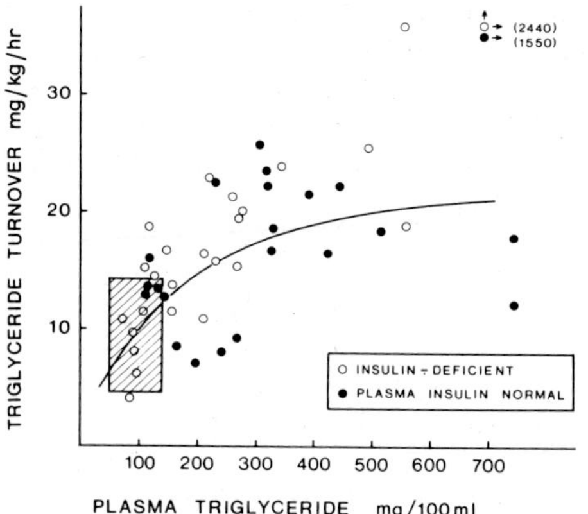

FIG. 1. Relationship between plasma triglyceride concentration and total turnover rate in 47 diabetic patients. The hatched area presents the distribution of both values in a selected normal population and the curve is extrapolation of the regression obtained in the normal subjects. The curve describes the rise of plasma triglyceride concentration on increasing production rate when the removal efficiency is not changed.

cient cases had a triglyceride removal defect. The triglyceride turnover rate of insulinopenic diabetics varied within a wide range from low normal to markedly increased values. The turnover rate was very similar in diabetic patients with subnormal circulating insulin and in non-diabetic subjects who showed an exaggerated insulin response to oral glucose (Fig. 2).

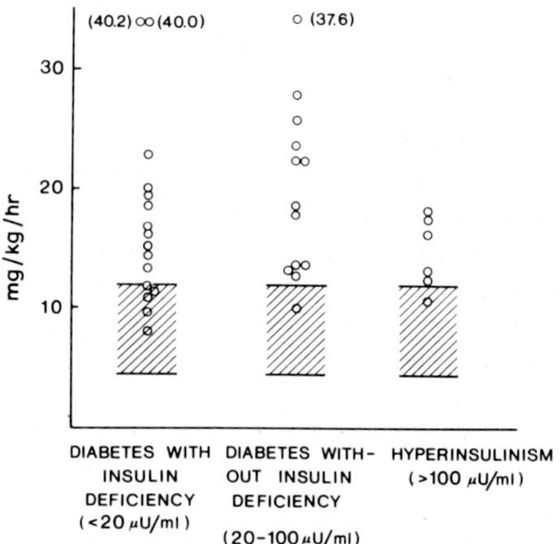

FIG. 2. Plasma triglyceride production rate in insulin-deficient diabetics, in patients with diabetes associated with normal plasma insulin level, and in non-diabetic persons with exaggerated insulin response to oral glucose.

The fractional turnover rate of plasma endogenous triglycerides in insulin-deficient and insulin-resistant diabetics is presented in Figure 3. Again, there is no difference between the 2 types of diabetes. The fractional removal may be decreased in cases with hypertriglyceridemia but this occurs with approximately similar frequency in subjects with decreased insulin values as in those with normal or excessive insulin.

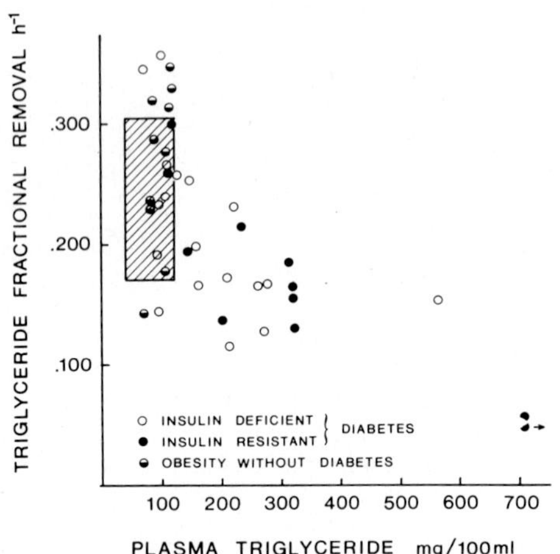

FIG. 3. Plasma endogenous triglyceride fractional removal rate in diabetic patients and in non-diabetic obese subjects. The hatched area represents the normal range.

CHANGES OF PLASMA TRIGLYCERIDE METABOLISM DURING TREATMENT OF DIABETES

It is known that when diabetes is brought under control by insulin, oral antidiabetic drugs or diet, the elevated plasma triglyceride values will in most cases decrease and often reach a completely normal range. Only in exceptional instances is the hypertriglyceridemia resistant to treatment of diabetes and responds only when some hypolipidemic drugs are added. According to our experience a severe diabetic hyperlipemia is more or less resistant to any form of treatment except a marked restriction of calories. The response seems to be quite unpredictable.

With the exception of dietary treatment and phenformin the control of diabetes is achieved only by increasing the amount of circulating insulin. It is therefore of interest to know whether the decrease of plasma triglyceride concentration on treatment of diabetes occurs due to an improved elimination or through reduced formation of plasma triglycerides. Triglyceride turnover has been determined before and after treatment in 9 diabetic patients who received either insulin or oral sulfonylureas. The results appear from Figures 4 and 5, which indicate that the triglyceride turnover (production) rate was decreased in all subjects whose plasma triglyceride level was lowered by the control of diabetes. The fractional removal rate, on the other hand, showed quite inconsistent changes which were not related to the extent of decrease of plasma triglyceride level. In 2

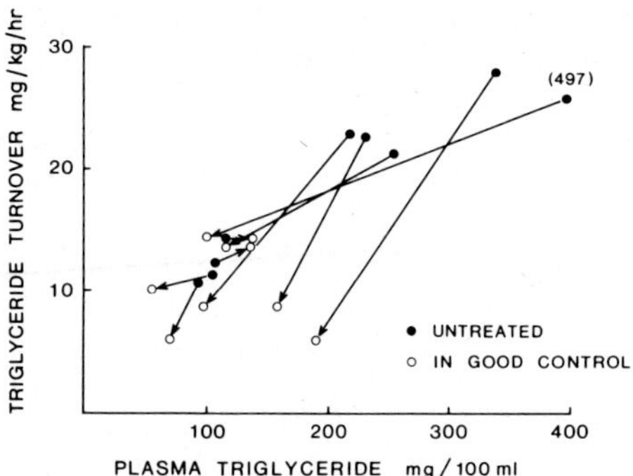

FIG. 4. Effect of adequate treatment of diabetes with either insulin or oral sulphonylureas on plasma triglyceride concentration and turnover rate.

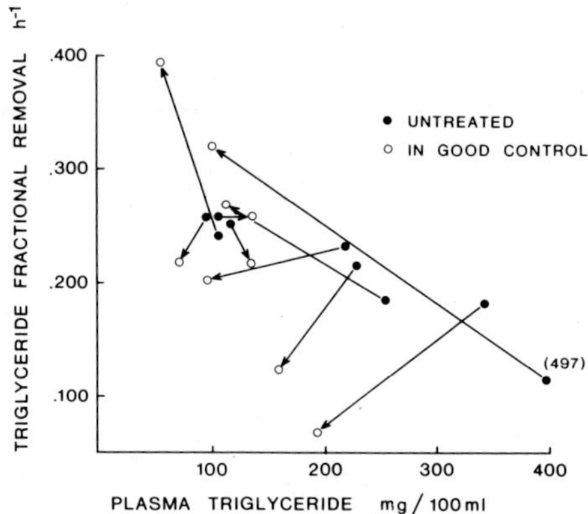

FIG. 5. Effect of treatment of diabetes with insulin or oral sulphonylureas on the fractional removal rate of endogenous plasma triglycerides.

subjects whose triglyceride concentration was not normalized by treatment the fractional removal was unexpectedly impaired in spite of a considerable reduction of hypertriglyceridemia.

It thus seems that adequate treatment of diabetes by increasing the blood insulin content diminishes circulating triglyceride pool mainly by reducing the production of plasma triglycerides.

E. A. NIKKILÄ

PLASMA ENDOGENOUS TRIGLYCERIDE METABOLISM IN ACTIVE ACROMEGALY

Patients with active acromegaly have either an excessive insulin response with a normal glucose tolerance or a normal or low insulin secretion and latent or manifest diabetes. These combinations offer a good opportunity to study the relationship between insulin secretory status and plasma triglyceride metabolism. For this reason we have examined the triglyceride metabolism in 8 cases of active acromegaly, 5 of which were insulin hypersecretors while 3 had decreased glucose tolerance and relative insufficiency of insulin release. All had high plasma growth hormone.

The results are demonstrated in Figure 6. Three patients had marked hypertriglyceridemia and all these also had excessive insulin levels. In these 3 cases the triglyceride production was significantly above normal and the fractional removal rate was decreased. The 3 patients with latent diabetes had normal plasma triglyceride concentration and fractional elimination rate while the production was slightly increased. One subject differed from the others by having a normal triglyceride level in plasma and a normal production and removal rate in spite of very high plasma insulin response to oral and intravenous glucose. This subject was an adolescent boy with gigantism and only slight acromegalic features. It is possible that the age accounts for the different behavior of triglyceride metabolism in this patient as compared to the rest of the material.

This small series suggests that hyperinsulinism (in the presence of excessive plasma growth hormone levels) stimulates the production of plasma endogenous triglycerides but does not increase their removal efficiency and thus gives rise to elevation of triglyceride concentration in plasma. High circulating growth hormone without hyperinsulinism does not influence the plasma triglyceride metabolism.

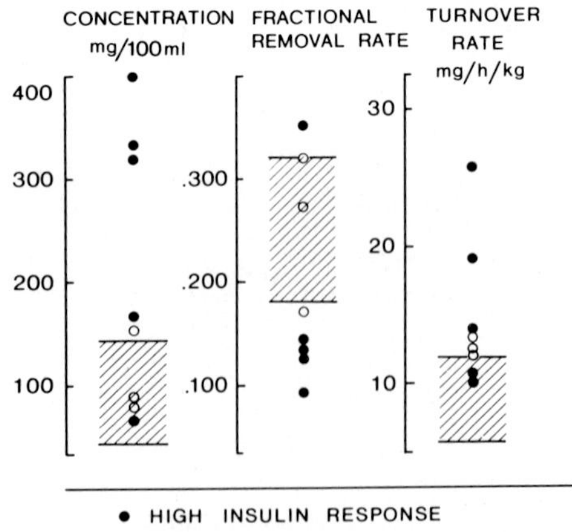

FIG. 6. Kinetic parameters of plasma triglyceride in 8 patients with active acromegaly. The subjects with abnormally high insulin response to oral glucose are shown separately from those with a normal or low insulin. None of the patients had manifest diabetes. The hatched area represents normal range.

PLASMA TRIGLYCERIDE TURNOVER IN A PATIENT WITH BETA CELL ADENOMA

Another opportunity to study the effect of high plasma insulin level on triglyceride metabolism is presented by patients with insulin-secreting adenoma of the pancreas. One such case, a man of 65, was recently examined in our department. He had extremely high fasting plasma insulin levels but only moderate hypoglycemia, indicating the presence of marked insulin resistance (Table 1). Plasma total triglyceride was abnormally low for his age and almost all was transported in low density lipoprotein (LDL) fraction. The total turnover rates of plasma triglyceride and of VLDL triglyceride were clearly less than normal but the fractional turnover rate of the latter fraction was much accelerated.

On the basis of this single experience hyperinsulinism in the presence of hypoglycemia (inhibited gluconeogenesis) decreases the production of VLDL triglycerides and stimulates their removal from the circulation. Apparently the transformation of VLDL to LDL also occurs more rapidly than under normal conditions but as the total VLDL synthesis is low there is no greater accumulation of LDL particles. It is probable that also the catabolism of LDL is accelerated in patients with insulinoma.

If this finding is confirmed in other patients with beta cell tumor it will suggest that insulin stimulates the secretion of triglycerides into plasma only in the presence of normal or increased blood glucose levels. This view is supported by the observation that exogenous insulin diminishes the plasma triglyceride level in normal subjects (Schlierf and Kinsell, 1965).

TABLE 1

Plasma triglyceride transport in a patient with active insulin-secreting adenoma of the pancreas
(Blood glucose 3.0 mM, plasma insulin 130 μU/ml)

Endogenous triglyceride	Total TG	VLDL TG	LDL TG
Concentration mg/100 ml	36	4.5	28
Fractional turnover rate hr^{-1}	0.132	1.360	–
Absolute turnover rate mg/kg/hr	2.2	2.8	–

TG = triglyceride

REMOVAL OF INTRAVENOUS FAT IN RELATION TO INSULIN SECRETION

Intravenous fat tolerance test with Intralipid has been introduced as a measure of the body's capacity to eliminate chylomicron triglycerides from the blood (Boberg et al., 1969). In order to determine the role of insulin secretion in this removal process we have compared the results of Intralipid test to maximal plasma insulin levels obtained during intravenous arginine stimulation. The subjects were diabetics or non-diabetic obese persons subsequently treated by subtotal fasting. The latter group was studied both with isocaloric diet and after one week's starvation to learn whether the known decrease of insulin secretion during caloric restriction could diminish the removal of intravenous fat.

In diabetic and non-diabetic subjects studied during a normal isocaloric diet there was no correlation between the fractional elimination of Intralipid (K value) on the one hand and the plasma insulin peak level in the intravenous arginine test on the other (Fig. 7). Patients with an excellent insulin response showed decreased clearance of the intravenous fat and vice versa. The complete independence of these 2 variables was even more clearly evident from the changes that occurred during starvation. As expected, the insulin response to arginine was much reduced in every subject during the fasting but simultaneously the fractional removal rate of Intralipid was increased in all cases except one (Fig. 8).

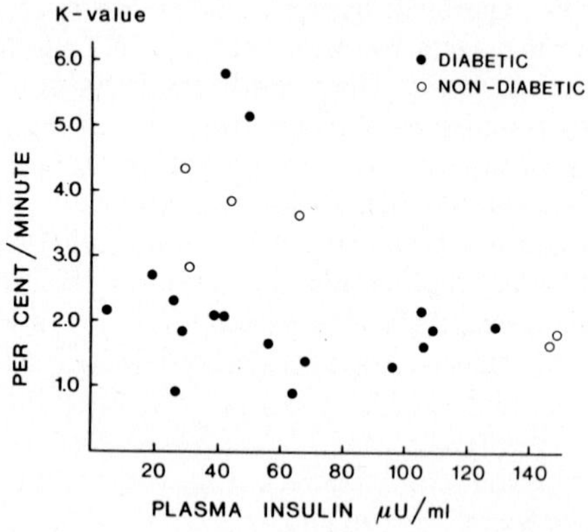

FIG. 7. Disappearance rate of Intralipid in relation to peak level of plasma insulin after intravenous arginine.

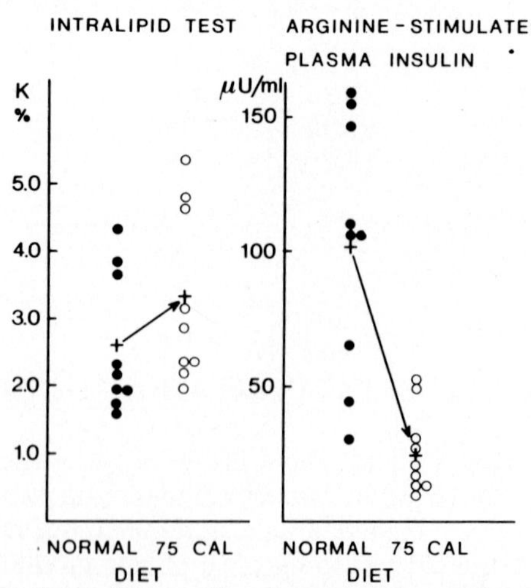

FIG. 8. Effect of 75-calorie diet on the disappearance of intravenous Intralipid and on arginine-stimulated plasma insulin peak level.

These observations could thus bring no evidence to support the hypothesis that plasma insulin levels influence the efficiency of the removal of exogenous particulate fat from the blood. This is in accordance with the conclusion reached above that insulin treatment of diabetics did not systematically improve the elimination of endogenous plasma triglycerides.

CONCLUSIONS

Insulin influences both production and removal of plasma triglycerides but still the relationship of insulin secretion to plasma triglyceride metabolism is complex in man. In untreated diabetics there is no obvious correlation between circulating insulin levels and the production, concentration or elimination of endogenous plasma triglycerides. In one-third of diabetics who have elevated plasma triglyceride level there is some degree of removal defect of endogenous triglycerides but the most common cause of hypertriglyceridemia in human diabetes is an increased release of triglycerides into circulation. When diabetes is brought under control the plasma triglyceride level decreases and this is accounted for by reduced formation rather than by improved removal of blood triglycerides.

In acromegalic patients with hyperinsulinism hypertriglyceridemia is common and is mainly caused by an enhanced production of plasma triglycerides. On the other hand, in a patient with active beta cell adenoma, hyperinsulinism was associated with a decreased formation and much accelerated fractional turnover of VLDL triglycerides.

The rate of elimination of intravenous Intralipid from the blood stream is not related to the extent of insulin secretion. Thus, during starvation the removal of intravenous fat is improved while the insulin secretion is much reduced.

ACKNOWLEDGEMENT

The turnover studies were carried out in collaboration with M. Kekki, M.D.

REFERENCES

BALASSE, E. O., BIER, D. M. and HAVEL, R. J. (1972): Early effects of anti-insulin serum on hepatic metabolism of plasma free fatty acids in dogs. *Diabetes, 21,* 280.

BASSO, L. V. and HAVEL, R. J. (1970): Hepatic metabolism of free fatty acids in normal and diabetic dogs. *J. clin. Invest., 49,* 537.

BOBERG, J., CARLSON, L. A. and HALLBERG, D. (1969): Application of a new intravenous fat tolerance test in the study of hypertriglyceridemia in man. *J. Atheroscler. Res., 9,* 159.

HEIMBERG, M., DUNKERLEY, A. and BROWN, T. O. (1966): Hepatic lipid metabolism in experimental diabetes. I. Release and uptake of triglycerides by perfused livers from normal and alloxan-diabetic rats. *Biochim. biophys. Acta (Amst.), 125,* 252.

KESSLER, J. I. (1962): Effect of insulin on release of plasma lipolytic activity and clearing of emulsified fat intravenously administered to pancreatectomized and alloxanized dogs. *Clin. Med., 60,* 747.

NIKKILÄ, E. A. (1973): Triglyceride metabolism in diabetes mellitus. *Progr. biochem. Pharmacol., 8,* 271.

NIKKILÄ, E. A. and KEKKI, M. (1973): Plasma triglyceride transport kinetics in diabetes mellitus. *Metabolism, 22*, 1.

REAVEN, G. M., LERNER, R. L., STERN, M. P. and FARQUHAR, J. W. (1967): Role of insulin in endogenous hypertriglyceridemia. *J. clin. Invest., 46,* 1756.

ROBINSON, D. S. (1970): The function of the plasma triglycerides in fatty acid transport. *Comprehens. Biochem., 18,* 51.

SCHLIERF, G. and KINSELL, L. W. (1965): Effect of insulin in hypertriglyceridemia. *Proc. Soc. exp. Biol. Med. (N.Y.), 120,* 272.

TOPPING, D. L. and MAYES, P. A. (1972): The immediate effects of insulin and fructose on the metabolism of the perfused liver. Changes in lipoprotein secretion, fatty acid oxidation and esterification, lipogenesis and carbohydrate metabolism. *Biochem. J., 126,* 295.

INDICES OF CARBOHYDRATE METABOLISM IN PATIENTS WITH ENDOGENOUS HYPERTRIGLYCERIDEMIA

S. SAILER

Department of Medicine, University of Innsbruck, Austria

A clinical observation, the frequent coexistence of endogenous hypertriglyceridemia and carbohydrate intolerance, suggests that these 2 symptoms are related to each other or even influence each other. Since hypertriglyceridemia and diabetes mellitus are well-known risk factors for the development of atherosclerosis, the relationship between endogenous hypertriglyceridemia and carbohydrate intolerance is of very high clinical significance. Further, the understanding of the pathophysiological mechanism of this interrelationship should form the basis of a successful treatment of these risk factors.

In order to investigate the frequency of impaired glucose tolerance, we studied 192 patients with endogenous hypertriglyceridemia (TG concentration > 300 mg%). Cases of hyperlipemia were classified according to Frederikson's criteria. The glucose tolerance test was considered abnormal ('diabetic') according to the criteria of Fajans and Conn (1959). The results are summarized in Table 1.

TABLE 1
Frequency of impaired glucose tolerance in 192 patients with endogenous hypertriglyceridemia

Type of hyperlipemia	N	'Diabetic' GTT	% 'Diabetics'
II_B	32	16	50
III	16	14	88
IV	124	58	47
V	20	14	70

The question arises whether this impaired glucose tolerance in patients with endogenous hypertriglyceridemia is caused by insulin deficiency or by insulin resistance. Reaven et al. (1967) observed a positive relationship between plasma insulin concentration and triglyceride increase produced by a high carbohydrate diet. They suggested that hypertriglyceridemia in most subjects results from an increase in hepatic triglyceride secretion rate secondary to exaggerated postprandial increases in plasma insulin concentration. In our patients with endogenous hypertriglyceridemia a correlation between triglyceride concentration and insulin area after the glucose load was only demonstrable in patients without glycosuria, whereas in patients with glycosuria the insulin response after glucose is very poor, as it is observed in insulin deficiency diabetes (Sailer et al., 1968). This observation was made also by Glueck et al. (1969). These data show, that the insulin concentration in the plasma of patients with endogenous hypertriglyceridemia was high in a quarter and low also in a quarter of the patients, the rest having normal insulin concentrations. Also Eaton and Nye (1973) could not demonstrate a correlation between triglyceride concentration and insulin level, basal or after a glucose load, in all patients with endogenous hypertriglyceridemia. Of course, these data do not support the hypothesis that hyperinsulinemia after a glucose load plays a major causal role in the development of endogenous hypertriglyceridemia.

It seems to be well established that the secretion rate of very low density lipoproteins by the liver is not much higher in patients with endogenous hypertriglyceridemia compared with normal persons (Ryan and Schwartz, 1965; Sailer et al., 1966; Havel, 1968; Eaton et al., 1969). In order to study a possible effect of hyperinsulinemia in the so-called carbohydrate induction of endogenous hypertriglyceridemia, we measured the incorporation of plasma glucose-C into plasma triglycerides in the fasting state and during a glucose load in normals and in patients with endogenous hypertriglyceridemia. In the fasting state, in normals and in patients with endogenous hypertriglyceridemia, no incorporation of plasma glucose-C into plasma TG-FA could be observed. Of the glycerol used for the esterification of plasma FFA into plasma TG 30–40% was derived from plasma glucose-C. There was no difference between normals and patients with endogenous hypertriglyceridemia. During a glucose load, in normals as well as in the patients, the major part of the glycerol-C used for the esterification of plasma FFA into plasma TG was derived from plasma glucose. Under these conditions, the synthesis of plasma TG-FA from plasma glucose is somewhat higher in patients with endogenous hypertriglyceridemia than in normal persons, but accounts quantitatively for less than 10% of the esterification rate of plasma FFA into plasma TG (Sandhofer et al., 1969). In other words, the de novo synthesis of plasma TG-FA from plasma glucose does not play any significant role in the plasma TG influx, even under a massive glucose load, neither in normals nor in patients with endogenous hypertriglyceridemia. Therefore, it seems very unlikely, that hyperglucosemia and hyperinsulinemia lead to an elevation of the concentration of endogenous plasma triglycerides by means of an increased secretion rate of very low density lipoproteins.

Very recently, Schlierf and Dorow (1973) studied the diurnal patterns of glucose, insulin, and plasma triglycerides in normals and in patients with endogenous hypertriglyceridemia. If the patients received 60 g of glucose every 2 hours during the night, the insulin concentration was, besides the elevation of blood glucose, about 5 times higher than without glucose feeding, in normals as well as in patients with endogenous hypertriglyceridemia. At the same time, no significant change in triglyceride concentration could be observed. On the other hand, a continuous infusion of nicotinic acid during the night did not alter the glucose or the insulin response, but lowered the concentration of FFA and of TG considerably. From these studies we might conclude that hyperglycemia and hyperinsulinemia cannot be regarded the major factors responsible for the regulation of the concentration of endogenous plasma triglycerides. These data tend to confirm previous findings that the infusion of insulin (Jones and Arky, 1965; Schlierf and Kinsell,

1965) or carbohydrate feeding (Havel, 1957) actually lowers triglyceride levels slightly during the course of several hours.

In summary, the impaired glucose tolerance in the majority of patients with endogenous hypertriglyceridemia is caused either by insulin resistance or, in other patients, by insulin deficiency. In spite of the fact that insulin deficiency leads to impaired removal of endogenous plasma triglycerides and to a decreased fractional esterification rate of FFA into plasma TG in the liver (Sailer et al., 1967; Woodside and Heimberg, 1972), there is little evidence that hyperglucosemia and hyperinsulinemia lead to endogenous hypertriglyceridemia from an increased secretion rate of endogenous plasma triglycerides since (1) in many patients with endogenous hypertriglyceridemia the insulin concentration in the plasma is very low (basal and after a glucose load); (2) impaired glucose tolerance and hyperinsulinemia is not confined to a certain lipoprotein pattern (type) of endogenous hypertriglyceridemia; (3) formation of plasma TG-FA from plasma glucose-C is not different in normals and patients with endogenous hypertriglyceridemia, even after a glucose load. The formation of plasma TG-FA from plasma glucose-C does not quantitatively play a significant role in normals or in patients with endogenous hypertriglyceridemia, even after a heavy glucose load; (4) diurnal patterns of glucose, insulin, and TG concentration do not show a correlation between glucose response, insulin concentration and triglyceride concentration, and (5) carbohydrate feeding or insulin lowers the TG level in man.

REFERENCES

EATON, R. P., BERMAN, M. and STEINBERG, D. (1969): Kinetic studies of plasma free fatty acid and triglyceride metabolism in man. *J. clin. Invest., 48,* 1560.

EATON, R. P. and NYE, W. H. R. (1973): The relationship between insulin secretion and triglyceride concentration in endogenous lipemia. *J. lab. clin. Med., 81,* 682.

FAJANS, S. S. and CONN, J. W. (1959): The early recognition of diabetes mellitus. *Ann. N.Y. Acad. Sci., 82,* 208.

GLUECK, C. J., LEVY, R. I. and FREDRICKSON, D. S. (1969): Immunoreactive insulin, glucose tolerance, and carbohydrate inducibility in types II, III, IV and V hyperlipoproteinemia. *Diabetes, 18,* 739.

HAVEL, R. J. (1957): Early effects of fasting and of carbohydrate ingestion on lipids and lipoproteins of serum in man. *J. clin. Invest., 36,* 855.

HAVEL, R. J. (1968): Triglyceride and very low density lipoprotein turnover. In: *Proceedings of the 1968 Deuel Conference on Lipids on the Turnover of Lipids and Lipoproteins, Carmel, Calif. 1968,* pp. 117–121. Editors: G. Cowgill, D. L. Estrich and P. D. Wood. U.S. Department of HEW, NIH, Bethesda, Md.

JONES, D. P. and ARKY, R. A. (1965): Effects of insulin on triglyceride and free fatty acid metabolism in man. *Metabolism, 14,* 1287.

REAVEN, G., LERNER, R. L., STERN, M. P., FARQUHAR, J. W. and NAKANISHI, R. (1967): Role of insulin in endogenous hypertriglyceridemia. *J. clin. Invest., 46,* 1756.

RYAN, W. G. and SCHWARTZ, T. B. (1965): Dynamics of plasma triglyceride turnover in man. *Metabolism, 14,* 1243.

SAILER, S., SANDHOFER, F. and BRAUNSTEINER, H. (1966): Umsatzraten für freie Fettsäuren und Triglyceride im Plasma bei essentieller Hyperlipämie. *Klin. Wschr., 44,* 1032.

SAILER, S., SANDHOFER, F. and BRAUNSTEINER, H. (1967): Beziehungen zwischen Blutzuckerspiegel, Umsatzraten der freien Fettsäuren und Fettsäureeinbau in Plasmatriglyceriden bei Diabetikern. *Klin. Wschr., 45,* 86.

SAILER, S., BOLZANO, K., SANDHOFER, F., SPATH, P. and BRAUNSTEINER, H. (1968): Triglyceridspiegel und Insulinkonzentration im Plasma nach oraler Glukosegabe bei Patienten mit primärer kohlenhydratinduzierter Hypertriglyceridämie. *Schweiz. med. Wschr.*, *98,* 1512.

SANDHOFER, F., BOLZANO, K., SAILER, S. and BRAUNSTEINER, H. (1969): Quantitative Untersuchungen über den Einbau von Plasmaglukose-Kohlenstoff in Plasmatriglyceriden und die Veresterungsrate von freien Fettsäuren des Plasmas zu Plasmatriglyceriden während oraler Zufuhr von Glukose bei primärer kohlenhydratinduzierter Hypertriglyceridämie. *Klin. Wschr.*, *47,* 1086.

SCHLIERF, G. and KINSELL, L. W. (1965): Effect of insulin in hypertriglyceridemia. *Proc. Soc. exp. Biol. Med. (N.Y.)*, *120,* 272.

SCHLIERF, G. and DOROW, E. (1973): Diurnal patterns of triglycerides, free fatty acids, blood sugar, and insulin during carbohydrate-induction in man and their modification by nocturnal suppression of lipolysis. *J. clin. Invest.*, *52,* 732.

WOODSIDE, W. F. and HEIMBERG, M. (1972): Hepatic metabolism of free fatty acids in experimental diabetes. *Israel J. med. Sci.*, *8,* 309.

BIOCHEMISTRY AND STRUCTURE OF DEGENERATIVE LESIONS IN DIABETES

THE POLYOL PATHWAY: A MODEL FOR BIOCHEMICAL MECHANISMS BY WHICH HYPERGLYCEMIA MAY CONTRIBUTE TO THE PATHOGENESIS OF THE COMPLICATIONS OF DIABETES MELLITUS

ALBERT I. WINEGRAD, ANTHONY D. MORRISON and REX S. CLEMENTS, Jr.

George S. Cox Medical Research Institute, Department of Medicine, University of Pennsylvania, Philadelphia, Pa., and the Department of Medicine, University of Alabama Medical Center, Birmingham, Ala., U.S.A.

Any discussion of the long-term complications of diabetes mellitus must recognize that what we presently term diabetes mellitus may prove to be a group of diseases with diverse etiologies. By our present diagnostic criteria all of these disorders would share the ability to induce an abnormality in insulin secretion with a resultant derangement in the regulation of plasma glucose fluctuations. It is possible that certain long-term complications are restricted to specific etiological forms of diabetes; however, from the data presently available, none of the long-term complications appears to be confined to what is presently considered genetically determined diabetes mellitus. It appears reasonable therefore to examine the metabolic abnormalities that are common to all diabetics to determine whether mechanisms exist by which they may contribute to the development of specific long-term complications.

Recent studies in which blood glucose has been continuously monitored throughout the day in both normal and diabetic subjects suggest that abnormalities in plasma glucose fluctuations in diabetics are grossly underestimated by the arbitrary standards of control that are now in common use (Molnar et al., 1972). The possibility that hyperglycemia itself may contribute to the pathogenesis of specific long-term complications has not received serious attention in the past, and cannot be dismissed on the basis of the data derived from clinical trials. Without exception the latter studies have been comparisons of patients with varying degrees of *abnormal* plasma glucose fluctuation; in addition, their design has given little attention to the role that commonly associated but independently determined genetic abnormalities (such as those affecting lipoprotein metabolism) may play in determining the clinical course (Bondy and Felig, 1971; Winegrad et al., 1973).

Recent evidence suggests that increased polyol pathway activity provides a model for biochemical mechanisms by which hyperglycemia may induce derangements in the metabolism of a number of tissues that are common sites of pathological changes in long-term diabetics. To our minds it is unlikely that increased polyol pathway activity will in itself provide a total explanation for the development of any of the long-term complications. However, the data available suggest that metabolic abnormalities resulting from increased polyol pathway activity could well be a significant factor in the pathogenesis of specific lesions, and could amplify the effects resulting from insulin deficiency or from independent but commonly associated genetic defects. These data should give pause to those who dismiss the pathogenetic significance of hyperglycemia even though the value of normalizing plasma glucose by means such as islet transplantation remains to be tested.

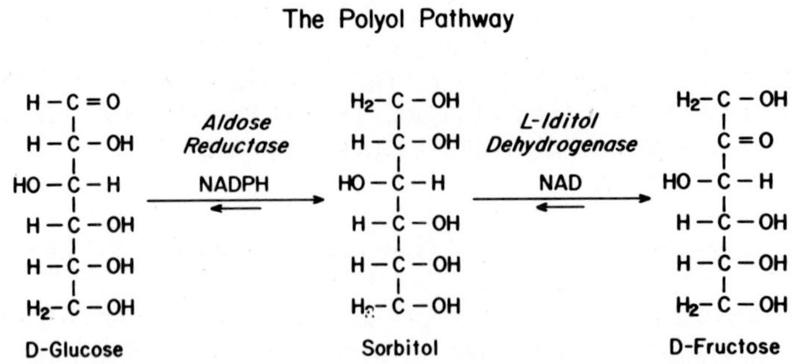

The Polyol Pathway

D-Glucose		Sorbitol		D-Fructose
H–C=O	*Aldose Reductase*	H_2–C–OH	*L-Iditol Dehydrogenase*	H_2–C–OH
H–C–OH	NADPH → / ←	H–C–OH	NAD → / ←	C=O
HO–C–H		HO–C–H		HO–C–H
H–C–OH		H–C–OH		H–C–OH
H–C–OH		H–C–OH		H–C–OH
H_2–C–OH		H_2–C–OH		H_2–C–OH

FIG. 1. Aldose reductase (alditol:NADP oxidoreductase) catalyzes the NADPH-dependent reduction of D-glucose and a wide range of aldose sugars to their polyol derivatives; the human enzyme has been purified to homogeneity from placenta (Clements and Winegrad, 1972). L-iditol dehydrogenase (sorbitol dehydrogenase) catalyzes the NAD-dependent oxidation of sorbitol to D-fructose. The polyol pathway has been shown to operate in an essentially irreversible fashion in sheep seminal vesicles (Hers, 1957), human erythrocyte (Travis et al., 1971; Morrison et al., 1970a), rabbit aortic intima and media (Morrison et al., 1972), and human placenta (Rodman et al., 1972).

The polyol pathway consists of 2 reactions by which free (i.e., non-phosphorylated) glucose is converted to D-fructose with the concomitant reduction of NAD^+ with reducing equivalents derived from NADPH. As shown in Figure 1, glucose is first reduced to its polyol derivative sorbitol; this reaction is catalyzed by aldose reductase which requires NADPH as a co-factor. Sorbitol is subsequently oxidized to D-fructose by an enzyme resembling hepatic cytoplasmic sorbitol dehydrogenase for which NAD^+ is the preferred co-factor. Although the individual reactions of the polyol pathway are potentially reversible, the conversion of glucose to fructose has been found to be an essentially irreversible process in those tissues in which it has been most thoroughly studied: sheep seminal vesicles (Hers, 1957), rabbit aortic intima and media (Morrison et al., 1972), human erythrocyte (Travis et al., 1971), and human placenta (Rodman et al., 1972). The essentially irreversible behavior of the polyol pathway has been explained on thermodynamic grounds since the usual difference in the redox states of the free NAD^+/NADH and $NADP^+$/NADPH couples in the cytoplasm of mammalian cells is such that reactions in which NADPH is utilized for the reduction of NAD^+ are associated with a large decrease in free energy (Atkinson, 1971). Professor Hers of Louvain first demonstrated that the polyol pathway is operative in mammalian tissues (Hers, 1957), and that it is responsible for the synthesis of seminal fluid and fetal plasma fructose. For a time aldose reductase was believed to be restricted to the accessory glands of the male genital tract and to the placenta of some mammalian species. However, by enzyme isolation and starch-gel electrophoresis, aldose reductase has been demonstrated in most rabbit and rat tissue and appears to be widely distributed in mammalian tissues (Clements et al., 1969a). In the human there is evidence that the polyol pathway is operative in seminal vesicles (Engel et al., 1970), placenta (Rodman et al., 1972; Clements and Winegrad, 1972), lens (Pirie and Van Heyningen, 1964), brain (Wray and Winegrad, 1966), peripheral nerve (Clements, unpublished observation), aortic intima and media (Clements et al., 1969b), and erythrocyte (Morrison et al., 1970a). It may be operative in other tissues as well. However, the specific cellular localization of polyol pathway activity within the organs of man or experimental animals has in most instances not been determined.

The physiological function of polyol pathway activity in tissues other than the seminal vesicles and placenta is obscure; because of this fact and the very high Km's for glucose exhibited by aldose reductases it has been suggested that outside of the placenta and seminal vesicles the polyol pathway is vestigial or normally metabolizes only sugars other than glucose (Van Heyningen, 1962). The latter is undoubtedly an erroneous conclusion since sorbitol is a normal constituent of tissues that contain aldose reductase activity.

In tissues in which the intracellular transport of glucose is not subject to insulin regulation and is not rate-limiting for glucose phosphorylation, the activity of the polyol pathway appears to be regulated in large part by the ambient glucose concentration. This has been shown to be the case in seminal vesicles (Hers, 1957, 1960), lens (Van Heyningen, 1962), peripheral nerve (Stewart et al., 1967; Gabbay et al., 1966), brain (Stewart et al., 1967), human erythrocyte (Travis et al., 1971; Morrison et al., 1970a), pancreatic islet (Morrison et al., 1970b), and aortic intima and media (Morrison et al., 1972; Clements et al., 1969b). In such tissues a rise in plasma or medium glucose concentration results in an increase in free intracellular glucose concentration such as that observed when paired samples of aortic intima and media are incubated with 5 mM and 50 mM glucose (Table 1). Insulin does not affect the volume of glucose distribution in

TABLE 1

Effect of medium glucose concentration on intracellular glucose concentration and polyol pathway activity in rabbit aortic intima and media. Data are derived from experiments in which paired samples of aortic tissue were incubated for 2 hours at 37°C in Krebs bicarbonate buffer, pH 7.4, containing 5 mM and 20 mM glucose, or 5 mM and 50 mM glucose (Morrison et al., 1972)

Medium glucose (mM)	Intracellular glucose (mM)	Aortic sorbitol (μM)	Aortic fructose (μM)	Fructose production (μmoles/kg/2 hr)
5	3.64 ± 0.28	11.5 ± 0.5	35.0 ± 2.3	216 ± 18
20	––	19.1 ± 0.7	60.7 ± 4.0	780 ± 81
50	26.48 ± 4.78	30.1 ± 3.1	84.9 ± 11.9	1430 ± 54

this tissue and the free intracellular glucose concentration in tissue incubated with 5 mM glucose averages 3.64 ± 0.28 mM; whereas in paired samples incubated with 50 mM glucose the intracellular glucose concentration averages 26.48 ± 4.78 mM. The effects of an increase in free intracellular glucose concentration on polyol pathway activity are readily explained by the kinetic characteristics of aldose reductase and sorbitol dehydrogenase. Thus the intracellular glucose concentration in aortic tissue incubated with a physiological glucose concentration (5 mM) is less than 1/10th the apparent Km for glucose of rabbit aortic aldose reductase (5.6×10^{-2} M) and of the aldose reductases isolated from other tissues (Morrison et al., 1972; Clements and Winegrad, 1972; Hayman and Kinoshita, 1965; Moonsammy and Stewart, 1967). Consequently a rise in intracellular glucose concentration would be expected to result in increased glucose reduction to sorbitol. Similarly the Km for sorbitol of aortic sorbitol dehydrogenase (0.7 mM) is more than 10 times the intracellular sorbitol concentration (0.04 mM) found in aortic tissue incubated with a physiological glucose concentration, and a rise in sorbitol concentration would result in increased sorbitol oxidation to fructose. Thus, as shown in Table 1, increasing the medium glucose concentration from 5 mM to 20 or 50 mM results in increased concentrations of both sorbitol and fructose in the aorta.

Increased concentrations of sorbitol and fructose have been demonstrated in many tissues from animals with experimental diabetes as well as in the lenses, peripheral nerves, and erythrocytes of human diabetes. However, it must be recognized that the tissue levels of sorbitol and fructose by themselves do not provide an accurate estimate of polyol pathway activity since tissues that contain this pathway may release free fructose into the plasma or incubation medium. This is illustrated by the fact that during a 2-hour incubation with 5 mM glucose rabbit aorta releases fructose that is 17 times the molar equivalent of the steady state sorbitol concentration (Table 1). Moreover, when the medium glucose concentration is increased to 20 mM or 50 mM there is a 3.5-fold and more than 6-fold increase in flux through the polyol pathway respectively; however, these increases in flux are not accompanied by proportional increases in aortic sorbitol and fructose concentrations (Table 1). These and similar data obtained with human erythrocytes (Travis et al., 1971; Morrison et al., 1970a) suggest that there is a relatively rapid turnover of endogenously synthesized sorbitol in a number of mammalian tissues. This appears to be the case in peripheral nerve, for Stewart et al. (1967) found that the administration of insulin to alloxan diabetic rats resulted in a striking fall in the elevated glucose, sorbitol, and fructose concentrations in the sciatic nerve within one hour. These observations are contrary to the common assumption that there is a very slow turnover of endogenously synthesized sorbitol in most mammalian tissues.

The initial evidence that increased polyol pathway activity resulting from hyperglycemia may have pathological consequences came from Van Heyningen's studies of experimental 'sugar' cataracts (Van Heyningen, 1959, 1962). Experimental diabetes in rats reproducibly results in the development of cataracts; the time required for cataract formation is inversely related to the degree of hyperglycemia. The significance of hyperglycemia as distinct from insulin deficiency was demonstrated by Patterson (1953) who found that cataract formation could be prevented by lowering the blood glucose by phloridzin administration. Van Heyningen (1959, 1962) called attention to the fact that experimentally-induced elevated plasma concentrations of D-glucose, D-galactose, or D-xylose, all of which are substrates for lens aldose reductase, are associated with cataract formation in the rat. Moreover, during the development of 'sugar' cataract the polyol derivative of the specific sugar present in high concentrations in the plasma appears in the lens. Sorbitol is a normal constituent of human and mammalian lens, but in human or experimental diabetes the sorbitol concentration in the lens has been found to be markedly elevated (Pirie and Van Heyningen, 1964). The association between hyperglycemia, increased polyol formation, and catact formation is well established. Kinoshita has observed the development of opacities in lenses maintained in organ culture with elevated glucose concentrations, and demonstrated that these changes can be minimized by the addition of an inhibitor of lens aldose reductase, cyclopentanediacetic acid (CPDA), to the incubation medium (Chylack and Kinoshita, 1969). More recently Kuck (1970) has reported that both aldose reductase and sorbitol dehydrogenase activities are absent in the lenses of mice of the CFW strain. It is of note that neither alloxan diabetes nor galactose feeding results in cataract formation in these mice despite the development of high intracellular concentrations of glucose or galactose in the lens.

The initial light microscopic studies of experimentally-induced diabetic and galactosemic cataracts suggested that the early changes were 'hydropic swelling' of the lens fibers which led to rupture of the hydropic cells and the appearance of interfibrillar clefts filled with protein debris. These observations by Friedenwald and Rytel (1966) were a major stimulus to the formulation of the osmotic hypothesis by Kinoshita (1965). This hypothesis attributes the association between increased polyol formation and cataractogenesis to the osmotic effects of the increased concentrations of sorbitol or other polyols in the lens.

It is known that tissues other than the liver usually lack mechanisms for the facilitated transport of sorbitol and other hexitols, and that even in the face of high concentration differences the rate of transport of these hexitols across the cell membrane is very slow. There are no quantitative data on the rate of turnover of sorbitol in the lens; however, in view of the significant concentration present in normal lens (1.5 μmoles/g in rats) most workers have assumed that it is very slow. The magnitude of the increased hexitol concentrations observed in the lenses of rats with alloxan diabetes or fed diets containing 40% galactose is sufficient to exert a significant osmotic effect (Chylack and Kinoshita, 1969; Kinoshita, 1965; Stewart et al., 1967). Kinoshita found that the water content of rabbit lenses incubated with elevated concentrations of glucose or galactose increased, at least initially, in parallel with the increases in lens sorbitol or galactitol content (Chylack and Kinoshita, 1969; Kinoshita, 1965). A number of derangements in active transport have been demonstrated in lenses in which experimental cataracts are developing (Kinoshita, 1965; Kinoshita et al., 1969). Kinoshita observed that increasing the medium osmolality minimized the defects in the active transport of K^+, amino acids, and free myoinositol in rabbit lenses incubated with high galactose concentrations. These observations have been interpreted as indicating the primacy of the osmotic effects of polyol accumulation with regard to cataract formation (Kinoshita, 1965; Kinoshita et al., 1969).

While there would seem little doubt that osmotic effects may contribute to the formation of 'sugar' cataracts, particularly under in vitro conditions, there are significant limitations to the osmotic hypothesis. Thus recent electron microscopic studies by Kuwabara et al. (1969) on the progression of cataracts induced by galactose feeding in rats indicate that even in its earliest phases this process involves much more than a simple swelling of the lens fibers. The earliest changes are seen in the anterior lens epithelium which shows a marked increase in free and membrane-bound ribosomes, and subsequently proliferates to form a multicellular layer. Some of the epithelial cells appear irregularly shaped and edematous at the outset. In addition, although in the early stages the cytoplasm of the lens fibers contains vacuoles, one of the most striking changes is the development of large intercellular cysts (Kuwabara et al., 1969). Clearly these fine structural changes require a more detailed biochemical explanation than that presently available. In addition, Stewart et al. (1968) have observed that when rats are fed a high galactose diet for 4 days and then transferred to a normal diet the lens galactitol level falls to very low levels within 4 to 7 days without any significant change in the elevated lens water content. The subsequent fall in lens water to normal levels correlates in time with the rise of the lens myoinositol content to a normal level rather than with changes in lens galactitol content. Similar observations have been made in peripheral nerve (Stewart et al., 1968). These data suggest that the increased water content of the lens in animals with elevated plasma aldose levels may not result solely from the osmotic effects of increased lens polyol concentrations. The relevance of experimental 'sugar' cataracts to those occurring in human diabetics requires clarification. It is generally agreed that increased polyol pathway activity may contribute to subcapsular vacuole formation and to the development of the 'snowflake' opacity observed in poorly controlled young diabetics. Whether it may provide an explanation for the increased frequency with which senile cataract extraction is performed in diabetics is disputed.

In considering the possible consequences of increased polyol pathway activity in other tissues there has been a tendency to approach the question in terms of the osmotic hypothesis. This is scarcely justified on the basis of the data available, since there is evidence that metabolic derangements resulting from increased polyol pathway activity need not be restricted to those predicted by the osmotic hypothesis. Thus in human erythrocytes polyol pathway activity accounts for approximately 1.8% of the glucose uptake at a physiological medium glucose concentration but may increase to 11% during incubation with 50 mM glucose (Travis et al., 1971). Under these conditions, the increased utilization of NADPH for glucose reduction to sorbitol results in increased pentose phosphate activity as a consequence of changes in the redox state of the $NADP^+$/NADPH couple. In addition, the markedly increased rate of sorbitol oxidation to fructose results in an increased free NADH/NAD ratio with resultant changes in the steady state levels of a number of glycolytic intermediates and a significant fall in erythrocyte 2,3-diphosphoglycerate (Morrison et al., 1970a). Thus, in the human erythrocyte, increased polyol pathway activity may significantly alter the redox state of both free pyridine nucleotide couples. It is of interest that Van Heyningen (1962) originally suggested that such changes might contribute to the development of experimental 'sugar' cataracts.

Studies in aortic intima and media provide further evidence of metabolic derangements that are not readily explained by the osmotic hypothesis (Morrison et al., 1972). As noted earlier, an increased medium glucose concentration results in increased aortic sorbitol and fructose concentrations and increased flux through the polyol pathway. The magnitude of the observed increases in aortic sorbitol is too small to exert a significant osmotic effect or to result in a detectable increase in water content. However, although aortic tissue incubated with 5 mM glucose for 3 hours maintains a relatively constant water content, incubation with 20 mM or 50 mM glucose for the same period results in easily detectable increases in water content that are similar in magnitude to those observed in the aortae of chronically hypertensive rats by Tobian et al. (1969). This increase in aortic water content is associated with a decrease in the inulin space, and appears to be related to increased polyol pathway activity. Similar increases in water content are observed during incubation with elevated concentrations of galactose, which is also a substrate for aortic aldose reductase, but not with fructose or mannitol. In addition, Dr. Morrision has observed that the addition of CPDA, which inhibits aortic aldose reductase, prevents the increase in aortic water content and all of the associated metabolic derangements observed in aortic tissue incubated with elevated glucose concentrations. The nature of these associated metabolic abnormalities is of interest since it points out the necessity to examine the consequences of increased polyol pathway activity with regard to the metabolic characteristics of each of the tissues which are sites of pathological changes in long-standing diabetics. The increase in aortic water content resulting from exposure to elevated glucose concentrations results in impaired oxygenation of the arterial wall at physiological oxygen tensions. The oxygen uptake of aortic tissue incubated with 20 mM or 50 mM glucose for 2 hours is significantly reduced when compared with tissue incubated with 5 mM glucose for the same period; in the latter case the oxygen uptake remains linear in medium saturated with 95% air during a 3-hour incubation and is unaltered by an increase in oxygen tension. In contrast, tissue incubated with 20 or 50 mM glucose initially exhibits an oxygen uptake similar to that of tissue incubated with 5 mM glucose which declines after the first half hour. This is associated with a significant increase in glycolysis and an increase in aortic lactate/pyruvate ratio. The oxygen uptake of tissues pre-incubated with elevated glucose concentrations can be restored to normal by increasing the oxygen tension of the medium to that of Krebs bicarbonate buffer saturated with 95% oxygen, 5% CO_2, or by increasing the osmolality of the incubation medium (which is already quite high) by the addition of 40 mM mannitol. These in vitro effects of exposure to elevated glucose concentrations may have in vivo counterparts since the water content of aortic tissue from alloxan diabetic rabbits has been found to be significantly greater than that of normal animals of the same age and sex, and aortic tissue from diabetic rabbits exhibits a reduced oxygen uptake at a physiological oxygen tension. The mechanism by which increased polyol pathway activity induces these alterations in aortic tissue exposed to elevated glucose concentrations remains to be clarified. Recent studies have demonstrated that increased polyol pathway activity results in a significant decrease in aortic free myoinositol content, and that the addition of 10 mM myoinositol prevents the increase in aortic water content and the decrease in oxygen uptake that usually results from incubation with elevated glucose concentrations. These effects have been shown to be non-osmotic in nature. These data have led us to speculate that the effects of increased polyol pathway activity in aortic intima and media may be mediated in part through changes in the metabolism of myoinositol or of the phosphoinositides.

It should be remembered that the intima and subjacent portions of the media in larger arteries are normally devoid of capillaries and are dependent upon diffusion from the lumen and from adventitial capillaries for the provision of their oxygen requirement. Hyperglycemia has emerged as a significant factor in the incidence of certain forms of occlusive arterial disease in recent epidemiological studies. In current speculation concerning factors that can adversely affect the normal function of the arterial wall it has frequently been noted that the respiration of the inner arterial wall is particularly susceptible to hypoxia resulting from impaired oxygen diffusion (Whereat, 1967; Haust, 1970; Robertson, 1968). Since the development of arterial disease in any given person may be determined by multiple factors, the consequences of the metabolic derangements resulting from exposure to elevated glucose concentrations may be determined by interaction with other genetic and environmental factors that operate in the production of arterial disease.

The significance of recent studies of the polyol pathway is primarily that it indicates the existence of at least one biochemical mechanism by which hyperglycemia may result in significant alterations in the metabolism of a number of mammalian tissues in which the intracellular transport of glucose is not subject to insulin regulation and is not limiting for glucose phosphorylation. In these tissues the regulation of polyol pathway activity is dependent upon a normal regulation of plasma glucose fluctuations. There is evidence that in specific tissues polyol pathway activity is also subject to hormonal regulation (Clements et al., 1969b; Mann, 1965), and the effects of sex and age remain to be clarified. The long-term consequences of abnormally increased polyol pathway activity must eventually be assessed in terms of the specific metabolic characteristics of the individual tissue at risk, and the additional independent factors that may be operative to adversely affect these tissues. A simplistic approach either to the mechanism(s) by which increased polyol pathway induces alterations in the metabolism of these tissues or to their possible long-term consequences is not justified by the data available. It is, however, clear that it is premature to dismiss the significance of hyperglycemia in the pathogenesis of the long-term complications of diabetes mellitus.

REFERENCES

ATKINSON, D. E. (1971): Adenine nucleotides as stoichiometric coupling agents in metabolism and as regulatory modifiers: the adenylate energy charge. *Metab. Pathways, 5,* 1.

BONDY, P. K. and FELIG, P. (1971): Relation of diabetic control to development of vascular complications. *Med. Clin. N. Amer., 55,* 889.

CHYLACK Jr., L. T. and KINOSHITA, J. H. (1969): A biochemical evaluation of a cataract induced in a high-glucose medium. *Invest. Ophthalmol., 8,* 401.

CLEMENTS Jr., R. S., WEAVER, J. P. and WINEGRAD, A. I. (1969a): The distribution of polyol:NADP oxidoreductase in mammalian tissues. *Biochem. biophys. Res. Commun., 37,* 347.

CLEMENTS Jr., R. S., MORRISON, A. D. and WINEGRAD, A. I. (1969b): Polyol pathway in aorta: regulation by hormones. *Science, 166,* 1007.

CLEMENTS Jr., R. S. and WINEGRAD, A. I. (1972): Purification of alditol:NADP oxidoreductase from human placenta. *Biochem. biophys. Res. Commun., 47,* 1473.

ENGEL, R. M. E., HOSKINS, D. D. and WILLIAMS-ASHMAN, H. G. (1970): Enzymes of the nonphosphorylative (sorbitol) pathway for fructose biosynthesis of primate seminal vesicles. *Invest. Urol., 7,* 333.

FRIEDENWALD, J. S. and RYTEL, D. (1966): Contribution to the histopathology of cataract. *Arch. Ophthalmol., 53,* 825.

GABBAY, H., MEROLA, L. O. and FIELD, R. A. (1966): Sorbitol pathway: presence in nerve and cord with substrate accumulation in diabetes. *Science, 151,* 209.

HAUST, M. D. (1970): Injury and repair in the pathogenesis of atherosclerotic lesions. In: *Atherosclerosis. Proceedings of the 2nd International Symposium.* Editor: R. J. Jones. Springer, Heidelberg.

HAYMAN, S. and KINOSHITA, J. H. (1965): Isolation and properties of lens aldose reductase. *J. biol. Chem., 240,* 877.

HERS, H. G. (1960): Le mécanisme de la formation du fructose séminal et du fructose foetal. *Biochim. biophys. Acta (Amst.), 37,* 127.

HERS, H. G. (1957): *Le Métabolisme du Fructose.* Editions Arscia, Bruxelles.

KINOSHITA, J. H. (1965): Cataracts in galactosemia. *Invest. Ophthalmol., 4,* 786.

KINOSHITA, J. H., BARBER, G. W., MEROLA, L. O. and TUNG, B. (1969): Changes in the levels of free amino acids and myoinositol in the galactose-exposed lens. *Invest. Ophthalmol., 8,* 625.

KUCK Jr., J. F. R. (1970): Response of the mouse lens to high concentrations of glucose or galactose. *Ophthal. Res., 1,* 166.

KUWABARA, T., KINOSHITA, J. H. and COGAN, D. G. (1969): Electron microscopic study of galactose-induced cataract. *Invest. Ophthalmol., 8,* 133.

MANN, T. (1965): *The Biochemistry of Semen and of the Male Reproductive Tract.* Wiley, New York.

MOLNAR, G. D., TAYLOR, W. F. and HO, M. M. (1972): Day-to-day variation of continuously monitored glycaemia: A further measure of diabetic instability. *Diabetologia, 8,* 342.

MOONSAMMY, G. I. and STEWART, M. A. (1967): Purification and properties of brain aldose reductase and L-hexonate dehydrogenase. *J. Neurochem., 14,* 1187.

MORRISON, A. D., CLEMENTS Jr., R. S., TRAVIS, S. B., OSKI, F. and WINEGRAD, A. I. (1970a): Glucose utilization by the polyol pathway in human erythrocytes. *Biochem. biophys. Res. Commun., 40,* 199.

MORRISON, A. D., WINEGRAD, A. I., FINK, C. J. and LACY, P. E. (1970b): Sorbitol synthesis in isolated rat pancreatic islets. *Biochem. biophys. Res. Commun., 38,* 491.

MORRISON, A. D., CLEMENTS Jr., R. S. and WINEGRAD, A. I. (1972): Effects of elevated glucose concentrations on the metabolism of the aortic wall. *J. clin. Invest., 51,* 3114.

MORRISON, A. D. and WINEGRAD, A. I. (1973): Reversal of the metabolic derangements observed in aortic tissue incubated with elevated glucose concentration by inhibiting polyol pathway activity. In: *Abstracts, VIII Congress of the International Diabetes Federation, Brussels 1973,* p. 177. Editors: J. J. Hoet and P. Lefebvre. International Congress Series No. 280, Excerpta Medica, Amsterdam.

PATTERSON, J. W. (1953): Effect of lowered blood sugar on the development of diabetic cataracts. *Amer. J. Physiol., 172,* 77.

PIRIE, A. and VAN HEYNINGEN, R. (1964): The effect of diabetes on the content of sorbitol, glucose, fructose and inositol in the human lens. *Exp. Eye Res., 3,* 124.

ROBERTSON Jr., A. L. (1968): Oxygen requirements of the human arterial intima in atherogenesis. *Progr. Biochem. Pharmacol., 4,* 305.

RODMAN, H. M., GUPTA, V. and LANDAU, B. R. (1972): The polyol pathway in human placenta (Abstract). *Diabetes, 21/Suppl. 1,* 329.

STEWART, M. A., SHERMAN, W. R., KURIEN, M. M., MOONSAMMY, G. I. and WISGERHOF, M. (1967): Polyol accumulations in nervous tissue of rats with experimental diabetes and galactosemia. *J. Neurochem., 14,* 1057.

STEWART, M. A., KURIEN, M. M., SHERMAN, W. R. and COTLIER, E. V. (1968): Inositol changes in nerve and lens of galactose fed rats. *J. Neurochem., 15,* 941.

TOBIAN, L., OLSON, R. and CHESLEY, G. (1969): Water content of arteriolar wall in renovascular hypertension. *Amer. J. Physiol., 216,* 22.

TRAVIS, S. F., MORRISON, A. D., CLEMENTS Jr., R. S., WINEGRAD, A. I. and OSKI, F. A. (1971): Metabolic alterations in the human erythrocyte produced by increases in glucose concentrations. The role of the polyol pathway. *J. clin. Invest., 50,* 2104.

VAN HEYNINGEN, R. (1959): Formation of polyols by the lens of rats with 'sugar' cataract. *Nature (Lond.), 184,* 194.

VAN HEYNINGEN, R. (1962): The sorbitol pathway in the lens. *Exp. Eye Res., 1,* 396.

WHEREAT, A. F. (1967): Recent advances in experimental and molecular pathology. Atherosclerosis and metabolic disorder in the arterial wall. *Exp. mol. Pathol., 7,* 233.

WINEGRAD, A. I., CLEMENTS Jr., R. S. and MORRISON, A. D. (1973): Oral antidiabetic agents: Limitations and hazards. In: *Controversy in Internal Medicine - II.* Editors: F. J. Ingelfinger, M. Finland, A. S. Relman and R. Ebert. W. B. Saunders Co., Philadelphia, In press.

WRAY, H. and WINEGRAD, A. I. (1966): Free fructose in human cerebrospinal fluid. *Diabetologia, 2,* 82.

ULTRASTRUCTURE AND GLUCOSE METABOLISM OF AN ISOLATED BLOOD CAPILLARY PREPARATION*

E. RASIO, M. BENDAYAN** and E. B. SANDBORN

Department of Medicine and Department of Anatomy, University of Montreal Medical School, Montreal, Quebec, Canada

There is little information regarding the sequence of events which are responsible for the morphological and functional alterations of blood capillaries in diabetes mellitus. The progressive accumulation of basement membrane material leads to, or coexists with, the loss of normal permeability. On the one hand, it has been proposed that high levels of circulating glucose can increase the synthesis of basement membrane collagen and alter its chemical composition so as to cause a defective filtration (Beisswenger and Spiro, 1973). On the other hand, it has been argued that the pathogenesis of the diabetic microangiopathy is not related to the metabolic disturbance induced by the deficiency of insulin action but represents a distinct primary lesion (Siperstein et al., 1968). In view of these conflicting ideas, the metabolism of vascular endothelium and the factors involved in its regulation deserve to be investigated more thoroughly. In mammals, blood capillaries are so intimately mingled with the other tissue structures that they cannot be isolated without damage. In the teleost fishes, however, blood capillaries are found to assemble in an almost pure form: the most favorable situation is encountered with the rete mirabile of the eel swimbladder. The aim of this study is (1) to describe the ultrastructure of this unique preparation of vascular endothelium, (2) to report the chemical composition of the basement membrane, and (3) to outline the tissue glucose utilization and its regulation by insulin and glucose added to the medium.

MATERIAL AND METHODS

The procedures of isolation of the blood capillaries from the rete mirabile of the swimbladder of the eel have been detailed elsewhere (Rasio, 1973). For the ultramicroscopic studies, the prerete artery to the swimbladder was perfused in situ with a lactate Ringer solution containing 5% dimethylsulfoxide (DMSO), followed by a 3-minute perfusion with a fixative solution containing 4% glutaraldehyde, 2% acrolein and 5% DMSO in a 0.2 M cacodylate buffer (Sandborn, 1970). The rete was removed from the swimbladder and

* This work was supported by grants from The Medical Research Council of Canada, DG 74 and MA 4222.

** M. Bendayan is a postgraduate student at the Medical School of the University of Montreal.

fixed for an additional 45 minutes in the same fixative. The techniques used for scanning and transmission electron microscopy have been described (Bendayan et al., 1974).

Basement membranes were isolated from blood-free capillaries by sonic disruption in 1 M NaCl; the collagen components were analyzed by methods already published (Spiro, 1967; Beisswenger and Spiro, 1973). The metabolic incubations were carried out in Krebs-Ringer bicarbonate buffer, pH 7.40, for 2 hours at 37°C. Under these conditions, the respiration of the capillary tissue is linear. Tissue sorbitol was measured by means of a fluorimetric enzymatic assay using sheep liver sorbitol dehydrogenase (Clements et al., 1969). Fructose in the medium was determined with an enzymatic procedure on perchloric filtrates (Travis et al., 1971). In studies of sugar transport, the intracellular penetration of sugar was calculated in double tracer incubations where water-^{3}H and sugar-^{14}C spaces were simultaneously determined. Intracellular water was assumed to represent the difference between the experimentally measured water-^{3}H space and an average inulin-^{14}C space as measured in a different set of experiments. A detailed account of the procedure will be published elsewhere (Rasio, 1974).

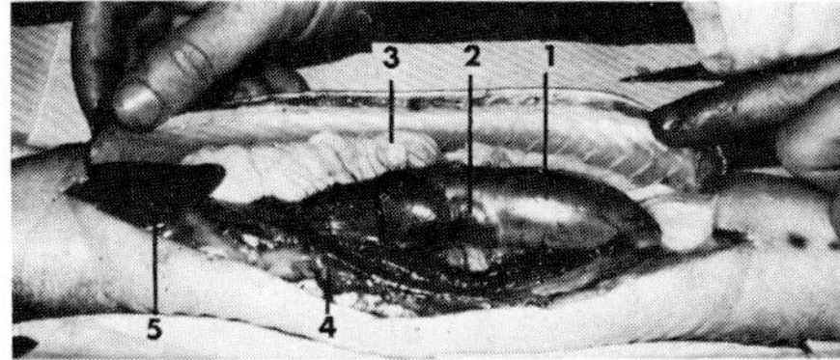

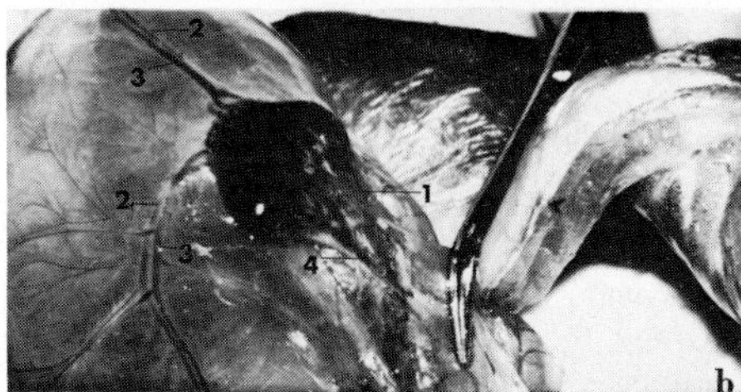

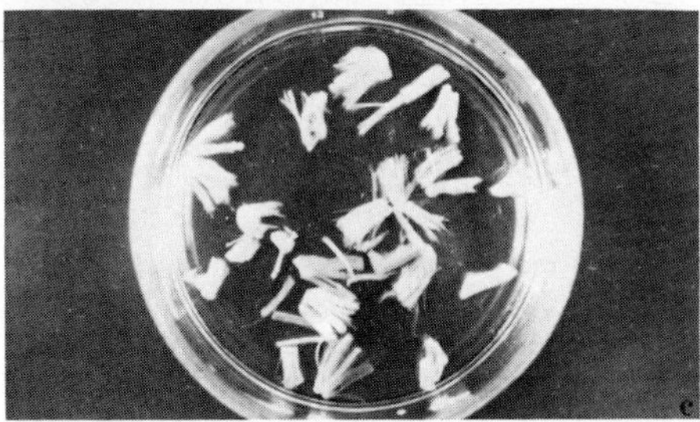

FIG. 1. a: The swimbladder (1) with its rete (2) appears between the ovaries (3) and the digestive tract (4); liver (5) is seen in rostral position. b: Vascular connections of the rete: (1) preretal artery, (2) postretal arteries, (3) preretal veins, (4) postretal vein. c: Stacks of capillaries free of blood and ready for incubation.

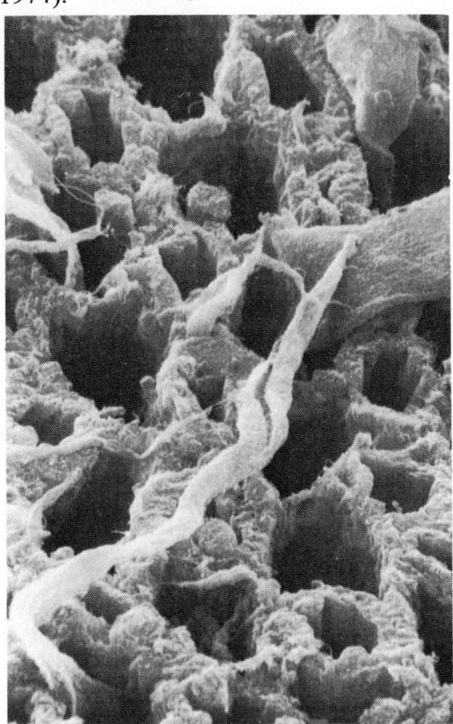

FIG. 2. Scanning electron micrograph of the rete showing the capillaries in transversal section and occasional collagen fibers. (X 2850.)

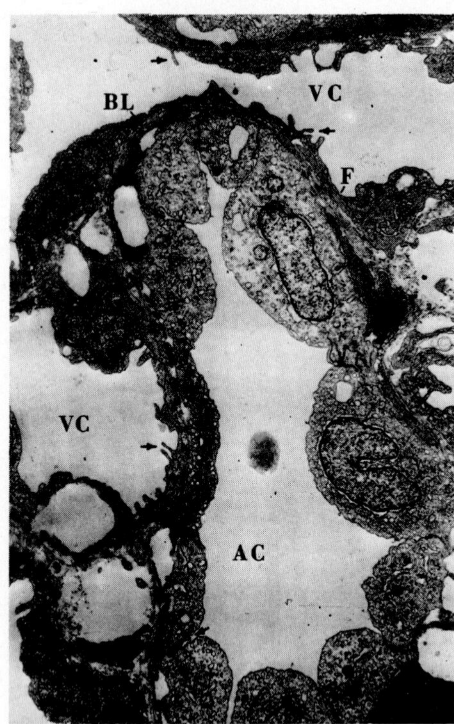

FIG. 3. Transmission electron micrograph. Cross-section of arterial and venous capillaries. The arterial capillary (AC) has a high endothelium (2–4 μ) and is very vacuolated. The endothelium of the venous capillary (VC) is lower, varying from 0.2 μ to 1 μ at the level of the nucleus. Pericytes (Per) are seen between the basal laminae (BL). Operculae (arrow) appear at the luminal borders of both capillaries. (X 3600.)

RESULTS

Morphology of the capillaries of the rete

The swimbladder is an oblong nacreous gas-filled sac with a well-developed network of capillaries in its connective tissue wall. It lies between the digestive tract and the ovaries. The rete mirabile or red body appears as a moderate-sized dark red mass on the swimbladder wall. The capillary network of the rete arises from the branches of the preretal artery. Two postretal arteries supply the blood to the swimbladder wall. The blood is then returned by 2 preretal veins to the rete from where it is carried to the hepatic portal vein by the postretal vein (Fig. 1). Scanning electron micrographs confirm the well-known close contact between the arterial and the venous capillaries of the rete which lie in parallel stacks. Collagen fibers appear in the space between the capillaries (Fig. 2).

In transmission electron microscopy, the arterial capillary endothelial cell is much thicker and more vacuolated than the venous. Operculae protrude from the luminal borders. Pericytes are seen quite often along the base of the arterial capillaries (Fig. 3).

The capillary cytoplasm (Figs 4 and 5) contains numerous mitochondria with both tubular and flattened cristae. Many filaments and microtubules are closely associated with the endoplasmic reticulum, the mitochondria and the desmosomes. Most striking is the variety of conformations of the smooth-surfaced membranes including the dumb-bell shaped, interconnected vesicles throughout the cytoplasm. The plasma membrane invaginates at the apex, the base and the intercellular aspects of the cells. Gap junctions form the apical part of the intercellular junctional complex, and, at a deeper level, several small desmosomal plaques are visible. The venous capillary endothelium (Fig. 5) has few fenestrations and some plasma membrane invaginations. Similar invaginations are evident in the pericyte, predominantly on the venous aspect of the capillary endothelial cells. Mitochondria in the pericyte have cristae which are mostly tubular but are sometimes seen as folds of the inner membrane.

The interconnections between the apical and basal vesicles in the arterial capillary endothelial cell form long tubular branching systems with alternating dilatations and constrictions (Figs 6 and 7). Those invaginations intrude deeply into the cytoplasm, reaching the cisternae of the endoplasmic reticulum. Some multivesicular bodies are present in the cytoplasm. In the gap junction, filamentous cross-over from the membrane of one cell to that of the other are commonly seen. Ribosomes are abundant in the pericytes and the venous capillaries (Fig. 7). Glycogen granules are present in greatest number in the arterial capillaries. A distinct basal lamina is recognizable between the venous endothelium and the arterial endothelium or the pericytes but appears only occasionally between arterial endothelium and pericytes. Collagen fibrils are observed between the basal laminae. Lipid droplets can reach a considerable size in the venous capillary (Fig. 8). Smaller dense granules are more common in both types of endothelial cells and pericytes.

Structure of basement membranes and amino acid composition

The fine fibrillar component of the basal lamina is the principal ultrastructural element seen in extracted membranes. A few collagen fibrils contaminate the preparation (Fig. 9). The amino acid composition of the basement membrane is given in Table 1.

Glucose utilization by the capillary tissue

The preparation of the tissue has been described (Rasio, 1973). The filamentous capillaries, free of blood, are shown in Figure 1. All results are given as mean values ± S.E.M. and are expressed per g wet weight of capillary tissue.

Pathways of glucose utilization In Krebs-Ringer bicarbonate buffer with glucose 5 mM, the glucose uptake averages 24.8 ± 1.0 μM/g/hr (N = 36), the lactic acid release 48.8 ± 2.1 μM/g/hr (N = 36), and the fructose release 0.363 ± 0.030 μM/g/hr (N = 8). In Krebs-Ringer bicarbonate buffer with glucose-^{14}C (U) 5 mM, the incorporation of glucose carbon into $^{14}CO_2$ is 2.75 ± 0.18 μM/g/hr (N = 26), into glycogen 0.588 ± 0.096 μM/g/2 hr (N = 12), into total lipid 0.576 ± 0.156 μM/g/2 hr (N = 12), into protein 0.192 ± 0.012 μM/g/2 hr (N = 16) and into basement membrane 0.033 ± 0.003 μM/g/2 hr (N = 14). The pathways of glucose utilization are outlined in Figure 10.

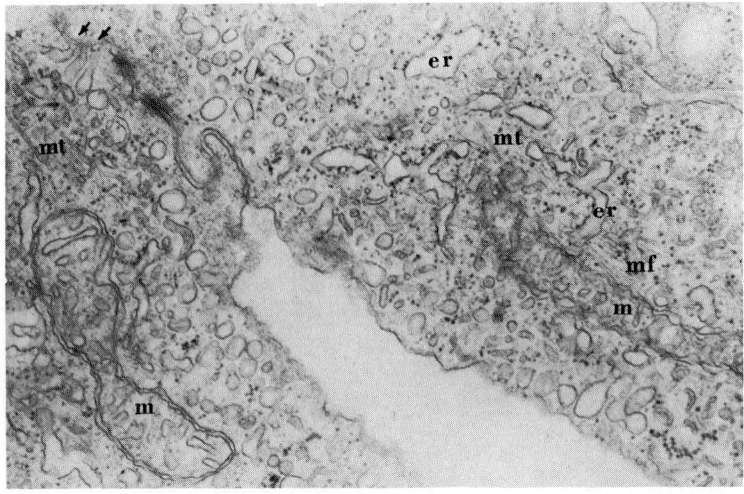

FIG. 4. Electron micrograph of a transverse section of arterial capillary cells presenting an intercellular junction with desmosomes. In the cytoplasm there is a large population of vesicles, some interconnected and some opening at the intercellular junction (arrow). Microtubules (mt) and microfilaments (mf) are closely associated with the endoplasmic reticulum (er) and the mitochondria (m). (X 16,700.)

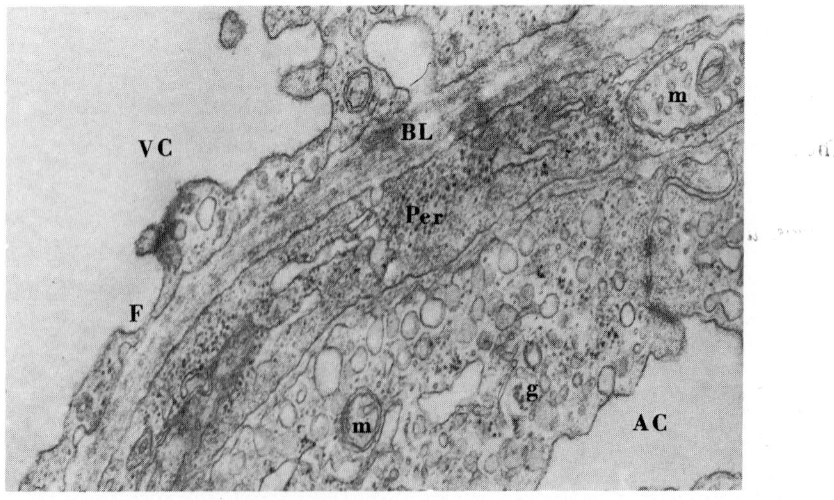

FIG. 5. Electron micrograph of the capillary endothelial cells. The basal laminae (BL) between the venous endothelial cell and the pericyte are well defined (400–600 Å). The fenestration (F) is closed by a diaphragm. Note vesicles in the endothelial cells and pericyte, glycogen granules (g) in the cytoplasm (X 25,600.)

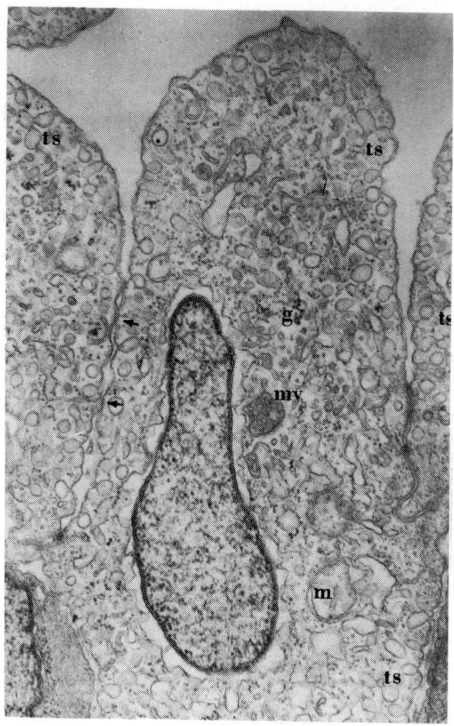

FIG. 6. Electron micrograph of the arterial endothelial cell. A great number of vesicles forming a branching tubular system (ts), open at the luminal or basal plasma membrane of the cell. Multivesicular body (mv), mitochondria (m) and glycogen granules (g) are present in the cytoplasm. Filaments cross over the intercellular junction (arrow). (X 14,500.)

Effect of the medium glucose concentration on the glucose utilization by capillary tissue In paired experiments where the medium glucose concentration is raised from 5 to 15 mM and from 5 to 30 mM, all the pathways of glucose utilization are increased in linear fashion and at different rates (Fig. 11). For each pathway, the mean values at 5, 15 and 30 mM are significantly different from one to the other ($0.05 > P > 0.01$). Tissue sorbitol rises from 29.3 ± 4.6 to 53.9 ± 7.1 nM/g/2 hr.

Effect of insulin on the glucose utilization by capillary tissue The addition of insulin (beef, 0.1 U/ml) to Krebs-Ringer bicarbonate medium containing glucose 5 mM, does not modify glucose uptake (27.9 ± 1.0 μM/g/hr vs. 26.4 ± 0.7 μM/g/hr in paired controls, N = 14), lactic acid production (53.8 ± 3.7 μM/g/hr vs. 52.9 ± 3.0 μM/g/hr in controls, N = 14) nor glucose carbon incorporation into $^{14}CO_2$ (2.66 ± 0.16 μM/g/hr vs. 2.66 ± 0.16 in controls, N = 14), into glycogen (0.468 ± 0.072 μM/g/2 hr in controls, N = 6) and into total lipid (0.240 ± 0.024 μM/g/2 hr vs. 0.248 ± 0.024 μM/g/2 hr in controls, N = 6). When capillaries are isolated from hyperglycemic alloxan-treated eels, the glucose uptake averages 28.1 ± 1.2 μM/g/hr, the lactate production 51.5 ± 3.3

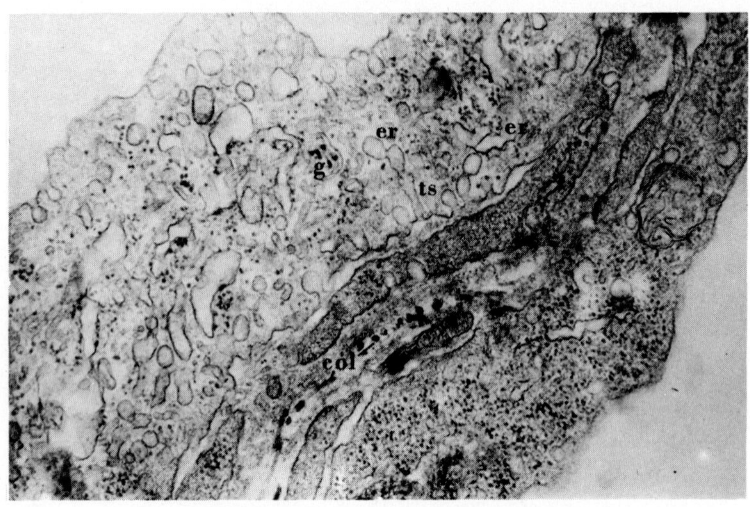

FIG. 7. Electron micrograph of the endothelial cells. The long tubular system (ts) reaches the endoplasmic reticulum (er). Microtubules and filaments are seen throughout the cytoplasm. Collagen fibers (col) appear in the interstitial space between the basal laminae. (X 19,000.)

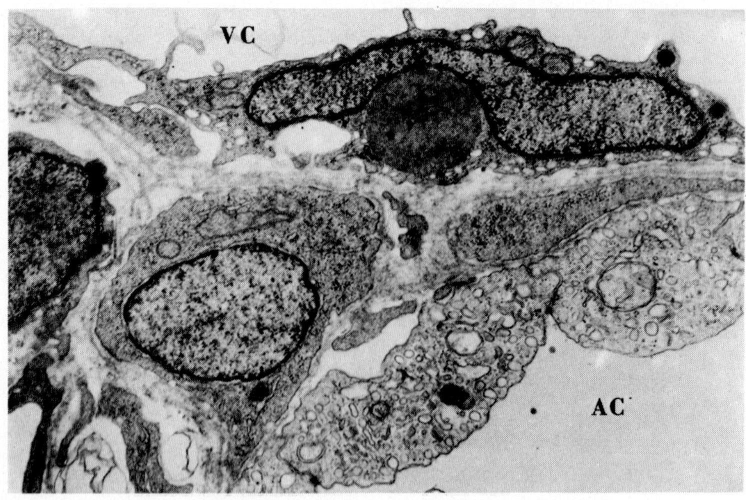

FIG. 8. Electron micrograph showing one large and many smaller dense granules, thought to be lipid droplets, in the cytoplasm of all types of cells. Note the large amount of mitochondria. (X 10,300.)

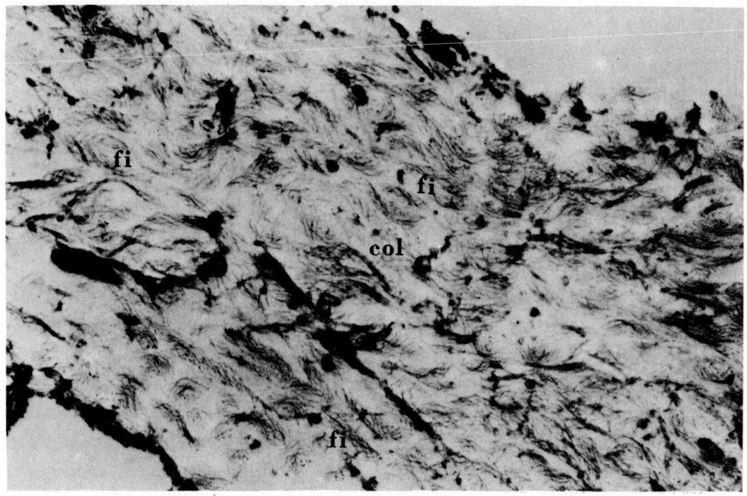

FIG. 9. Electron micrograph of isolated basement membrane material with its fine fibrillar structure (fi) and collagen fibers (col). (X 23,000.)

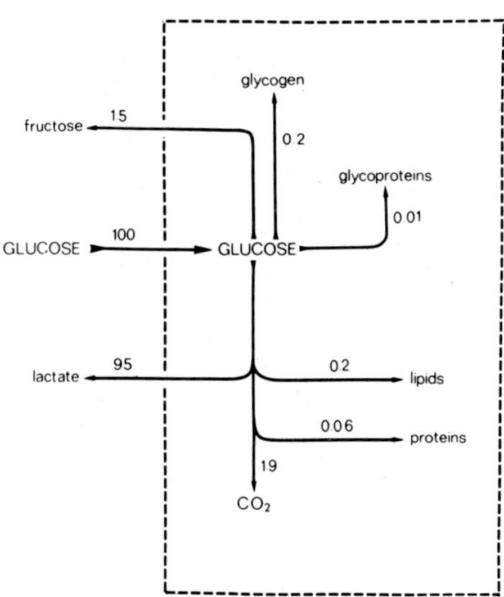

FIG. 10. Qualitative and quantitative aspects of glucose utilization by capillary tissue. Numbers indicate glucose conversion as percentage of glucose uptake.

TABLE 1

Composition of capillary basement membranes

Component	Amount
	Residues/1000 total amino acid residues
Hydroxyproline	42.3
Aspartic acid	76.4
Threonine	37.2
Serine	51.6
Glutamic acid	102.5
Proline	87.4
Glycine	211.1
Alanine	80.2
Valinc	37.5
Half-cystine	18.4
Methionine	15.9
Isoleucine	25.7
Leucine	50.6
Tyrosine	16.2
Phenylalanine	25.5
Hydroxylysine	9.0
Lysine	41.3
Histidine	14.1
Arginine	55.3
Tryptophan	2.9
Glc-Gal-Hyl	3.8
Gal-Hyl	0.8
Glucose	4.0
Galactose	5.5
Mannose	3.4
Fucose	0.7
Glucosamine	6.0

There are 448 micromoles of total amino acids in 100 mg of the dry protein. In addition, 27 micromoles/100 mg of an unknown component was seen on amino acid analyzer.

μM/g/hr and the glucose carbon incorporation into $^{14}CO_2$ 3.14 ± 0.40 μM/g/hr (N = 12). These values do not differ from corresponding values obtained with capillaries from normal eels and are not modified by the addition of fish insulin (0.1 U/ml) to the medium: 29.2 ± 0.9 μM/g/hr for glucose uptake, 54.1 ± 3.7 μM/g/hr for lactate production and 3.33 ± 0.32 μM/g/hr for glucose carbon incorporation into $^{14}CO_2$ (N = 12, paired experiments).

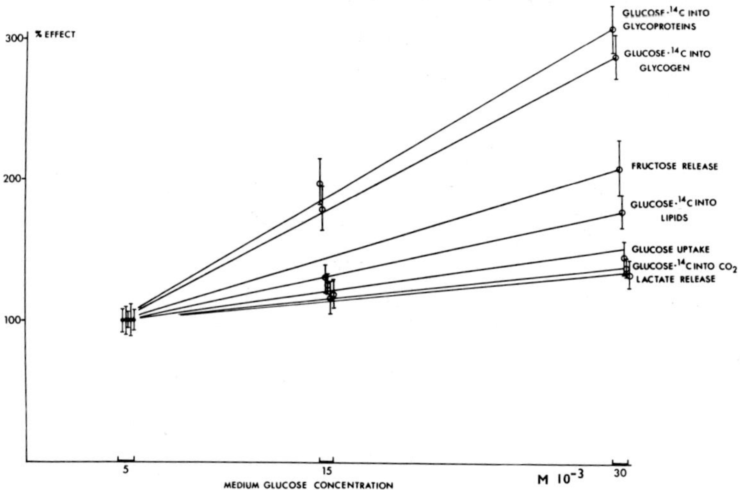

FIG. 11. Effects of glucose concentration in the medium on glucose utilization by capillary tissue. Mean values ± S.E.M. N = 8 to 18.

The passage of glucose across the cell membrane of vascular endothelium

After a 2-hour incubation in Krebs-Ringer bicarbonate buffer with glucose 5 mM, at 37°C, the water-^{3}H space is 68.5 ± 1.5 μl/100 mg wet weight (N = 22), the 3-O-methyl ^{14}C-glucose space is 67.3 ± 1.1 μl/100 mg wet weight (N = 20), the sorbitol-^{3}H space is 62.8 ± 1.1 μl/100 mg wet weight (N = 10) and the inulin-^{14}C space 44.9 ± 1.3 μl/100 mg wet weight (N = 14).

For all the tracers, equilibrium with tissue water is achieved after a one-hour incubation. Figure 12 shows that insulin (fish, 0.1 U/ml) added to the medium, does not modify the initial rate of 3-O-methyl ^{14}C-glucose entry into intracellular water.

In Figure 13, it can be seen that after the equilibration of 3-O-methyl ^{14}C-glucose 5 mM or L-glucose-^{14}C 5 mM in tissue water, the addition to the medium of D-glucose to a final concentration of 30 mM does not significantly reduce the intracellular level of the labelled sugars. Phlorizin 10^{-7} or 10^{-5} M does not modify glucose uptake, lactic acid production and glucose carbon incorporation into $^{14}CO_2$ (Table 2).

DISCUSSION

The blood capillaries isolated from the rete mirabile of the swimbladder of the eel may represent a useful preparation for the study of the pathogenesis of various human capillary disorders in general and of the diabetic microangiopathy in particular. This assumption rests on the following considerations. Firstly, the ultrastructure of both venous and arterial capillaries of the rete shows similar characteristics as the capillaries of the same variety in mammalian tissues (Majno, 1965). The analogies apply to the endothelial cells with their large population of cytoplasmic vesicles, to the intercellular junctions with

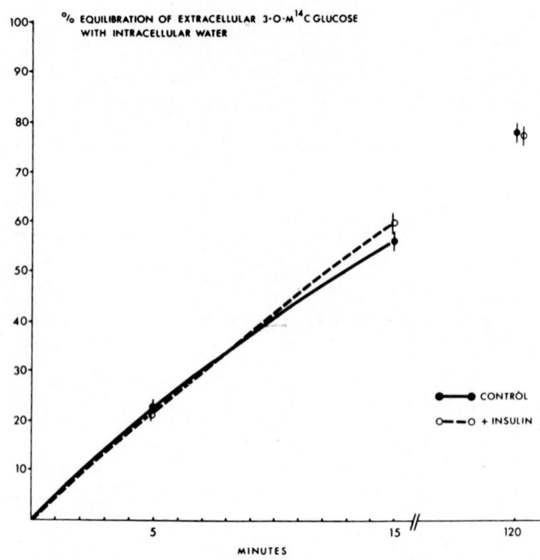

FIG. 12. Effect of insulin (fish, 0.1 U/ml) on the rate of 3-O-methyl ^{14}C-glucose entrance in intracellular water of capillary tissue. Mean values ± S.E.M. N = 8.

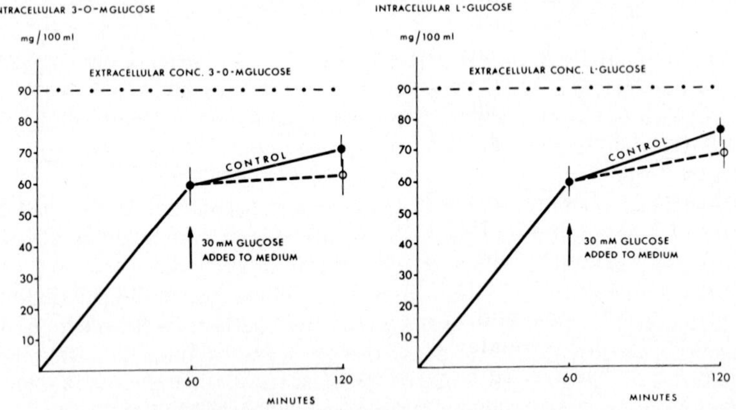

FIG. 13. Extrusion of intracellular 3-O-methyl-glucose and L-glucose by extracellular D-glucose in capillary tissue. Mean values ± S.E.M. N = 8.

their occluding zonules, to the basement membrane with its finely fibrillar structure and to the pericytes which lie between leaflets of this membrane. A more detailed description of the capillaries of the rete will be published (Bendayan et al., 1974).

Secondly, the amino acid composition of the isolated basement membrane is typically that of the collagen family of proteins: there is a high content of glycine; hydroxylysine and hydroxyproline are present; the amounts of carbohydrates and cysteine are substantial. Analyses of the amino acid residues indicate a striking similarity with the base-

TABLE 2
Effect of phlorizin on glucose utilization by capillaries

Phlorizin	Glucose uptake	Lactate release	^{14}C-glucose into CO_2
M		μmoles/g/hr	
0	26.1 ± 2.9	41.9 ± 3.1	0.476 ± 0.58
10^{-7}	27.3 ± 2.6	43.4 ± 3.2	0.474 ± 0.27
10^{-5}	27.9 ± 2.0	43.1 ± 3.3	0.444 ± 0.42

Glucose concentration 5 mM. N = 8.
Mean values ± S.E.M.

ment membranes of lung capillaries of the dog (Kefalides and Denduchis, 1969). In respect to bovine and human glomerular basement membranes, there is less hydroxylysine, hydroxyproline and hydroxylysine-linked disaccharide and more proline and lysine (Spiro, 1967; Beisswenger and Spiro, 1973). This could be due to less hydroxylation and less glycosydation of the protein components.

Thirdly, hyperglycemia can be induced in the eel by the intravascular injection of alloxan. It should be pointed out that a spontaneous diabetes has been reported in the carp, a teleost fish like the eel; remarkably, the disease induces pathological changes in the beta cell and in blood capillary vessels which are almost identical to those seen in human diabetes (Nakamura et al., 1971; Yokote, 1970).

Finally, on a functional point of view, the rete can be considered as a lung-type organ where high oxygen pressures are built in arterial blood by virtue of a Bohr effect on venous blood (Berg and Steen, 1968). There are other advantages to the rete: the arteries and veins at both poles can be catheterized, thus allowing counter-current perfusion studies of the isolated vascular organ. Because the capillaries are straight, unbranched and parallel and because arterial and venous capillaries alternate in a highly regular arrangement, many difficulties encountered in measuring permeability in tissue capillary beds can be avoided. It is concluded from the above considerations that the rete mirabile of the eel swimbladder is a unique preparation of blood capillaries in that it allows the simultaneous study of the structure, the permeability and the metabolism of the vascular endothelium in any given experimental condition. As an initial step towards this multifacetted investigation, a study of glucose metabolism has been undertaken.

Glycolysis is the major pathway of glucose utilization: more than 95% of the glucose consumed is released as lactate in the medium. Glucose oxydation to CO_2 accounts for 25% of the energy production rate, for a theoretical oxygen requirement of about 65 μl/g/hr. The respiration can be related to the presence of mitochondria in both pericytes and endothelial cells.

Emphasis has recently been put on the presence of sorbitol in tissues other than seminal vesicles where it has long since been recognized (Hers, 1960). It has been found that the polyol pathway is widely distributed in mammalian tissues, such as the lens (Van

Heyningen, 1962), the aorta (Clements et al., 1969), the erythrocyte (Travis et al., 1971), the pancreatic beta cell (Morrison et al., 1970), the nervous tissue (Gabbay et al., 1966) and the placenta (Rodman et al., 1972). The polyol pathway is also operative in the capillaries of the rete: the release of free fructose in the medium represents 1.5% of the glucose uptake (Rasio et al., 1972). Other pathways of glucose utilization include glucose carbon incorporation into glycogen, total lipid, protein and collagen. Glycogen and lipid stores are visible in the cytoplasm of the endothelial cells.

Glucose utilization is not regulated by insulin added in vitro nor is it modified when capillaries are isolated from alloxan-treated eels. On the other hand, all the pathways of glucose utilization are stimulated by increasing the levels of glucose in the medium. The over-utilization of glucose is prominent in the conversion of carbon to glycogen, lipid, sorbitol and collagen. It has been shown that elevated ambient glucose concentrations result in increased polyol pathway activity in many insulin-insensitive tissues. This is associated with an increase in the water content or alteration in the redox potential of the cells. Such derangements may provide a mechanism by which hyperglycemia contributes to the development of specific tissue diseases (Travis et al., 1971; Gabbay et al., 1966; Morrison et al., 1972). With capillaries of the rete, when glucose concentration in the medium is raised from 5 to 30 mM, there is a 2-fold increase in glucose flux through the polyol pathway. Further studies will have to determine whether high levels of intracapillary sorbitol as a consequence of increased glucose concentration in the extracellular space can lead to cellular edema and impairment of the permeability of the vascular membrane.

When capillaries are incubated in a medium with glucose 30 mM, the incorporation of glucose carbon into basement membrane collagen is 3 times higher than in a medium with glucose 5 mM. It has been shown that glomerular basement membranes in diabetic subjects contain more hydroxylysine and more of its glycosydically-linked disaccharide unit (Beisswenger and Spiro, 1973). The overproduction of units rich in carbohydrate could interfere with the layering of the peptide chains and thereby contribute to the increased porosity of the membrane. It is not known at present if the increased flux of glucose carbon in glycoproteins of the rete capillaries during incubations with high medium glucose concentrations is indicative of the same specific chemical alteration as described in diabetic glomerular basement membranes.

The fact that glucose utilization depends on the ambient glucose concentration and does not respond to insulin suggests that the intracellular passage of glucose is not a rate-limiting factor in glucose utilization by blood capillaries. Phlorizin at concentrations known to inhibit sugar transport in kidney and small intestine has no effect on glucose uptake, glycolysis, and CO_2 production. Furthermore, fish insulin added in vitro does not change the initial rate of glucose entrance in cellular water. Finally the addition of glucose 30 mM to the extracellular milieu cannot displace 3-O-methylglucose nor L-glucose from the the cellular water where both sugars had been previously equilibrated. From these preliminary studies and from other experiments in progress, it appears that there is no saturation nor competition for the process of intracellular glucose passage. It is conceivable, therefore, that in diabetes mellitus increased levels of extracellular glucose as a result of insulin deficiency may cause overutilization of glucose by capillary tissue along pathways such as those leading to glycoproteins, sorbitol, glycogen, lipids and so forth. It may prove worthwhile studying whether or not the accumulation of such products can alter the normal structure and permeability of the vascular endothelium.

ACKNOWLEDGEMENTS

The cooperation of Dr. A. D. Morrison and A. I. Winegrad for the study of the polyol pathway and of Dr. R. G. Spiro and Dr. N. Kalant for studies of the basement membrane, is gratefully acknowledged. The authors thank Miss M. P. Dea and Miss C. Venne for their technical assistance.

REFERENCES

BEISSWENGER, P. J. and SPIRO, R. G. (1973): Studies of the human glomerular basement membrane. Composition, nature of the carbohydrate units and chemical changes in diabetes mellitus. *Diabetes, 22,* 180.

BENDAYAN, M., SANDBORN, E. B. and RASIO, E. (1974): The capillary endothelium in the rete mirabile of the swimbladder of the eel (Anquilla anguilla). Functional and ultrastructural aspects. *Canad. J. Physiol.,* submitted for publication.

BERG, T. and STEEN, J. B. (1968): The mechanism of oxygen concentration in the swimbladder of the eel. *J. Physiol. (Lond.), 195,* 631.

CLEMENTS Jr., R. S., MORRISON, A. D. and WINEGRAD, A. I. (1969): Polyol pathway in aorta: regulation by hormones. *Science, 166,* 1007.

GABBAY, K. H., MEROLA, L. O. and FIELD, R. A. (1966): Sorbitol pathway: presence in nerve and cord with substrate accumulation in diabetes. *Science, 151,* 209.

HERS, H. G. (1960): L'aldose-reductase. *Biochim. biophys. Acta, 37,* 120.

KEFALIDES, N. A. and DENDUCHIS, B. (1969): Structural components of epithelial and endothelial basement membranes. *Biochemistry, 8,* 4613.

MAJNO, G. (1965): Ultrastructure of the vascular membrane. In: *Handbook of Physiology, Circulation, Vol. III,* Chapter 64, pp. 2293–2375. Editors: W. F. Hamilton and P. Dow. American Physiological Society, Washington, D.C.

MORRISON, A. D., WINEGRAD, A. I., FINK, C. J. and LACY, P. E. (1970): Sorbitol synthesis in isolated rat pancreatic islets. *Biochem. biophys. Res. Commun., 38,* 491.

MORRISON, A. D., CLEMENTS Jr., R. S. and WINEGRAD, A. I. (1972): Effect of elevated glucose concentrations on the metabolism of the aortic wall. *J. clin. Invest., 51,* 3114.

NAKAMURA, M., YAMADA, K. and YOTOTE, M. (1971): Ultrastructural aspects of the pancreatic islets in carps of spontaneous diabetes mellitus. *Experientia (Basel), 27,* 75.

RASIO, E. A., MORRISON, A. D. and WINEGRAD, A. I. (1972): Demonstration of polyol pathway activity in an isolated capillary preparation. *Diabetes, 21/Suppl. 1,* 330.

RASIO, E. (1973): Glucose metabolism in an isolated blood capillary preparation. *Canad. J. Biochem., 51,* 701.

RASIO, E. (1974): The passage of glucose across the cell membrane of isolated blood capillaries. To be published.

RODMAN, H. M., GUPTA, V. and LANDAU, B. R. (1972): The polyol pathway in human placenta. *Diabetes, 21/Suppl. 1,* 329.

SANDBORN, E. B. (1970): Materials and methods. In: *Cells and Tissues by Light and Electron Microscopy, Vol. 1,* pp. 1–3. Academic Press, New York, N.Y.

SIPERSTEIN, M. D., UNGER, R. H. and MADISON, L. L. (1968): Studies of muscle capillary basement membranes in normal subjects, diabetic and prediabetic patients. *J. clin. Invest., 47,* 1973.

SPIRO, R. G. (1967): Studies on the renal glomerular basement membrane. Preparation and chemical composition. *J. biol. Chem., 244,* 602.

TRAVIS, S. F., MORRISON, A. D., CLEMENTS Jr., R. S., WINEGRAD, A. I. and OSKI, F. A. (1971): Metabolic alterations in the human erythrocyte produced by increases in glucose concentration. The role of the polyol pathway. *J. clin. Invest., 50,* 2104.
VAN HEYNINGEN, R. (1962): The sorbitol pathway in the lens. *Exp. Eye Res., 1,* 396.
YOKOTE, M. (1970): Sekoke disease, spontaneous diabetes in carp found in fish farms. I. Pathological studies. *Bull. Freshwater Fisheries Res. Lab., 20,* 39.

RENAL GLOMERULAR BASEMENT MEMBRANE SUBUNITS*

ROBERT G. SPIRO

Department of Biological Chemistry and Medicine, Harvard Medical School, and the Elliott P. Joslin Research Laboratory, Boston, Mass., U.S.A.

The morphological alterations observed in the renal glomerulus in diabetes are characterized by a thickening of the basement membrane of the capillary loops and the deposition of an excess of similar material in the mesangium (Farquhar et al., 1959; Kimmelstiel et al., 1962; Bloodworth, 1963). These changes may be manifestations of a generalized microangiopathy. In order to elucidate the biochemical basis of this renal pathology, the glomerular basement membrane has been the subject of intensive studies in our laboratory for a number of years.

These investigations have so far revealed that both excessive and chemically altered basement membrane material is deposited in the diabetic glomerulus (Beisswenger and Spiro, 1970, 1973) and that the activity of the basement membrane synthesizing machinery, as measured by a kidney glucosyltransferase, is elevated in the diabetic state (Spiro and Spiro, 1971). The finding that early insulin treatment of diabetic rats could restore the level of this enzyme to normal values suggested that at least some steps in the assembly of the basement membrane are under the direct or indirect control of this hormone.

Studies on basement membrane isolated from both bovine (Spiro, 1967a) and human (Beisswenger and Spiro, 1973) glomeruli have indicated that it belongs to the collagen family of proteins but differs in important respects from fibrillar collagens, particularly in its higher content of sugar, hydroxylysine and half-cystine residues (Table 1).

The carbohydrate of the basement membrane is distributed between 2 distinct types of units, one consisting of a glucosylgalactose disaccharide linked to hydroxylysine (2-O-α-D-glucopyranosyl-O-β-D-galactopyranosylhydroxylysine) and the other represented by a branched heteropolysaccharide made up of sialic acid, fucose, galactose, mannose and N-acetylglucosamine attached to asparagine residues on the peptide chains (Spiro, 1967b, c). Approximately 80% of the hydroxylysine and 6% of the asparagine residues are substituted by carbohydrate in this manner.

The diabetic membrane differs most conspicuously from the normal by an increase in its hydroxylysine content as well as in the number of glucosylgalactose disaccharides attached to this amino acid (Table 1). While the concomitant decrease in lysine (with the sum of lysine and hydroxylysine remaining constant) suggested that increased hydroxyl-

* This work was supported by a grant from the American Heart Association, Grant AM 17325 from the National Institutes of Health and by the Adler Foundation, Rye, New York.

TABLE 1
Comparison of normal and diabetic human glomerular basement membrane with skin tropocollagen

Constituent†	Basement membrane (human)*		Skin tropocollagen (calf)
	Normal	Diabetic	
	Residues/1000 total amino acid residues		
Glycine	214	238[⊕]	320
Hydroxyproline	81	88[⊕]	94
Hydroxylysine	25	30+	7
Lysine	25	20+	27
Aspartic acid	66	62	45
Tyrosine	16	14+	3
Half-cystine	20	20	–§
Glucose	18	23+	1
Galactose	20	25+	2
Mannose	5	5	–
Hexosamines	10	10	–

* From Beisswenger and Spiro, 1973.
† Only values for key amino acids and sugars are given.
⊕ Values significantly different from normal with $P < 0.05$.
\+ Values significantly different from normal with $P < 0.01$.
§ Dash indicates that less than 1 residue per 1000 amino acid residues is present.

ation of lysine with subsequent glycosylation may take place in the diabetic state, the finding of altered levels of a few other amino acids, including glycine and hydroxyproline, raised the possibility that the diabetic changes might be the result of an altered subunit composition of the membrane. To explore the latter alternative, an attempt has been made to isolate and characterize the subunits of the basement membrane.

While the renal glomerular basement membrane can be readily solubilized by digestion with bacterial collagenase to yield glycopeptides and peptides, and a study of such proteolytic fragments has provided valuable structural information (Spiro, 1967b), a more discriminating method of solubilization not involving the cleavage of peptide bonds had to be employed for the purpose of subunit separation.

The basement membrane does not dissolve in buffered salt solution but can be solubilized to a limited extent by extraction at room temperature with sodium dodecyl sulfate at pH 7.0 (Table 2) to yield protein having a more polar composition than the whole membrane, with a lower content of glycine, hydroxyproline, hydroxylysine and glucosylgalactosyl disaccharide, and a higher content of the sugars uniquely associated with the heteropolysaccharide unit, such as N-acetylglucosamine and mannose (Hudson and Spiro,

1972a). After reduction and alkylation, a marked enhancement of the solubility of the membrane is noted and a fraction representing about 80% of its weight may be obtained with an amino acid and saccharide composition very similar to the native membrane (Table 2).

TABLE 2

*Comparison of the composition of the material solubilized by sodium dodecyl sulfate extraction of the native and reduced-alkylated bovine glomerular basement membrane**

Constituent†	Whole membrane (unextracted)	Sodium dodecyl sulfate solubilized+ Native membrane	Sodium dodecyl sulfate solubilized+ Reduced-alkylated membrane
	Residues/1000 total amino acid residues		
Glycine	212	115	189
Hydroxyproline	77	17	75
Hydroxylysine	22	5	23
Lysine	27	41	25
Aspartic acid	66	85	70
Tyrosine	17	28	19
Half-cystine	23	29	27§
Glucose	17	6	16
Galactose	22	13	21
Mannose	6	10	6
Hexosamines	12	20	11
(Per cent of membrane weight)	(100)	(22)	(79)

* From Hudson and Spiro, 1972 a, b.
† Only values for key amino acids and sugars are given.
\+ Extracted for 36 hours at room temperature.
§ Determined as S-carboxymethylcysteine.

Polyacrylamide gel electrophoresis of the reduced or reduced-alkylated glomerular basement membrane in sodium dodecyl sulfate has revealed the presence of a large number of components ranging in molecular weight from 25,000 to 220,000 in addition to some material which is too large to penetrate the gel (Hudson and Spiro, 1972b) (Fig. 1). These components have been fractionated first by gel filtration according to size, then by ion exchange chromatography on DEAE- and CM-cellulose according to charge, and finally by polyacrylamide electrophoresis in sodium dodecyl sulfate, again according

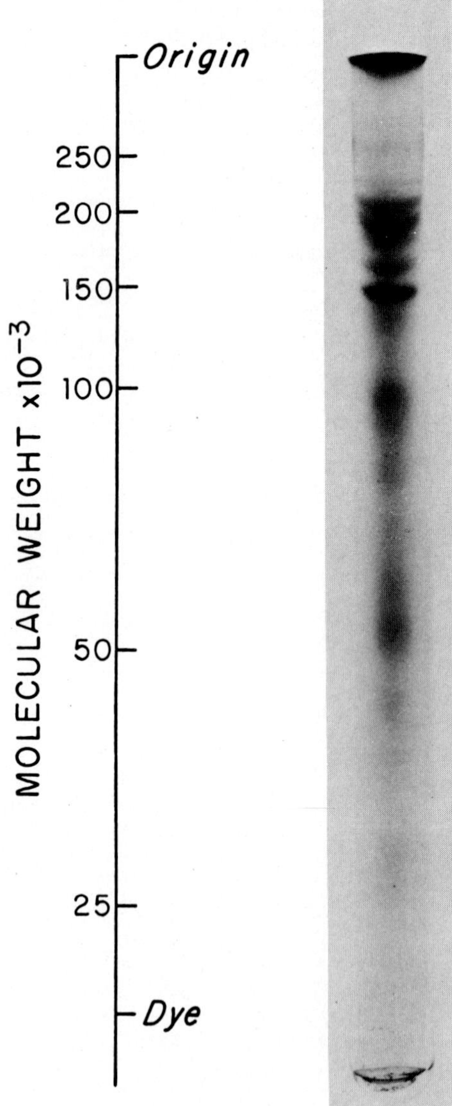

FIG. 1. Migration of subunits of reduced glomerular basement membrane during polyacrylamide-gel electrophoresis in sodium dodecyl sulfate. Molecular weight of components can be determined from scale which is based on electrophoretic movement of reduced standard proteins.

to size, to yield to date about 50 distinct molecular species (Sato and Spiro, unpublished data).

A great variation in the composition of the subunits obtained in this manner was evident (Table 3). Even components of apparently identical molecular weight which would migrate to the same position on polyacrylamide electrophoresis of the unfractionated membrane were found to have quite different amino and sugar contents. Some subunits had a high glycine, hydroxyproline and hydroxylysine content, while others had lower levels of these amino acids and greater amounts of lysine, aspartic acid, half-cystine, and tyrosine. A reciprocal relationship was observed between the number of hydroxylysine and lysine residues so that the sum of these 2 amino acids remained fairly constant (Table 3).

As indicated by their hydroxylysine and glucosamine content, most components were found to contain carbohydrate in the form of disaccharides and heteropolysaccharides although in quite different proportions (Table 3). A small number of subunits obtained by sodium dodecyl sulfate extraction of the unreduced membrane, however, appear to contain their carbohydrate solely in the form of heteropolysaccharide units (Levine and Spiro, unpublished data).

TABLE 3
*Composition of several purified subunits of the bovine glomerular basement membrane**

Constituent†	Subunit+						
	A	B	C	D	E	F	G
(Molecular weight)§	(160,000)		(140,000)	(95,000)		(67,000)	(63,000)
	Residues/1000 total amino acid residues						
Glycine	289	178	173	304	103	116	218
Hydroxyproline	109	57	35	123	15	12	70
Hydroxylysine	42	20	15	39	4	4	22
Lysine	14	27	31	14	38	42	23
Aspartic acid	48	69	75	50	90	92	61
Tyrosine	9	12	18	8	17	22	19
Half-cystine⊕	11	25	30	9	34	43	23
Glucosamine	4	11	15	4	30	27	5

* T. Sato and R. G. Spiro, unpublished data.
† Only values for key amino acids and sugars are given.
+ The subunits are designated arbitrarily by letters A through G; no fixed designation has yet been established.
§ Molecular weight determined by polyacrylamide gel electrophoresis.
⊕ Determined as S-carboxymethylcysteine.

These studies suggest that the glomerular basement membrane is a highly cross-linked structure in which peptide chains varying in size as well as in the proportion of helical (collagen-like) and polar segments which they contain are layered over each other (Fig. 2). Although disulfide bonds appear to be the major cross-links, other interchain linkages are likely to occur, as some very high molecular weight material remains after reduction and alkylation of the membrane. However, a search for lysine or hydroxylysine-derived cross-links such as occur in fibrillar collagens and elastins employing tritiated sodium borohydride as a labeling agent has failed to detect appreciable amounts of these in the basement membrane (Sato and Spiro, unpublished data).

It is of interest that a soluble protein has now been found in the form of the Clq component of human complement (Yonemasu et al., 1971; Reid et al., 1972) which is believed to contain discrete collagen-like and polar regions, such as have been proposed for the peptide chains of the basement membrane (Spiro, 1970).

It is evident from the present investigations that if only a few basic biosynthetic subunits of the basement membrane exist, their identity is masked by the extensive heterogeneity of the components described. This heterogeneity is almost certainly partly due to the multiple postribosomal enzymatic steps operative in basement membrane synthesis including hydroxylation of lysine and proline, assembly of both types of carbohydrate units and the establishment of cross-links between peptide chains (Spiro, 1969). However, physiological degradative processes could also contribute to this remarkable polydispersity and could be brought about by the action of neutral proteases, such as have been found in leukocytes, which are capable of digesting basement membrane (Janoff and Zeligs, 1968). Products of such proteolysis would tend to be attached to the parent structure by disulfide bonds and only become recognizable after chemical cleavage of these bonds in the isolated membrane preparation.

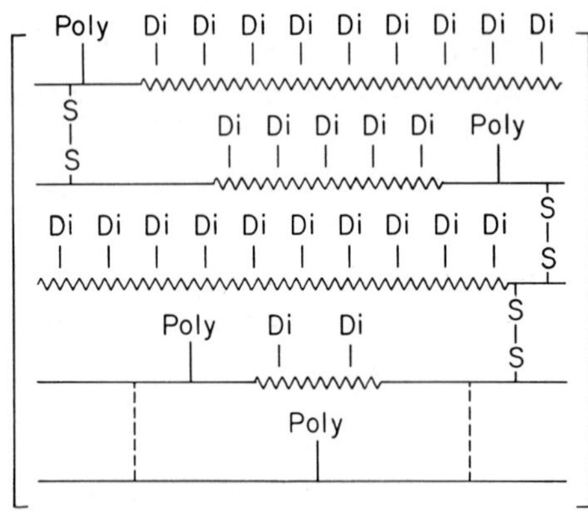

FIG. 2. Diagrammatic representation of a section of the glomerular basement membrane. The positions of disaccharide (Di) and heteropolysaccharide (Poly) units on the peptide chains are shown. It may be noted that the relative proportions of the 'collagen-like' (jagged lines) and more polar segments (straight lines) of the peptide chains vary greatly. Interchain disulfide bonds are indicated but some other as yet undetermined covalent cross-links may also exist. A small number of peptide chains which are quite polar in nature are attached to the membrane by non-covalent bonds (dashed lines).

This proposed subunit make-up of the glomerular basement membrane in which peptide chains containing varying lengths of collagen-like and polar regions coexist may provide a basis for understanding the compositional changes observed in the diabetic membrane. A preferential production in diabetes of subunits rich in collagen-like regions would account for the increased hydroxylysine, glucosylgalactose disaccharide, glycine and hydroxyproline levels, as well as the decreased amounts of lysine and tyrosine observed in the diseased membrane. Differences in other amino acids and sugars would not necessarily be expected, since in compositional studies conducted on the whole membrane changes would only be observed in constituents which vary most strikingly among subunits. Enhanced production of these disaccharide-rich subunits could account for the altered character of the diabetic basement membrane, as the increased number of these bulky saccharide units could interfere sterically with the packing of the peptide chains and thereby lead to increased permeability of the membrane in this disease.

A careful evaluation of the subunit composition of the diabetic membrane will provide the necessary information to assess the validity of this hypothesis.

REFERENCES

BEISSWENGER, P. J. and SPIRO, R. G. (1970): Human glomerular basement membrane: Chemical alterations in diabetes mellitus. *Science, 168,* 596.

BEISSWENGER, P. J. and SPIRO, R. G. (1973): Studies on the human glomerular basement membrane. Composition, nature of the carbohydrate units and chemical changes in diabetes mellitus. *Diabetes, 22,* 180.

BLOODWORTH Jr., J. M. B. (1963): Diabetic microangiopathy. *Diabetes, 12,* 99.

FARQUHAR, M. G., HOPPER Jr., J. and MOON, H. D. (1959): Diabetic glomerulosclerosis: Electron and light microscopic studies. *Amer. J. Pathol., 35,* 721.

HUDSON, B. G. and SPIRO, R. G. (1972a): Studies on the native and reduced alkylated renal glomerular basement membrane. Solubility, subunit size and reaction with cyanogen bromide. *J. biol. Chem., 247,* 4229.

HUDSON, B. G. and SPIRO, R. G. (1972b): Fractionation of glycoprotein components of the reduced alkylated renal glomerular basement membrane. *J. biol. Chem., 247,* 4239.

JANOFF, A. and ZELIGS, J. D. (1968): Vascular injury and lysis of basement membrane in vitro by neutral protease of human leukocytes. *Science, 161,* 702.

KIMMELSTIEL, P., KIM, O. J. and BERES, J. (1962): Studies on renal biopsy specimens with the aid of the electron microscope. I. Glomeruli in diabetes. *Amer. J. clin. Pathol., 38,* 270.

REID, K. B. M., LOWE, D. M. and PORTER, R. R. (1972): Isolation and characterization of C1q, a subcomponent of the first component of complement, from human and rabbit sera. *Biochem. J., 130,* 749.

SPIRO, R. G. (1967a): Studies on the renal glomerular basement membrane. Preparation and chemical composition. *J. biol. Chem., 242,* 1915.

SPIRO, R. G. (1967b): Studies on the renal glomerular basement membrane. Nature of the carbohydrate units and their attachment to the peptide portion. *J. biol. Chem., 242,* 1923.

SPIRO, R. G. (1967c): The structure of the disaccharide unit of the renal glomerular basement membrane. *J. biol. Chem., 242,* 4813.

SPIRO, R. G. (1969): Glycoproteins: Their biochemistry, biology and role in human disease. *New Engl. J. Med., 281,* 991, 1043.

SPIRO, R. G. (1970): Biochemistry of basement membranes. In: *Chemistry and Molecular Biology of the Intercellular Matrix, Vol. I,* pp. 511–534. Editor: E. A. Balazs. Academic Press, London.

SPIRO, R. G. and SPIRO, M. J. (1971): Effect of diabetes on the biosynthesis of the renal glomerular basement membrane. Studies on the glucosyltransferase. *Diabetes, 20,* 641.

YONEMASU, K., STROUD, R. M., NIEDERMEIER, W. and BUTLER, W. T. (1971): Chemical studies on C1q; a modulator of immunoglobulin biology. *Biochem. biophys. Res. Commun., 43,* 1388.

STRUCTURE AND BIOCHEMISTRY OF DEGENERATIVE LESIONS IN DIABETES MELLITUS. PATHOGENESIS OF DIABETIC NEUROPATHY

J. D. WARD

Royal Infirmary, and University of Sheffield, United Kingdom

I regard the nerve in a diabetic as quite different from all other tissues and in reviewing recent work into the pathogenesis of diabetic nerve damage I would like you to bear this important difference in mind. The structural and biochemical changes that we know occur in diabetic nerve vary from time to time and have a definite capacity for return towards normal. It is this known capacity for significant recovery that distinguishes nerve in the diabetic from almost all other tissues, where steady progressive degenerative change seems to be the rule.

STRUCTURAL CHANGES IN DIABETIC NERVE

Here we must consider the myelin sheath, axon, Schwann cell and basement membrane. The most obvious structural change on microscopy is segmental demyelination, beautifully demonstrated by Thomas and Lascelles (1966) in individually teased nerve fibres. This change is seen in most diabetic nerves examined, is much more marked in nerves from patients with significant clinical neuropathy and is more pronounced in diabetic animals who have been poorly controlled (Preston, 1967). However, there is no information in man to indicate whether this change is prominent at an early stage in the life of a diabetic or consistently present in all those diabetics who do not have signs of clinical neuropathy. I personally feel that it is important to establish at what sort of stage in a diabetic's life physical changes develop in the nerves. There is a distinct capacity for recovery in this condition for a prominent feature in such nerves is remyelination and histological studies suggest that demyelination and remyelination are occurring continuously, with a tendency to more demyelination when metabolic control of the diabetic state is poor.

Now since the myelin sheath is made up of a spiral wrapping of the Schwann cell surface membrane around the axon it has always been assumed that segmental demyelination indicated a primary fault in the Schwann cell itself. However, work on segmental demyelination in non-diabetic nerve suggests that such demyelination may result from either a primary disturbance of Schwann cell function or may be secondary to axonal disturbance (Thomas, 1971; Dyck, 1971). At present it is undecided whether demyelination in diabetes is primary or secondary: I would give my vote to primary Schwann cell dysfunction.

Electron microscopic studies have revealed other changes in nerve. Bischoff (1973)

again demonstrated that segmental demyelination was a prominent feature but axonal disintegration was also seen in nearly 30% of his cases with small fibres particularly affected. The Schwann cells appeared to contain cytoplasmic inclusions suggestive of fat droplets, but it is not clear if these differ substantially from similar inclusions known to occur with increasing age. However, similar droplets have been observed in Schwann cells from diabetic dogs where very interestingly Schwann cell damage was occasionally noted in the absence of fibre damage and vice versa (Bloodworth, 1973).

Some thickening of the basement membrane around the Schwann cell and axon seems to occur in diabetic nerve – human, dog and hamster – but quantitative studies similar to those in blood vessels from other tissues have not been made and no biochemical analysis of this basement membrane has been carried out. In the present state of knowledge it is not possible to state where the primary insult occurs in the diabetic nerve. No doubt there is a close and dynamic interrelationship between the Schwann cell, its membrane and the axon, and without a full understanding of these relationships it will remain difficult to do other than speculate.

In some of these histological studies changes have been observed in the small blood vessels supplying nerve changes exactly the same as those described in small vessels elsewhere in the body. However, extensive occlusion of these vessels does not occur and I would take this opportunity of stating that there is no structural evidence whatsoever to support the concept that diffuse vascular disease is the basic cause of damage to the diabetic nerve. Moreover, the clinical features of relapses and remissions along with known structural variations are not easily explained on a vascular basis. A biochemical hypothesis seems much more likely.

BIOCHEMICAL CHANGES IN DIABETIC NERVE

In all biochemical studies of diabetic peripheral nerve extracts of whole nerve have been used and there is very little information available regarding the biochemistry of individual sections of nerve. As with structural changes chemical relationships probably exist between different parts of nerve.

Abnormalities of myelin lipids in diabetes have been reviewed at a previous congress and need only be briefly summarized (Eliasson, 1966; Eliasson and Samet, 1969).

1. Triglyceride, cholesterol and phospholipid synthesis is decreased.
2. A shift of fatty acid spectrum towards unsaturated acids.
3. Depressed incorporation of fatty acids into myelin.
4. Glycogen production is almost nil.
5. Insulin does not increase incorporation of glucose or acetate into lipid.
6. Insulin does seem to facilitate acetate incorporation towards the normal direction.

More recent myelin lipid analysis by Pratt (1969) has revealed a 62% decrease in triglyceride and a 76% increase in cholesterol, but in commenting on this difference in cholesterol concentration it should be stressed that there are differences between animals of different ages, with differing severity of metabolic disease and even in the part of nerve analysed. In detailed fatty acid analysis of diabetic nerve, young animals had a decrease of palmitate, oleate and linoleate with an increase in stearate and polyunsaturated acids, while in the adult only oleate was increased and linoleate decreased.

There seems no doubt that the myelin of diabetic nerve is biochemically different in a number of respects from normal myelin, but none of this helps to tell us why the nerve is brought to this state. Abnormal myelin would suggest that the cell producing it – the Schwann cell – is at fault. Protein electrophoresis and sedimentation of myelin have been performed in one case of human diabetic neuropathy and sedimentation properties were quite different from those of normal myelin, suggesting a serious structural disintegration (Palo et al., 1972). It is thought that myelin proteins are synthesized in the cytoplasm of the Schwann cell and this study would again suggest Schwann cell dysfunction – but primary or secondary?

Perhaps the most interesting biochemical change detected in diabetic nerve in recent years is the accumulation of products of the sorbitol pathway. As there is a 'workshop' devoted to this pathway I will merely review the known facts with respect to nerve:

1. This pathway and its enzymes are present in peripheral nerve, spinal cord and brain.
2. In diabetic nerve sorbitol and fructose accumulate very rapidly as the blood glucose (and nerve glucose) rises (Stewart et al., 1966).
3. Concentrations are directly related to the level of the blood glucose.
4. Concentrations of these products are returned towards normal by control of the blood glucose (Ward et al., 1972).
5. Diabetic nerve manufactures more sorbitol and glucose than normal nerve per unit of supplied glucose (Gabbay, 1969).

The most important question relating to the sorbitol pathway is whether such concentrations of these compounds are harmful to peripheral nerve and if so whether there is any evidence as to how they harm the nerve. There is some evidence that the sorbitol pathway may be related to the Schwann cell – the association of the sorbitol producing enzyme aldose reductase with it (Gabbay and O'Sullivan, 1968), and the demonstration of fructose accumulation in transected nerve at a time when it is known that Schwann cells are proliferating (Stewart et al., 1965). However, this is not direct proof of a damaging effect.

Animals fed galactose accumulate galacticol in their nerves and there is a reduction in electrical nerve conduction (Gabbay, 1972). In rats with high blood levels of myoinositol again motor nerve conduction is impaired, and this fact is always taken as an indication of structural change in nerve (segmental demyelination) (Clements et al., 1973). Here is strong evidence that other sugar alcohols can lead to nerve dysfunction and presumably nerve damage, and this would support the suggestion that in diabetic nerve sorbitol is likewise harmful. I must stress that in both these studies nerves were not examined histologically so segmental demyelination is only inferred. Since it is known that sorbitol accumulation may be kept at a minimum by control of the blood glucose, then here is direct evidence that a complication of the diabetic state may be avoided by simple blood glucose control. As I said earlier, diabetic nerve is different from other tissues, for this claim cannot be made elsewhere in the body.

It has been suggested that sugar alcohols may damage cells by exerting unusual osmotic pressure. However, from the concentrations of sorbitol known to occur in nerve an undue osmotic pressure would not be expected, and in all the electron microscope work so far performed on nerve there is no suggestion of structural changes likely to be due to the affects of undue osmotic pressure (Thomas, personal communication).

The aim of this panel has been to discuss structure and biochemistry, so I have not mentioned the function of peripheral nerve which is to transmit electrical impulses. The study of the passage of an impulse down a nerve is an enormously complex subject and we have very little information regarding the diabetic nerve. The flow of ions in and out of myelin and the axon as well as the electrical potential of the myelin itself must all be considered. Eliasson (1969) has produced some evidence to suggest that the diabetic nerve fibre has a reduced electrical resistance especially at the internode, and has suggested that 'leaky' myelin at the internodes might well be the cause of reduced conduction velocity. I raise this matter to remind you that the answer to the problem of change in the diabetic nerve may lie in such functional abnormalities.

Structure and biochemistry have one important link here, and that is in *function.* Whether segmental demyelination is primary or secondary is yet to be decided, but it is the most prominent finding in diabetic nerve and its presence leads to a delay in electrical nerve conduction. We know that nerve conduction is worse in poorly controlled patients and animals and improves when blood glucose is returned to normal (Gregersen, 1967; Gregersen, 1968; Ward et al., 1971). These facts are in parallel with what we know of segmental demyelination itself. Biochemically we know that sorbitol accumulation is controlled by lowering the blood glucose and as there is a strong suggestion that sugar alcohols lead to nerve damage we can link structure and biochemistry and say that control of the metabolic state prevents damage to the diabetic nerve.

Before summarizing I would like to introduce a concept, namely *vulnerability.* It is known that all nerves with segmental demyelination are vulnerable to insults such as anoxia and trauma, and presumably other unidentified insults. Hence the diabetic nerve is vulnerable. If this vulnerability can be kept at a minimum (by good control of the blood glucose) then significant deterioration in nerve function due to other insults would be unlikely to occur.

SUMMARY

1. Diabetic nerve is different from other nerves and from other diabetic tissues.
2. Segmental demyelination is a prominent finding, *but*
3. Is the Schwann cell primarily or secondarily affected?
4. Lipid droplets occur in the Schwann cell; axons may disintegrate and basement membrane can be thickened. How are they interrelated?
5. Myelin lipid shows a number of quantitative and qualitative abnormalities.
6. Products of the sorbitol pathway accumulate in diabetic nerve and can be limited by blood glucose control.
7. There is evidence that sugar alcohols lead to damage of peripheral nerve. Finally
8. The cause of damage to diabetic nerve is *metabolic, not* vascular.
9. Diabetic nerve damage can be significantly minimized by blood glucose control.

REFERENCES

BISCHOFF, A. (1973): Ultrastructural pathology of peripheral nervous system in early diabetes. In: *Early Diabetes, Suppl. 2 to Advances in Metabolic Disorders,* p. 441. Academic Press, New York and London.

BLOODWORTH, J. M. B. (1973): In: *Early Diabetes, Suppl. 2 to Advances in Metabolic Disorders,* p. 471. Academic Press, New York and London.

CLEMENTS, R. S., De JESUS, P. V. and WINEGRAD, A. I. (1973): Raised plasma myoinositol levels in uraemia and experimental neuropathy. *Lancet, i,* 1137.

DYCK, P. J. (1971): The concept of secondary segmental demyelination. In: *Abstracts, II International Congress on Muscle Disorders, Perth, November 1971,* p. 74. Editors: B. A. Kakulas and A. S. J. Dixon. International Congress Series No. 237, Excerpta Medica, Amsterdam.

ELIASSON, S. G. (1966): Lipid synthesis in peripheral nerve from alloxan diabetic rats. *Lipids, 1,* 237.

ELIASSON, S. G. (1969): Properties of isolated nerve fibres from alloxanized rats. *J. Neurol. Neurosurg. Psychiat., 32,* 525.

ELIASSON, S. G. and SAMET, J. M. (1969): Alloxan induced neuropathies: lipid changes in nerve and root fragments. *Life Scis, 8,* 493.

GABBAY, K. H. and O'SULLIVAN, J. B. (1968): The sorbitol pathway: Enzyme localisation and content in normal and diabetic nerve and cord. *Diabetes, 17,* 239.

GABBAY, K. H. (1969): Factors affecting the sorbitol pathway in diabetic nerve. *Diabetes, 18,* 336.

GABBAY, K. H. (1972): Nerve conduction defects in galactose fed rats. *Diabetes, 21,* 295.

GREGERSEN, G. (1967): Diabetic neuropathy: Influence of age, sex, metabolic control and duration of diabetes on motor conduction velocity. *Neurology, 17,* 972.

GREGERSEN, G. (1968): Variations in motor conduction velocity produced by acute changes in the metabolic state in diabetic patients. *Diabetologia, 4,* 273.

PALO, J., SAVOLAINEN, H. and HALTIA, M. (1972): Proteins of peripheral nerve in diabetic neuropathy. *J. neurol. Scis, 16,* 193.

PRATT, J. H., BERRY, J. S., KAYE, B. and GOETZ, S. C. (1969): Lipid class and fatty acid composition of rat brain and sciatic nerve in alloxan diabetes. *Diabetes, 18,* 556.

PRESTON, G. M. (1967): Peripheral neuropathy in the alloxan diabetic rat. *J. Physiol., 189,* 49.

STEWART, M. A., PASSONNEAU, J. V. and LOWRY, O. H. (1965): Substrate changes in peripheral nerve during ischaemia and Wallerian degeneration. *J. Neurochem., 12,* 719.

STEWART, M. A., SHERMAN, W. R. and ANTHONY, S. (1966): Free sugars in alloxan diabetic rat nerve. *Biochem. biophys. Res. Commun., 22,* 488.

THOMAS, P. K. and LASCELLES, R. G. (1966): The pathology of diabetic neuropathy. *Quart. J. Med., 35,* 489.

THOMAS, P. K. (1971): Morphological basis for alterations in nerve conduction in peripheral neuropathy. *Proc. Roy. Soc. Med., 64,* 295.

WARD, J. D., FISHER, D. J., BARNS, C. G., JESSOP, J. D. and BAKER, R. W. R. (1971): Improvement in nerve conduction following treatment in newly diagnosed diabetics. *Lancet, i,* 428.

WARD, J. D., BAKER, R. W. R. and DAVIES, B. H. (1972): Effect of blood sugar control on the accumulation of sorbitol and fructose in nervous tissue. *Diabetes, 21,* 1173.

THE NATURAL HISTORY OF BASEMENT MEMBRANE DISEASE IN DIABETES MELLITUS*

JOSEPH R. WILLIAMSON, NANCY VOGLER and CHARLES KILO

Departments of Pathology and Internal Medicine, Washington University School of Medicine, St. Louis, Mo., U.S.A.

Although capillary basement membrane thickening clearly occurs with much greater frequency in the diabetic than in the general population, the pathogenesis, the natural history, and the pathophysiological significance of capillary basement membrane disease are poorly understood. The prevalence of basement membrane disease reported by different investigators varies considerably and the nature of the relationship of basement membrane disease to carbohydrate intolerance is still strongly debated. In our opinion most if not all of the published observations and disparate results can be reconciled in light of what is known of the natural history of the mode of onset and rate of progression of carbohydrate intolerance in juvenile-onset and maturity-onset diabetics.

In this discussion of the natural history of diabetic basement membrane disease we will consider 2 questions.

1. What is the time relationship between the development of carbohydrate intolerance and the onset and progression of basement membrane disease, as evidenced by basement membrane thickening in quantitative electron microscopic studies?

2. How do basement membranes thicken?

In order for any study to yield reliable information regarding the precise nature of the relationship between basement membrane disease and carbohydrate intolerance, 3 important requirements must be met. First, the date of onset of carbohydrate intolerance must be known with some accuracy. Second, reliable, sensitive methods must be used for quantitating basement membrane thickening. Third, the assessment of basement membrane thickening in diabetics must be based on comparison with control subjects carefully matched by age and sex to the diabetics. The importance of the last seemingly obvious requirement, attested to by the magnitude of age-related basement membrane thickening and sex differences in basement membrane width in normal subjects (Kilo et al., 1972), can hardly be overemphasized since many published reports are remiss on this point.

Perhaps the major problem in studies of the natural history of basement membrane disease is in dating, with any degree of certainty, the onset of carbohydrate intolerance which may precede the clinical diagnosis of diabetes by many years. Most of the published reports documenting basement membrane disease in diabetes mellitus have been based on studies of maturity-onset diabetics in whom mild to moderate carbohydrate intolerance may be present for years, even decades, before the diagnosis of diabetes is

* These studies have been supported by USPHS grant No. HL 13694, and by gifts from the Upjohn Company, Eli Lily Company, and the St. Louis Diabetes Association.

established. Thus it is quite hazardous to draw any conclusions from such studies regarding which comes first, basement membrane disease or carbohydrate intolerance.

In the so-called juvenile-onset diabetic, the duration of asymptomatic carbohydrate intolerance prior to the time diabetes is diagnosed is generally considered to be much shorter than for the maturity-onset diabetic. Even so, Fajans et al. (1970) and Fajans (1971) have shown that in children and in young adults asymptomatic carbohydrate intolerance may also be present for many years before progressing to overt diabetes. In any case, by focusing our attention on juvenile-onset diabetics for studies of the relationship between carbohydrate intolerance and basement membrane disease, we can eliminate 20–40 years of uncertainty in dating the onset of carbohydrate intolerance.

On the basis of the published reports of Pardo et al. (1972), Osterby-Hansen (1965), and our own studies on 92 juvenile-onset insulin-requiring diabetics, the first statement we would make in answer to question number 1 is that basement membrane disease is virtually non-existent in capillaries of skeletal muscle and glomeruli of diabetics under age 20 in whom the duration of diabetes is less than 6 months at the time of biopsy. In the series of Pardo et al. (1972) there are 4 such individuals all of whose muscle capillary basement membranes are within normal limits. We have 9 such individuals, only 1 of whom has basement membrane thickening (on the basis of 95% confidence limits (Kilo et al., 1972; Williamson et al., 1973)) giving a prevalence of 11%, compared to 12% for age- and sex-matched control subjects. Osterby-Hansen (1965) has similar data based on renal biopsies of newly diagnosed juvenile diabetics.

In subjects under age 20 with a known duration of diabetes of 4 years or less, the prevalence of muscle capillary basement membrane disease is still only 20–25% as reported by 3 different investigators (Pardo et al., 1972; Danowski et al., 1972; and our own data). The agreement is quite good even though different methods of fixation were used and basement membrane width was measured by different techniques. Observations of these same investigators support our second statement in response to question number 1 which is that the prevalence and severity of basement membrane disease increase with longer known duration of carbohydrate intolerance. Our own data on the prevalence of basement membrane disease and duration of carbohydrate intolerance are shown in Table 1. The increasing prevalence of basement membrane thickening with longer known dura-

TABLE 1

Prevalence of muscle capillary basement membrane thickening (BMT) in insulin-requiring diabetics under the age of 20 at the time diabetes was diagnosed

Duration of diabetes (years)	Number of subjects	% with BMT*
0–0.5	9	11
0.5–4	18	22
5–9	30	35
10–19	24	42
20	11	82

* Basement membrane thickening was evaluated on the basis of 95% age- and sex-adjusted confidence limits for mean basement membrane width and for standard deviations (Kilo et al., 1972; Williamson et al., 1973).

tion of diabetes is consistent with clinical experience that the prevalence and severity of other complications (retinopathy, nephropathy, and neuropathy) also increase with longer known duration of diabetes.

It is of interest that the basement membranes of 2 of the 11 subjects with diabetes of 20 years known duration or longer are still within normal limits. Although this suggests that other factors in addition to carbohydrate intolerance may be of importance in the pathogenesis of basement membrane disease, it may also be that these 2 subjects are better controlled than the others.

The failure of many investigators to demonstrate an association between known duration of diabetes and the prevalence and magnitude of basement membrane disease is attributable, at least in part, to the much higher prevalence of basement membrane thickening at the time diabetes is first diagnosed in older subjects. As shown in Table 2,

TABLE 2

Prevalence of muscle capillary basement membrane thickening (BMT) in newly diagnosed diabetics of different ages

Age at diagnosis	Number of subjects	% with BMT*
0–19	10	10
20–39	20	35
40–59	39	44
60–80	16	50

* Basement membrane thickening was evaluated on the basis of 95% age- and sex-adjusted confidence limits for mean basement membrane width and for standard deviations (Kilo et al., 1972; Williamson et al., 1973).

over 40% of newly diagnosed diabetics between ages 40 and 59 already have demonstrable basement membrane disease at the time diabetes is first diagnosed. For the reasons already discussed, such figures or statistics cannot be accepted as evidence that basement membrane disease precedes carbohydrate intolerance.

The likelihood that other as yet unidentified factors influence basement membrane disease, in addition to duration of carbohydrate intolerance, is suggested by the data shown in Figure 1. No basement membrane thickening is discernible in the newly diagnosed group of zero years duration (nor is there any evidence of basement membrane thickening in this group in an analysis of variance). On the other hand significant basement membrane thickening ($T = 2.07$, < 0.05) is already evident in some diabetics in whom the average duration of disease is approximately 2 years. Very little progression of basement membrane disease occurs during the next 10 years, however, in those subjects still under age 20. It is of interest that in the 7 and 13 years duration groups, the onset and most of the known duration of diabetes are prepubertal. In contrast basement membrane disease continues to progress in the 7 and 13 year groups comprised of subjects over age 20. In both of these groups the onset of diabetes is much later than for the under 20 age groups and most of the known duration of diabetes is postpubertal.

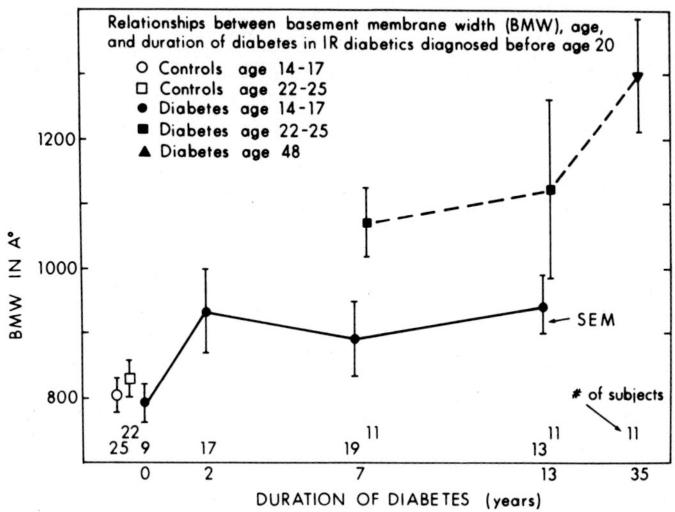

Fig. 1. Relationship between basement membrane width (BMW), age, and duration of diabetes in insulin-requiring diabetics diagnosed before age 20.

It is of interest that these observations are similar to clinical experience that in subjects with the same known duration of diabetes, the prevalence of retinopathy tends to be higher in those subjects in whom diabetes was diagnosed later in life (Caird et al., 1969). It is of particular interest therefore that among subjects with a known duration of diabetes of approximately 13 years, retinopathy is present in 4 of the 11 (36%) subjects over age 20 but is not present in any of the 13 subjects under age 20 ($X^2 = 5.67$, $P < 0.025$). Retinopathy was also present in 5 of the 11 subjects with diabetes of over 20 years duration. Basement membrane thickening was demonstrable in 78% of subjects with retinopathy. The significance of these observations is far from clear. However, they suggest that further studies of juvenile diabetics may provide important clues to the pathogenesis of basement membrane disease in diabetes.

The second question we would like to consider very briefly is 'How does basement membrane thicken?' Morphological and statistical evidence from many published reports (reviewed in Kilo et al., 1972) indicate that the capillary bed is not uniformly affected by basement membrane disease. The excessive accumulation of basement membrane tends to be segmental in distribution. By that we mean that there are longitudinal segments of vessels with thick membranes contiguous with longitudinal segments of vessels with perfectly normal basement membrane. There are also focal asymmetrical accumulations of basement membrane; however, their contribution to the overall accumulation of basement membrane would appear to be much less important than the segmental accumulations (Kilo et al., 1972; Williamson et al., 1973). The segmental and focal character of basement membrane disease suggests that local or regional factors, e.g. vasospasm, ischemia, or leakage of plasma factors which might influence synthesis or degradation of basement membrane, may play an important role in the pathogenesis of basement membrane disease.

In some instances thickened basement membranes appear to be laminated. This observation, coupled with experimental evidence that regenerating capillaries tend to grow back inside the basement membrane sheath of pre-existing capillaries (the cellular elements of which have been lost due to necrosis) to which they add their own newly synthesized basement membrane, has led Vracko and Benditt (1970) to postulate that basement membrane thickening is a quantum event reflecting endothelial cell death. This is a most intriguing hypothesis and it seems very likely that basement membrane thickening may indeed take place in this manner in both normal subjects and diabetics. On the other hand, in our experience, thickened basement membranes are much more often unilaminar than multilaminar which suggests that basement membrane thickening may be accomplished by other mechanisms in addition to that proposed by Vracko and Benditt.

CONCLUSIONS

1. Basement membrane disease is virtually non-existent in newly diagnosed diabetics under age 20 and is uncommon in those in whom the known duration of diabetes is less than 4 years.
2. Diabetic retinopathy and basement membrane disease are influenced by as yet unidentified age-related factors and by duration of carbohydrate intolerance.
3. Basement membrane disease tends to be segmental in character, which suggests that local or regional factors may play an important role in the pathogenesis.

REFERENCES

CAIRD, F. I., PIRIE, A. and RAMSELL, T. G. (1969): The natural history of diabetic retinopathy. In: *Diabetes and The Eye,* pp. 72–100. Blackwell Scientific Publications, Oxford and Edinburgh.

DANOWSKI, T. S., FISHER, E. R., KHURANA, R. C., NOLAN, S. and STEPHAN, T. (1972): Muscle capillary basement membrane in juvenile diabetes mellitus. *Metabolism, 21,* 1125.

FAJANS, S. S., FLOYD Jr., J. C., CONN, J. W. and PEK, S. (1970): The course of asymptomatic diabetes of children, adolescents, and young adults. In: *Early Diabetes,* pp. 377–384. Editors: R. A. Camerini-Davalos and J. S. Cole. Academic Press, New York, N.Y.

FAJANS, S. S. (1971): What is diabetes? Definition, diagnosis, and course. In: *Medical Clinics of North America,* pp. 793–805. Editors: P. Felig and P. K. Bondy. W. B. Saunders, Philadelphia, Pa.

KILO, C., VOGLER, N. and WILLIAMSON, J. R. (1972): Muscle capillary basement membrane changes related to aging and to diabetes mellitus. *Diabetes, 21,* 881.

OSTERBY-HANSEN, R. (1965): A quantitative estimate of the peripheral glomerular basement membrane in recent juvenile diabetes. *Diabetologia, 1,* 97.

PARDO, V., PEREZ-STABLE, E., ALZAMORA, D. B. and CLEVELAND, W. W. (1972): Incidence and significance of muscle capillary basal lamina thickness in juvenile diabetes. *Amer. J. Pathol., 68,* 67.

VRACKO, R. and BENDITT, E. P. (1970): Capillary basal lamina thickening. Its relationship to endothelial cell death and replacement. *J. Cell Biol., 47,* 281.

WILLIAMSON, J. R., VOGLER, N. J. and KILO, C. (1973): Early capillary basement membrane changes in subjects with diabetes mellitus. In: *Vascular and Neurological Changes in Early Diabetes,* pp. 363–367. Editors: R. A. Camerini-Davalos and H. S. Cole. Academic Press, New York, N.Y.

DIABETIC RETINOPATHY: NATURAL HISTORY, PATHOLOGY AND THERAPY

THE PLACE AND THE EFFECT OF PITUITARY ABLATION FOR DIABETIC RETINOPATHY

RUSSELL FRASER, E. M. KOHNER*, G. F. JOPLIN, F. H. DOYLE, A. M. HAMILTON* and R. K. BLACH*

Departments of Medicine and Diagnostic Radiology, Royal Postgraduate Medical School and Retinal Diagnostic Unit, Moorfields Eye Hospital, London, United Kingdom

In 1930 Houssay and Biasotti demonstrated the amelioration of diabetes which follows pituitary ablation, and when cortisol became available for postoperative maintenance, hypophysectomy became possible in man. In 1955 Luft et al. first did therapeutic hypophysectomy to curb the progress of severe active diabetic retinopathy, at a time when no other treatments were available. Since then, well over a thousand patients with diabetic retinopathy have had various types of pituitary ablation done to arrest the progress of retinopathy. A recent series of reports was collected in the Airlie House Symposium of 1968 (Goldberg and Fine, 1969). Since then 5 year follow-up examinations have become available, and also the alternative treatment, photocoagulation, has become established. So we must reassess the place of pituitary ablation.

WHY SHOULD PITUITARY ABLATION HELP?

Pituitary ablation (PA) removes several insulin antagonists, especially growth hormone; it decreases insulin requirements by nearly half (Joplin et al., 1965) and also reduces the tendency of the diabetic's blood sugar to rise during his normal overnight fast (Oakley et al., 1967a). Obviously, it will also curb the growth hormone overproduction which Hansen (1970, 1971) has shown to be a diabetic feature, and one eliminated only by meticulous blood sugar-managed diabetic control, stricter than any used in clinical management. We found that after pituitary ablation the amelioration of the retinopathy was correlated with the completeness of the elimination of growth hormone secretion (Wright et al., 1969) and we and others have also found that the retinopathy response is better after complete rather than slight ablation (Joplin et al., 1967; Pearson et al., 1969; Teuscher et al., 1966). PA also keeps the cortisol and thyroxine supply down to maintenance levels – this too may be of importance in ameliorating diabetic retinopathy.

DATA AVAILABLE TO ASSESS PITUITARY ABLATION FOR DIABETIC RETINOPATHY

Diabetic retinopathy is well known to vary in severity, in the rate of its progress and also

* Supported by grants from the Wellcome Trust.

in the main signs to be seen in the fundus. So objective methods of evaluating its treatment are obviously necessary, and also a control series selected by a random procedure to assess the rate of progress without any specific treatment. Visual acuity determination to record preservation of sight is clearly the most important criterion, provided the follow-up continues long enough. This also has to be supplemented by assessment of the retinopathy features, in order to appraise which features do or do not respond to the treatment. For this purpose, we have used the Hammersmith Grading System (Oakley et al., 1967b). This is a photographic method in which each eye's status is graded by comparison with a standard set of reference photographs for each of the following retinopathy features – (1) haemorrhages and microaneurysms, (2) new vessels, (3) fibrous retinitis proliferans, and (4) hard exudates.

In the following review of how PA can influence diabetic retinopathy, we shall draw mostly on our experience at Hammersmith, accumulated in a collaborative study involving both ophthalmologists and physicians; but we shall indicate where other workers confirm or disagree with our findings (Joplin et al., 1965; Joplin et al., 1967; Kohner et al., 1971, 1972). In earlier years, PA was performed for the full range of diabetic retinopathy encountered, provided sight was in some degree impaired but not yet clearly lost; and unless uraemia (blood urea > 75 mg/100 ml) or severe cardiovascular disease obviously precluded it. Later, as the characteristics of the irreversible and the reversible eyes became more clearly defined, only cases showing severe but still reversible retinopathy have been chosen. During the last year we have excluded subjects over 45 years of age or with any uraemia (i.e. blood urea > 50 mg/100 ml).

First, to assess which features can or cannot improve after pituitary ablation, we shall examine the 1-year outcome of the main diabetic retinopathy features among our patients in whom maximal ablation was obtained. Secondly, we shall assess the effects of PA by contrasting the outcome seen among our series of 52 patients randomly allocated either to PA or to being followed as controls (Kohner et al., 1972). The only other such randomly allocated trial which has been published, that by Lundbaek et al. (1969), shows similar trends. Finally, we shall follow the results seen in the 2 groups of patients for whom we now feel PA is most indicated, i.e., those without significant fibrous retinitis proliferans but with either (1) new vessels on the disc, or (2) 'florid' diabetic retinopathy, i.e., severe widespread new vessels. From our subjects followed over 5 years after an adequate pituitary ablation, we have selected those who originally showed these retinal features in one or more eyes and will present their general and visual outcome.

FEATURES PITUITARY ABLATION DOES NOT MODIFY

Figure 1 shows the Hammersmith Grading for various retinopathy features before and at 1-year follow-up after maximal pituitary ablation. This shows on the one hand that PA, even when maximal by endocrine testing, does not alter the extent of hard exudates or of fibrous retinitis proliferans. Thus, we can recognise that PA has no place in the treatment of hard exudates or maculopathy, nor would it be expected to reverse fibrous retinitis proliferans. Therefore, we exclude from this treatment patients with both eyes irreversible by these features, or with either visual acuity under 6/24 or fibrous retinitis proliferans threatening the macula.

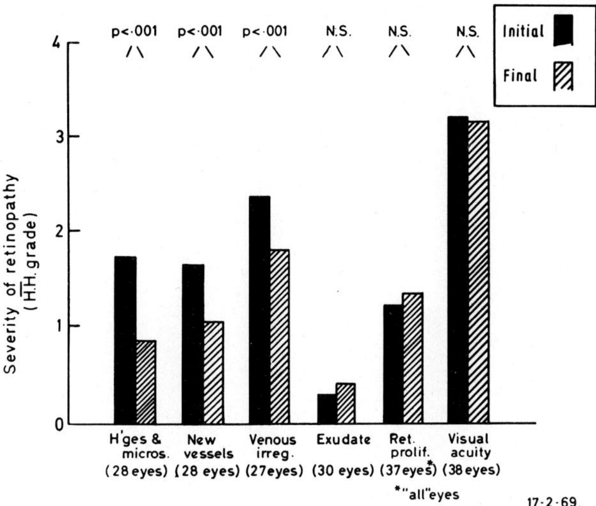

FIG. 1. Hammersmith grading of various diabetic retinopathy features before and at one year after maximal pituitary ablation (From Oakley et al., 1967b, by courtesy).

WHERE CAN PITUITARY ABLATION HELP?

The same Figure 1 shows that PA can lessen haemorrhages and microaneurysms, new vessels and venous abnormalities; but also that it usually lessens them rather than that it eliminates them. When is this rather drastic treatment worth trying? Figure 2 compares the visual acuity of patients from our randomised trial who had new vessels arising from the disc at their first visit. It shows that by the sixth year the mean visual acuity was still between 6/6 and 6/12 for the treated subjects, but less than 6/60 for the control series, all but one of whom were blind.

We can also look at a wider sampling of all our 45 patients (66 eyes) whose initial photographs showed new vessels on the disc, before their pituitary implants done from 1960 to 1969 (Fig. 3). Here we contrast the different grades of pituitary ablation. Figure 3 shows that the visual acuity of those only slightly ablated behaves rather like that of our control subjects of Figure 2; but the others with more complete ablation had their sight preserved beyond 4 years follow-up. The associated assessments of their retinopathy features also show the retinopathy responses behind this. Among the maximally ablated, regression was seen in the new vessel grading, and in addition there was no tendency to an increase of the fibrous retinitis proliferans, a feature seen among those but slightly ablated.

We have also assessed the preservation of eyesight found among subjects followed over 5 years beyond pituitary ablation for either disc new vessels or florid diabetic retinopathy (Table 1). With 'florid' retinopathy, we find that sight has been preserved in over 75% (Fig. 4). We are at present collecting our control data on the outcome from such florid retinopathy without pituitary ablation – from some earlier patients followed without ablation, and some subjects more recently treated by photocoagulation. The present indications are that sight is not preserved in these patients (Hamilton et al., 1973). It is

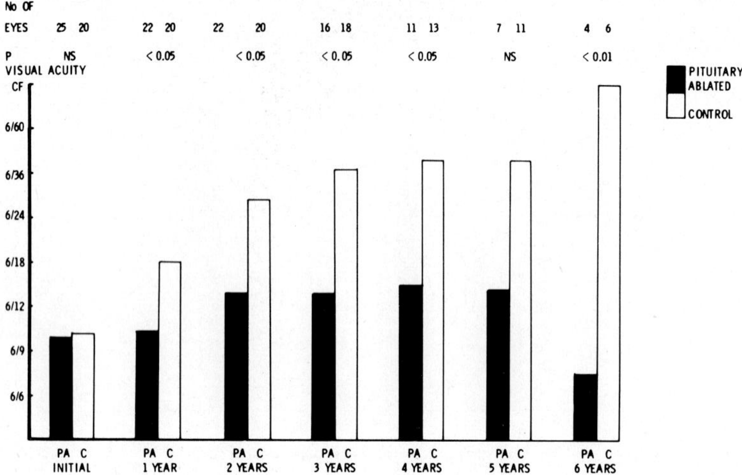

FIG. 2. Progress of the mean visual acuity among patients with new vessels on the disc, randomly selected for pituitary ablation or control (From Kohner et al., 1972, by courtesy).

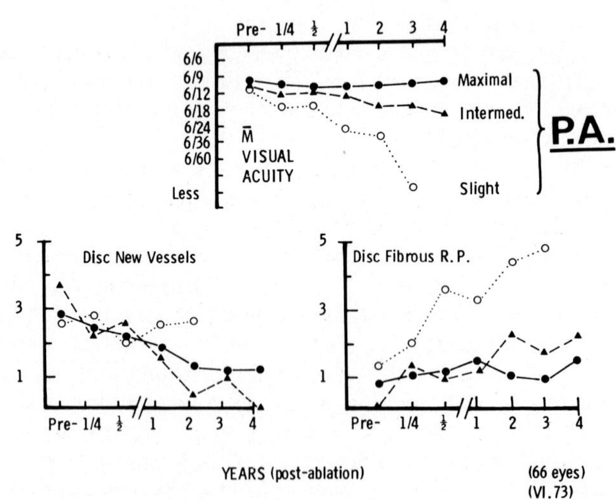

FIG. 3. Comparison of 45 patients (66 eyes) with new vessels arising from the optic disc, grouped according to the degree of pituitary ablation achieved (maximal, intermediate or slight), as regards the subsequent progress of visual acuity, the mean grading of new vessels on the disc and the mean grading for the associated retinitis proliferans (Adapted from Panisset et al., 1971, by courtesy).

TABLE 1

Preservation of eyesight (visual acuity > 6/24) after adequate pituitary ablation over 5 years ago, for reversible proliferative diabetic retinopathy including new vessels

	Sample		% Sight preserved		
	Patients	Eyes	Mean Follow-up (years)	Patients	Eyes
'Florid'*	10	12	4.5	100%	75%
'Treatable'+	27	41	4.4	81%	78%

* Defined as extensive new vessels (grade 4 or worse Hammersmith Grading in at least 2 photographic fields).
\+ Defined as similar lesser new vessels without inevitable threats to eyesight (VA over 6/24 and no fibrous retinitis proliferans threatening the macula).

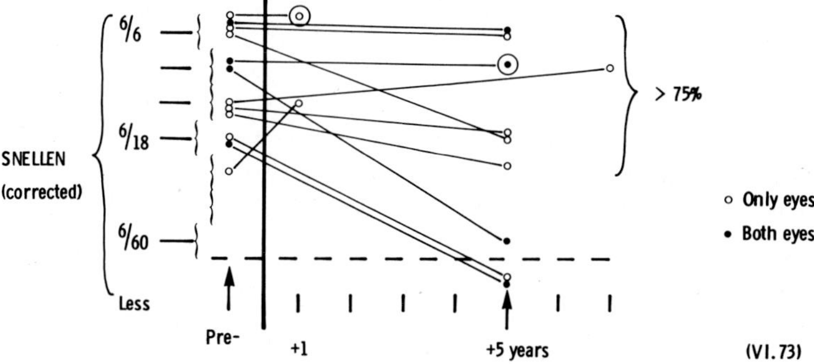

FIG. 4. Progress in visual acuity among 10 patients (12 eyes) followed over 5 years after adequate pituitary ablation for 'florid' retinopathy.

already recognised that new vessels from the disc in diabetic retinopathy seriously worsen the prognosis (Kohner et al., 1971).

Finally, there is data available from a follow-up beyond 5 years among our subjects in whom maximal pituitary ablation was achieved for a reversible diabetic retinopathy including new vessels of less than 'florid' severity, often but not always involving the disc (Fig. 5). Again, preservation of sight beyond 5 years is the usual outcome; a comparable outcome has been reported by Field (personal communication). Thus, reversible diabetic retinopathy may have its remission accelerated by pituitary ablation and then sight preservation is the usual expectation after 5 years, provided the subjects also have reasonably good diabetic supervision, and they have been suitably selected having at least one reversible eye. Good results can be expected even in those with new vessels of 'florid' extent or arising from the disc.

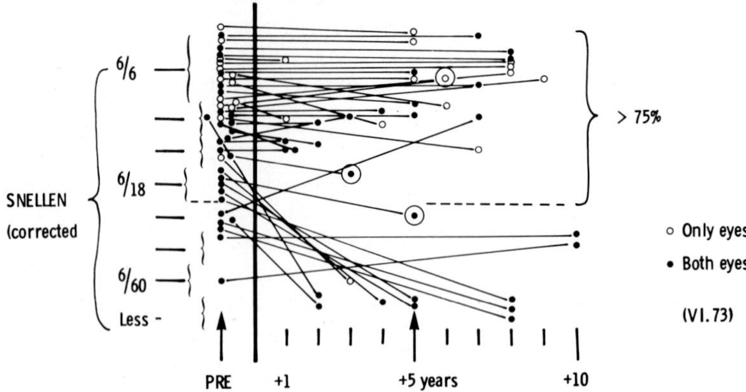

FIG. 5. Progress in visual acuity followed over 5 years after maximal pituitary ablation for 'treatable' diabetic retinopathy (i.e. with new vessels less than 'florid'; 27 patients, 41 eyes).

But what of the patient's general health? Many hypopituitary patients have now been managed for years on the available maintenance therapy with apparently good preservation of health. In the early years of managing these diabetic patients, it seemed that satisfactory general health could be maintained with the usual steroid and thyroxine maintenance. However, we must remember that they have been selected as subjects showing in their retinae a rapidly advancing diabetic microangiopathy, and presumably their other vessels are also affected. Our patients, followed for 5 years, have revealed a disturbingly high incidence of late (after one and a half years) cardiovascular or renal deaths. Many developed hypertension and/or uraemia (Fig. 6). We are at present ascertaining corresponding figures for our control series. Clearly, it is wise to recognise the serious prognostic import of proliferative diabetic retinopathy, and unwise to advise pituitary ablation to save sight, except in young subjects free of uraemia and of signs of serious cardiovascular disease.

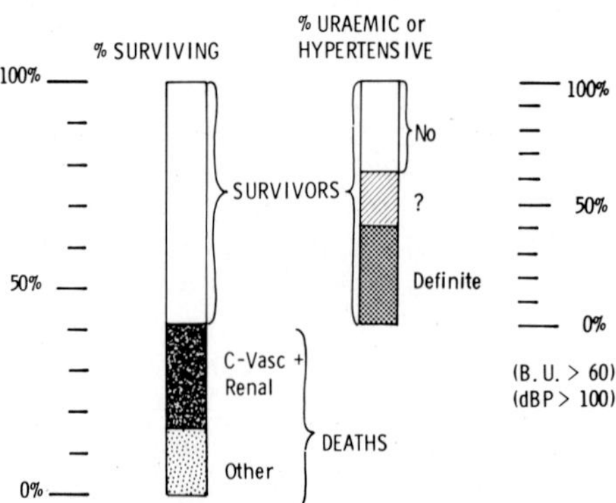

FIG. 6. The percentage survival with and without hypertension (diastolic blood pressure > 100) or uraemia (blood urea > 60 mg/100 ml), at 5 years after adequate pituitary ablation for 'florid' or other treatable diabetic retinopathy (37 patients).

SUMMARY AND CONCLUSIONS

1. Adequate (or maximal) pituitary ablation ameliorates haemorrhages, microaneurysms, new vessels and venous abnormalities in diabetic retinopathy but leaves unaltered fibrous retinitis proliferans and hard exudates.
2. At 5 years after adequate pituitary ablation, among diabetic subjects with originally reversible new vessels either arising from the disc or of 'florid' extent, eyesight is preserved in over 75% of eyes, but over 60% of subjects have either been lost from a cardiovascular/renal 'late' death or developed signs of increased uraemia or hypertension.
3. Therefore, only subjects with reversible retinopathy including new vessels either of 'florid' extent or arising from the disc, should be considered for PA, and only if they are young and of normal renal function. PA can usually preserve their eyesight over 5 years, but their risks from cardiovascular/renal disease are still high.

ACKNOWLEDGEMENTS

For help in the collection and analysis of this data we are indebted to many colleagues, notably to Professor David Hill, Mr. Hung Cheng, Dr. Nigel Oakley and to Miss Barbara Sutcliffe. We are also greatly indebted to the Wellcome Trust for their support in the many aspects of this work.

REFERENCES

GOLDBERG, M. F. and FINE, S. L. (1969): *Symposium on the Treatment of Diabetic Retinopathy*, pp. 1–853. Editors: M. R. Goldberg and S. L. Fine. United States Public Health Service Publication 1890.

HAMILTON, A. M., KOHNER, E. M., BLACH, R. K., CHENG, H., BOWBYES, J., JOPLIN, G. F. and FRASER, T. R. (1973): Florid diabetic retinopathy. In preparation.

HANSEN, A. P. (1970): Abnormal serum growth hormone response to exercise in juvenile diabetics. *J. clin. Invest., 49,* 1467.

HANSEN, A. P. (1971): Normalization of growth hormone hyperresponse to exercise in juvenile diabetics after 'normalization' of blood sugar. *J. clin. Invest., 50,* 1806.

HOUSSAY, B. A. and BIASOTTI, A. (1930): Hypophysectomie et diabète pancreatique. *Arch. int. Pharmacodyn., 38,* 250.

JOPLIN, G. F., FRASER, T. R., HILL, D. W., OAKLEY, N. W., SCOTT, D. J. and DOYLE, F. H. (1965): Pituitary ablation for diabetic retinopathy. *Quart. J. Med., 35,* 443.

JOPLIN, G. F., OAKLEY, N. W., HILL, D. W., KOHNER, E. M. and FRASER, T. R. (1967): Diabetic retinopathy. II. Comparison of disease remission induced by various degrees of pituitary ablation by Y-90. *Diabetologia, 3,* 406.

KOHNER, E. M., DOLLERY, C. T., FRASER, T. R. and BULPITT, C. J. (1970): Effect of pituitary ablation on diabetic retinopathy studied by fluorescence angiography. *Diabetes, 19,* 703.

KOHNER, E. M., PANISSET, A., CHENG, H. and FRASER, T. R. (1971): Diabetic retinopathy: New vessels arising from the optic disc. 1. Grading system and natural history. *Diabetes, 20,* 816.

KOHNER, E. M., JOPLIN, G. F., BLACH, R. K., CHENG, H. and FRASER, T. R. (1972): Pituitary ablation in the treatment of diabetic retinopathy. (A randomised trial). *Trans. ophthal. Soc. U.K., XCII,* 79.

LUFT, R., OLIVECRONA, H. and SJÖGREN, B. (1955): Hypophysectomy in man: Experiences in severe diabetes mellitus. *J. clin. Endocr., 15,* 391.

LUNDBAEK, K., MALMROS, R., ANDERSEN, H. C., RASMUSSEN, J. H., BRUNTSE, E., MADSEN, P. H. and JENSEN, V. A. (1969): Hypophysectomy for diabetic angiopathy: A controlled clinical trial. In: *Symposium on the Treatment of Diabetic Retinopathy, Chapter 25,* pp. 291–311. Editors: M. F. Goldman and S. L. Fine. United States Public Health Service Publication 1890.

OAKLEY, N. W., WRIGHT, A. D., FRASER, T. R. and HASLAM, R. M. (1967a): Fasting blood sugar and serum growth hormone in hypopituitary diabetics. *Lancet, 1,* 523.

OAKLEY, N. W., HILL, D. W., JOPLIN, G. F., KOHNER, E. M. and FRASER, T. R. (1967b): Diabetic retinopathy. I. The assessment of severity and progress by comparison with a set of standard fundus photographs. *Diabetologia, 3,* 402.

PANISSET, A., KOHNER, E. M., CHENG, H. and FRASER, T. R. (1971): Diabetic retinopathy: New vessels arising from the optic disc. II. Response to pituitary ablation by yttrium 90 implant. *Diabetes, 20,* 824.

PEARSON, O. H., THOMAS, C. I., KAUFMAN, B., SHEALY, C. N., COLLINS Jr., W. F., JANE, J. and JACKSON, C. C. R. (1969): Pituitary ablation in the treatment of diabetic retinopathy. In: *Symposium on the Treatment of Diabetic Retinopathy, Chapter 28,* pp. 331–339. Editors: M. F. Goldberg and S. L. Fine. United States Public Health Service Publication 1890.

TEUSCHER, A., FANKHAUSER, S., GIRAND, J. and WYSS, F. (1966): The significance of endocrine activity in hypophysectomized diabetics. *Helv. med. Acta, 33,* 29.

WRIGHT, A. D., KOHNER, E. M., OAKLEY, N. W., HARTOG, M., JOPLIN, G. F. and FRASER, T. R. (1969): Serum growth hormone levels and the response of diabetic retinopathy to pituitary ablation. *Brit. med. J., 2,* 346.

DIABETIC RETINOPATHY – NATURAL COURSE*

MATTHEW D. DAVIS, F. L. MYERS, R. L. ENGERMAN,
G. DE VENECIA and G. H. BRESNICK

Department of Ophthalmology, University of Wisconsin, Madison, Wis., U.S.A.

Our responsibility in this panel discussion is to present the common ophthalmoscopic features of 'diabetic retinopathy' and to illustrate the typical course followed. We have followed several hundred patients for periods of one to several years with serial stereoscopic fundus photography. Strong clinical impressions have resulted, but we are not yet satisfied with our attempts at quantitation of photographic findings and shall restrict this presentation to a qualitative description of what we consider to be characteristic fundus findings. Similar observations have been made by many other workers and we claim no priority for the concepts to be discussed. Furthermore, we cannot provide convincing direct evidence for most of the pathogenetic inferences to be drawn and they must be considered speculative.

All physicians are familiar with the lesion generally considered to be most characteristic of diabetic retinopathy, the capillary microaneurysm. It is often difficult to be certain whether a specific red dot is an aneurysm or a punctate hemorrhage, but for clinical purposes this distinction is not necessary and we may conveniently refer to punctate red spots as 'punctate hemorrhages and/or microaneurysms'. Actually, most such lesions are probably aneurysms, especially those that show a central light reflex and/or remain unchanged in appearance over periods of many months. When the wall of the aneurysm becomes thickened, a white ring may be seen surrounding the red dot which represents blood in the lumen of the aneurysm. As the wall of the aneurysm becomes thicker and more opaque, the red dot with a white ring around it becomes a white dot, since the blood within the lumen of the aneurysm, if a lumen is still present, is completely obscured.

Patients do not develop visual symptoms on the basis of microaneurysms, unless leakiness of their walls leads to retinal edema which extends into the macula. Such edema is the most common cause of decreased visual acuity in non-proliferative diabetic retinopathy. That retinal edema originates from microaneurysms (and/or adjacent capillaries) with excessively permeable walls can be deduced from the fundus appearance with stereoscopic ophthalmoscopy. Characteristically, a group of several aneurysms can be seen near the center of a disc-shaped zone of thickened retina. Since this thickened retina retains

* Supported in part by Grant EY00342 from the National Institutes of Health, U.S. Public Health Service.

near normal transparency, it cannot be easily appreciated without a stereoscopic examining method. Typically, a ring of hard exudates can be seen surrounding the zone of edematous retina. The morphology of this complex of lesions strongly suggests that the lipid comprising the hard exudate came from the plasma through the walls of the aneurysms and was deposited at the edge of the edematous zone, where, it seems, the fluid, electrolytes and other small molecules which leaked out with the lipid have been resorbed into the circulation through capillary walls having more nearly normal permeability. These areas of retinal edema can be seen anywhere in the posterior one-third to one-half of the retina, but symptoms are produced only when the macula is involved.

The appearance described above is typical of adult-onset diabetics with non-proliferative retinopathy. In younger patients with proliferative diabetic retinopathy, it is much less common to see the typical rings of hard exudate, although macular edema is not uncommon. When macular edema has been present for a long time (probably several months), clear cystoid spaces become visible in the retina.

Another arrangement of lesions characteristic of diabetic retinopathy consists of a few red spots, presumably microaneurysms, and one or more tiny, barely visible, dilated retinal vessels arranged around one or two faint 'soft exudates', or cotton-wool patches. Ashton and Harry (1963), and subsequently others, have demonstrated that these ill-defined white spots in the inner retinal layers are areas of focal ischemia caused by closure of small zones of the capillary bed. Trypsin digest preparations of such areas demonstrate the central zone of occluded capillaries, which show loss of endothelial cells and intramural pericytes. The adjacent microaneurysms are also very clearly demonstrated as are the dilated vessels, barely visible in fundus photographs. These dilated vessels, generally termed 'shunt vessels', as suggested by Cogan and Kuwabara (1963), show marked hypertrophy and hypercellularity. Cogan and Kuwabara suggested that the intramural pericytes may have a vasomotor function, and put forward the hypothesis that a selective loss of such cells in diabetic retinopathy may lead to shunt vessel formation with diversion of blood flow from adjacent areas of the capillary bed and their subsequent atrophy. However, the 'shunt vessels' have not been convincingly demonstrated clinically or histopathologically prior to the development of occluded capillaries. Moreover, most observers agree that flow through such vessels appears slower than normal, not more rapid, as would be expected if they were functioning as shunts. At the present time it seems more likely that capillary closure is the earlier lesion. The hypertrophic vessels seem to represent vasoproliferation, perhaps in response to ischemia resulting from capillary closure, perhaps as a direct result of rheological disturbances. Presumably, such vessels frequently represent hypertrophy of pre-existing channels, but, at least occasionally, they seem best interpreted as actual intraretinal neovascularization. The term 'intraretinal microvascular abnormalities' has been suggested for these vessels (Davis et al., 1969) and, although cumbersome, provides a designation which at least has the virtue of making no assumptions regarding their origin or functional role.

Until a better theory is suggested, we believe both microaneurysms and intraretinal microvascular abnormalities are best explained as proliferation of endothelium as the result of deficient blood flow.

The typical irregularities in the retinal veins generally designated 'beading' also seem best explained as vasoproliferation. These venous changes occur typically after the development of microaneurysms, 'shunt vessels' and cotton-wool patches, and their development suggests that new vessels may soon make their appearance on the inner surface of the retina.

Although proliferation of endothelial cells seems to be an important part of diabetic retinopathy early in its evolution, the term 'proliferative diabetic retinopathy' is conventionally reserved for eyes in which newly formed blood vessels and/or fibrous tissue are present on the inner surface of the retina or further forward in the vitreous cavity. Such vessels frequently arise from the optic disc or along the course of the larger retinal veins. Initially they appear 'bare', but semi-opaque 'fibrous' tissue often becomes visible adjacent to them within a few months. The new vessels typically follow a cycle of proliferation and regression. Regression is usually only partial, but occasionally a new vessel network may disappear completely, leaving a varying amount of fibrous tissue in its wake. The new vessels and fibrous tissue create strong adhesions between the retina and the vitreous.

New vessels may proliferate and regress over a period of several years, while vision remains good. Eventually, however, in most eyes with proliferative diabetic retinopathy contraction of the vitreous and/or the fibrous tissue accompanying the vessels occurs, pulling some of the new vessels forward into the vitreous cavity. Vitreous hemorrhage frequently begins at this time and typically recurs periodically over the next several years. If adhesions between the retina, new vessels and vitreous are strong, detachment of the retina often occurs, frequently involving the macula. Vitreous hemorrhage and retinal detachment are the 2 major causes of visual impairment in the proliferative stage of diabetic retinopathy.

Although the course described above is considered 'typical', it is important to emphasize that prediction of the course which will be followed in any individual eye is very difficult. Which eyes will show marked regression of new vessels and when such regression will begin cannot be accurately assessed. For this reason, cause and effect conclusions regarding any individual eye are not justified. An eye that does well *following* any type of treatment cannot be assumed to have done well *because* of the treatment. Prospective, randomized controlled studies are necessary for evaluation of treatment of diabetic retinopathy.

In summary, from the clinical point of view, 4 processes appear to be occurring in diabetic retinopathy:

1. Increased permeability of vessels.
2. Closure of capillaries (and larger vessels).
3. Proliferation of endothelium.
4. Contraction of fibrous tissue and/or vitreous.

The interrelationships of these processes are not entirely clear, but for the present it seems reasonable to look upon this common and distressing manifestation of diabetes as a gradually increasing failure of retinal circulation during which some poorly understood stimulus leads to an attempt at compensating vasoproliferation. This in turn, because of anatomic peculiarities of the eye, often leads to vitreous hemorrhage, retinal detachment and blindness.

REFERENCES

ASHTON, N. and HARRY, J. (1963): The pathology of cotton wool spots and cytoid bodies in hypertensive retinopathy and other diseases. *Trans. ophthalmol. Soc. U.K.*, *83*, 91.

COGAN, D. G. and KUWABARA, T. (1963): Capillary shunts in the pathogenesis of diabetic retinopathy. *Diabetes, 12,* 293.

DAVIS, M. D., NORTON, E. W. D. and MYERS, F. L. (1969): The Airlie classification of diabetic retinopathy. In: *Symposium on the Treatment of Diabetic Retinopathy, Chapter 2,* pp. 7–22. Editors: M. F. Goldberg and S. L. Fine. U. S. Government Printing Office, Washington, D.C.

THE CONTRIBUTION OF FLUORESCENCE ANGIOGRAPHY TO THE UNDERSTANDING OF DIABETIC RETINOPATHY*

C. T. DOLLERY and EVA M. KOHNER

Departments of Clinical Pharmacology and Medicine, Royal Postgraduate Medical School, London, United Kingdom

Fluorescence angiography (Novotny and Alvis, 1961) has made 3 major contributions to the understanding of diabetic retinopathy. The first of these has been an improvement in the clinical recognition of vascular changes, especially those in the capillary bed (Kohner et al., 1967). The second has been measurements of the rate of change of capillary lesions by repeated examinations of the same area. Fluorescence angiography has also made it possible to examine the validity of a number of hypotheses concerning the pathogenesis of retinal vascular changes in diabetes.

Techniques used to obtain fluorescence angiograms of the retina are well established (Wise et al., 1971), and this account is confined to the information derived from such studies.

THE RECOGNITION OF MICROVASCULAR LESIONS

Thorough examination of the retina by means of the ophthalmoscope and slit lamp make it possible to identify a great many of the features of diabetic retinopathy during a routine clinical examination. However, individual normal capillaries cannot be resolved by these techniques and thus it is extremely difficult to detect areas where the capillaries are not perfused. It can also be difficult to differentiate small rounded blot haemorrhages from microaneurysms. Many more microaneurysms are visible on fluorescence angiograms than on colour pictures (Novotny and Alvis, 1961; Scott et al., 1964; Norton and Gutman, 1965; Oosterhuis and Lammens, 1965). Microaneurysms can occur in any part of the capillary bed but pathological descriptions suggest that they are most numerous at the venous end of capillaries. The retinal veins drain from the deep capillary bed and it might be anticipated that the majority of microaneurysms would be in this layer. Stereoscopic fluorescence angiograms of the macula region do not support this view, as aneurysms are present in both deep and superficial layers.

One of the most striking findings on fluorescence angiograms of diabetics is the frequency of areas of capillary non-perfusion. These are often present in early cases although in this instance the size of the areas involved is small. In patients with severe retinopathy large areas of retina, sometimes 2 or 3 disc diameters across, may not be perfused.

* This work was supported by the Wellcome Trust.

Arterial lesions and arteriosclerosis in diabetic retinopathy have long been recognised (Ashton, 1953) but fluorescence angiograms have revealed a number of additional features. Arteries that cross areas of capillary closure often leak fluorescein into their wall. These vessels sometimes have pouches on each side which probably represent pruned-off side branches. Minute arterioles feeding areas of cotton wool spots are usually extremely narrowed or occluded and they frequently leak fluorescein.

Venous dilatation and beading with formation of bizarre venous loops are common features of patients with severe retinopathy and are readily detected with the ophthalmoscope. An additional abnormality demonstrated by fluorescence angiography is diffuse leakage of fluorescein from some of these abnormal segments of large veins.

Small tufts of new vessels are particularly readily detected by fluorescence angiography because in common with other types of neovascularisation they leak fluorescein profusely. Abnormal dilating intraretinal capillaries which later evolve into a new vessel system may also sometimes be detected by their leakage on fluorescence angiograms.

Although the detection of these additional features by fluorescence angiography is of value in improving clinical description of the disease, their main use is in serial studies to evaluate the rate of progression.

THE RATE OF CHANGE OF VASCULAR ABNORMALITIES IN DIABETES

It is difficult to derive a quantitative measurement of the severity of diabetic retinopathy. There are many different features, not all of which may be present and not all of which progress at the same rate. Grading systems using colour photographs have been devised at Hammersmith Hospital (Oakley et al., 1967) and proposals for a grading system were put forward at the O'Hare meeting in 1969. These methods can be used for evaluating the rate of progression of the disease, but they are insensitive. More precise and sensitive methods have been devised by studying the rate of progression of individual features such as microaneurysms and cotton wool spots over a period of time.

Kohner and Dollery (1970) obtained a series of fluorescence angiograms of the same area of retina in diabetic patients over periods up to 3 years. They identified the individual aneurysms present in the defined area on the first occasion, and examined subsequent photographs to see whether each individual feature was still present or had disappeared. From this examination they were able to derive the rate of disappearance of the microaneurysms. Similarly, by observing the appearance of new aneurysms, they could measure the rate of formation. The measurement proved to be reproducible and the rate of disappearance was similar in patients with moderate and severe retinopathy, although the former had more microaneurysms per mm^2 of retina than the latter. The disappearance rate was faster in the first few months of observation than later when it averaged about 0.9 and 1% per month respectively. Thus retinal microaneurysms proved to be long-lived structures. The longevity of capillary aneurysms in diabetes might be because the damage to the capillary bed is irreversible. However, a study of a group of patients who had pituitary ablation showed a much higher rate of microaneurysms (4.1% per month), suggesting that the slow rate of disappearance in the other patients was because vascular damaging factors persisted, rather than that the aneurysms themselves could not be remodelled and disappear.

Further evidence for a slow rate of turnover of capillary abnormalities in diabetes has come from the serial study of areas of capillary closure and cotton wool spots. The area of cotton wool spots on a colour photograph can be measured at intervals over a period of time. In treated malignant hypertensives the average time for the area of cotton wool spots to shrink to half its initial value was 36 weeks (n = 4). However, in diabetic patients under 40 years, the rate of progression was a great deal slower, the average time to reach half the initial area being approximately 30 weeks (n = 5). In patients treated by pituitary ablation the rate of disappearance of cotton wool spots was much higher, the half disappearance time being 2 months (Kohner et al., 1969).

The explanation for this finding may be related to the speed of revascularisation of the capillary bed and the macrophages which phagocytose the swollen and disrupted axons of nerve fibre which compose the cotton wool spots. In hypertension which is treated successfully the capillary bed is restored to normal within a few weeks. In diabetes areas of capillary closure often persist unchanged for months or years. If pituitary ablation allows some degree of restoration of capillary perfusion in the area of cotton wool spot, this could explain the higher rate of disappearance of these lesions in such patients.

The particular value of these 2 techniques is that they are sensitive indicators of the response to treatment and as new methods of treating retinopathy are devised they are likely to be of particular value in assessing them. Unfortunately neither is of any use in evaluating destructive treatments like photocoagulation.

EVIDENCE CONCERNING THE PATHOGENESIS OF DIABETIC RETINOPATHY

A number of 'vascular' theories of the origins of particular retinopathy features have been proposed. As many of the features of diabetic retinopathy resemble those resulting from partial obstruction of the central retinal vein, or diminished flow to the eye as a result of common carotid artery obstruction, it has been suggested that diabetic retinopathy is due to impaired blood flow through the retina. It has been proposed that large tortuous residual capillaries crossing areas of capillary closure represent 'shunts' which are draining away the capillary flow from the surrounding vessels and cause them not to be perfused (Cogan and Kuwabara, 1963).

A vascular theory for the origin of new vessels has been suggested. New vessels arise in conditions such as retrolental fibroplasia and branch vein occlusion in which the circulation to an area of retina has been interrupted. The hypothesis has been advanced that new vessels represent a frustrated growth of collaterals as a result of an adjacent area of partial retinal ischaemia. Fluorescence angiography has been of value in studying all of these hypotheses.

Direct measurement of retinal blood flow in diabetes by means of a flow meter is not possible as the vessels are too small and inaccessible. Two indirect methods of measuring flow have been proposed. The first is to measure mean transit time in a retinal artery and adjacent vein (Bulpitt and Dollery, 1970), and the second is to measure the velocity of flow in a retinal artery from a cinefluorescent angiogram taken at a high framing speed. So far useful data has only emerged from the first method. Measurements of mean transit time cannot be translated into measurements of flow unless an estimate is available of the vascular volume between the arterial and venous sampling points. Bulpitt and Dollery (1970) suggested that as an approximation the cross-sectional areas of the artery and vein at the point the dye concentrations were measured should be used for this purpose. Using this method, they were able to show that the 'retinal blood flow' in patients with anaemia was almost double that of normal individuals. The same method has been applied to diabetics where the mean transit time figures were found to be similar to those in normal individuals (Kohner, 1971). However, as the average diameter of retinal veins in diabetics was slightly greater than in normals the estimates of flow were in many cases higher than those of normal individuals. There are a number of potential errors and uncertainties in application of the mean transit time method to a circulation which contains leaking vessels, and may have leakage into the wall of the vessel at the site of observation. Despite these uncertainties it seems very unlikely that the total blood flow through the diabetic retinal circulation is diminished below normal, at least in early cases, although local flow may be unevenly distributed. Thus the diminished flow theory of the pathogenesis of diabetic retinopathy does not find any support in these observations.

The large irregular residual capillary channels that Cogan and Kuwabara (1963) referred to as shunts are present in some, but not all, areas of capillary closure. In one or two instances they appear to be acting as high flow structures in that the transit time through them is appreciably more rapid than through the surrounding capillary bed. However, in most instances they fill at the same speed or more slowly than surrounding capillaries and it is impossible to accept that they could be acting as shunts. Furthermore, when arteriovenous malformations form in the retinal circulation, the feeding and draining vessels hypertrophy and a very high flow to such structures can be readily detected by fluorescence angiography.

New vessels in the retina usually arise in 1 of 5 situations (Kohner and Dollery, 1973). The first group arise from the capillary bed and are initially difficult to distinguish from dilated capillaries in the normal position. Later their arrangement becomes more irregular and they begin to leak fluorescein. The second group often arise as small rosettes near or on large veins. The third group take the form of arborising arcades often arising from the neighbourhood of a large vein. There is frequently a small arterial feeding channel which can be detected on a fluorescence angiogram. Flow through these large structures is usually slow. The fourth group of new vessels usually arise from large veins and may form large venous loops. They may regress if the main channel of the vein to which they are attached reopens. A fifth type arise from retinal arteries in the periphery and these may form a rosette or arborising patterns similar to those arising from retinal veins. New vessel systems usually arise in patients whose retina shows widespread capillary damage. However, it is difficult to relate new vessel systems to specific disorders of the vascular bed. The first type frequently originate near the edge of an area of capillary non-perfusion and the third type often arborise over an area of closed capillary. However, the second and fourth types which originate from the large veins do not appear to have any specific relationship to poorly perfused areas of capillary, although substances in the blood flowing through these veins may stimulate vasoproliferation.

Although new vessels are often compared with collaterals, the differences are more striking than the resemblances. Collaterals are usually direct, they join vein to vein or artery to artery, they run through the existing vascular bed and flow from them is usually rapid, and they do not leak fluorescein. New vessels are disorderly; they grow forward from the normal vascular bed, they do not connect channels of the same type, flow through them is usually slow, and they leak fluorescein profusely. It is noteworthy that after a branch retinal vein occlusion collaterals and new vessels may co-exist and they are readily differentiated from one another.

The stimulus to new vessel proliferation is not known but appears to arise from inadequately perfused retinal tissue. The chemical factors responsible for disorderly new vessels may be similar to those concerned with collateral development but as yet there is no evidence to support this view. Thus fluorescein angiography has not supported any of the 'vascular' theories of the causation of diabetic retinopathy, and this remains a mystery.

REFERENCES

ASHTON, N. (1953): Arteriolar involvement in diabetic retinopathy. *Brit. J. Ophthalmol., 37,* 282.

BULPITT, C. J. and DOLLERY, C. T. (1970): Retinal cine-angiography. *Brit. J. Kinematography, Sound & Television,* p. 14.

COGAN, D. B. and KUWABARA, T. (1963): Capillary shunts in the pathogenesis of diabetic retinopathy. *Diabetes, 12,* 293.

KOHNER, E. M., DOLLERY, C. T., PATERSON, J. W. and OAKLEY, N. W. (1967): Arterial fluorescein studies in diabetic retinopathy. *Diabetes, 16,* 1.

KOHNER, E. M., DOLLERY, C. T. and BULPITT, C. J. (1969): Cotton wool spots in diabetic retinopathy. *Diabetes, 16,* 691.

KOHNER, E. M. and DOLLERY, C. T. (1970): The rate of formation and disappearance of retinal microaneurysms in diabetes. *Europ. J. clin. Invest., 1,* 167.

KOHNER, E. M. (1971): The effect of diabetes on retinal vascular function. *Acta diabet. lat., 8/Suppl. 1,* 135.

KOHNER, E. M. and DOLLERY, C. T. (1973): Diabetic Retinopathy in Complications of Diabetes Mellitus. Editors: H. Keen and J. Jarrett. Arnold, in press.

NORTON, E. W. D. and GUTMAN, F. (1965): Diabetic retinopathy studied by fluorescein angiography. *Ophthalmologica, 150,* 5.

NOVOTNY, H. R. and ALVIS, D. L. (1961): Method of photographing fluorescence in circulating blood in the human retina. *Circulation, 24,* 82.

OAKLEY, N. W., HILL, D. W., JOPLIN, G. F., KOHNER, E. M. and FRASER, R. (1967): A grading system for diabetic retinopathy. *Diabetologia, 3,* 402.

OOSTERHUIS, J. A. and LAMMENS, A. J. (1965): Fluorescein photography of the ocular fundus. *Ophthalmologica (Basel), 140,* 210.

SCOTT, D. J., DOLLERY, C. T., HILL, D. W., HODGE, J. V. and FRASER, R. (1964): Fluorescein studies of diabetic retinopathy. *Brit. med. J., 1,* 811.

WISE, G. N., DOLLERY, C. T. and HENKIND, P. (1971): Fluorescein fundus photography. In: *The Retinal Circulation.* Harper & Rowe, New York.

DIABETIC RETINOPATHY: PATHOLOGY*

PAUL HENKIND**

Department of Ophthalmology, Albert Einstein College of Medicine/Montefiore Hospital and Medical Center, Bronx, New York, N.Y., U.S.A.

Before entering into a consideration of the pathology of diabetic retinopathy, I should like to pose a question. Is there a specific diabetic retinopathy? Perhaps the best answer is that provided by Larsen (1960): 'The individual fundus lesion seen in diabetics is not specific to diabetes. Similar lesions may occur in several other diseases, but in diabetics the general ophthalmoscopic picture is so characteristic that the fundus changes can be considered as a clinical entity, the diabetic retinopathy'. The difficulty for the ocular pathologist is similar to that faced by the clinician, most of the retinal lesions found on ordinary light microscopy are suggestive of, but not specific for diabetes (Cunha-Vaz, 1972). We may ask, why is this so? One explanation is that diabetic retinopathy is basically a vasculopathy, and retinal vessels can undergo only a limited number of responses or alterations. Indeed, the majority of retinal vascular responses is seen in the diabetic. There are, however, certain clues which point to a retinopathy being diabetic in origin and these can be considered briefly: (1) *Laterality* – diabetic retinopathy is overwhelmingly a bilateral condition. If only one eye is involved, one should look for another cause of the 'diabetic' retinopathy. (2) *Symmetry* – diabetic retinopathy is often symmetrical, involving similar portions of both fundi, and being of approximately equal severity in both eyes. Asymmetry of retinopathy in a diabetic occurs when there is unilateral carotid artery disease (Gay and Rosenbaum, 1966), previous chorioretinal or optic nerve disease (Aiello et al., 1968), and perhaps, in cases of unilateral high myopia or ocular hypertension. (3) *Location* – diabetic retinopathy is basically a posterior pole disease with the retinal periphery usually being spared. This is opposite to the situation encountered in sickle cell disease and the dysproteinemias, disorders which generally involve the anterior retina either selectively or predominantly. Central retinal vein occlusion, in certain stages, sometimes mistaken for diabetic retinopathy, involves both the anterior and posterior retina in hemorrhagic processes. (4) *Progression* – diabetic retinopathy may be reversible or it may wax and wane, but in general it is a progressive disorder. The first 3 points, laterality, symmetry, and location may be as important clues for the ocular pathologist as for the clinician. The fourth point, progression, is basically a clinical feature.

* Supported in part by Grant # EY-00613-03 from the National Institute of Health.
** Professor and Chairman, Department of Ophthalmology.

This presentation deals with the pathology of human diabetic retinopathy, its relationship to similar human retinal disorders and experimental diabetic retinopathy.

The lesions seen in the diabetic retina by conventional light and electron microscopy can be divided into vascular and non-vascular entities, the latter most likely dependent upon the former for their development. Alterations in the vascular bed are most readily studied by light microscopic examination of retinal 'digests'. The nature of the retinal vascular basement membrane (a property apparently of central nervous system vessels and not of other blood vessels) permits the isolation of the entire retinal vascular tree from the surrounding neural and glial cells (Kuwabara and Cogan, 1960). Using such preparations, stained appropriately, one can examine the angioarchitecture of the retinal vascular bed and the integrity of the endothelial cells and intramural pericytes (mural cells) of the vessels. Digest preparations reflect the in vivo retinal vascular situation as demonstrated by fluorescein angiography (Kohner and Henkind, 1970).

In Table 1 are listed the vascular alterations described for diabetic retinopathy. Both the clinical and histopathologic features are noted, and an attempt is made to determine the specificity of the lesion for the diabetic process. Of the 9 alterations listed in the table, 7 can be observed clinically if we are allowed the liberty of including the findings

TABLE 1
Retinal vascular alterations in diabetes

Alteration	Ophthalmoscopy	Histopathology
1. Microaneurysms	Characteristic, not specific	Possibly specific
2. Venous dilatation	Common, not specific	Unknown
3. Venous beading, etc.	Characteristic, not specific	Unknown specificity
4. Arteriovenous 'shunts'	Characteristic, not specific (seen by fluorescein angiogram)	Characteristic, not specific
5. Arterial changes	Not specific	Not specific
6. Neovascularization (retinitis proliferans)	Characteristic, not specific	Unknown specificity
7. Capillary closure	Characteristic, not specific (seen by fluorescein angiogram)	Not specific
8. Intramural cell degeneration	Not seen	Possibly specific
9. Vascular basement membrane change	Not seen	Possibly specific

of fluorescein angiography (1–7), and 5 of these are very suggestive of diabetic retinopathy (1, 3, 4, 6, 7), but not one is pathognomonic of the disease. The histopathologic correlates of these clinical findings are, with the possible exception of the microaneurysms and arteriovenous shunts, non-specific. Toussaint (1968) feels that the topography of the diabetic retinal microaneurysms and the accompanying intramural pericyte degeneration are specific findings which separate such aneurysms from those seen in conditions such as venous thrombosis, Eales' disease, sickle cell disease, pulseless disease (aortic arch syndrome), carotid artery insufficiency, and hyperviscosity diseases (Garner and Ashton, 1972; Wise et al., 1971). In all of these conditions there is impairment of retinal blood flow. There are, however, no reports of clinical pathologic correlations of posterior pole retinal microaneurysms in patients without diabetes, thus making it, at this time, impossible to state authoritatively that such aneurysms are histologically unlike those seen in diabetes. The intraretinal arteriovenous shunts, noted initially by Cogan and Kuwabara (1963), and almost certainly developed from the pre-existing retinal capillary bed, are more commonly seen in diabetic retinopathy than in any other condition. Similar A-V pathways have been noted in retinal digests of long-standing glaucomatous eyes, and clinically, by fluorescein angiography, in Leber's multiple miliary aneurysms (G. N. Wise, personal communication). The most specific feature is the fact that these are indeed arteriovenous intercommunications and not A-A shunts as seen after branch retinal artery occlusion, or V-V shunts which are seen after retinal vein occlusion.

The 2 histopathologic features noted in the table (8, 9) are possibly specific for diabetes mellitus. While there has been some controversy over the role of the intramural pericyte in diabetic retinopathy (de Oliveira, 1966), there is abundant evidence that these cells are selectively involved in the diabetic process (Yanoff, 1966; Speiser et al., 1968). The function of these cells in health or disease is still a matter of speculation. Vascular basement membrane thickening is certainly a common finding in diabetic retinopathy and is most readily demonstrated by PAS (periodic acid-Schiff) staining. Recent quantitative ultrastructural studies (Sosula et al., 1972) suggest that thickening of the retinal capillary basement membrane is a very early finding in experimental diabetes, but this needs confirmation. Not noted in the table, but certainly worth mentioning, is the work of Cunha-Vaz (1972) who suggests that the initial vascular involvement in diabetic retinopathy is related to endothelial cell dysfunction.

Table 2 is a modification of his material. Endothelial cell proliferation, mainly on the venous side of the circulation, was also noted in retinae from patients with polycythemia, leukemia, myeloma, Eales' disease, macroglobulinemia, and central retinal vein thrombosis. Areas of capillary bed closure were observed in digests of retinas from patients with scleroderma, hypertension, pernicious anemia, and central retinal vein obstruction.

The non-vascular alterations described for diabetic retinopathy are listed in Table 3. Of the 5 alterations listed, 4 are clinical features (1–4) and 3 are characteristic of, but not specific for diabetes (1–3). In our opinion, all of the findings, with the possible exception of the histochemical alterations, are secondary to microvascular disease. The typical hemorrhages of diabetic retinopathy are so-called dot and blot hemorrhages. Histologically they appear as aggregates of red blood cells in the inner nuclear and outer plexiform layers of the retina. The lack of a vascular basement membrane around these red cells distinguishes them from the clinically similar microaneurysms. Identical hemorrhages are seen in cases of retinal vein occlusion, and perhaps in venous stasis retinopathy due to carotid artery disease. The presence of superficial, flame-shaped hemorrhages seen clinically, or their histological counterpart, linear hemorrhages in the nerve fiber layer of the

TABLE 2
*Evolution of retinal vascular lesions in diabetes**

Stages	Ophthalmoscopy	Pathology: Small vessels, Venous side	Pathology: Small vessels, Arterial side	Pathology: Large vessels
1. Initial	Rare aneurysm	Endoth. prol. ++ Aneurysm ++	Endoth. deg. +	Vein ±
2. Intermediate	Numerous aneurysms hemorrhages exudate	Endoth. prol. ++ Aneurysm++	Endoth. deg. ++ Focal cap. clos.	Vein ±
3. Advanced	Same lesions as in stage 2	Endoth. deg. +++ Aneurysm +++ A-V shunts Large area cap. clos.		Vein ++ Artery +
4. Final	Same lesions plus retinitis proliferans	Endoth. deg. ++++ Aneurysm +++ Generalized cap. clos.		Vein ++ Artery +++

* Modified from Cunha-Vaz (1972).
Endoth. prol. = Endothelial cell proliferation
Endoth. deg. = Endothelial cell degeneration
Cap. clos. = Capillary closure

retina, is not typical of the diabetic process, but instead suggests underlying hypertensive disease.

Deep, circumscribed, yellowish exudates are seen in diabetic retinopathy, and also in non-diabetics with Coats' disease, senile macular degeneration, and retinal vein obstruction. Peripheral retinal angiomas may also give an exudative picture at the macular which might be mistaken for the diabetic process. The exudates typically occupy the outer retina, lying mainly within the outer plexiform layer, but also involve the nuclear layers. The exudative material is rich in lipid and mucopolysaccharide, but in early lesions there may be more albuminous material. Toussaint (1968) has noted that more superficially located exudates, in the nerve fiber, ganglion cell, and inner plexiform layers, appear less dense, but seem to be comprised of the same material. He feels that all of these exudates develop in areas of retinal capillary dysfunction. In addition to the above described exudates which seem to push aside the normal surrounding cells of the retina, there are degenerative foci in the outer plexiform layer. These foci (plages de dégénérence, Toussant, 1968) which give a 'swiss cheese' appearance to histologic sections of the posterior retina, stain intensely with PAS, variably with lipid stains, and only faintly with eosin. The exact clinical counterpart of these lesions is unknown.

TABLE 3
Retinal non-vascular alterations in diabetes

Alteration	Ophthalmoscopic appearance	Histopathology
1. Hemorrhage	Characteristic, not specific	Not specific
2. Exudate	Characteristic, not specific	Not specific
3. Cotton-wool spots	Characteristic, not specific	Not specific
4. Macular edema	Not specific, best seen by fluorescein angiography	Probably not specific
5. Histochemical reaction	Invisible	Possibly specific

Only recently has it been appreciated that cotton-wool spots can occur in diabetics without concomitant hypertension. Such spots, which develop at the posterior pole of the retina, predominantly in the distribution of the radial peripapillary capillaries (Henkind, 1972), are the result of focal ischemia (Ashton et al., 1966). Histologically one finds foci of swollen nerve fibers with a central cluster of cell-like bodies. These have been called 'cytoid' bodies, and are in reality terminal swellings of Cajal. To date, there has been no study to determine whether the cotton-wool spots seen in the non-hypertensive diabetic differ in ultrastructure or histochemical reaction from the cotton-wool spots seen in the hypertensive individual.

Macular edema has recently been emphasized as 'an overlooked complication of diabetic retinopathy' (Patz et al., 1973). This feature is best appreciated by contact lens and slit lamp examination or by fluorescein angiography, and can occur in diabetics with seemingly mild background retinopathy. Presumably the edema results from leakage of fluid into the macular from surrounding altered macular capillaries. Clinicopathologic correlations have not yet been performed, but would presumably show cystoid spaces in the macular region.

Toussaint (1968) outlines the histochemical findings of normal compared to diabetic retinae. The marked differences occur in the reaction of the Müller fibers in the diabetic when stained with acid phosphatase, and the positive staining with ATPase of both plexiform layers in the diabetic compared to the normal retina.

There seems to be little question that there is a diabetic retinopathy, and that its pathogenesis is intimately associated with the diabetic state. The factor which initiates the retinal vascular response leading to the various stages of diabetic retinopathy is as yet unknown. Hormonal, chemical, neural, and vascular factors have all been implicated or postulated as inciting agents of diabetic retinopathy, generally without confirmation. The most important retinal problem, proliferative vasculopathy or retinitis proliferans, has been noted in conditions such as retrolental fibroplasia, Eales' disease, retinal vein occlusion, sickle cell disease, dysproteinemias, Behçet's disease, and malaria, among others. Each of these disorders has a different etiology, but the retinal vascular response or involvement ends up the same. While it may not be fruitful to equate the other conditions with diabetic retinopathy, it does seem logical to look for the common factors that cause retinal neovascularization. Perhaps the tumor angiogenic factor of Folkman et al. (1971) will prove to be the factor X of Wise (1956), which is responsible for retinal neovascularization.

Concerning experimental diabetic retinopathy, both spontaneously diabetic animals and induced diabetic animals have been intensively studied over the past decade by a variety of clinical and histological methods. To date, there is still not a uniformly satisfactory experimental model which mimics human diabetic retinopathy. The most important lesion, retinitis proliferans, has not been demonstrated in spontaneously diabetic animals, nor in long-term induced diabetic animals, with the possible exception of the rat (Toussaint, 1968). It is evident that much experimental work still remains to be done.

REFERENCES

AIELLO, L. M., BEETHAM, W. P., BALODIMOS, M. D., CHAZAN, B. I. and BRADLEY, R. F. (1968): Ruby laser photocoagulation in treatment of diabetic proliferating retinopathy. Preliminary report. In: *Symposium on the Treatment of Diabetic Retinopathy,* p. 437. Public Health Service Publication No. 1890.

ASHTON, N., DOLLERY, C. T., HENKIND, P., HILL, D. W., PATERSON, J. W., RAMALHO, P. S. and SHAKIB, M. (1966): Focal retinal ischemia. *Brit. J. Ophthal., 50,* 281.

COGAN, D. G. and KUWABARA, T. (1963): Capillary shunts in the pathogenesis of diabetic retinopathy. *Diabetes, 12,* 293.

CUNHA-VAZ, J. G. (1972): Diabetic retinopathy. Human and experimental studies. *Trans. ophthal. Soc. U.K., 92,* 111.

FOLKMAN, J., MERLER, E., ABERNATHY, C. and WILLIAMS, G. (1971): Isolation of a tumor factor responsible for angiogenesis. *J. exp. Med., 133,* 275.

GARNER, A. and ASHTON, N. (1972): Ophthalmic artery stenosis and diabetic retinopathy. *Trans. ophthal. Soc. U.K., 92,* 101.

GAY, A. J. and ROSENBAUM, A. L. (1966): Retinal artery pressure in asymmetric diabetic retinopathy. *Arch. Ophthal., 75,* 758.

HENKIND, P. (1972): Radial peripapillary capillaries. Past, present and future. In: *Fluorescein Angiogram Symposium, Tokyo,* in press.

KOHNER, E. M. and HENKIND, P. (1970): Correlation of fluorescein angiogram and retinal digest. *Amer. J. Ophthal., 69,* 403.

KUWABARA, T. and COGAN, D. G. (1960): Studies of retinal vascular patterns. Part 1. Normal architecture. *Arch. Ophthal., 64,* 904.

LARSEN, H. W. (1960): Diabetic retinopathy. An ophthalmoscopic study with a discussion of the morphologic changes and pathogenetic factors in this disease. *Acta ophthal., Suppl. 60.*

DE OLIVEIRA, L. N. F. (1966): Pericytes in diabetic retinopathy. *Brit. J. Ophthal., 50,* 134.

PATZ, A., SCHATZ, H., BERKOW, J. W., GITTELSOHN, A. M. and TICHO, U. (1973): Macula edema – an overlooked complication of diabetic retinopathy. *Trans. Amer. Acad. Ophthal. Otolaryng., 77,* 34.

SOSULA, L., BEAUMONT, P., HOLLOWS, F. C. and JONSON, K. M. (1972): Dilatation and endothelial proliferation of retinal capillaries in streptozotocin-diabetic rats. Quantitative electron microscopy. *Invest. Ophthal., 11,* 926.

SPEISER, S., GITTELSOHN, A. M. and PATZ, A. (1968): Studies on diabetic retinopathy. B. Influence of diabetes on intramural pericytes. *Arch. Ophthal., 80,* 332.
TOUSSAINT, D. (1968): Contribution à l'étude anatomique et clinique de la rétinopathie diabétique chez l'homme et chez l'animal. *Path. europ., Brussels.*
WISE, G. N. (1956): Retinal neovascularization. *Trans. Amer. Ophthal. Soc., 54,* 729.
WISE, G. N., DOLLERY, C. T. and HENKIND, P. (1971): *The Retinal Circulation.* Harper and Row, New York.
YANOFF, M. (1966): Diabetic retinopathy. *New Engl. J. Med., 274,* 1344.

ASSESSMENT OF THE SEVERITY OF DIABETIC RETINOPATHY IN RELATION TO MORPHOLOGICAL FUNDUS CHANGES AND VISUAL DISTURBANCES

HANS-WALTHER LARSEN

Department of Ophthalmology, Gentofte Hospital, Hellerup, Denmark

Before entering the problems of photocoagulation I shall make an assessment of the severity of diabetic retinopathy in relation to morphological fundus changes and visual disturbances. In order to evaluate this, it is necessary to consider the non-proliferative stage and the proliferative stage of diabetic retinopathy separately, and for each stage put forward the question: which morphological fundal changes damage vision and to what degree do these changes reduce central or peripheral vision, or both?

In the non-proliferative stage of diabetic retinopathy, so-called *simple diabetic retinopathy* or *background retinopathy*, visual disturbances are usually due to macular edema or hard exudates in the macular area. Macular edema (Fig. 1), which is due to a leakage from damaged vessels in the macular and perimacular area, usually gives rise to a moderate reduction of central vision, but this reduction of vision is reversible if the edema disappears, unless it has been of long standig.

A certain amount of edema is usually present, when hard exudates develop. Hard exudates (Fig. 2) tend to accumulate in the macular and the perimacular area and give rise to central or paracentral scotomas, which in most instances are irreversible and persist

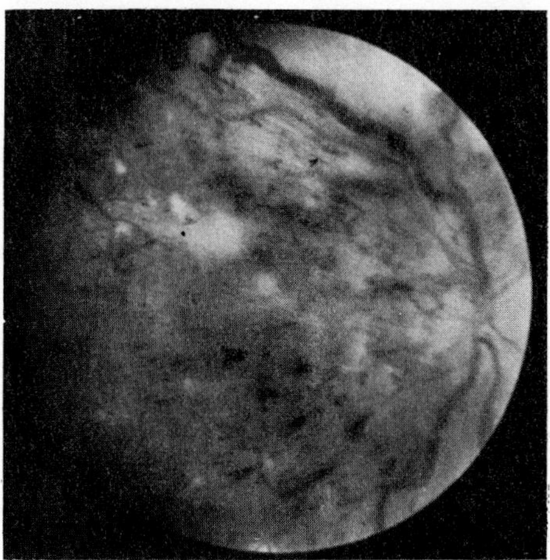

FIG. 1. Diabetic retinopathy with macular edema.

even after the hard exudates have disappeared again. Hard exudates are usually more prominent in maturity-onset diabetics than in juvenile diabetics. A reduction in central vision due to simple diabetic retinopathy is therefore far more common in older diabetics. Microaneurysms (Fig. 3) and retinal hemorrhages do cause small scotomas, but usually not major visual disturbances, unless they are located in the fovea centralis.

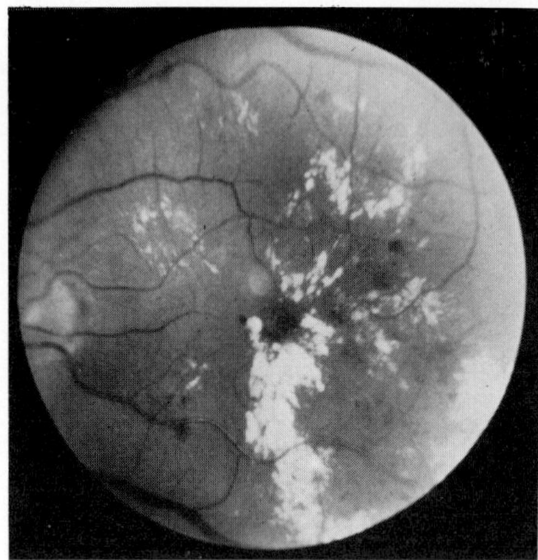

FIG. 2. Simple diabetic retinopathy with hard exudates in the macular area.

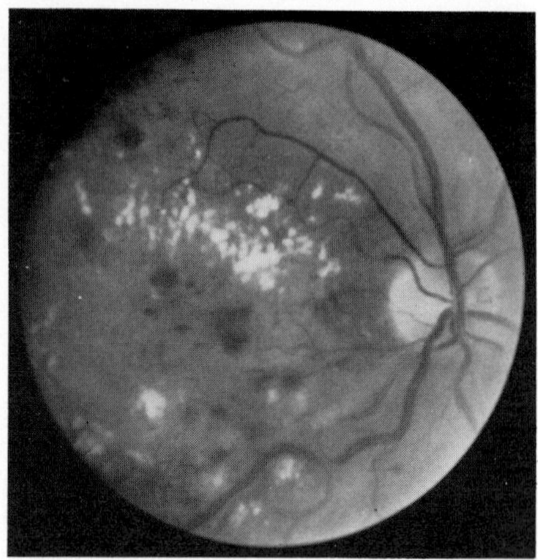

FIG. 3. Simple diabetic retinopathy with hemorrhages in the macula causing reduction of central vision.

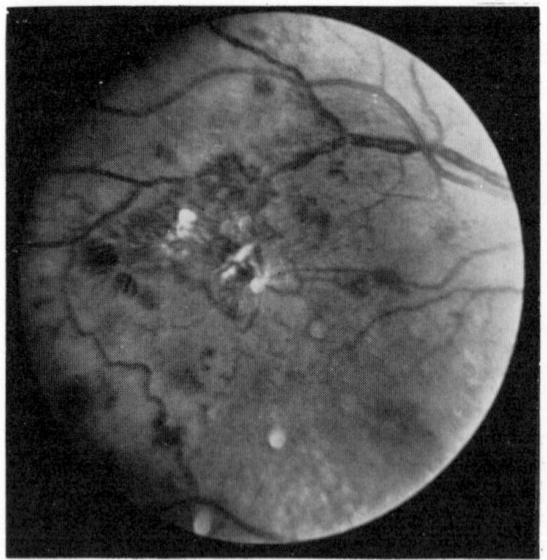

FIG. 4. Proliferative diabetic retinopathy, early stage, with neovascularization outside the macular area.

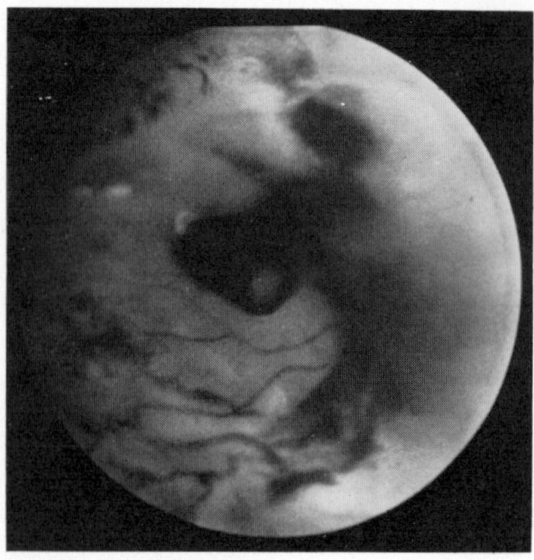

FIG. 5. Preretinal and vitreous hemorrhage.

As mentioned, simple retinopathy therefore may give rise to a reduction of central vision, causing inability to read, but usually does not give rise to major disturbances of the peripheral vision. Even if central vision is severely reduced these patients are able to walk around and take care of themselves.

In the early stage of *proliferative diabetic retinopathy,* visual disturbances are less dependent on the localization (Fig. 4) and extent of neovascularization, but more dependent on preretinal (Fig. 5) and vitreous hemorrhage. In particular, vitreous hemorrhages may seriously damage vision. In the late stages, of course, the localization (Fig. 6) and extent of fibrous tissue proliferation and any localized (Fig. 7) or more diffuse retinal detachment determine the degree of visual damage.

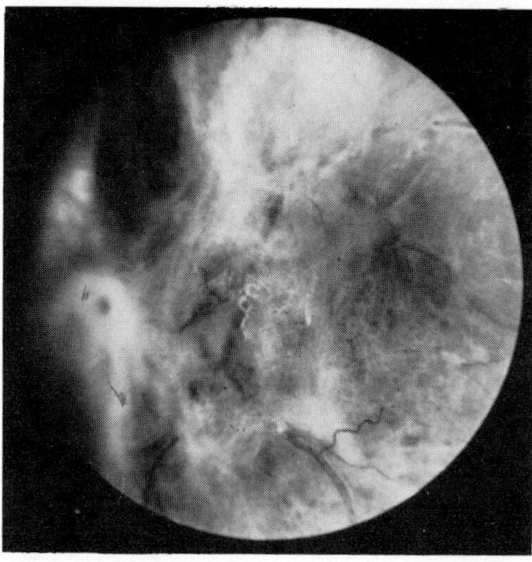

FIG. 6. Proliferative diabetic retinopathy, advanced stage, with extensive veils of fibrous tissue.

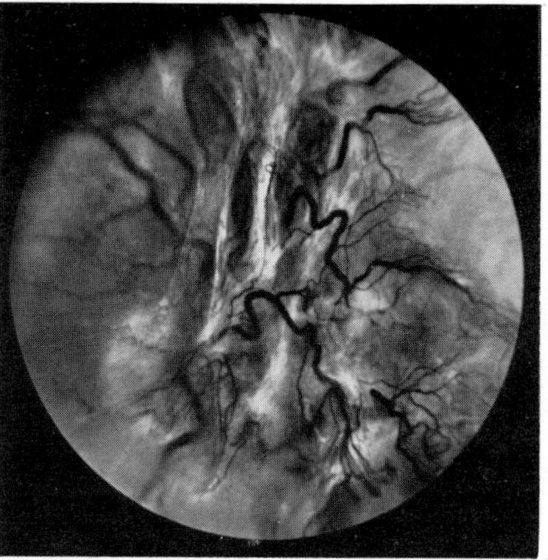

FIG. 7. Proliferative diabetic retinopathy, late stage, with localized retinal detachment.

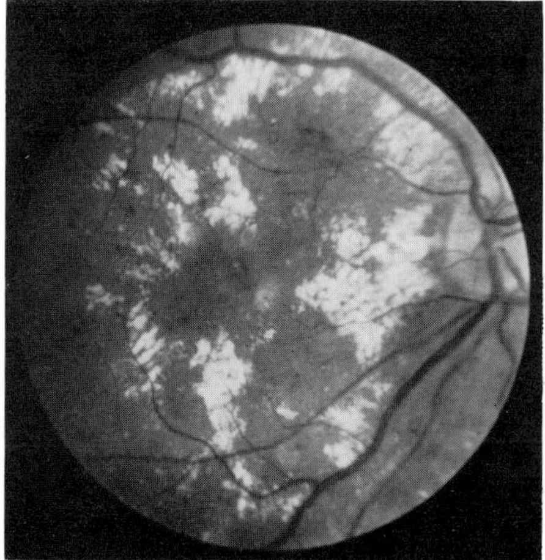

FIG. 8. Simple diabetic retinopathy, right eye, before light coagulation treatment.

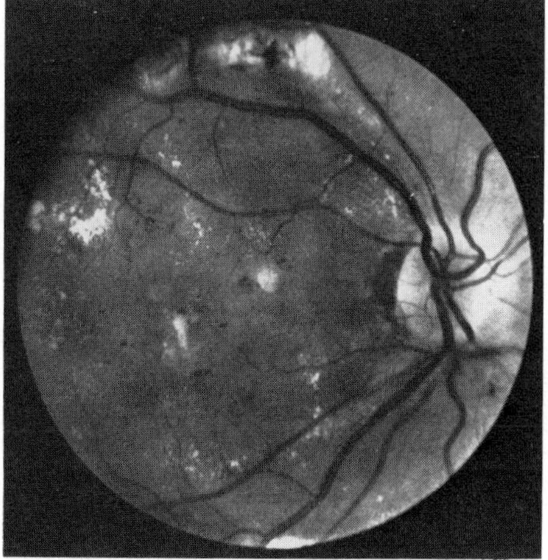

FIG. 9. Same eye as Figure 8, 2 years after treatment.

The proliferative stage of diabetic retinopathy is always serious in relation to vision, because not only central but also peripheral vision may be damaged severely within a few years, and especially by vitreous hemorrhage. Cases with neovascularization outside the disc and the macular area, however, have a better prognosis than cases with neovascularization extending from the optic disc.

The proliferative stage of diabetic retinopathy is seen more often in juvenile diabetics with long-standing diabetes than in maturity-onset diabetics. The condition gives rise to major medicosocial problems, because of working incapacity, when not only the central but also the peripheral vision is severely damaged.

About 75% of cases with reduced visual acuity from diabetic retinopathy show simple retinopathy, while the remaining 25% show proliferative retinopathy.

INDICATIONS AND CONTRAINDICATIONS FOR LIGHT COAGULATION

For many years, research has been deeply involved in developing methods to stop the progression of retinopathy in order to preserve vision. Dr. Fraser (this Volume, pp. 431–438) mentioned pituitary ablation as one of the methods.

Light coagulation is another method. The aim of light coagulation treatment is to seal leaking points in the fundus in order to prevent or reduce macular edema and hard exudates, or to coagulate newly formed vessels in the fundus, so as to prevent major hemorrhages and extensive connective tissue proliferation. In the non-proliferative stage of diabetic retinopathy or simple retinopathy the most commonly accepted indications for light coagulation are macular edema and hard macular exudates. The treatment should, however, start before central vision has been reduced too much and irreversibly damaged. In advanced cases with hard exudates it is possible to reduce the number of exudates, but the scotomas will still remain.

In the proliferative stage of diabetic retinopathy the main indication for light coagulation is the presence of newly formed vessels in the retina, lying preretinally or intravitreally, and containing little or no connective tissue.

Fibrous tissue proliferations should not be treated with light coagulation, unless containing numerous newly formed vessels, because treatment will often result in fibrous contraction, which may provoke retinal detachment; another contraindication is vitreous hemorrhage.

Light coagulation treatment of the proliferative stage of diabetic retinopathy should therefore be done in the early stages to prevent vitreous hemorrhage and fibrous tissue proliferation.

ARGON LASER VERSUS XENON ARC LIGHT COAGULATION

Two main types of light coagulators are available for treatment of fundus disorders: the argon laser and the xenon light coagulator.

Until a few years ago, the xenon arc light coagulator was the only light coagulator available. The emitted light from the xenon arc light coagulator consists of a continuum in the visible part of the spectrum with some peak lines in the infrared spectrum. Emitted light below 400 nm is cut off by ultraviolet absorbing optics. About 90% of the visible light is transmitted through the ocular structures into the fundus.

When the light is focused on the retina, it becomes absorbed in the retinal and choroidal pigment and the light is thus transformed into heat. During the light coagulation the temperature in the treated area of the fundus rises to about 70°C, while the increase in temperature of the other ocular structures does not exceed 1–2°C and therefore is of little importance.

A photocoagulation effect is only possible when the retina is in contact with the retinal and choroidal pigment. In order to destroy preretinal neovascularization by the xenon arc light coagulator, it is thus necessary to release enough energy, not only to produce coagulation of the retina in its full thickness, but also to heat up that part of the vitreous, which contains the pathological vessels, so that they can be destroyed. In many instances, therefore, xenon arc light coagulation will damage the nerve fiber layer and produce arcuate scotomas. If the neovascularization extends more than about 10 diopters or 3 mm in front of the retina, light coagulation is not possible with the xenon arc light coagulator.

It was therefore a step forward, when the argon laser was introduced into therapy a few years ago. The emitted light from the argon laser consists of a narrow peak between 488 and 515 nm. The light is absorbed not only in the retinal and choroidal pigment, but also in the hemoglobin of the vessels. The argon laser is thereby able to coagulate and occlude the vessels, even if they are not in contact with the retina.

With the argon laser, we are able to treat areas in the fundus between 50 and 1,000 μ in diameter, while the xenon arc light coagulator cannot operate satisfactorily with an aperture less than 3 degrees, corresponding to 1,000 μ in the fundus. The argon laser is therefore in several respects superior to the xenon arc light coagulator.

RESULTS OF TREATMENT BY LIGHT COAGULATION

During the last 10 years, numerous papers have been presented on the favorable results of light coagulation in diabetic retinopathy. Most series, however, are not controlled studies, and the results are therefore still difficult to evaluate. I will therefore not submit any statistics on the results, but just mention that controlled trials are in progress both in the USA, in England and in Scandinavia. The results of these controlled studies will perhaps be available within 3–4 years. Until then, it is only possible to pass on an impression, held by many of those concerned with the light coagulation treatment of diabetic retinopathy: that macular edema and hard exudates react favorably to treatment in many cases; that early stages of neovascularization also react favorably to light coagulation, especially those cases with proliferations lying outside the disc and macular area; that more advanced cases of neovascularization react less favorably or even become worse, due to shrinkage of fibrous tissue and, eventually, retinal detachment.

The effect of light coagulation in diabetic retinopathy is illustrated in Figures 8–15. Figures 8 and 9 show a case of simple diabetic retinopathy before treatment, and the same eye 2 years later. For comparison Figures 10 and 11 show the other eye of the same patient before treatment and two years later. It is evident that the treated eye has become much better than the non-treated eye. Figures 12 and 13 show the favorable result in a case of proliferative retinopathy with neovascularization extending from the disc before treatment and 4 years after treatment, and Figures 14 and 15 show a case with neovascularization in the fundus periphery before treatment and 3 years later.

Finally, I must point out that light coagulation should be considered a palliative treatment. It cannot prevent neovascularization occurring at other sites in the fundus. The patients must therefore still be followed at 3–6 months intervals and treated again if new proliferations occur. Nevertheless, in many cases light coagulation is of value in preserving vision for a shorter or longer period.

We must admit, however, that light coagulation cannot be the final answer in the treatment of diabetic retinopathy. Future research must therefore concentrate on the prevention of diabetic retinopathy.

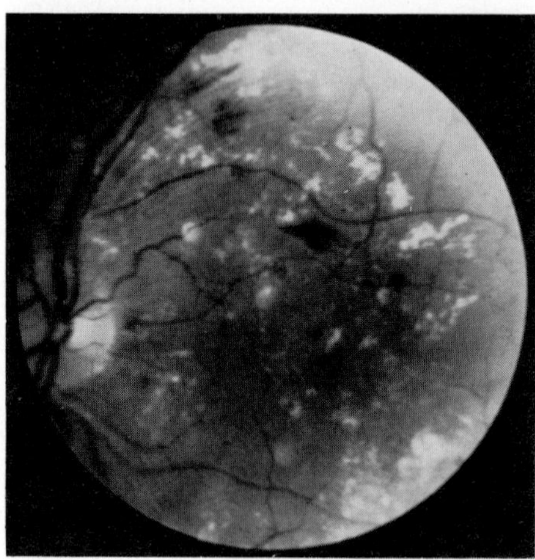

FIG. 10. Non-treated left eye from same patient as Figure 8, before treatment of right eye.

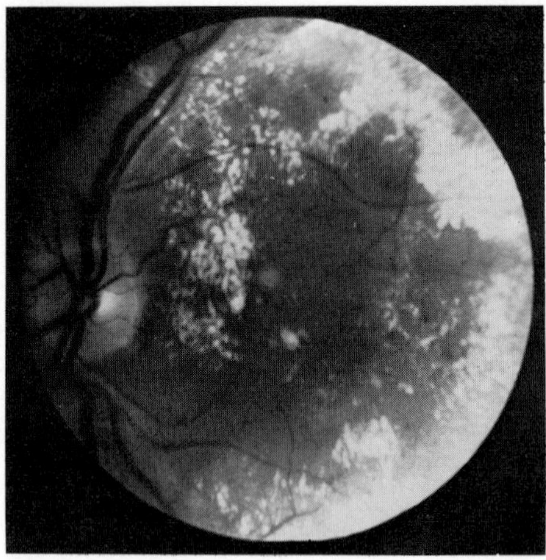

FIG. 11. Same non-treated eye as Figure 10, 2 years later.

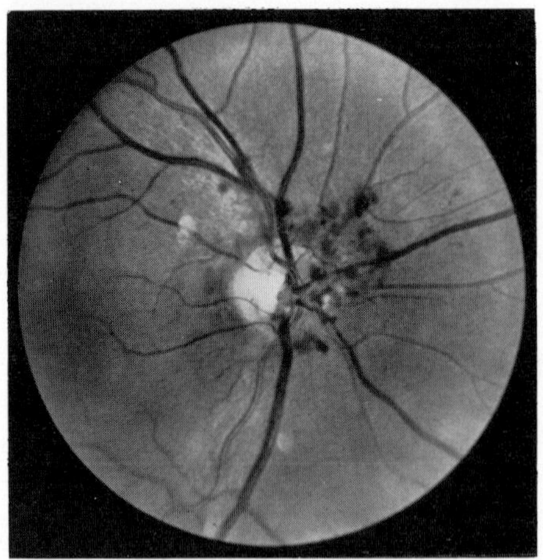

FIG. 12. Proliferative diabetic retinopathy before light coagulation treatment.

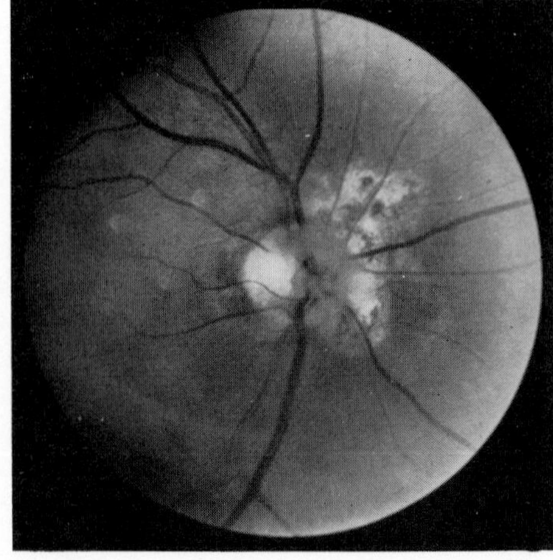

FIG. 13. Same eye as Figure 12, 4 years later.

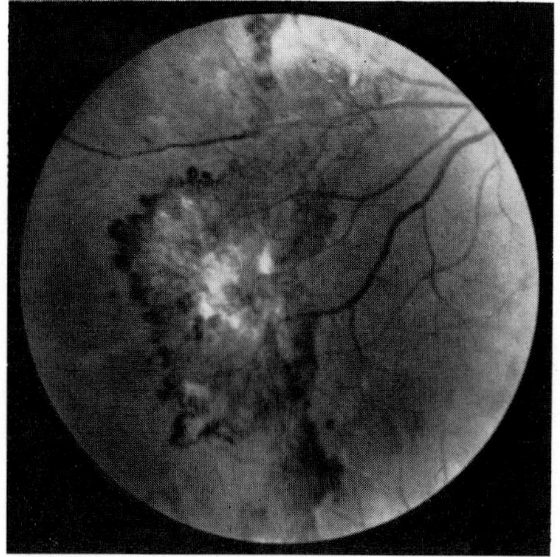

FIG. 14. Proliferative diabetic retinopathy before light coagulation treatment.

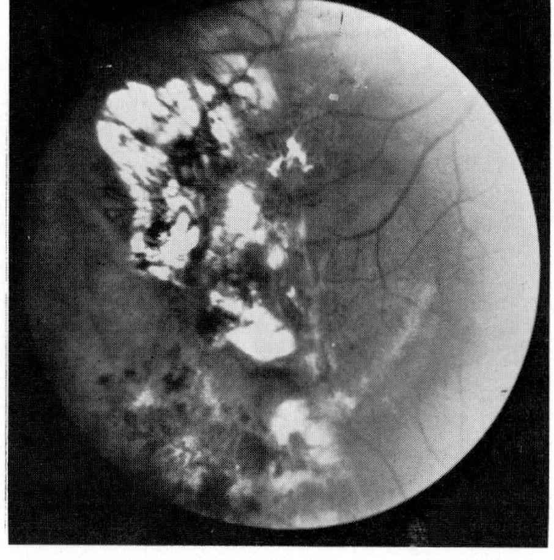

FIG. 15. Same eye as Figure 14, 3 years later.

REFERENCES

AMALRIC, P. and BIAU, C. (1967): Rétinopathie diabétique. La diathermocoagulation et la photocoagulation dans le traitement de la rétinopathie diabétique. *Arch. Ophtal. (Paris), 27,* 567.

GUINAN, P. (1967): Treatment of proliferative diabetic retinopathy. *Brit. J. Ophthal., 51,* 289.

IRVINE, A. R. and NORTON, E. W. D. (1971): Photocoagulation for diabetic retinopathy. *Amer. J. Ophthal., 71,* 437.

MCMEEL, J. W. (1967): *Treatment of Proliferative Diabetic Retinopathy*. Wilmer Meeting, April 1967.

MEYER-SCHWICKERATH, G. R. E. (1959): Lichtkoagulation. *Klin. Mbl. Augenheilk., Suppl. 33.*

MEYER-SCHWICKERARTH, G. R. E. and SCHOTT, K. (1968): Diabetic retinopathy and photocoagulation. *Amer. J. Ophthal., 66,* 597.

OKUN, E. (1968): The effectiveness of photocoagulation in the therapy of proliferative diabetic retinopathy (a controlled study in 50 patients). *Trans. Amer. Acad. Ophthal. Otolaryng., 72,* 246.

OKUN, E and CIBIS, P. A. (1966): The role of photocoagulation in the therapy of proliferative diabetic retinopathy. *AMA Arch. Ophthal., 75,* 337.

PATZ, A., SCHATZ, H. and RYAN, S. J. (1971): Argon laser photocoagulation for treatment of advanced diabetic retinopathy. *Trans. Amer. Acad. Ophthal. Otolaryng., 76,* 984.

RIASKOFF, S. (1972): Die diabetische Retinopathie und ihre Behandlung mit Lichtkoagulation. *Docum. Ophthal. (Den Haag), 32,* 1.

RUBINSTEIN, K. and MYSKA, V. (1972): Treatment of diabetic maculopathy. *Brit. J. Ophthal., 56,* 1.

SPALTER, H. F. (1971): Photocoagulation of circinate maculopathy in diabetic retinopathy. *Amer. J. Ophthal., 71,* 242.
WESSING, A. (1972): Über Technik und Indikation für die Lichtkoagulation bei diabetischer Retinopathie. *Klin. Mbl. Augenheilk., 160,* 274.
WETZIG, P. D. and JEPSON, C. N. (1967): Further observations on the treatment of diabetic retinopathy by light-coagulation. *Trans. Amer. Acad. Ophthal. Otolaryng., 71,* 902
ZETTERSTRÖM, B. (1972): The value of photocoagulation in diabetic retinopathy. *Acta Ophthal. (Kbh.), 50,* 351.
ZWENG, H. C., LITTLE, H. L. and PEABODY, R. R. (1971): Argon laser photocoagulation of diabetic retinopathy. *AMA Arch. Ophthal., 86,* 395.
ZWENG, H. C., LITTLE, H. L. and PEABODY, R. R. (1972): Further observations on argon laser photocoagulation of diabetic retinopathy. *Trans. Amer. Acad. Ophthal. Otolaryng., 76,* 990.

THE FETO-MATERNAL UNIT IN DIABETES

INTRODUCTORY REMARKS

JOSEPH J. HOET

Department of Medicine, University of Louvain, Belgium

The purpose of this panel is to integrate into the daily delivery of health care recent data on the realignments of fuels during pregnancy, obtained through clinical investigation and by the appropriate animal models.

Besides the genetic factors, the changes of the *milieu interieur* of the mother during pregnancy may influence the birth weight and birth size in the human even when these parameters remain in the physiological range. The duration of pregnancy, birth rank of the infant, maternal stature, maternal weight and maternal weight gain during pregnancy are correlated with normal birth weight. This indicates that the hormonal balance of the mother will influence the adaptation of the fetus. The hormonal balance of the mother depends upon the interaction of sexual and polypeptide hormones, the placenta or the fetus, as well as the metabolic status due to the food intake by the mother (de Gasparo and Hoet, 1971).

To achieve growth and maturity in the limits of the physiological range, the fetus draws the essential nutriments from the mother whose metabolic adaptation will be a continuous sequence of 'accelerated starvation' with food deprivation and 'facilitated anabolism' when food is ingested.

The studies to date indicate that the secretory reaction of the fetal endocrines will be pertinent to the inflow of maternal nutriments and that the fetus is glucose-dependent. It is therefore apposite that the realignment of the metabolic fuels in the pregnant mother as well as the fetal reaction to derangements of this realignment should be explored. The growth and the maturity of the fetus might not then remain in the physiological range.

In infants of diabetic mothers without vascular complication or major infection there seems to be ample supply of nutriments, and the blood sugar of the mother has been shown to influence fetal growth and fetal weight (Hoet, 1969). Other nutriments, like amino acids, may play a key role in maintaining anabolism imposed by fetal growth. The fetal pancreas will react to the stimulus of the nutriments derived from the mother and fetal hyperinsulinemia has been shown to be conducive to the growth of heavy birth weight newborn infants.

In order for this overgrowth to occur, other endocrine fetal organs, hypophysis and adrenals as well as other hormones (estrogens), have to acquire a new secretory response (de Gasparo and Hoet, 1971). They influence in their turn the secretory potentialities of the endocrine pancreas and will therefore have at least a permissive action in the fetal overgrowth. In infants of diabetic mothers with vascular complications the overflow of nutriments derived from the mother is impaired. This impairment will in turn inhibit normal growth.

Ethical reasons preclude a systematic analysis in human subjects, hence the importance of animal studies. The pancreatic secretion of the newborn indicates how sensitive this organ is to various metabolic fuels, especially amino acids. With these new concepts, better therapeutic goals can be achieved and increasingly sophisticated tests can be used to assess the maturity and viability which may differ from organ to organ (e.g. lung, kidney, adrenals).

On the basis of this new knowledge about the metabolic behavior of the mother and the dependent, non-autonomous fetus, adequate advice can be given concerning the proper amount of fat, proteins and carbohydrates to be administered as well as their schedule during the day and early night. Exercise and application of insulin treatment during the day and early night also will have to be aligned. This integrated advice will be given on the a priori assumption that reducing the blood sugar and concomitant parameters to physiological levels will gear the metabolic fuels and the hormonal secretion so that a healthy close to normal neonate may be born. However, the control of the mother may not be easy to achieve and the viability of the infant not simple to assess. Therefore the diabetic mother should be under close supervision from the physician and the obstetrician with the neonatalogist being informed of the evolution of pregnancy and the possible delivery date.

Frequent blood sugars (4 to 5 times), continuous adaptation of the insulin requirements and of physical exercises as well as the use of the different tests for the fetal organ's viability require sophisticated team work, which can only be achieved in specialized centres where an expertise has been acquired and is readily available at all times.

The patient should be followed on a 3 to 4 times a week basis and taken into hospital for the last weeks of pregnancy. The hospital has to offer the facilities for a standardized diet, frequent meals, exercises and very regular round the clock insulin therapy. Induction of delivery has to be possible at all times. However, with proper regulation, delivery could be delayed till the 39th week, so preventing the possible deleterious long-term effects of prematurity.

The panel agreed that, on the basis of the data presented, everything in the diabetic has to be foreseen: the planning of pregnancy, the perfect equilibrium before and during pregnancy, as well as the timing of the delivery. Nothing should be improvised with regard to the diabetic mother.

From the study of pregnancy in the diabetic, the panel made several clinical deductions:

1. In view of the uncommensurable complications of pregnancy in a diabetic woman with vascular disease, the young girls with insulin-dependent diabetes have to be under tight control from the onset of their disease. Early diagnosis and irreproachable treatment is mandatory to prevent or reduce the vascular complications which will have a deleterious effect upon the pregnancy.
2. Tight control of the diabetes will immediately improve the survival rate of the infants. It is the one instance where good control of the blood sugar will prevent the deleterious consequences of diabetes. On an a priori basis, this suggests that the prevention of long-term complications of diabetes can be achieved by early diagnosis and normalization of the blood sugar.
3. With better therapeutic goals, better results will be obtained. However, if fetal survival is one parameter of the effect of the appropriate treatment, it is the long-term follow-up which is indicative of good application of therapy. However, it is not yet known what kind of long-term follow-up is needed. This is mandatory and definitely work for the

future: what are the causes of congenital malformations, what long-term effect has ketonemia upon the brain, what are the causes of brain damage and is there permanent damage to the fetal pancreas when it is overstimulated at the fetal stage?

4. The treatment adhered to hitherto may have to be revised in a few years time when beta cell derived from cultures may be used to achieve still better control.

The success of having a normal infant born to a diabetic woman is the result of integrated team work, where present clinical investigations are applied to the delivery of health care and where the physician, obstetrician and pediatrician collaborate with a devoted diabetic woman and her husband. The panel concluded that, especially in the diabetic, preventive medicine starts during life before birth.

REFERENCES

HOET, J. J. (1969): Normal and abnormal foetal weight gain. In: *Ciba Foundation Symposium on Foetal Autonomy, 1969,* pp. 186–213. Editors: G. E. W. Wolstenholme and Meave O'Connor. Churchill, London.

DE GASPARO, M. and HOET, J. J. (1971): Normal and abnormal foetal weight gain. In: *Proceedings of the VIIth Congress of the International Diabetes Federation, Buenos Aires, 1970,* p. 667. Editor: R. R. Rodriguez. International Congress Series No. 231, Excerpta Medica, Amsterdam.

A MONKEY MODEL OF HUMAN PREGNANCY COMPLICATED BY GLUCOSE INTOLERANCE

RONALD A. CHEZ and DANIEL H. MINTZ

Pregnancy Research Branch, National Institute of Child Health and Human Development, National Institutes of Health, Bethesda, Md., and Department of Medicine, University of Miami School of Medicine, Miami, Fla., U.S.A.

We are in complete accord with Alexander Pope's dictum 'The Proper Study of Mankind is Man'. Having thus aligned ourselves, let us expand this rationality by also affirming that the use of man as an experimental model is proscribed by ethical considerations. These 2 truths have resulted in the search for animal models by scientific investigators. In some instances, naturally occurring diseases which simulate disease in man have been identified; in other instances, artificially induced diseases have been utilized (Cornelius, 1969; Jones, 1969).

With regard to diabetes mellitus specifically, glucose-intolerant states have been found or achieved in many species including the dog, Chinese hamster, horse, rat, sand rat, mouse, cat and simians (Cornelius, 1969; DiGiacomo et al., 1971; Jones, 1969; Kirk et al., 1972; Howard, 1971, 1972; Lang, 1966; Pitkin et al., 1970; Rerup, 1970). For some of us, the subhuman primate has an emotional appeal because of its apparent phylogenetic proximity. Actually, old world monkeys are a divergent evolutionary branch from man. However, monkeys possess important biological assets when the research study conditions require pregnancy as well as a pathologic state. Their litter size is one. The length of gestation is 5–6 months. The functional maturity of the newborn equates to that of humans. The morphological/functional characteristics of the placenta of both the Rhesus monkey and the baboon are more analogous to the human than to other species of laboratory animals (Adolph, 1970).

In the past several years, fetal physiologists have centered their attention on both the pregnant Rhesus monkey and the pregnant sheep to ask questions pertinent to human gestation. We have had the privilege of being monkey midwives through our relationship of many years with Dr. Donald L. Hutchinson. Recently the work has been directed primarily at maternal-fetal-neonatal carbohydrate metabolism.

The Rhesus monkey has an anatomic legacy which allows ease of access to the fetal circulation without interrupting the integrity of the amniotic sac. The placenta is bidiscoid. The 2 lobes are connected by interplacental vessels which contain fetal blood. This relationship permits sequential sampling of fetal blood via cannulation without direct manipulation of the fetus. Using this surgical approach, we have asked questions about fetal responsiveness (Reynolds et al., 1954) to directly applied stimuli and placental substrate transfer. Specifically, we have used this technique to assess in vivo carbohydrate metabolism in the Rhesus monkey third trimester fetus and the premature newborn of both normal and streptozotocin-induced glucose-intolerant mothers.

The proof/disproof of an animal model of man is the ability to extrapolate data to man. During the years of our work, human data on carbohydrate metabolism in pregnancy have accumulated from the enhanced availability and use of blood aliquots obtained from abortuses, scalp samples in labor, and the umbilical cord at birth. In almost every instance the data from the 2 species equates. This paper will detail these findings.

Blood samples from the human and monkey fetus and newborn are relatively small in volume secondary to the techniques used in obtaining them as well as the circulating blood volume; microtechniques are essential. Present laboratory methodology permits the measurement of insulin, growth hormone, glucagon, glucose, and free fatty acid concentrations using microtechniques. Applying this research protocol and these laboratory procedures, the following similarities have been found between the human and Rhesus monkey, *Macaca mulatta* (monkey references are starred).

MID-THIRD TRIMESTER FETUS IN A GLUCOSE-TOLERANT MOTHER

1. Maternal fasting hyperinsulinemia and an enhanced insulin response to intravenously administered glucose are present in both human and monkey pregnancy (Pitkin et al., 1970*; Spellacy and Goetz, 1963).
2. There is a relative barrier to the unidirectional maternal to fetal placental transfer of insulin, growth hormone, and glucagon (Adam et al., 1969, 1972; Chez et al., 1970*, 1973b*; Gitlin et al., 1965; Johnston et al., 1972; Josimovich and Knobil, 1961*; King et al., 1971; Mintz et al., 1969*). Minimal unidirectional fetal to maternal placental transfer of these hormones is present in the monkey (Chez et al., 1970*. 1973b*; Josimovich and Knobil, 1961*; Mintz et al., 1969*; Pitkin and Reynolds, 1969*).
3. The transfer of glucose across the placenta is secondary to the driving force of the plasma glucose concentration gradient between mother and fetus. A direct relationship exists between maternal, fetal, and amniotic fluid concentrations of glucose (Chez et al., 1972*; Chinard et al., 1956*: Spellacy et al., 1973). A possibility of a placental saturation level in man has been postulated (Beard et al., 1971) but it is not present in the monkey (Chez et al., 1973a*).
4. The basal fetal levels of plasma glucose, glucagon, insulin, and free fatty acids are similar (Chez et al., 1972*; Gentz et al., 1969; Mintz et al., 1969*; Spellacy et al., 1973; Thorell, 1970). Fetal plasma growth hormone levels are low in the monkey and equivalent to the findings in humans by some investigators (Spellacy et al., 1973) but not by others (Kaplan et al., 1972).
5. Granules containing insulin are present in the fetal pancreatic beta cell (Osman Hill, 1926*; Robb, 1961). There is no change in basal fetal plasma insulin concentrations after an intravenous glycemic stimulus (Chez and Mintz, 1973; Mintz et al., 1969*; Obenshain et al., 1970). Although there is no change in monkey fetal plasma insulin with an oral glycemic stimulus, intravenous arginine or theophylline infusion, there is an increment of plasma insulin after the intravenous injection of tolbutamide, glucagon, dibutyryl cyclic AMP, theophylline and glucose, and an infusion of mixed amino acids (Chez et al., 1970*, 1971*; Mintz et al., 1969*, 1972*). As of this writing, the presence of these findings in the human fetus has not been documented.

PREMATURE NEWBORN OF GLUCOSE-TOLERANT MOTHER ON THE FIRST DAY OF LIFE

1. There is a delayed or attenuated insulin response to intravenous glucose. The response is biphasic in the human and monophasic in the monkey (Chez and Mintz, 1973; Mintz et al., 1969*).
2. Relative to fetal levels, the plasma free fatty acid concentration is elevated (Chez et al., 1970*; Gentz et al., 1969).
3. The intravenous administration of mixed amino acids, tolbutamide, theophylline with glucose, and glucagon is associated with a prompt increase in plasma insulin concentrations (Chez et al., 1970*; Grasso et al., 1968, 1970; Mintz et al., 1969*, 1972*).
4. Induced hyperglycemia does not suppress plasma growth hormone levels (Cornblath et al., 1965; Mintz et al., 1969*).

MID-THIRD TRIMESTER FETUS AND PREMATURE NEWBORN FROM GLUCOSE-INTOLERANT MOTHER (DIABETES MELLITUS IN THE HUMAN, STREPTOZOTOCIN TREATMENT IN THE MONKEY)

1. Fetal macrosomia, placental hyperplasia, polyhydramnios, and third trimester intrauterine death occur (Farquhar, 1959; Mintz et al., 1972*; Peel, 1955).
2. Fetal and newborn hyperinsulinemia are present. Pancreatic beta cell hyperplasia is found in histologic examination (Chez and Mintz, 1973; Jørgensen et al., 1966; Mintz et al., 1972*).
3. There is prompt insulin release when glucose is administered intravenously to the fetus as well as an insulin responsiveness to the infusion of a dilute mixture of amino acids; the latter is not yet confirmed in the human. A prompt plasma insulin response to an intravenous glycemic stimulus in the newborn is found (Chez and Mintz, 1973; Mintz et al., 1972*; Mølsted-Pedersen and Jørgensen, 1972).

Having thus provided evidence to support our hypothesis that an animal model of carbohydrate metabolism in normal and glucose-intolerant human pregnancy does exist, we now wish to provide perspective.

Scientifically, diabetes mellitus is not just glucose intolerance. Rather, it is a continuum of pathologic phenomena with various times of onset and incidence rates for each individual. There is no evidence that either the streptozotocin-induced glucose intolerant state nor the naturally occurring glucose intolerant state reported in an occasional older monkey equates to the disease in man. Biologically, the Rhesus monkey has the potential of being as heterogeneous in its stock as man. There are differences in the ecological environment and diet of the species and differences in the physiological and structural ontogeny of the newborn. Practically, there are important considerations of supply, cost, docility, housing needs, breeding capacity, acute experimental conditions, and a relatively limited blood volume.

These comments do not invalidate or disparage existing and presently evolving work in these or other studies. They serve merely to emphasize the requirements governing all scientific investigation: to be conscious of limitations, rigorous in defining the variables, and circumspect about interpretation.

REFERENCES

ADAM, P. A. J., TERAMO, K., RAÏHA, N., GITLIN, D. and SCHWARTZ, R. (1969): Human fetal insulin metabolism early in gestation. *Diabetes, 18,* 409.

ADAM, P. A. J., KING, K. C., SCHWARTZ, R. and TERAMO, K. (1972): Human placental barrier to I^{125}-glucagon early in gestation. *J. clin. Endocr., 34/5,* 773.

ADOLPH, E. F. (1970): Physiological stages in the development of mammals. *Growth, 34/2,* 113.

BEARD, R. W., TURNER, R. C. and OAKLEY, N. W. (1971): An investigation into the control of blood glucose in fetuses of normal and diabetic mothers. In: *Proceedings of the Second Congress on Perinatal Medicine,* p. 114. Editors: P. J. Huntingford, R. W. Beard, F. E. Hytten and J. W. Scopes. Karger, Basel.

CHEZ, R. A. and MINTZ, D. H. (1973): The development and function of the human endocrine pancreas. In: *The Endocrine Milieu of Pregnancy, Puerperium, and Childhood,* p. 17. Editor: R. B. Jaffe. Ross Laboratories, Columbus, Ohio.

CHEZ, R. A., MINTZ, D. H., HORGER III, E. O. and HUTCHINSON, D. L. (1970): Factors affecting the response to insulin in the normal subhuman pregnant primate. *J. clin. Invest., 49/8,* 1517.

CHEZ, R. A., MINTZ, D. H. and HUTCHINSON, D. L. (1971): Effect of theophylline on glucagon and glucose-mediated plasma insulin response in subhuman primate fetus and neonate. *Metabolism, 20/8,* 805.

CHEZ, R. A., MINTZ, D. H. and HUTCHINSON, D. L. (1972): Carbohydrate metabolism in primate pregnancy. In: *Proceedings of the Fourth International Congress of Endocrinology,* p. 1157. Editor: R. Scow. International Congress Series No. 273, Excerpta Medica, Amsterdam.

CHEZ, R. A., MINTZ, D. H., REYNOLDS, W. A. and HUTCHINSON, D. L. (1973a): Maternal-fetal plasma carbohydrate relationships in monkey pregnancy. *Amer. J. Obstet. Gynec.,* in press.

CHEZ, R. A., MINTZ, D. H., MIRSKY, A. I. and HUTCHINSON, D. L. (1973b): Fetal glucagon metabolism in the monkey (Macaca mulatta). *Amer. J. Obstet. Gynec.,* in press.

CHINARD, F. P., DANESINO, V., HARTMANN, W. L., HUGGETT, A. St. G., PAUL, W. and REYNOLDS, S. R. M. (1956): The transmission of hexoses across the placenta in the human and the Rhesus monkey. *J. Physiol., 132/3,* 289.

CORNBLATH, M., PARKER, M. L., REISNER, S. H., FORBES, A. E. and DAUGHADAY, W. H. (1965): Secretion and metabolism of growth hormone in premature and full term infants. *J. clin. Endocr., 25/3,* 209.

CORNELIUS, C. E. (1969): Animal models – A neglected medical resource. *New Engl. J. Med., 281/17,* 934.

DiGIACOMO, R. F., MYERS, R. E. and BAEZ, L. R. (1971): Diabetes mellitus in a Rhesus monkey (Macaca mulatta): A case report and literature review. *Lab. anim. Sci., 21/4,* 572.

FARQUHAR, J. W. (1959): The child of the diabetic woman. *Arch. Dis. Childh., 34/1,* 76.

GENTZ, J. C. H., WARRNER, R., PERSSON, B. E. H. and CORNBLATH, M. (1969): Intravenous glucose tolerance, plasma insulin, free fatty acids and beta-hydroxybutyrate in underweight newborn infants. *Acta paed. scand., 58/5,* 481.

GITLIN, D., KUMATE, J. and MORALES, C. (1965): Metabolism and maternofetal transfer of human growth hormone in pregnant women at term. *J. clin. Endocr., 25/12,* 1599.

GRASSO, S., SAPORITO, N., MESSINA, A. and REITANO, G. (1968): Serum-insulin response to glucose and amino acids in the premature infant. *Lancet, 2/1,* 755.

GRASSO, S., SAPORITO, N., MESSINA, A. and REITANO, G. (1970): Effect of theophylline, glucagon, theophylline plus glucagon on insulin secretion in the premature infant. *Diabetes, 19/10,* 837.

HOWARD Jr., C. F. (1971): New technique for inducing diabetes mellitus in monkeys. *Primate News, 9/3,* 3.

HOWARD Jr., C. F. (1972): Spontaneous diabetes in the colony of Celebes apes. *Primate News, 10/9,* 3.

JOHNSTON, D. I., BLOOM, S. R., GREENE, K. R. and BEARD, R. W. (1972): Failure of the human placenta to transfer pancreatic glucagon. *Biol. Neonate, 21/3,* 375.

JONES, T. C. (1969): Mammalian and avian models of disease in man. *Fed. Proc., 28/1,* 162.

JØRGENSEN, K. R., DECKERT, T., PEDERSEN, L. M. and PEDERSEN, J. (1966): Insulin, insulin antibody and glucose in plasma of newborn infants of diabetic women. *Acta endocr. (Kbh.), 52/3,* 1966.

JOSIMOVICH, J. B. and KNOBIL, E. (1961): Placental transfer of I^{131}-insulin in the Rhesus monkey. *Amer. J. Physiol., 200/3,* 471.

KAPLAN, S. L., GRUMBACH, M. M. and SHEPARD, T. H. (1972): The ontogenesis of human fetal hormones. *J. clin. Invest., 51/12,* 3080.

KING, K. C., ADAM, P. A. J., SCHWARTZ, R. and TERAMO, K. (1971): Human placental transfer of human growth hormone-I^{125}. *Pediatrics, 48/8,* 534.

KIRK, J. H., CASEY, H. W. and HARWELL Jr., J. F. (1972): Diabetes mellitus in two Rhesus monkeys. *Lab. anim. Sci., 22/3,* 245.

LANG, C. M. (1966): Impaired glucose tolerance in the squirrel monkey (Saimiri sciuresis). *Proc. Soc. exp. Biol. Med. (N.Y.), 122/1,* 84.

MINTZ, D. H., CHEZ, R. A. and HORGER III, E. O. (1969): Fetal insulin and growth hormone metabolism in the subhuman primate. *J. clin. Invest., 48/1,* 176.

MINTZ, D. H., CHEZ, R. A. and HUTCHINSON, D. L. (1972): Subhuman primate pregnancy complicated by streptozotocin-induced diabetes mellitus. *J. clin. Invest., 51/4,* 837.

MØLSTED-PEDERSEN, L. and JØRGENSEN, K. R. (1972): Aspects of carbohydrate metabolism in newborn infants of diabetic mothers. *Acta Endocr. (Kbh.), 71/5,* 1972.

OBENSHAIN, S. S., ADAM, P. A. J., KING, K. C., RAÏHA, N., RAIVO, K., TERAMO, K. and SCHWARTZ, R. (1970): Human fetal insulin response to sustained maternal hyperglycemia. *New Engl. J. Med., 283/7,* 566.

OSMAN HILL, W. C. (1926): A comparative study of the pancreas. *Proc. zool. Soc. (Lond.),* 581.

PEEL, J. H. (1955): Management of the pregnant diabetic. *Brit. med. J., 2/2,* 870.

PITKIN, R. M. and REYNOLDS, W. A. (1969): Insulin transfer across the hemochorial placenta. *Obstet. Gynec., 33/5,* 626.

PITKIN, R. M., VAN ORDEN, D. E. and REYNOLDS, W. A. (1970): Plasma insulin response and glucose tolerance in pregnant Rhesus monkeys. *Endocrinology, 86/2,* 435.

PITKIN, R. M. and REYNOLDS, W. A. (1970): Diabetogenic effects of streptozotocin in Rhesus monkeys. *Diabetes, 19/2,* 85.

RERUP, C. C. (1970): Drugs producing diabetes through damage of the insulin secreting cells. *Pharmacol. Rev., 22/4,* 485.

REYNOLDS, S. R. M., PAUL, W. M. and HUGGETT, A. St. G. (1954): Physiological study of the monkey fetus in utero. *Bull. Johns Hopk. Hosp., 95/7,* 256.

ROBB, P. (1961): The development of the islets of Langerhans in the human fetus. *Quart. J. exp. Physiol., 46/5,* 335.

SPELLACY, W. N. and GOETZ, F. C. (1963): Plasma insulin in normal late pregnancy. *New Engl. J. Med., 268/18,* 988.

SPELLACY, W. N., BUHI, W. C., BRADLEY, B. and HOLSINGER, K. K. (1973): Maternal, fetal and amniotic fluid levels of glucose, insulin and growth hormone. *Obstet. Gynecol., 41/3,* 323.

THORELL, J. I. (1970): Plasma insulin levels in normal foetuses. *Acta endocr. (Kbh.), 63/2,* 134.

FACILITATED ANABOLISM IN LATE PREGNANCY: SOME NOVEL MATERNAL COMPENSATIONS FOR ACCELERATED STARVATION*

NORBERT FREINKEL, BOYD E. METZGER, MENACHEM NITZAN, ROBERT DANIEL, BARBARA Z. SURMACZYNSKA and THEODORE C. NAGEL

Center for Endocrinology, Metabolism, and Nutrition and the Departments of Medicine and Biochemistry, Northwestern University Medical School, Chicago, Ill., U.S.A.

Theoretical considerations as well as certain observations in normal women (Bleicher et al., 1964) prompted us to suggest in 1964 that the pattern of metabolic response to dietary deprivation in late pregnancy should conform to 'accelerated starvation' (Freinkel, 1965). Our hypothesis was advanced at the Fifth Congress of the International Diabetes Federation during a panel on Diabetes in Pregnancy chaired by the man who pioneered all the inquiries into that area, the late Professor Joseph P. Hoet (Freinkel, 1965). We proposed 'accelerated starvation' on the assumption that the transition to endogenous fuels, whenever food is withheld, must occur more rapidly in the mother since she has to supply not only her own needs but also those of the developing conceptus. Moreover, we indicated that products of fat metabolism alone, even if they crossed the placenta freely, as is the case for ketones (Scow et al., 1958; Sabata et al., 1968), could not support fetal growth since nitrogen as well as 3- to 6-carbon building blocks would be required for the anabolism of proteins, complex carbohydrates and glyceride-glycerol. Thus, we speculated that the fasting pregnant mother also would be unable to conserve her endogenous fuels other than fat with the same parsimony that characterizes starvation under non-gravid conditions (Freinkel, 1965).

Six years later, at another panel during the Seventh Congress of the International Diabetes Federation we were able to review the substantive evidence that had accumulated in support of the concept of 'accelerated starvation' (Freinkel et al., 1971). More rapid activation of net lipolysis during dietary deprivation in gravid animals had been documented with isolated fat pads in vitro (Freinkel et al., 1970; Knopp et al., 1970; Chernick and Novak, 1970) as well as with direct measurements of FFA and glycerol in plasma and tissues (Knopp et al., 1970; Chernick and Novak, 1970; Freinkel, 1969; Herrera et al., 1969). Increased muscle catabolism had been demonstrated on the basis of relative changes in muscle mass and urinary losses of relevant electrolytes such as potassium and phosphorus (Herrera et al., 1969). Inordinately exaggerated rises in plasma and urinary ketones with fasting in pregnancy had attested to the accelerated rate of ketogenesis (Herrera et al., 1969; Scow et al., 1964; Felig and Lynch, 1970). Finally, aug-

* Supported in part by Research Grant AM-10699 and Training Grant AM-05071 from the National Institute of Arthritis and Metabolic Diseases; and by Clinical Research Center Grant RR-48 from the Division of Research Resources, National Institutes of Health, Bethesda, Maryland.

mented gluconeogenic potential had been delineated with isotopic studies in vivo (Herrera et al., 1969), perfused livers in vitro (Metzger et al., 1970, 1973), and the finding of heightened urinary nitrogen losses during early fasting in gravid humans (Felig and Lynch, 1970) as well as laboratory animals (Herrera et al., 1969). The 'accelerated starvation' had been ascribed in part to the continuing removal of glucose and amino acids by the fetus, leading to the reduction of these moieties as well as of circulating insulin in maternal plasma. It was suggested that the pattern was also abetted directly or indirectly by the endocrine principles which were being elaborated unremittingly by the placenta, and that the new equilibrium would necessitate increased insulinogenesis at all times (Freinkel et al., 1970, 1971).*

In 1973, therefore, substantial evidence attests to the fact that nitrogen and lipid catabolism occur more rapidly during fasting in pregnancy and that these quantitative exaggerations of the response to dietary deprivation justify the designation 'accelerated starvation'. However, that term also has certain implications for the fed state. In the least it would mean that the pregnant animal starts off from a different metabolic baseline whenever she eats than her non-gravid counterpart. In theory, at the time of eating, tissues from the gravid animal should (a) contain more abundant fatty acids, (b) be utilizing more fat products, (c) have experienced more antecedent catabolism, and (d) perhaps be in more precariously balanced nitrogen equilibrium.

In this paper, we should like to focus on recent studies on the interrelationships among maternal fuels during the fed state in late pregnancy. For our purposes, we have confined ourselves to the longest period of dietary deprivation that the mother normally encounters, namely overnight fast, and to the simplest of all fuels, namely glucose. We have specifically attempted to see whether there are novel mechanisms, above and beyond the usual, by which the mother could replete her tissue reserves in anticipation of the next wave of 'accelerated starvation'. In other words, we have been seeking mechanisms of facilitated anabolism as the converse of 'accelerated starvation'.

To approach this question, simple glucose solutions (100 g glucose as Dextrofizz) were given at 8.00 a.m., after 14 hour overnight fast, to (a) normal pregnant women in week 30–40 of gestation, (b) the same subjects 5–8 weeks postpartum, and (c) nulliparous, age-matched volunteers. Specimens were secured before and after these dietary challenges and analyzed for glucose (Hoffman, 1937), immunoreactive insulin (IRI) (Herrera et al., 1969), free fatty acids (FFA) (Marshal and Hoover, 1971), total amino acids (Palmer and Peters, 1965), triglycerides (Kessler and Lederer, 1965), and cholesterol (Levine and Zak, 1964). Basal values for these parameters are summarized in Table 1. As has been observed previously, women in late pregnancy after overnight fast ('0' time) displayed lower values

* Some qualitatively unique features have also been recognized since then (Freinkel et al., 1972). For example, it has become apparent that there are some restraints to muscle catabolism during fasting in pregnancy since maternal plasma amino acids are unable to keep up with glucogenic potential (Metzger et al., 1971; Felig et al., 1972) so that hypoglycemia prevails as the fast is extended (Herrera et al., 1969; Scow et al., 1964; Felig and Lynch, 1970). Similarly, a far greater proportion of the nitrogen which is evolved during intrahepatic gluconeogenesis from amino acids emerges in a potentially reutilizable form as ammonia (or glutamine) rather than as urea (Metzger et al., 1970, 1973), and therefore may be salvaged for pyrimidine biosynthesis (Shambaugh et al., 1971). Thus, the 'accelerated starvation' need not be wholly profligate (Freinkel et al., 1972).

TABLE 1
*Basal values for plasma metabolites and insulin in young women after overnight fast**

	Non-gravid (16)	Late pregnancy (36)	P
Glucose (mg/100 ml)	87.5 ± 1.6	80.3 ± 1.2	< 0.001
Insulin (μU/ml)	9.0 ± 0.9	12.6 ± 0.7	< 0.01
Amino acids (mmoles/l)	3.82 ± 0.13	3.18 ± 0.11	< 0.001
FFA (μmoles/l)	626 ± 42	725 ± 21	< 0.05
Triglyceride (mg/100 ml)	76.2 ± 7.0	181 ± 10	< 0.001
Cholesterol (mg/100 ml)	163 ± 8.7	205 ± 5.7	< 0.001

* All basal specimens of blood were secured in duplicate between 8.00 and 9.00 a.m. after a 14 hour fast. Subjects were recumbent for at least 30 minutes prior to securing blood specimens and throughout subsequent challenges with oral glucose. 'Late pregnancy' denotes normal women in week 30–40 of gestation.

for plasma glucose (Bleicher et al., 1964; Silverstone et al., 1961; Hagen, 1961) and amino acid nitrogen (Bonsnes, 1947; Christensen et al., 1957), and higher concentrations of plasma FFA (Bleicher et al., 1964; Burt, 1960; Kalkhoff et al., 1964), insulin (Bleicher et al., 1964; Leake and Burt, 1962; Spellacy and Goetz, 1963), triglycerides (Scow et al., 1964; Oliver and Boyd, 1955; Svanborg and Vikrot, 1965), and cholesterol (Scow et al., 1964; Oliver and Boyd, 1955; Svanborg and Vikrot, 1965) than non-gravid subjects.

INTERRELATIONSHIPS BETWEEN GLUCOSE, IMMUNOREACTIVE INSULIN (IRI) AND FFA IN LATE PREGNANCY

Figure 1 depicts the changes in glucose, insulin, and FFA following oral administration of 100 g glucose after overnight fast during week 30–40 of pregnancy and again 5–8 weeks postpartum. The data reaffirm what has been known for a number of years: glucose increments are higher and more prolonged antepartum than following delivery (Spellacy and Goetz, 1963; O'Sullivan and Mahan, 1964; Beck and Wells, 1969; Kalkhoff et al., 1970), and attended by more marked increases in IRI (Spellacy and Goetz, 1963; Beck and Wells, 1969; Kalkhoff et al., 1970). (Ongoing collaborative studies between Dr. Richard L. Phelps in our laboratory and Dr. Arthur H. Rubenstein of the University of Chicago would tend to exclude inappropriate amounts of proinsulin as the basis for the hyperinsulinemia.) However, certain additional points which have not been emphasized previously warrant comment. Firstly, the absolute rise in plasma glucose following ingestion of glucose is not significantly greater at 15 minutes antepartum and only marginally so at 30 minutes whereas the increment in insulin is already significantly higher at 15 minutes. The hyperresponsiveness of the insulin secretory mechanism in gestation is in accord with the inferences derived from intravenous challenges with glucose and other

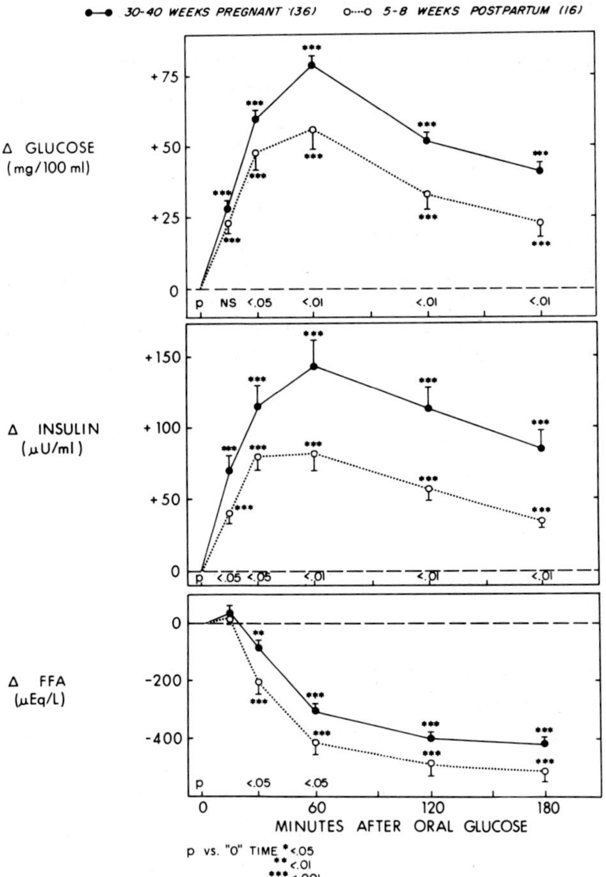

FIG. 1. Effect of pregnancy on the response of plasma glucose, immunoreactive insulin and FFA to oral glucose. Oral glucose (100 g) was administered at 8.00 a.m. after 14 hours overnight fast to 36 normal women during 30–40 weeks of gestation and again to 16 of them 5–8 weeks postpartum. Mean ± S.E.M. values for the subsequent changes in plasma glucose, insulin, and FFA are shown. The asterisks denote the significance of the changes at each time point (P vs. '0 minutes': * = < 0.05, ** = < 0.01, and *** = < 0.001) and have been derived on the basis of paired t analyses with fasting values in individual subjects. The P values at the bottom of each panel denote the significance of the differences between antepartum and postpartum changes at each time point on a paired t basis.

secretogogues (Bleicher et al., 1964; Kalkhoff et al., 1964; Yen et al., 1971). However, the failure of this 'extra' insulin to blunt the early (15 minute) increment in plasma glucose following oral glucose may suggest that the liver as well as the periphery is relatively resistant to insulin after overnight fast in late pregnancy. That premise is based on the supposition that (1) the liver constitutes the first metabolic target for both the absorbed glucose and the insulin released by stimulated secretion; and (2) the early rise of blood sugar reflects glucose that has survived the immediate insulin-mediated extraction and disposition within the liver (Perley and Kipnis, 1967). Secondly, the early decline of FFA following glucose ingestion, i.e., at 15 and 30 minutes, is significantly less antepartum than postpartum despite comparable increases in plasma glucose. Presumably, therefore, net interruption of ongoing lipolytic events by glucose and insulin may be somewhat slower antepartum. In the least, since tissue and extracellular FFA tend to be in equilibrium and plasma FFA are higher antepartum, it appears that ingested glucose is made available to tissues which are already, and perhaps continuingly, metabolizing FFA to an increased extent.

The relationship between the basal levels of plasma FFA at the time of glucose ingestion and the integrated subsequent changes in plasma glucose (i.e. 'glucose area') were examined to assess whether the heightened and more prolonged antepartum availability of FFA could be playing a role in impeding glucose flux. The results are summarized in Figure 2. Fasting FFA and net glucose area displayed a significant correlation ($r = 0.503$; $P < 0.01$).

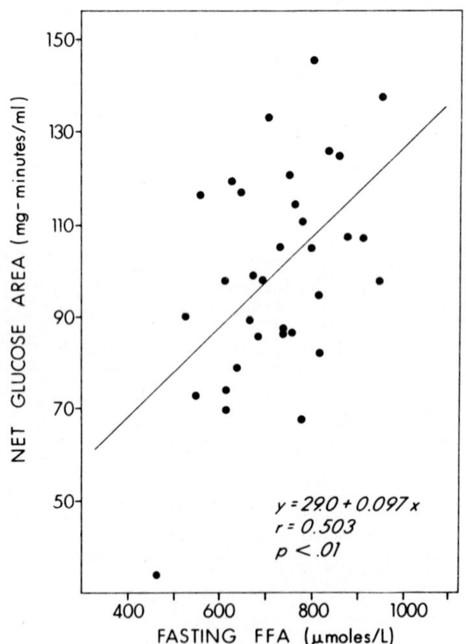

FIG. 2. The relationship between the hyperglycemic response to glucose during pregnancy and fasting FFA. Regression equations were derived relating fasting FFA at the time of glucose ingestion to the integrated changes in plasma glucose ('net glucose area') during the subsequent 180 minutes. Subjects were normal women in week 30–40 of pregnancy.

ACUTE EFFECTS OF ORAL GLUCOSE ON PLASMA TRIGLYCERIDES AND CHOLESTEROL IN LATE PREGNANCY

Carbohydrate-induced triglyceridemia in non-diabetics has been varyingly associated with impedance to glucose utilization, more active and larger adipocytes, hyperlipacidemia, and hyperinsulinemia (Reaven et al., 1967; Bernstein et al., 1972; Eaton and Nye, 1973; Schlierf and Dorow, 1973). The presence of all these phenomena in late pregnancy prompted us to monitor plasma triglycerides and cholesterol in our subjects (Metzger et al., 1973). Changes from baseline values following 100 g oral glucose are summarized in Figure 3.

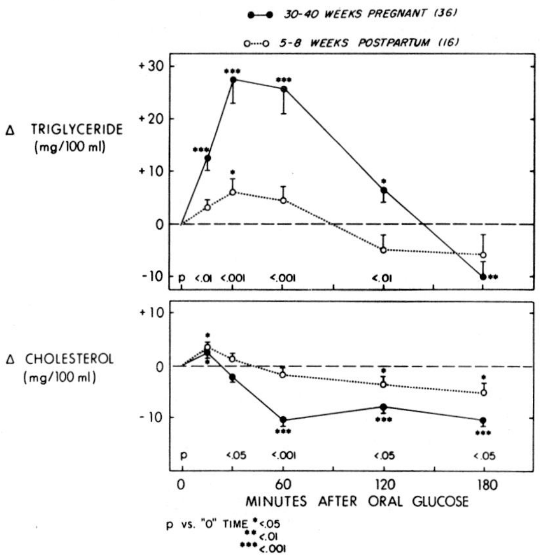

FIG. 3. Effect of pregnancy on the acute response of plasma triglycerides and cholesterol to oral glucose. Subjects with normal carbohydrate tolerance were challenged with 100 g oral glucose after overnight fast. Subsequent changes in plasma triglycerides and cholesterol have been presented and analyzed statistically as in Figure 1.

Triglycerides displayed dramatic ante- vs. postpartum differences following oral glucose. Antepartum, profound and highly significant increases in plasma triglycerides were seen at 15, 30, and 60 minutes with a subsequent fall to levels significantly below baseline by 180 minutes. Comparable acute excursions in triglycerides were not seen postpartum; triglyceride values tended to remain near baseline save for a minor and marginally significant increment at 30 minutes. Examination of plasma cholesterol indicates that the antepartum increases in triglycerides reflected increased endogenous biosynthesis rather than a 'pile up' due to deficient lipoprotein clearance (Fig. 3). Although marginally significant increments in plasma cholesterol were seen antepartum as well as postpartum within 15 minutes following the administration of glucose, values fell to a small but highly significant extent at 60, 120 and 180 minutes antepartum (Fig. 3). The diverging triglyceride/cholesterol relationships suggested selective increases in the entry of lipoproteins of lower density into the circulation. Analysis of 30-minute plasmas by flotation-ultracentrifugation, heparin-Mg^{++} precipitation, and agarose gel electrophoresis (with staining for pre-beta lipoproteins) corroborated that the acute changes were confined almost wholly to the very low density lipoprotein (VLDL) fraction. In this regard, recent evidence indicates that the fasting lipemia of non-diabetic human pregnancy also cannot be explained by impaired lipid removal (Knopp and Arky, 1972).

To derive more precise insights into the determinants of the acute carbohydrate-induced endogenous triglyceridemia, the 36 antepartum subjects whom we had examined were subdivided into 2 groups. Subjects were classified as 'responders' and 'non-responders', depending on whether or not they displayed triglyceride increments exceeding basal values by 10% or more at any time during oral glucose tolerance. By this criterion, there were 22 'responders' and 14 'non-responders'. The former did not differ from the latter either in terms of body weight, or in their changes in plasma cholesterol, glucose, or FFA following glucose administration. However, one major difference emerged. The 'responders' elaborated more insulin (Fig. 4), and presumably therefore required more insulin to arrest net lipolysis, attenuate hyperlipacidemia and dispose of the same amount of glucose. This relative insulin resistance can be inferred from the significant correlation which we found for all 36 subjects between antepartum fasting plasma insulin and the net triglyceride area following glucose administration ($r = 0.465; P > 0.01$).

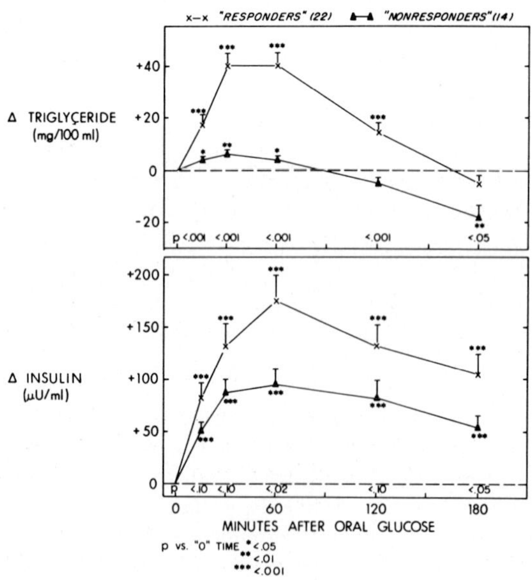

FIG. 4. Relationship between plasma insulin and acute rise in plasma triglycerides following oral glucose in late pregnancy. The 36 antepartum subjects shown in Figure 3 have been subdivided into 'responders' and 'non-responders' on the basis of their acute increment in triglyceride following oral glucose. For details, see text.

Regardless of mediation, the findings suggest a novel means whereby some of the excess carbohydrate in the diet can be retained by the mother and excluded from immediate access to the fetus. In contrast to the ready transplacental transfer of glucose, triglycerides seem to traverse the placenta poorly (Coltart, 1972). Thus, the incorporation of an increased proportion of dietary glucose into VLDL provides a mechanism for excluding the glucose from the fetus at a time of dietary surfeit and retaining it for subsequent recall as glycerol during fasting. Within this formulation, while some of the dietary glucose might be used for the de novo biosynthesis of fatty acids, more of it would be trapped as glyceride-glycerol during the esterification of intrahepatic fatty acids. The fatty acids from the resultant VLDL could be subsequently deployed to replete adipose stores, a process which would consume more glucose to provide glyceride-glycerol for re-esterification within depot fat. In essence, the heightened turnover of fat would facilitate maternal anabolism in the fed state by enabling a sugar moiety, namely glycerol, to be stored for subsequent recall and transplacental passage when food is withheld.

EFFECTS OF ORAL GLUCOSE ON PLASMA GLUCAGON

Maternal anabolism would be facilitated further if there were mechanisms for attenuating glycogenolysis, gluconeogenesis, and muscle catabolism above and beyond heightened insulin alone. A search for such a mechanism prompted studies to secure the first characterization of glucagon dynamics during human pregnancy (Daniel et al., 1972) since the alpha cell is another site which may be responsive to the flux of glucose and insulin (Vance et al., 1968; Unger, 1971). Accordingly, blood specimens were collected with Trasylol and EDTA and analyzed for plasma immunoreactive glucagon (IRG) with antibody 30 K and recent immunoassay modifications (Santeusanio et al., 1972) in collaboration with Drs. Roger Unger and Gerald Faloona.

Basal values for IRG, glucose, and insulin after 14 hour overnight fast in 25 pregnant women (during week 30–40 of gestation), in 16 women postpartum, and in 26 nulliparous volunteers are summarized in Table 2. As previously reported (vide supra) plasma glucose was lower and insulin higher in the pregnant than in the non-gravid subjects. Plasma IRG appeared unaltered by pregnancy when compared to the nulliparous group. However, a small but significant decrement in basal IRG was seen in the postpartum population (Table 2). The pair-matched net changes in IRG that occurred when 16 of the pregnant subjects were challenged with 100 g glucose and again 5–8 weeks postpartum are summarized in Figure 5. As before, the deviations from baseline for glucose and insulin were greater ante- than postpartum, so that net glucose and insulin areas, integrated over 180 minutes, were approximately 35% and 45% greater respectively during pregnancy. To what extent is gestational hyperreactivity of the beta cell associated with some altered secretory function of the alpha cell? As can be seen, antepartum as well as postpartum, the administration of glucose elicited the predicted reductions in plasma IRG. Significant decrements were observed from 30 minutes onward following glucose administration postpartum. However, as has *not* been reported previously, the decrements in plasma IRG were more pronounced antepartum. On a pair-matched basis, they were significantly greater at 120 and 180 minutes in association with the concurrently enhanced increments in plasma glucose and insulin. Thus, whereas maximal decline of IRG was only 15.3% postpartum, it averaged 28.6% in the same subjects antepartum.

TABLE 2
*Basal relationships of plasma glucose, insulin and glucagon in normal women after overnight fast**

	Plasma		
	Glucose mg/100 ml	Insulin μU/ml	Glucagon pg/ml
A. Antepartum (25)	80 ± 1.5	13.0 ± 1.0	60 ± 3.0
B. Postpartum (16)	87 ± 1.4	8.2 ± 0.6	43 ± 3.3
C. Nullipara (26)	88 ± 0.8	6.0 ± 0.3	64 ± 5.8
P			
A vs. B	< 0.01	< 0.001	< 0.001
A vs. C	< 0.001	< 0.001	N.S.
B vs. C	N.S.	< 0.01	< 0.01

* Specimens were secured as described in Table 1. 'Antepartum' denotes week 30–40 of gestation; 'Postpartum' refers to some of the same women re-examined 5–8 weeks following delivery; 'Nullipara' denotes non-gravid, nulliparous volunteers in the same age group.

The data are consistent with the view that, in pregnancy, as under non-gravid conditions, glucagon secretion may be subject to feed-back suppression directly or indirectly by insulin-mediated glucose flux. Indeed, the phenomenon appears to be exaggerated during gestation so that alpha cells are 'turned off' more markedly by glucose in pregnancy as beta cells are 'turned on' to a greater extent. The present findings corroborate our earlier observations in humans that heightened beta cell activity preponderates in the gestational hyperplasia of pancreatic islets (Daniel et al., 1972), and they are also concordant with preliminary findings in the pregnant rat (Saudek and Knopp, 1973; Metzger et al., unpublished observations).

Another form of 'facilitated anabolism', therefore, seems operative, since the disparate and relatively unopposed augmentation of insulin would favor retention and storage of dietary glucose in the mother not only as glycogen but also as the triglycerides, cited above. It should be recalled that glucagon deficiency may be associated with rapid induction of hyperlipemia (Paloyan and Harper, 1961) and it has been postulated (Eaton and Kipnis, 1969) that reciprocal changes in insulin and glucagon are complementary in carbohydrate-induced increases in the formation of VLDL.

EFFECTS OF ORAL GLUCOSE ON PLACENTAL HORMONES

Since the earliest characterization of human chorionic somatomammotropin (HCS), it had been felt that the prevailing plasma levels of this hormone were unaffected by acute

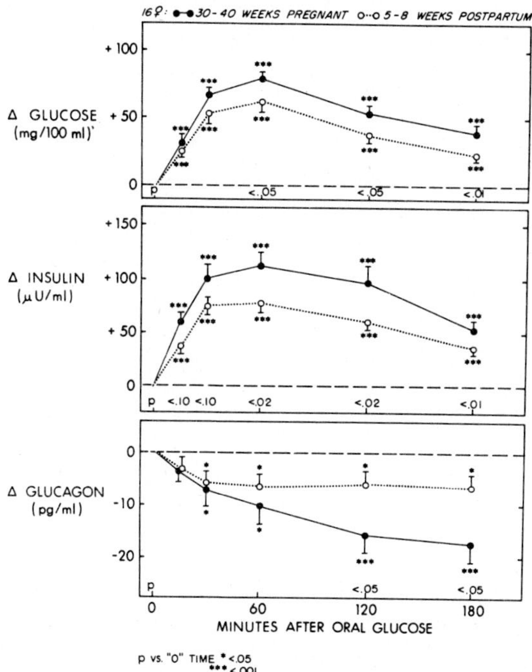

FIG. 5. Effects of pregnancy on the response of plasma glucose, insulin, and glucagon to oral glucose in subjects with normal carbohydrate tolerance. Oral glucose (100 g) was administered after overnight fast to 16 normal women during 30–40 weeks of gestation and again 5–8 weeks postpartum. Mean ± S.E.M. values for subsequent changes in plasma glucose, insulin, and glucagon are presented and analyzed for statistical significance as in Figure 1.

changes in the concentration of circulating maternal fuels (see Freinkel, 1965, and Freinkel et al., 1971, for review of literature). However, several recent observations seem to conflict with this dogma. Firstly, Burt et al. (1970) noted progressive 'decreases in the concentration of HPL amounting to 400–500 μg/ml' during the first 30 minutes following intravenous administration of 25 g glucose 'under basal conditions after 15 hour fast' at or near term. Subsequently, Spellacy et al. (1971) also observed that '27 pregnant women' who had been fasted overnight displayed significant reductions of HCS averaging 500 μg/ml within 5 minutes following 25 g glucose intravenously and coincident with an increase in blood glucose averaging 163 mg% above pretest levels. Although others have been unable to reproduce these effects of intravenous glucose (Ajabor and Yen, 1972), we were prompted to evaluate changes in plasma HCS in situations which more nearly parallel the usual metabolic experience of the pregnant female. Thus, we analyzed for plasma HCS (Samaan et al., 1966) in 33 normal subjects whose basal HCS averaged 8.4 ± 0.45 μg/ml when they were given 100 g glucose by mouth after overnight fast during week 30–40 of pregnancy. As summarized in Figure 6, minor (albeit significant on a pair-matched basis) reductions of plasma HCS were evident at 30 minutes ($P < 0.01$)

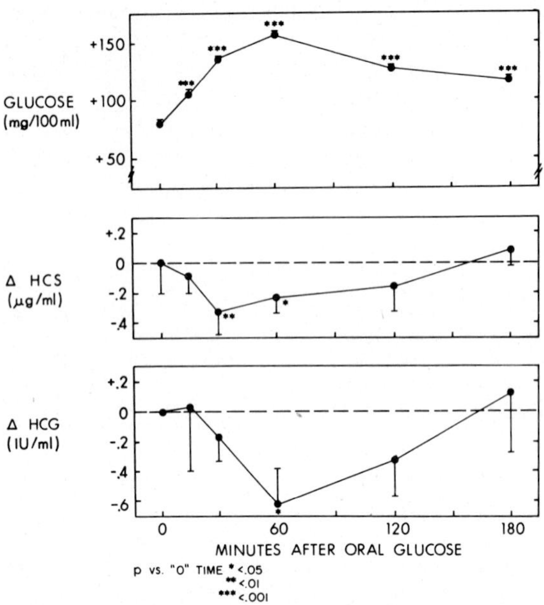

FIG. 6. Effect of oral glucose on plasma levels of human chorionic somatomammotropin (HCS) and human chorionic gonadotropin (HCG) in late pregnancy. Absolute values for plasma glucose (Mean ± S.E.M.) in 33 normal women given 100 g oral glucose during week 30–40 of pregnancy are shown in the upper panel. Concomitant changes in plasma HCS and HCG are expressed as deviations (± S.E.M.) from the initial fasting levels of 8.4 ± 0.45 μg/ml and 12.9 ± 1.6 I.U./ml respectively. The asterisks denote statistical significance of these changes on the basis of paired t analyses as in Figure 1.

and 60 minutes ($P < 0.05$) following glucose administration. Comparable experiences were also encountered during oral glucose tolerance tests in 14 gestational diabetics although a statistically significant correlation between the decrement in HCS and the increment in plasma glucose could not be demonstrated in either group.

The possibility that the seeming fall in HCS was simply due to heightened plasma dilution via the osmotically obligated 'extra' glucose could not be supported by direct measurements. It was rendered less likely by concurrent analyses for plasma human chorionic gonadotropin (HCG) which were instituted on the assumption that HCS and HCG should change in parallel if dilution alone were responsible. However, the temporal relationships proved to be entirely different. Whereas glucose also tended to reduce plasma HCG, the HCG decrements in normal subjects reached nadir levels at later times than HCS (Fig. 6, lower panel), and, in gestational diabetics, the reductions of HCG did not achieve statistical significance at any time. Thus, the small drop in plasma HCS that is seen in normals and some gestational diabetics following oral glucose during late pregnancy appears to be a real phenomenon. As yet it cannot be said whether it results from reductions in placental elaboration of hormone or transitory increases in hormone degradation. One cannot even directly implicate glucose per se. However, regardless of mediation, the data would suggest that maternal tissues may be confronted by slightly smaller concentrations of HCS whenever plasma glucose rises following alimentation. Since HCS has been shown to exhibit contrainsulin actions in normal subjects when administered in a fashion that simulates pregnancy (Beck and Daughaday, 1967; Kalkhoff et al., 1969), and since HCS also displays lipolytic properties in vitro (Turtle and Kipnis, 1967), the effect of glucose upon HCS which we have described may constitute yet another example of 'facilitated anabolism'. If HCS exerts moment-to-moment impact upon metabolic integration, attenuation of its anti-anabolic actions could occur in the immediate postprandial period when carbohydrate economy preponderates.

SUMMARY AND CONCLUSIONS

Heretofore, we have emphasized that the developing fetus poses exaggerated catabolic implications for the mother when food is withheld, especially in late pregnancy. We have stressed that maternal adaptations to dietary deprivation must then occur at a more rapid rate and that the resultant metabolic profile can be designated as 'accelerated starvation' (Freinkel, 1965; Freinkel et al., 1971). The present studies have focused on another aspect of gestational changes in metabolism, namely, the features that may selectively favor maternal repletion and anabolism when food is ingested. Three new examples of such facilitated anabolism have been delineated. Firstly, we have shown that a larger proportion of the ingested glucose appears to be converted into circulating triglyceride, a mechanism which, in view of the relative impermeability of the placenta to esterified fats, would assure retention of some of the carbohydrate excess by the mother for later recall. Secondly, we have shown that the exaggerated hyperglycemia and heightened outpouring of insulin by the mother following glucose ingestion effects a more profound suppression of plasma glucagon during pregnancy. This per se could facilitate the carbohydrate-induced triglyceridemia as well as assure an intrahepatic setting conducive to maximal glycogenesis. Finally, we have demonstrated that very small, although significant, reductions in plasma human chorionic somatomammotropin (HCS) attend the immediate period following glucose ingestion. Thus, insofar as tissue metabolism on a moment-to-moment basis may be modified by the contrainsulin properties of this hormone, such restraints would appear to be momentarily diminished whenever hyperglycemia prevails. We have designated these integrated interactions as examples of 'facilitated anabolism', and we have attempted to use the term as descriptive of hitherto unrecognized mechanisms by which maternal anabolism could be abetted in ways other than the traditional insulin-fuel interrelationships. Their quantitative importance remains to be assigned but they would present adjuvant modalities by which the fed mother in late pregnancy could again prepare for the exaggerated threats that characterize her metabolic homeostasis when food is withheld.

ACKNOWLEDGEMENTS

We are indebted to Dr. Robert T. Marshall, Dr. Richard L. Phelps, and Dr. Henry J. Ruder for assistance in various phases of these studies and to Professor Claude Cohen for help with statistical and computer analyses.

REFERENCES

AJABOR, L. N. and YEN, S. S. C. (1972): Effect of sustained hyperglycemia on the levels of human chorionic somatomammotropin in mid-pregnancy. *Amer. J. Obstet. Gynec., 112,* 908.

BECK, P. and DAUGHADAY, W. H. (1967): Human placental lactogen: Studies of its acute metabolic effects and disposition in normal man. *J. clin. Invest., 46,* 103.

BECK, P. and WELLS, S. A. (1969): Comparison of the mechanisms underlying carbohydrate intolerance in subclinical diabetic women during pregnancy and during postpartum oral contraceptive steroid treatment. *J. clin. Endocr., 29,* 807.

BERNSTEIN, R. S., GRANT, N., CRESPIN, S. R. and KIPNIS, D. M. (1972): Altered fat cell metabolism in endogenous hypertriglyceridemia (abstract). *Clin. Res., 20,* 541.

BLEICHER, S. J., O'SULLIVAN, J. B. and FREINKEL, N. (1964): Carbohydrate metabolism in pregnancy. V. The interrelations of glucose, insulin and free fatty acids in late pregnancy and postpartum. *New Engl. J. Med., 271,* 866.

BONSNES, R. W. (1947): The plasma amino acid and amino nitrogen concentration during normal pregnancy, labor, and early puerperium. *J. Biol. Chem., 168,* 345.

BURT, R. L. (1960): Plasma nonesterified fatty acids in normal pregnancy and puerperium. *Obstet. Gynec., 15,* 460.

BURT, R. L., LEAKE, N. H. and RHYNE, A. L. (1970): Human placental lactogen and insulin-blood glucose homeostasis. *Obstet. Gynec., 36,* 233.

CHERNICK, S. and NOVAK, M. (1970): Effect of insulin on FFA mobilization and ketosis in fasting pregnant rats. *Diabetes, 19,* 563.

CHRISTENSEN, P. J., DATE, J. W., SCHONHEYDER, F. and VOLQVARTZ, K. (1957): Amino acids in blood plasma and urine during pregnancy. *Scand. J. clin. lab. Invest., 9,* 54.

COLTART, T. M. (1972): Effect on fetal liver lipids of ^{14}C glucose administered intravenously to the mother. *J. Obstet. Gynaec. Brit. Cwlth., 79,* 639.

DANIEL, R., NITZAN, M., METZGER, B. E., FALOONA, G., UNGER, R. and FREINKEL, N. (1972): β cell/α cell imbalance in pregnancy (abstract). *Clin. Res., 20,* 552.

EATON, R. P. and KIPNIS, D. M. (1969): Effect of glucose feeding on lipoprotein synthesis in the rat. *Amer. J. Physiol., 217,* 1153.

EATON, R. P. and NYE, W. H. R. (1973): The relationship between insulin secretion and triglyceride concentration in endogenous lipemia. *J. lab. clin. Med., 81,* 682.

FELIG, P. and LYNCH, V. (1970): Starvation in human pregnancy: Hypoglycemia, hypoinsulinemia, and hyperketonemia. *Science, 170,* 990.

FELIG, P., KIM, Y. J., LYNCH, V. and HENDLER, R. (1972): Amino acid metabolism during starvation in human pregnancy. *J. clin. Invest., 51,* 1195.

FREINKEL, N. (1965): Effects of the conceptus on maternal metabolism during pregnancy. In: *On the Nature and Treatment of Diabetes,* pp. 679–691. Editors: B. S. Leibel and G. A. Wrenshall. International Congress Series No. 84, Excerpta Medica, Amsterdam.

FREINKEL, N. (1969): Homeostatic factors in fetal carbohydrate metabolism. In: *Fetal Homeostasis,* pp. 85–140. Editor: R. M. Wynn. Appelton, Century Crofts, New York, N.Y.

FREINKEL, N., HERRERA, E., KNOPP, R. H. and RUDER, H. J. (1970): Metabolic realignments in late pregnancy: A clue to diabetogenesis? In: *Early Diabetes,* pp. 205–219. Editors: R. A. Camerini-Davalos and H. S. Cole. Academic Press, New York, N.Y.

FREINKEL, N., METZGER, B. E., HERRERA, E., AGNOLI, F. and KNOPP, R. (1971): The effects of pregnancy on metabolic fuels. In: *Proceedings of the VII Congress of the International Diabetes Federation, Buenos Aires, August 23–28, 1970,* pp.

656–666. Editor: R. R. Rodriguez. International Congress Series No. 231, Excerpta Medica, Amsterdam.

FREINKEL, N., METZGER, B. E., NITZAN, M., HARE, J. W., SHAMBAUGH III, G. E., MARSHALL, R. T., SURMACZYNSKA, B. Z. and NAGEL, T. C. (1972): 'Accelerated starvation' and mechanisms for the conservation of maternal nitrogen during pregnancy. *Israel J. med. Sci., 8,* 426.

FREINKEL, N., METZGER, B. E., NITZAN, M., HARE, J. W., SHAMBAUGH III, G. E., MARSHALL, R. T., SURMACZYNSKA, B. Z. and NAGEL, T. C. (1972): 'Accelerated starvation' and mechanisms for the conservation of maternal nitrogen during pregnancy. In: *The Impact of Insulin on Metabolic Pathways,* pp. 252–292. Editor: E. Shafrir. Academic Press, New York, N.Y.

HAGEN, A. (1961): Blood sugar findings during pregnancy in normals and possible pre-diabetics. *Diabetes, 10,* 438.

HERRERA, E., KNOPP, R. H. and FREINKEL, N. (1969): Carbohydrate metabolism in pregnancy. VI. Plasma fuels, insulin, liver composition, gluconeogenesis and nitrogen metabolism during late gestation in the fed and fasted rat. *J. clin. Invest., 48,* 2260.

HOFFMAN, W. S. (1937): A rapid photoelectric method for the determination of glucose in blood and urine. *J. Biol. Chem., 120,* 51.

KALKHOFF, R., SCHALCH, D. S., WALKER, J. L., BECK, P., KIPNIS, D. A. and DAUGHADAY, W. H. (1964): Diabetogenic factors associated with pregnancy. *Trans. Ass. Amer. Phycns, 77,* 270.

KALKHOFF, R. K., RICHARDSON, B. L. and BECK, P. (1969): Relative effects of pregnancy, human placental lactogen and prednisolone on carbohydrate tolerance in normal and subclinical diabetic subjects. *Diabetes, 18,* 153.

KALKHOFF, R. K., JACOBSON, M. and LEMPER, D. (1970): Progesterone, pregnancy and the augmented plasma insulin response. *J. clin. Endocr., 31,* 24.

KESSLER, G. and LEDERER, H. (1965): Fluorometric measurement of triglycerides. In: *Automation in Analytical Chemistry,* p. 341. Editor: L. T. Skeggs. Mediad, New York, N.Y.

KNOPP, R. H., HERRERA, E. and FREINKEL, N. (1970): Carbohydrate metabolism in pregnancy. VIII. Metabolism of adipose tissue isolated from fed and fasted pregnant rats during late gestation. *J. clin. Invest., 49,* 1438.

KNOPP, R. H. and ARKY, R. A. (1972): Role of postheparin lipolytic activity (PHLA) in the type IIB lipemia of normal and diabetic pregnancy (abstract). *Clin. Res., 20,* 549.

LEAKE, N. H. and BURT, R. L. (1962): Insulin-like activity in serum during pregnancy. *Diabetes, 11,* 419.

LEVINE, J. B. and ZAK, B. (1964): Automated determination of serum total cholesterol. *Clin. Chim. Acta, 10,* 381.

MARSHALL, R. T. and HOOVER, N. (1971): An improved semi-automated method for assaying plasma free fatty acid levels. In: *Advances in Automated Analysis,* p. 491. Editors: E. C. Barton et al. Thurman Associates, Miami, Fla.

METZGER, B. E., AGNOLI, F. and FREINKEL, N. (1970): Effect of sex and pregnancy on formation of urea and ammonia during gluconeogenesis in the perfused rat liver. *Hormone Metabol. Res., 2,* 367.

METZGER, B. E., HARE, J. W. and FREINKEL, N. (1971): Carbohydrate metabolism in pregnancy. IX. Plasma levels of gluconeogenic fuels during fasting in the rat. *J. clin. Endocr., 33,* 869.

METZGER, B. E., NITZAN, M., DANIEL, R. and FREINKEL, N. (1973): Acute carbohydrate-induced hypertriglyceridemia in human pregnancy: A model for Type IV hyperlipoproteinemia? (abstract). *Clin. Res., 21,* 734.

METZGER, B. E., AGNOLI, F. S., HARE, J. W. and FREINKEL, N. (1973): Carbohydrate metabolism in pregnancy. X. Metabolic disposition of alanine by the perfused liver of the fasting pregnant rat. *Diabetes, 23,* 601.

OLIVER, M. F. and BOYD, G. S. (1955): Plasma lipid and serum lipoprotein patterns during pregnancy and puerperium. *Clin. Sci, 14,* 15.

O'SULLIVAN, J. B. and MAHAN, C. M. (1964): Criteria for the oral glucose tolerance test in pregnancy. *Diabetes, 13,* 278.

PALMER, D. W. and PETERS Jr., T. (1965): Simple automatic determination of amino groups in serum/plasma using trinitrobenzene sulfonate. In: *Automation in Analytical Chemistry,* p. 324. Editor: L. T. Skeggs. Mediad, New York, N.Y.

PALOYAN, E. and HARPER Jr., P. V. (1961): Glucagon as a regulating factor of plasma lipids. *Metabolism, 10,* 315.

PERLEY, M. J. and KIPNIS, D. M. (1967): Plasma insulin responses to oral and intravenous glucose: Studies in normal and diabetic subjects. *J. clin. Invest., 46,* 1954.

REAVEN, G. R., LERNER, R. L., STERN, M. P. and FARQUHAR, J. W. (1967): Role of insulin in endogenous hypertriglyceridemia. *J. clin. Invest., 46,* 1756.

SABATA, V., WOLF, H. and LAUSMANN, S. (1968): The role of free fatty acids, glycerol, ketone bodies and glucose in the energy metabolism of the mother and fetus during delivery. *Biol. Neonate, 13,* 7.

SAMAAN, N., YEN, S. C. C., FRIESEN, H. and PEARSON, O. H. (1966): Serum placental lactogen levels during pregnancy and in trophoblastic disease. *J. clin. Endocr., 23,* 1303.

SANTEUSANIO, F., FALOONA, G. R. and UNGER, R. H. (1972): Suppression effect of secretin upon pancreatic alpha cell function. *J. clin. Invest., 51,* 1743.

SAUDEK, C. D. and KNOPP, R. H. (1973): Glucagon deficiency in rat pregnancy (abstract). *Clin. Res., 21,* 637.

SCHLIERF, G. and DOROW, E. (1973): Diurnal patterns of triglycerides, free fatty acids, blood sugar, and insulin during carbohydrate-induction in man and their modification by nocturnal suppression of lipolysis. *J. clin. Invest., 52,* 732.

SCOW, R. O., CHERNICK, S. S. and SMITH, B. B. (1958): Ketosis in the rat fetus. *Proc. Soc. exp. Biol. Med. (N.Y.), 98,* 833.

SCOW, R. O., CHERNICK, S. S. and BRINLEY, M. S. (1964): Hyperlipemia and ketosis in the pregnant rat. *Amer. J. Physiol., 206,* 796.

SHAMBAUGH III, G. E., METZGER, B. E. and FREINKEL, N. (1971): Glutamine-dependent carbamyl phosphate synthetase in placenta and fetal structures of the rat. *Biochem. biophys. Res. Commun., 42,* 155.

SILVERSTONE, F. A., SOLOMONS, E. and RUBRICIUS, J. (1961): Rapid intravenous glucose tolerance test in pregnancy. *J. clin. Invest., 40,* 2180.

SPELLACY, W. N. and GOETZ, F. C. (1963): Plasma insulin in normal late pregnancy. *New Engl. J. Med., 268,* 988.

SPELLACY, W. N., BUHI, W. C., SCHRAM, J. D., BIRK, S. A. and McCREARY, S. A. (1971): Control of human chorionic somatomammotropin levels during pregnancy. *Obstet. Gynec., 37,* 567.

SVANBORG, A. and VIKROT, O. (1965): Plasma lipid fractions, including individual phospholipids, at various stages of pregnancy. *Acta med. scand., 178,* 615.

TURTLE, J. R. and KIPNIS, D. M. (1967): The lipolytic action of human placental lactogen on isolated fat cells. *Biochim. biophys. Acta (Amst.), 144,* 583.

UNGER, R. H. (1971): Glucagon physiology and pathophysiology. *New Engl. J. Med., 285,* 443.

VANCE, J. E., BUCHANAN, K. D., CHALLONER, D. K. and WILLIAMS, R. H. (1968): Effect of glucose concentration on insulin and glucagon release from isolated islets of Langerhans of the rat. *Diabetes, 17,* 187.

YEN, S. S. C., TSAI, C. C. and VELA, P. (1971): Gestational diabetogenesis: Quantitative analyses of glucose-insulin interrelationship between normal pregnancy and pregnancy with gestational diabetes. *Amer. J. Obstet. Gynec., 111,* 792.

REGULATION OF INSULIN AND HGH SECRETION IN THE PREMATURE INFANT

S. GRASSO, A. MESSINA, G. DISTEFANO, R. VIGO and G. REITANO

Department of Morbid Anatomy, General Pathology, and Pediatrics, University of Catania, Catania, Italy

The presence of human growth hormone (HGH) and insulin in the umbilical cord and fetal blood indicates that the fetal pituitary and pancreas produce HGH and insulin, respectively. Little is known, however, about the secretion of these hormones or their physiological effects.

As early as at 9 weeks of gestation, Pavlova et al. (1968) have measured HGH in the human fetal pituitary, and have found the total amount to be 1 μg. This rapidly increases, being 9.9 μg in 15–16 weeks old fetuses. Several authors (Kaplan, 1972; Gailani et al., 1970) have confirmed these observations by demonstrating that explants of the human pituitary synthesize and store HGH as early as at 8–9 weeks of gestation. Plasma concentrations in older fetuses and in umbilical cord plasma at term are higher than those found in the adult (Turner et al., 1971; Joassin et al., 1967).

After the 10th week of gestation the human fetal pancreas contains insulin, which rises during pregnancy to much above adult levels, being 12.7 ± 3.2 U/g between 34 and 40 weeks of gestation whereas in the adult it is 2.1 ± 0.3 U/g (Like and Orci, 1972; Steinke and Driscoll, 1965; Rastogi et al., 1970). Van Assche (1970) calculated that the relative amount of islet tissues of 40 normal fetuses, 20 weeks old or older, is 5.1 ± 1.6% (range from 1.9 to 9.8). This is considerably higher than the mean value of 1.5% established for the islet cell mass of the human adult pancreas. The average ratio of beta cells in the same fetuses is 40 ± 7.5% (range from 27 to 57). This result is lower than that of normal adults. Plasma insulin may be detected by the 14th to 16th week of gestation (Adam et al., 1969; Thorell, 1970). Neither maternal nor fetal HGH and insulin cross the placenta (Adam et al., 1969; King et al., 1971).

The studies that we report evaluate the insulin and HGH response to a variety of stimuli in the premature infant; we also review the literature on this subject.

MATERIAL AND METHODS

The subjects of these studies were healthy premature infants. Only those with a birth weight of less than 2500 g were included. The gestational age was calculated from the date of the first day of the last menstrual period and from clinical signs which show the maturity or immaturity of the infant (Battaglia et al., 1967; Usher et al., 1966). In the first 24 hours of life, before feeding was initiated, a polyethylene catheter was inserted into the umbilical vein to withdraw blood samples and administer infusions.

Serial levels of serum insulin, blood glucose, and serum HGH were measured after the administration of glucose, a mixture of 9 essential amino acids, and a combination of this mixture plus glucose or glucose with glucagon. Each infant received only one of these substances.

L-amino acids (Carlo Erba, Milan, Italy) were obtained in crystalline form as pure amino acids except for arginine, histidine and lysine which were obtained as hydrochlorides. The composition of 2.5 g of the mixture was: arginine 330 mg, lysine 380 mg, phenylalanine 330 mg, leucine 390 mg, methionine 240 mg, valine 300 mg, histidine 120 mg, isoleucine 230 mg, and threonine 180 mg. The mixture was made up in 25 ml normal saline.

The blood glucose was measured by a specific glucose oxidase method (Sigma Chemical Co., St. Louis, Mo., U.S.A.). Serum insulin and HGH were determined by radioimmunoassay methods (Hales and Randle, 1963; Schalch and Parker, 1964).

RESULTS AND DISCUSSION

The blood levels of glucose, insulin, and HGH in the first 24 hours of life in 166 premature infants are shown in Figure 1. Of these 166 children all had insulin measured, 154 had insulin and glucose measured, and 98 had measurements of insulin, glucose and HGH. These observations are essentially similar to those reported by other authors (Joassin et al., 1967; Baens et al., 1963; Gentz et al., 1969). The mean (± S.E.M.) blood glucose of these infants was 43 ± 1 mg/100 ml. Twenty-six infants (17%) had a blood glucose less than 30 mg/100 ml. The mean serum insulin was 11 ± 0.6 μU/ml and varied from 2 to 42 μU/ml. No correlation was found between blood glucose and serum insulin. The mean value of serum HGH was 31 ± 2 ng/ml and was extremely variable, ranging from 6 to 116 ng/ml. It has been found that the high concentration of this hormone falls almost to adult levels (0 to 5 ng/ml) during the following 8 weeks (Cornblath et al., 1965). Premature neonates tend to have higher plasma HGH levels for a longer period after delivery than do full-term neonates (Cornblath et al., 1965).

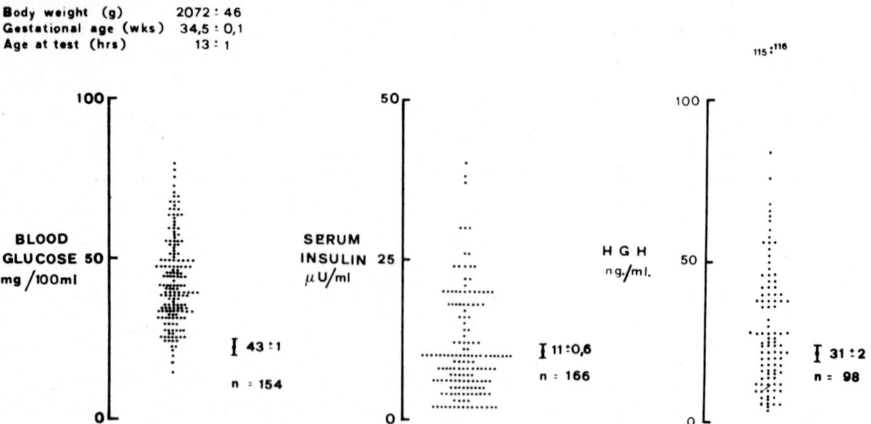

FIG. 1. Blood glucose, serum insulin and HGH levels in the first 24 hours of life in premature infants.

Figure 2 deals with something that has been demonstrated in vitro in the human fetal pancreas (Espinosa et al., 1970; Milner et al., 1972; Fujimoto and Williams, 1972) and pancreases of fetuses and newborns of other species such as monkeys, sheep or rats (Mintz et al., 1969; Bassett and Thornburn, 1971; Lambert et al., 1969; Asplund et al., 1969). That is, that glucose is a poor stimulant of insulin secretion throughout the fetal life and also during the neonatal period. In our infants, after receiving an infusion of 1.25 g of glucose for 30 minutes, the serum insulin only rose from 10.6 ± 1.4 μU/ml at time 0 to 18.6 ± 2.6 and 19.6 ± 3.8 μU/ml at 30 and 60 minutes. Unlike in older children and adults (Roth et al., 1963), where the HGH concentration is decreased by hyperglycemia, it rose gradually from a mean basal level of 26.3 ± 5.2 ng/ml to 72.2 ± 18.2 and 74.6 ± 15.4 at 60 and 90 minutes remaining at a level of 58.6 ± 12.4 at 120 minutes.

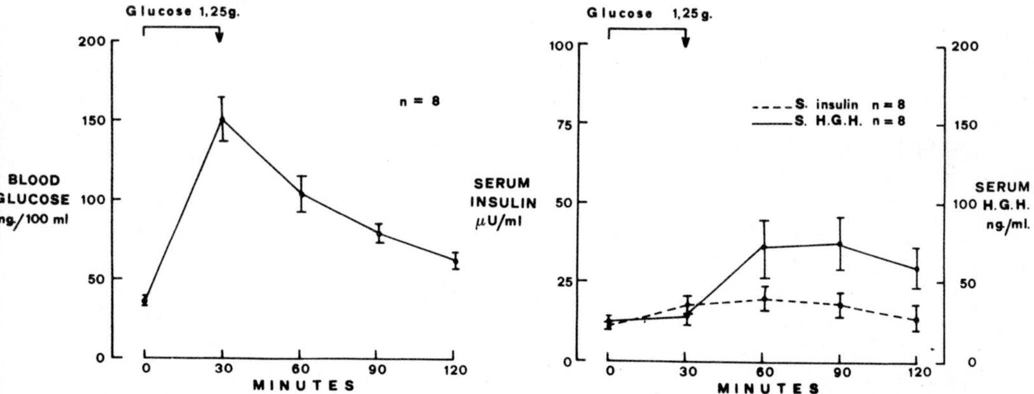

FIG. 2. Levels (mean ± S.E.M.) of blood glucose, serum insulin, and HGH in the premature infant following a 30-min. infusion of glucose (1.25 g). The body weight was 2215 ± 74.38 g.

An explanation for the poor insulin response to glucose remains uncertain and several hypotheses have been offered. Recent investigations have suggested that the insulin release may be modulated by the intracellular accumulation of cyclic 3′,5′-AMP within the beta cell (Malaisse et al., 1967). It has been suggested that the low effectiveness of glucose in the fetal pancreas could be due to an inadequate intracellular accumulation of this cyclic nucleotide (Fujimoto and Williams, 1972; Lambert et al., 1967; Grasso et al., 1970). In vivo, in the premature infant (Grasso et al., 1970) and monkey fetus (Chez et al., 1971), and in vitro with fetal human (Fujimoto and Williams, 1972; Heinze and Steinke, 1972; Milner et al., 1971) and rat (Lambert et al., 1967) pancreatic explants, it has been demonstrated that methylxanthines (theophylline and caffeine) and glucagon, agents known to increase cyclic AMP in the beta cells (Turtle and Kipnis, 1967), stimulate insulin release. Glucose becomes a powerful stimulant in the presence of ineffective doses of methylxanthines or of glucagon (Lambert et al., 1967; Grasso et al., 1970; Chez et al., 1971). However, direct evidence for a deficient cyclic AMP system is required for the verification of this hypothesis.

On the other hand Heinze and Steinke (1971) have shown that in the rat there is a marked difference between fetal and adult islets in their in vitro glucose metabolism.

Their findings could suggest a metabolic explanation for the difference in glucose-induced insulin release.

Another possible explanation arises from the observation that the fetal blood sugar is normally low (70–80% of that of the mother) and falls to lower levels during the neonatal period (Cornblath and Schwartz, 1966). It is therefore possible that the fetal pancreas has not recognized glucose as a stimulant for insulin release since it has not been stimulated by supranormal blood sugar concentrations. This hypothesis seems to be confirmed by the observation that infants of diabetic mothers display hyperplasia of the islets (Steinke and Driscoll, 1965), high levels of circulating insulin, and increased beta

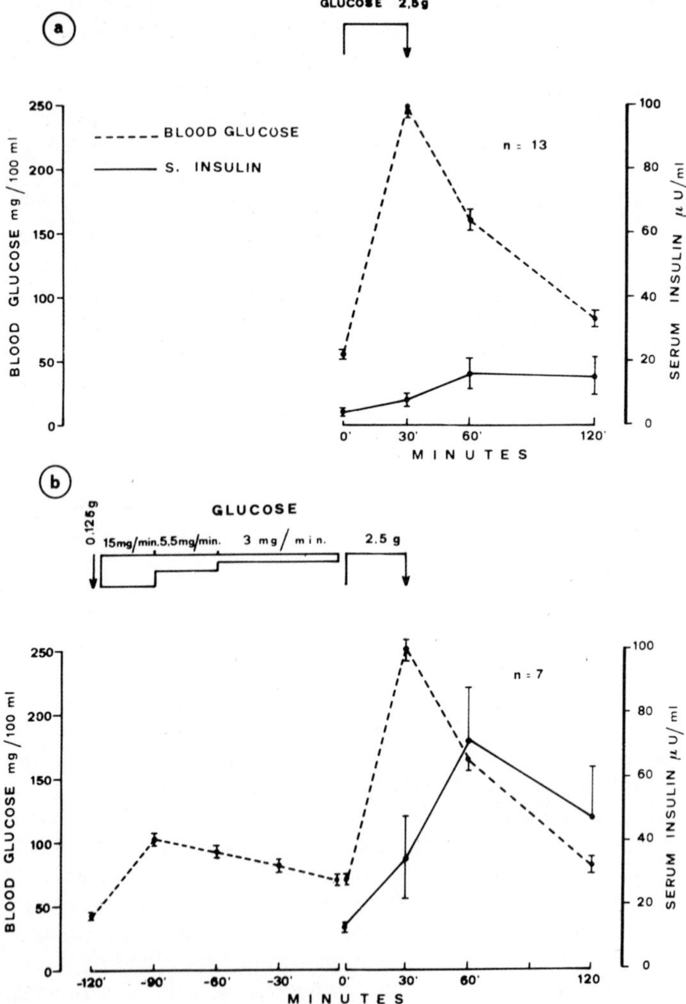

FIG. 3. Effects of a 30-min. infusion of glucose (2.5 g) in the premature infant (a) and (b) on blood glucose and serum insulin. In (b), before the acute glucose infusion, glucose was administered to raise the basal blood glucose level from 42 ± 4 to 68.8 ± 3.7 mg/100 ml. The body weight of these infants was 2168.75 ± 93.5 g.

cell response to glucose as compared to normal neonates (Jørgensen et al., 1966; Falorni et al., 1972). To explain these findings the hypothesis of maternal hyperglycemia-fetal hyperinsulinism has been advanced (Pedersen et al., 1954) and it seems that the following experiment proves this. As described above, if glucose is injected acutely, it is a poor stimulus of insulin secretion (Fig. 3a), but if an infusion of glucose administered for 120 minutes to raise the blood glucose of the infant from 42 ± 4 to 68.8 ± 3.7 mg/100 ml precedes the acute injection of glucose, the latter injection becomes a potent stimulus of insulin secretion. Serum insulin rose from a value of 12.8 ± 2.3 μU/ml to 35 ± 12.6 and 71.2 ± 16.9 μU/ml at 30 and 60 minutes. It declined to 47.2 ± 15.6 μU/ml at 120 minutes (Fig. 3b).

Quite opposite to glucose we have observed that a mixture of essential amino acids is a potent stimulus of insulin release in the premature infant (Grasso et al., 1968, 1973). In fact the infusion of 2.5 g of the above-mentioned mixture of amino acids for 30 minutes caused a rapid rise of serum insulin from a control value of 14 ± 2 μU/ml to a peak value of 100 ± 16 μU/ml at 30 minutes. It declined to 87 ± 26 μU/ml at 60 minutes, but was still high (mean 39 ± 7 μU/ml) above control level at the end of the experiment in all but one of the subjects. The blood glucose increased gradually from a control value of 36 ± 4 to 73 ± 4 mg/100 ml at 120 minutes (Fig. 4). We have also seen that the simultaneous administration of an ineffective dose of this mixture of amino acids (1.25 g) with glucose (1.25 g) caused a rapid and marked increase in serum insulin levels. Mean serum insulin rose from a control level of 9 ± 0.9 μU/ml to a peak of 75 ± 21 μU/ml at 30 minutes. It was still 73 ± 13 μU/ml at 60 minutes and then declined to 37 ± 6 μU/ml at 120 minutes (Fig. 5). Moreover, intravenous administration of this mixture of amino acids with and

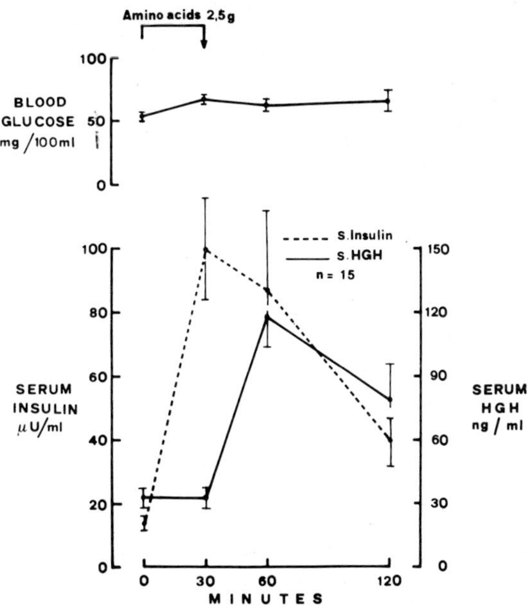

FIG. 4. Levels (mean ± S.E.M.) of blood glucose, serum insulin and HGH in the premature infant following a 30-min. infusion of a mixture of amino acids (2.5 g). The body weight was 2123 ± 109 g.

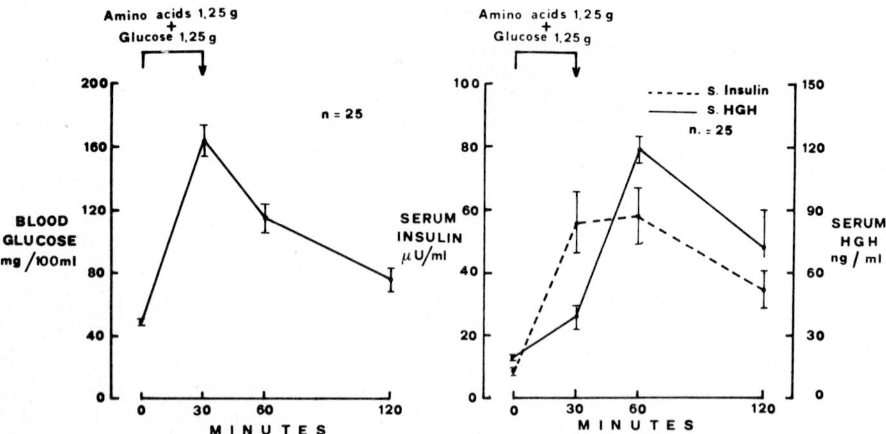

FIG. 5. Levels (mean ± S.E.M.) of blood glucose, serum insulin and HGH in the premature infant following a 30-min. infusion of amino acids (1.25 g) and glucose (1.25 g). The body weight was 2094 ± 61 g.

without glucose also induced a release of HGH into the blood. Maximal serum levels of HGH were reached 1 hour after the beginning of this infusion. With the mixture of amino acids alone the level rose from 33 ± 4 to 118 ± 15 ng/ml. With amino acids plus glucose the level rose from 20 ± 2 to 119 ± 6 ng/ml (Figs 4 and 5). Thus the endocrine response to intravenously administered amino acids, both with and without glucose, induces the release of insulin and HGH, but, unlike the adult where HGH secretion is rapidly suppressed by hyperglycemia, in the premature infant the HGH remains elevated.

That amino acids stimulate insulin release in the fetus and in the newborn has subsequently been demonstrated in vivo and in vitro. We have shown that arginine and arginine plus glucose stimulate insulin secretion in the premature infant (Reitano et al., 1971). Milner et al. (1972) have reported that in vitro this amino acid causes insulin release from human fetal islets. Mintz et al. (1972) infused monkey fetuses with a mixture of amino acids equal to that used by us, and obtained results similar to ours in premature infants. They also noted that fetuses from diabetic mothers required a 10-fold lower concentration of amino acids for a similar response.

Our experience deals with premature infants only, using a particular mixture of amino acids, but we suspect that, in the uterus, amino acids with glucose are the appropriate stimulus for insulin and HGH secretion. In fact, during pregnancy, the fetus receives a continuous supply of glucose and amino acids, plus a variety of other essential nutrients. The concentration of plasma amino acids is elevated in the fetus and slightly depressed in the maternal plasma (Lindblad, 1971). Glucose passes across the placental barrier and any fluctuation of the maternal blood glucose level is rapidly mirrored by that of the fetus (Cordero et al., 1970).

Recently we have learnt that insulin is synthesized as a single-chain polypeptide, proinsulin, most of which is converted to insulin within the beta cell (Steiner and Oyer, 1967). Studies have also shown that proinsulin is present in adult human blood. Recent studies by Gorden et al. (1972) and by Gorden and Roth (1969) have shown that the immunoreactive portion of serum insulin can be resolved by gel filtration into 2 components. One component is indistinguishable from crystalline pancreatic insulin (insulin component or little insulin); the second component, with higher molecular weight, may closely resemble proinsulin (proinsulin-like component or big insulin). Many questions concerning the extrapancreatic significance of proinsulin, in terms of biological activity, remain unanswered (Gorden et al., 1972; Rubenstein et al., 1972). As yet little information has been obtained about these components in the pancreas and in the blood of the newborn.

Rastogi et al. (1970) found the amount of proinsulin in 16 pancreases of human fetuses (aged 11–24 weeks) to vary from 0.26 to 1.6% of the total immunoreactive insulin. The same authors found that in adult pancreatic extract the proinsulin constituted 1.5% of the total immunoreactive insulin. We have analyzed blood samples taken from 4 premature infants at the end of a 120-minute infusion of glucose with glucagon (Table 1). The 2 components were separated using the method of Gorden and Roth (1969) and assayed for immunoreactive insulin by a double-antibody technique (Hales and Randle, 1963) using human insulin standards and antiserum against human insulin. The serum concentration of insulin was high (from 73.8 to 527.4 μU/ml) and the percentage of proinsulin varied from 3.8 to 8.3%. From this it is clear that the beta cell of the premature infant can release a large amount of insulin under the appropriate stimulus and that the proinsulin-insulin converting system functions adequately.

In conclusion the data reported in this paper, along with that in the literature, confirm that insulin and HGH are actively secreted by the pancreas and the pituitary of the newborn respectively, even though they respond to different stimuli from the adult. Information about their physiological effect is scarce. We think, however, that these hormones are probably metabolically active and that their main function is to stimulate the utilization of amino acids for the synthesis of protein during a time of very active growth.

TABLE 1

Percentage of 'big insulin' after a 120-minute infusion of glucose (4 g) plus glucagon (250 μg) in the premature infant during the first 24 hours of life

	Total insulin	'Little insulin'	'Big insulin'	%
1.	343.8	329.0	14.8	4.3
2.	527.4	507.2	20.2	3.8
3.	201.5	178.0	13.5	6.7
4.	73.8	67.7	6.1	8.3

REFERENCES

ADAM, P. A. J., TERAMO, K., RAIHA, N., GITLIN, D. and SCHWARTZ, R. (1969): Human fetal insulin metabolism early in gestation: response to acute elevation of the fetal glucose concentration and placental transfer of human insulin-I-131. *Diabetes, 18,* 409.

ASPLUND, K., WESTMAN, S. and HELLERSTROM, C. (1969): Glucose stimulation of insulin secretion from the isolated pancreas of foetal and newborn rats. *Diabetologia, 5,* 260.

VAN ASSCHE, F.A. (1970): *The Fetal Endocrine Pancreas. A Quantitative Morphological Approach.* Thesis. Katholieke Universiteit, Leuven, Belgium.

BAENS, G. S., LUNDEEN, E. and CORNBLATH, M. (1963): Studies of carbohydrate metabolism in the newborn infant. VI. Levels of glucose in blood in premature infants. *Pediatrics, 31,* 580.

BASSETT, J. M. and THORNBURN, G. D. (1971): The regulation of insulin secretion by the ovine foetus in utero. *J. Endocr., 50,* 59.

BATTAGLIA, F. C. and LUBCHENCO, L. O. (1967): A practical classification of newborn infants by weight and gestational age. *J. Pediat., 71,* 159.

CHEZ, R. A., MINTZ, D. H. and HUTCHINSON, D. L. (1971): Effect of theophylline on glucagon and glucose-mediated plasma insulin response in subhuman primate fetus and neonate. *Metabolism, 20,* 805.

CORDERO Jr., L., JEH, S., GRUNT, G. A. and ANDERSON, G. G. (1970): Hypertonic glucose infusion during labor. Maternal-fetal blood glucose relationships. *Amer. J. Obstet. Gynec., 107,* 295.

CORNBLATH, M., PARKER, M. L., REISNER, S. H., FORBES, A. E. and DAUGHADAY, W. H. (1965): Secretion and metabolism of growth hormone in premature and full-term infants. *J. clin. Endocr., 25,* 209.

CORNBLATH, M. and SCHWARTZ, R. (1966): Disorders of carbohydrate metabolism in infancy. In: *Major Problems in Clinical Pediatrics, Vol. III.* W. B. Saunders, Philadelphia, Pa.

ESPINOSA, M. M. A., DRISCOLL, S. G. and STEINKE, J. (1970): Insulin release from isolated human fetel pancreatic islets. *Science, 168,* 1111.

FALORNI, A., FRACASSINI, F., MASSI-BENEDETTI, F. and AMICI, A. (1972): Glucose metabolism, plasma insulin, and growth hormone secretion in newborn infants with erytroblastosis fetalis compared with normal newborns and those to diabetic mothers. *Pediatrics, 49,* 682.

FUJIMOTO, W. Y. and WILLIAMS, R. H. (1972): Insulin release from cultured fetal human pancreas. *Endocrinology, 91,* 1133.

GAILANI, S. D., NUSSBAUM, A., McDOUGALL, W. J. and McLIMANS, W. F. (1970): Studies on hormone production by human fetal pituitary cell cultures. *Proc. Soc. exp. Biol. Med. (N.Y.), 134,* 27.

GENTZ, J. C. H., WARRNER, R., PERSSON, B. H. E. and CORNBLATH, M. (1969): Intravenous glucose tolerance, plasma insulin, free fatty acids and β-hydroxybutyrate in underweight newborn infants. *Acta paediat. scand., 58,* 481.

GORDEN, P. and ROTH, J. (1969): Plasma insulin: Fluctuation in the "big" insulin component in man after glucose and other stimuli. *J. clin. Invest., 48,* 2225.

GORDEN, P., ROTH, J., FREYCHET, P. and KAHN, R. (1972): The circulating proinsulin-like components. *Diabetes, 21/Suppl. 2,* 673.

CRASSO, S., MESSINA, A., SAPORITO, N. and REITANO, G. (1970): Effect of theophylline, glucagon and theophylline plus glucagon on insulin secretion in the premature infant. *Diabetes, 19,* 837.

GRASSO, S., SAPORITO, N., MESSINA, A. and REITANO, G. (1968): Serum-insulin response to glucose and aminoacids in the premature infant. *Lancet, 2,* 755.

GRASSO, S., MESSINA, A., DISTEFANO, G., VIGO, R. and REITANO, G., (1973): Insulin secretion in the premature infant. Response to glucose and aminoacids. *Diabetes, 22,* 349.

HALES, C. N. and RANDLE, P. J. (1963): Immunoassay of insulin with insulin-antibody precipitate. *Biochem. J., 88,* 137.

HEINZE, E. and STEINKE, J. (1971): Glucose metabolism of isolated pancreatic islets: Difference between fetal, newborn and adult rats. *Endocrinology, 88,* 1259.

HEINZE, E. and STEINKE, J. (1972): Insulin secretion during development: Response of isolated pancreatic islets of fetal, newborn and adult rats to theophylline and arginine. *Hormone metabol. Res., 4,* 234.

JOASSIN, G., PARKER, M. L., PILDES, R. S. and CORNBLATH, M. (1967): Infants of diabetic mothers. *Diabetes, 16,* 306.

JØRGENSEN, K. R., DECKERT, I., PEDERSEN, L. M. and PEDERSEN, J. (1966): Insulin, insulin antibody and glucose in plasma of newborn infants of diabetic women. *Acta endocr. (Kbh.), 52,* 154.

KAPLAN, S. L., GRUMBACH, M. M. and SHEPARD, T. H. (1972): The ontogenesis of human fetal hormones. I. Growth hormone and insulin. *J. clin. Invest., 51,* 3080.

KING, K. C., ADAM, P. A. J., SCHWARTZ, R. and TERAMO, K. (1971): Human placental transfer of human growth hormone I-125. *Pediatrics, 48,* 534

LAMBERT, A. E., JEANRENAUD, B. and RENOLD, A. (1967): Enhancement by caffeine of glucagon–induced and tolbutamide–induced insulin release from isolated foetal pancreatic tissue. *Lancet, 1,* 819.

LAMBERT, A. E., JUNOD, A., STAUFFACHER, W., JEANRENAUD, B. and RENOLD, A. E. (1969): Organ culture of fetal rat pancreas: I. Insulin release induced by caffeine and by sugars and some derivatives. *Biochim. biophys. Acta (Amst.), 184,* 529.

LIKE, A. A. and ORCI, L. (1972): Embryogenesis of the human pancreatic islets: a light and electron microscopic study. *Diabetes, 21/suppl. 2,* 511.

LINDBLAD, B. S. (1971): The plasma aminogram in "small for date" newborn infants. In: *Metabolic Processes in the Foetus and Newborn Infant,* p. 111. Editors: M. P. Jonxis, H. K. A. Visser and J. A. Troelstra. H. E. Stenfert Kroese, Leiden.

MALAISSE, W. J., MALAISSE-LAGAE, F. and MAYHEW, D. (1967): A possible role for the adenylcyclase system in insulin secretion. *J. clin. Invest., 46,* 1724.

MILNER, R. D. G., ASHWORTH, M. A. and BARSON, A. J. (1972): Insulin release from human foetal pancreas in response to glucose, leucine and arginine. *J. Endocr., 52,* 497.

MILNER, R. D. G., BARSON, A. J. and ASHWORTH, M. A. (1971): Human foetal pancreatic insulin secretion in response to ionic and other stimuli. *J. Endocr., 51,* 323.

MINTZ, D. H., CHEZ, R. A. and HORGER III, E. O. (1969): Fetal insulin and growth hormone metabolism in the subhuman primate. *J. clin. Invest., 48,* 176.

MINTZ, D. H., CHEZ, R. A. and HUTCHINSON, D. L. (1972): Subhuman primate pregnancy complicated by streptozotocin–induced diabetes mellitus. *J. clin. Invest., 51,* 837.

PAVLOVA, E. B., PRONINA, T. S. and SKEBELSKAYA, Y. B. (1968): Histostructure of adenohypophysis of human fetuses and contents of somatotropic and adrenocorticotropic hormones. *Gen. comp. Endocr., 10,* 269.

PEDERSEN, J., BOJSEN–MOLLER, B. and POULSEN, H. E. (1954): Blood sugar in newborn infants of diabetic mothers. *Acta endocr. (Kbh.), 15,* 33.

RASTOGI, G. K., LETARTE, J. and FRASER, T. R. (1970): Immunoreactive insulin content of 203 pancreases from foetuses of healthy mothers. *Diabetologia, 6,* 445.

RASTOGI, G. K., LETARTE, J. and FRASER, T. R. (1970): Proinsulin content of pancreas in human fetuses of healthy mothers. *Lancet, 1,* 7.

REITANO, G., GRASSO, S., DISTEFANO, G. and MESSINA, A. (1971): The serum

insulin and growth hormone response to arginine and to arginine with glucose in the premature infant. *J. clin. Endocr., 33,* 924.
ROTH, J., GLICK, S. M., YALOW, R. S. and BERSON, S. A. (1963): Secretion of human growth hormone: physiologic and experimental modification. *Metabolism, 12,* 577.
RUBENSTEIN, A. H., BLOCK, M. B., STARR, J., MELANI, F. and STEINER, D. F. (1972): Proinsulin and C-peptide in blood. *Diabetes, 21/Suppl. 2,* 661.
SCHALCH, D. S. and PARKER, M. L. (1964): A sensitive double antibody immunoassay for human growth hormone in plasma. *Nature (Lond.), 203,* 1141.
STEINER, D. F. and OYER, P. E. (1967): The biosynthesis of insulin and probable precursor of insulin by a human islet cell adenoma. *Proc. nat. Acad. Sci. USA, 57,* 473.
STEINKE, J. and DRISCOLL, S. G. (1965): The extractable insulin content of pancreas from fetuses and infants of diabetic and control mothers. *Diabetes, 14,* 573.
THORELL, J. I. (1970): Plasma insulin levels in normal human foetuses. *Acta endocr. (Kbh.), 63,* 134.
TURNER, R. C., SCHNEELOCH, B. and PATERSON, P. (1971): Changes in plasma growth hormone and insulin of the human foetus following hysterotomy. *Acta endocr. (Kbh.), 66,* 577.
TURTLE, J. R. and KIPNIS, D. M. (1967): An adrenergic receptor mechanism for the control of cyclic 3′,5′ adenosine monophosphate synthesis in tissues. *Biochem. biophys. Res. Commun., 28,* 797
USHER, R., McLEAN, F. and SCOTT, K.E. (1966): Judgement of fetal age: II. Clinical significance of gestational age an objective method for its assessment. *Pediat. Clin. N. Amer., 13,* 835.

INTERRELATIONSHIP OF BIRTH WEIGHT WITH K VALUE AND PLASMA INSULIN SECRETION PATTERN IN NEWBORN INFANTS WITH ERYTHROBLASTOSIS FETALIS. A COMPARISON WITH INFANTS OF NORMAL AND OF DIABETIC MOTHERS*

LARS MØLSTED-PEDERSEN and JØRGEN PEDERSEN

Diabetes Center, Departments of Obstetrics and Gynecology (Y) and Neonatal Pediatrics (GN) Rigshospitalet, Copenhagen, University of Copenhagen, Denmark

Newborn infants of diabetic mothers (IDM) display a pronounced hyperinsulinism at birth, as is well-known. Generally, this hyperinsulinism is explained by the (maternal) hyperglycemia-(fetal) hyperinsulinism theory which runs as follows: Maternal hyperglycemia results in fetal hyperglycemia, and, hence, in hypertrophy of fetal islet tissue with insulin hypersecretion. The theory, in turn, will explain several characteristics of the neonates, e.g. their external configuration, overweight at birth, body composition and organ size and function (Pedersen, 1967). Therefore, the fact that hyperinsulinism at birth has been detected in infants with erythroblastosis fetalis (IEF) is of considerable theoretical interest, since this hyperinsulinism is not explicable by the hyperglycemia-hyperinsulinism theory. Several studies of IEF have been published over the last 10 years. For recent investigations and a survey of the literature the reader is referred to Falorni et al. (1972) and Mølsted-Pedersen et al. (1973).

Mølsted-Pedersen (1972) found a strong positive correlation of K value and insulinism with birth weight in normal infants as well as in IDM. Recently a similar positive correlation in IEF has been mentioned by Mølsted-Pedersen et al. (1973). Therefore, this investigation compares the insulinism in IEF, infants of normal mothers and IDM with due regard to the infants' birth weight.

MATERIAL AND METHODS

Intravenous glucose tolerance tests were performed on average 3 hours after birth in 60 infants of normal mothers, 50 IDM (white class A: 16, white classes B-F: 34 infants) and 18 IEF. The infants were fasted from birth. The glucose (0.5 g/kg) was administered through the umbilical vein in most of the infants and blood samples were drawn through a newly inserted catheter in the umbilical vein every 10 minutes during the subsequent 60 minutes. Plasma glucose was determined by a glucose oxidase method in an autoanalyzer. The K values were calculated on the basis of the absolute glucose values obtained in the interval 20–60 minutes after the glucose injection.

In part of the total material plasma insulin was also determined prior to and during the

* This investigation was supported by grants from the Danish Landsforeningen for Sukkersyge and Nordisk Insulinfond.

intravenous glucose tolerance test. The plasma insulin concentration was measured as immunologically detectable insulin (IDI) by the method of Hales and Randle using ^{125}I-insulin as tracer.

From this material in which K value as well as plasma insulin concentration were known, 11 infants of normal mothers and 10 IDM (white classes B-F) were selected in order to obtain a mean birth weight in each group comparable with that of about 3,000 g for the 17 IEF. This was preferably done by selection of babies with a low birth weight. In Table 1 the mean and range of birth weights and gestational ages in the 3 groups of infants are listed. Furthermore, from this material the infants of normal mothers whose plasma insulin concentrations during the i.v. glucose load were most similar to that of the 17 IEF were also selected. This could be accomplished simply by the selection of the total group of 15 normal infants with a birth weight surpassing 3,500 g. The mean birth weight of the normal infants was 4,050 g and the mean K value was 1.24 (Fig. 2).

For further information concerning the infants and the methodology, see: Mølsted-Pedersen (1972), Mølsted-Pedersen and Jørgensen (1972) and Mølsted-Pedersen et al. (1973). Student's t-test with the 5% level as the limit of significance was used in the statistical evaluation.

RESULTS

Table 1 shows relevant data for 3 groups of infants, of which those of the normal infants and the IDM were selected with respect to birth weight. Consequently the 3 groups of infants had approximately the same mean and ranges of birth weight. The gestation times, however, were different. In relation to gestation time the birth weight of normal infants and of IEF was normal, whereas the IDM were overweight. The K values of the IEF were in-between those of infants of normal mothers and IDM. Likewise the mean fasting plasma insulin concentration 3 hours after birth was significantly higher in the IEF than in the normal group, 28 and 16 μU/ml respectively ($t = 3.28$, $P<0.005$).

Figure 1 shows plasma insulin concentrations during the i.v. glucose tolerance test. The pattern of insulin secretion was similar in the normal infants and IEF. After an initial peak during the very first minutes (not shown in Fig. 1, since too few measurements were performed) the concentrations rose evenly through the first 40 minutes. In the IEF a maximum was reached in 40–60 minutes. In the control group the increase was not significant (or maximal) until after 50 minutes. Furthermore, throughout the experimental period the insulin concentration remained significantly higher in the IEF. The increase in plasma insulin concentration from 0 to 10 minutes after the start of the glucose infusion (ΔI) was 30 μU/ml in IEF as compared with 4 μU/ml in the controls. This difference was statistically significant ($t = 3.53$, $P < 0.005$). In IDM ΔI was still higher (Table 1); in this group the fasting plasma insulin concentration cannot be relied upon because of insulin antibodies whereas changes in insulin concentration are reliable. Figure 1 shows the maximum insulin concentration is reached as early as 10 minutes after the start of the i.v. glucose load thereafter declining to a so-called monophasic pattern.

Figure 2 shows the insulin secretion pattern after a glucose injection in the selected group of 15 normal full-term infants with a mean birth weight of 4,050 g and a mean K value of 1.24. It is approximately similar to that of the IEF group with a mean birth weight of 2,980 g, a mean gestation time of 261 days and a mean K value of 1.29 (Table 1).

TABLE 1

Clinical data for 3 groups of infants with similar birth weight (see text for details)

Group of infants	Number of infants	Birth weight (g) Mean	Birth weight (g) Range	Gestational age (days) Mean	Gestational age (days) Range	Umbilical venous plasma 3 hours after birth: Glucose (mg/100 ml)	Insulin (μU/ml)	ΔI* (μU/ml)	K value (%/min.)
Normal	11	3100	(2600–3500)	271	(247–293)	60	16	4	0.78
Erythroblastosis fetalis	17	2980	(2200–3600)	261	(229–278)	62	28	30	1.29
Diabetic mothers	10	3135	(2150–3900)	251	(232–263)	33	–	59	2.40

ΔI* = Plasma insulin concentration 10 minutes after the i.v. glucose load minus fasting insulin concentration.

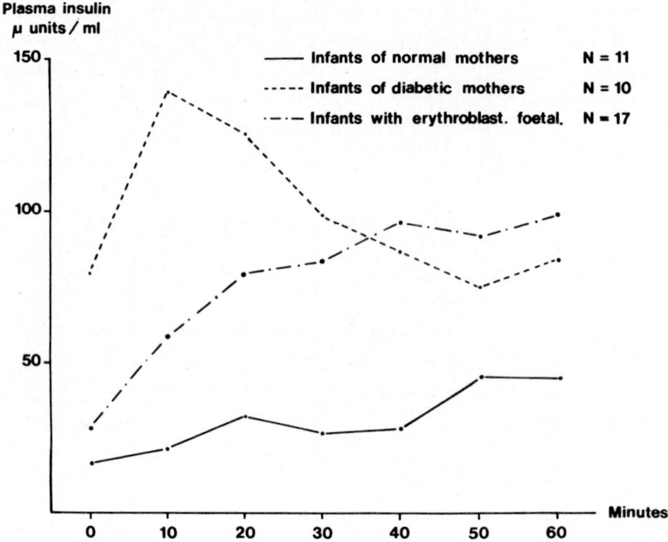

FIG. 1. Plasma insulin concentration during i.v. glucose tolerance test in 3 groups of infants with similar mean birth weights (cf. Table 1).

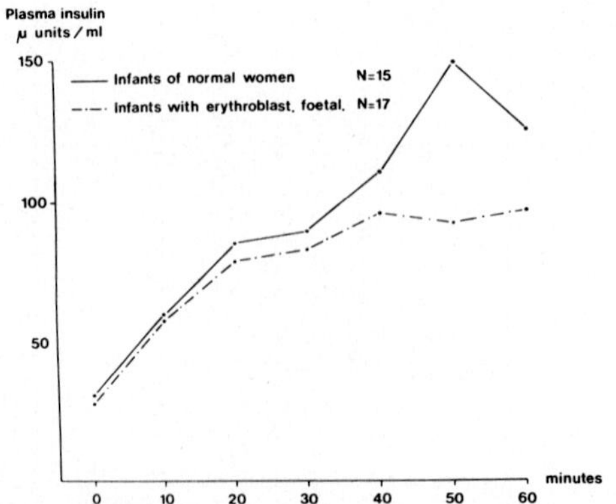

FIG. 2. Similar pattern of plasma insulin concentration during i.v. glucose tolerance test in normal infants (mean K value 1.24, mean birth weight 4,050 g) and infants with erythroblastosis (mean K value 1.29, mean birth weight 2,980 g).

For Figure 3 the total material was used. The regression line demonstrating the positive correlation between birth weight and K value for the group of 18 IEF is shown together with the corresponding lines for 60 infants of non-diabetic mothers, 16 IDM (white class A) and 34 IDM (white classes B-F). The slope of the regression line of the IEF differed significantly from zero ($t = 2.18$, $P < 0.05$) and the equation for the regression line was: $Y = -1.43 + 0.000897\,X \pm 0.637\,s$. The equations for the regression lines of normal infants and IDM have been previously mentioned (Mølsted-Pedersen, 1972). Whereas neither the slopes nor the intercepts of the regression lines for normal infants and IDM (white class A) differ significantly, those for IEF and IDM (white classes B-F) do differ significantly from those of normals. The regression line of the IEF is placed in-between those of IDM (white classes B-F) and IDM (white class A).

For Table 2 the IEF were divided into 2 groups consisting of the 10 infants with mild (Hb at birth $\geqslant$ 14 g/100 ml) and the 8 infants with moderate severe (Hb 11 g to 13.5 g/100 ml, 5 infants) and severe disease (Hb $<$ 11 g/100 ml, 3 infants), respectively. It is noteworthy that although the mean birth weight was the same in the 2 groups the mean K values differed, being lower in the group of infants with mild disease. The difference, however, was not statistically significant.

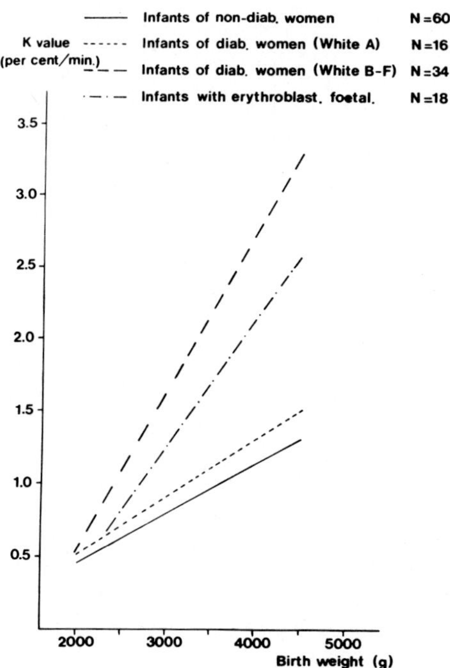

FIG. 3. Correlation between birth weight and K value in 4 groups of infants (total material).

TABLE 2

K value in relation to the concentration of hemoglobin in umbilical cord blood at birth in 2 groups of infants with erythroblastosis fetalis (Note the similar mean birth weight)

Hb (g/100 ml) Range	Hb (g/100 ml) Mean	Number of infants	Birth weight mean (g)	K value mean (%/min)
⩾14	16.6	10	3000	1.08
<14	10.7	8	3005	1.47

DISCUSSION

The elevated fasting insulin concentration and response following a glucose load together with the significantly higher disappearance rate of glucose in terms of the K value in IEF as compared to normal infants with a corresponding birth weight show the degree of hyperinsulinism in IEF (Table 1, Fig. 1). Apparently the insulin secretion pattern of IEF was like an exaggerated normal pattern differing from that seen in IDM (white classes B-F) (Fig. 1). This impression is underlined by the fact that the course as well as the level of the insulin concentration and mean K value after a glucose load were similar to those found in 15 normal full-term infants who, however, had an average birth weight of 4,050 g (Fig. 2). Thus, to define more precisely the hyperinsulinism of IEF, the K value and insulin secretion pattern of IEF with a birth weight of 3,000 g and a gestation time of 261 days were similar to those of normal full-term infants with a birth weight of 4,000 g. It should be mentioned, however, that Falorni et al. (1972) have found a monophasic insulin secretion pattern, characteristic of IDM, in 6 IEF with severe hemolytic disease. Verification of this observation would suggest the pattern of insulin secretion to be a consequence of the degree and duration of the fetal hyperinsulinism. In normal infants (and IDM white class A) small alterations of the K value correspond to large differences of birth weight (Fig. 3). As has been discussed (Pedersen and Mølsted-Pedersen, 1971; Mølsted-Pedersen, 1972) the positive correlation is not so close and the regression line different in IDM (white classes B-F). Their K values are far too great at a given birth weight compared with normal infants. Actually the mean K value of the IDM corresponds to a mean birth weight of 7,000 g in normal infants. Likewise the positive correlation between K value and birth weight of IEF has been 'disturbed'. If the mean K value (1.26) of the IEF is interpolated on the regression line for normal infants the IEF should have weighed about 4,350 g. This means that factors other than the normal glycemia-insulin growth, or weight impulse, have dominated (Pedersen and Mølsted-Pedersen, 1971).

In reality the birth weights of the IEF were normal in relation to their gestational age. Therefore, no effect on birth weight from their hyperinsulinism can be seen. This is thought to be due to the supposed lack of maternal hyperglycemia in IEF. On the contrary IDM are overweight (fat) in relation to their gestational age. Besides being born with hyperinsulinism they have also been exposed to maternal hyperglycemia.

Table 2 demonstrates the existence of a positive correlation between the severity of erythroblastosis fetalis in terms of Hb concentration at birth and the K values or hyperinsulinism. The K values are not proportional to the birth weight, but do correspond with the Hb concentration. This tendency discloses the perhaps not so astonishing fact that the hyperinsulinism seems to be related to the disease state.

According to our investigations and those in the literature IEF are born with hyperinsulinism. In some respects such infants are similar to, but in several respects dissimilar to IDM. Although IEF have an elevated plasma insulin concentration at birth and show neonatal hypoglycemia more frequently than do normal infants, it seems clear that the hyperinsulinism is less pronounced compared with IDM. Furthermore, the insulin response following an i.v. glucose load represents an exaggerated normal response and is fundamentally different in our series of IEF from that in IDM. Likewise, the hyperplasia of the pancreatic islet tissue is less marked in IEF as contrasted with IDM, and, noteworthy, in IEF there is a complete lack of the characteristic eosinophilic infiltration around the hypertrophic islets observed in IDM. Finally, the birth weight of IEF is normal in relation to their gestational age unlike the overweight in IDM. It should be mentioned that maternal hyperglycemia seems improbable in IEF, but to our knowledge their maternal pregnancy blood glucose level has not been systematically investigated (cf. Falorni et al., 1972; Mølsted-Pedersen et al., 1973).

Thus, most probably, the hyperinsulinism of IEF is of different genesis as that in infants of diabetic mothers. The cause and the mechanism of hyperinsulinism in IEF seem to be positively correlated with the severity of the erythroblastosis. One hypothesis holds that substances in the hemolyzed blood are directly or indirectly responsible (Steinke et al., 1967), another hypothesis suggests that higher plasma amino acid concentrations, due to increased hemolysis, may stimulate the insulin secretion (Mølsted-Pedersen et al., 1973). So far the problem is unsolved.

SUMMARY

The total number of subjects comprised 60 infants of non-diabetic mothers, 50 infants of diabetic mothers (white class A: 16 infants; white classes B-F: 34 infants) and 18 infants with erythroblastosis fetalis, in whom K values and, in most infants, the plasma insulin concentration during an i.v. glucose load were determined 3–6 hours after birth. The hemolytic disease was mild in 10, moderately severe in 5 and severe in 3 infants. In order to make the comparison valid the previously published material has been rearranged to achieve similar mean birth weights in the different infant groups.

In infants with erythroblastosis the mean fasting insulin concentration as well as the insulin concentration at each time during the i.v. glucose load and the disappearance rate of glucose (K value) were significantly higher than in the control group with similar birth weight. The pattern of the plasma insulin concentration during the i.v. glucose load was similar to that observed in the normal group (an exaggerated normal response), but different from the characteristic monophasic pattern in infants of diabetic mothers with a similar birth weight. Also plasma insulin and K values were higher in infants of diabetic mothers.

A control group of 15 normal infants was selected in such a way that the course and the level of the plasma insulin concentration during the i.v. glucose load were similar to those of the infants with hemolytic disease. The K values appeared to be similar in the 2 groups of infants. The mean birth weight and the mean gestation time, however, were only 3,000 g and 261 days, respectively, in the infants with erythroblastosis as contrasted with 4,050 g in the control group of normal full-term infants.

The regression lines demonstrating the positive correlation of birth weight with K value for all the groups were compared. The slopes and the intercepts for infants of diabetic mothers (white classes B-F) and for infants with erythroblastosis were similar. Both regression lines differed from those of infants of diabetic mothers (white class A) and normal infants which, on the other hand, were not significantly different.

The erythroblastotic infants who had a mean birth weight of 3,000 g should, in relation to their mean K value, have weighed 4,350 g if they had been normal infants.

Although both groups of infants have considerable hyperinsulinism, infants of diabetic mothers are overweight, whereas infants with erythroblastosis have a normal birth weight. This is thought to be due to a supposed lack of maternal hyperglycemia in the latter. After division of the infants with hemolytic disease into 2 groups with different Hb concentrations but similar mean birth weights the K value was observed to be insignificantly higher in the group with the lower Hb concentration.

The cause of hyperinsulinism in infants with erythroblastosis is so far unknown, but is probably different from the mechanism in the infants of diabetic mothers.

REFERENCES

FALORNI, A., FRACASSINI, F., MASSI-BERNADETTI, F. and AMICI, A. (1972): Glucose metabolism, plasma insulin, and growth hormone secretion in newborn infants with erythroblastosis fetalis compared with normal newborns and those born to diabetic mothers. *Pediatrics, 49,* 682.

MØLSTED-PEDERSEN, K. (1972): Aspects of carbohydrate metabolism in newborn infants of diabetic mothers. I. Intravenous glucose tolerance tests. *Acta endocr. (Kbh.), 69,* 174.

MØLSTED-PEDERSEN, L. and JØRGENSEN, K. R. (1972): Aspects of carbohydrate metabolism in newborn infants of diabetic mothers. III. Plasma insulin during intravenous glucose tolerance test. *Acta endocr. (Kbh.), 71,* 115.

MØLSTED-PEDERSEN, L., TRAUTNER, H. and JØRGENSEN, K. R. (1973): Plasma insulin and K values during intravenous glucose tolerance test in newborn infants with erythroblastosis foetalis. *Acta paed. scand., 62,* 11.

PEDERSEN, J. (1967): *The Pregnant Diabetic and Her Newborn. Problems and Management.* Munksgaard, Copenhagen.

PEDERSEN, J. and MØLSTED-PEDERSEN, L. (1971): Diabetes mellitus and pregnancy. The hyperglycaemia-hyperinsulinism theory and the weight of the newborn baby. In: *Proceedings of the 7th Congress of the International Diabetes Federation, Buenos Aires, 1971,* pp. 678–685. Editor: R. R. Rodriguez. International Congress Series No. 238, Excerpta Medica, Amsterdam.

STEINKE, J., GRIES, F. A. and DRISCOLL, S. G. (1967): In vitro studies of insulin inactivation with reference to erythroblastosis fetalis. *Blood, 30,* 359.

JUVENILE DIABETES, TOTAL DIABETES, BRITTLE DIABETES

EXPERIMENTAL MODELS FOR THE STUDY OF JUVENILE DIABETES*

PETER H. WRIGHT

Department of Pharmacology, Indiana University Medical Center,
Indianapolis, Ind., U.S.A.

This will not be an exhaustive account or an extensive assessment of all the experimental models which have been or are being used in the study of diabetes. It will, however, emphasize those models which have in the past provided or are now providing information for the elucidation of clinical problems associated with juvenile diabetes.

Diabetes, especially among young patients, has long been known to run in families (Pavy, 1885) but 'is in many respects a geneticist's nightmare (Neel et al., 1965)'. Onset of juvenile diabetes is acute and it is frequently taught that the appearance of symptoms is preceded by some form of 'stress'. Danowski (1957), for example, reported that many of his patients (42%) had histories of recent infections but White (1959) found 'infections of severity' in few of her cases (10%). Specific infections such as mumps (Kremer, 1947) have been mentioned but respiratory diseases are most frequently implicated (Brown, 1956). As a result of a very recent epidemiological study, Gamble and Taylor (1969) have suggested that the Coxsackievirus-B_4 might be an important etiological agent. Whatever the precipitating agent may be, the disease appears suddenly and progresses rapidly to a fatal outcome unless appropriate treatment with insulin, fluids and electrolytes is commenced. This first and any later attacks of ketoacidosis very closely resemble those seen in untreated pancreatectomized animals and have long been attributed to insulin deficiency. However, it has been shown recently that the onset of diabetic ketoacidosis, even with continuing if inadequate treatment with insulin, is accompanied by a marked increase in the level of circulating glucagon (Muller et al., 1973). In fact, Unger (1971) considers that inappropriately high glucagon relative to insulin secretion and 'blindness' of the alpha cells to the suppressive effects of glucose upon glucagon secretion constitute characteristic features of the juvenile diabetic, and that insulin deficiency per se is not solely responsible for his condition.

Immediately following recovery from the initial attack of ketoacidosis, the juvenile diabetic may require only small doses of insulin for the control of his disease (White, 1959). Tolbutamide is then said to have an insulogenic effect (Steinke et al., 1961) and the islets of Langerhans show histological evidence of insulin secretory activity (Gepts, 1965). Within a few months to a few years at most, however, this 'honeymoon period' is over, all evidence of pancreatic insulin secretory activity disappears and the patient

* This study was supported by Grants No. PHS AM 13237 and AM 16534 from the National Institutes of Health, and by The Upjohn Company, Kalamazoo, Mich.

becomes entirely dependent upon exogenous sources of the hormone. Unfortunately, treatment of the juvenile diabetic with insulin and appropriate dietary regimes has not lived up to the high hopes of those who first used insulin over 50 years ago. In the first place it has proved difficult to mimic with exogenous insulin the close metabolic control normally exerted by the pancreatic islets. Secondly, and possibly related, is the appearance of debilitating and even fatal complications in later life.

No syndrome, induced or appearing spontaneously, in experimental animals completely mimics all the features of human juvenile diabetes, but many, starting with that first induced by pancreatectomy of the dog by von Mering and Minkowski (1889), have exhibited specific features comparable with those seen in man. In the account which follows, some of the specific features of the human disease which have been reproduced experimentally will be considered.

INSULIN DEFICIENCY SYNDROMES

Insulin secretion in vivo can be prevented by removal or destruction of islet cells in the pancreas or it can be nullified by neutralization of endogenous insulin after its secretion from the pancreas. All 3 of these methods have been used experimentally.

Total pancreatectomy

This method, which is seldom used now, did prove useful for the study of insulin deficiency in animals such as the dog, cat and pig which have discrete pancreatic glands, but it has seldom been used for smaller and more easily accessible species such as the rat, rabbit and guinea pig whose pancreatic tissues are more diffusely distributed and more difficult to remove. The syndromes which follow pancreatectomy do vary from species to species but all can be treated successfully with insulin and pancreatic dietary supplements, and most are characterized by the appearance of fatal ketoacidosis if such treatment is withheld.

Destruction of insulin-secreting cells

Alloxan (Lukens, 1948) and streptozotocin (Arison et al., 1967; Brodsky and Logothetopoulos, 1969) have specific destructive effects upon the beta cells of the islets of Langerhans. Both induce a biphasic response in the injected animal; the blood sugar concentration first rises rapidly, then falls after a few hours to normal or hypoglycemic levels before rising permanently. Their modes of action are still not known but they do differ. Thus, for example, only streptozotocin will induce diabetes in the guinea pig (Collins-Williams et al., 1950; Brodsky and Logothetopoulos, 1969) and destroy insulin-secreting tissues in man (Gillman et al., 1957; Murray-Lyon et al., 1968; Blackard et al., 1970). In common with one another these 2 drugs have diabetogenic effects dependent upon dosage (Lukens, 1948; Junod et al., 1969), induce syndromes in rats and other animals which are not usually characterized by ketonuria (Lukens, 1948; Junod et al., 1967), and cause specific destruction of beta cells without any concomitant reactive inflammatory response (Duff, 1945; Brodsky and Logothetopoulos, 1969). These 2 drugs have been and are being used extensively to study the effects of insulin deficiency in experimental animals.

Neutralization of endogenously secreted insulin

Guinea pig anti-insulin serum after intravenous or intraperitoneal injection induces transient hyperglycemia in a variety of experimental animals (Moloney and Coval, 1955; Wright, 1965). When infused intravenously (Armin et al., 1960) or injected intraperitoneally (Anderson et al., 1963) into rats in large doses it induces a fatal syndrome which is very similar to that seen after pancreatectomy of the rat (Scow, 1957).

The diabetic syndromes induced by these 3 methods do differ from one another, even within the same species of experimental animal. Thus Lukens (1948) has likened alloxan diabetes to the syndrome induced in some animals by partial pancreatectomy; alloxan-diabetic animals will frequently live for long periods without insulin therapy and do not commonly exhibit ketonuria. If the alloxan-diabetic animal is pancreatectomized, however, it rapidly becomes ketotic and dies unless insulin is administered (Thorogood and Zimmermann, 1945). Ketonuria can also be induced in rats if large doses of streptozotocin are given (Junod et al., 1969). Although the degree of insulin deficiency induced by these various methods will affect the severity of the syndrome produced, it is also now apparent that induced changes in glucagon secretion may have an influence. Thus Muller et al. (1971) have recently shown that in the untreated alloxan-diabetic dog levels of circulating glucagon are high and diminish after insulin administration, and that shortly after injection of anti-insulin serum into the rat there is also an increase in serum glucagon concentration. Further studies of glucagon secretion and its relationship to insulin secretion in these and comparable experimental models may therefore help in our understanding of the part played by this hormone in the juvenile diabetic syndrome.

INSULITIS

This topic will be considered in more detail elsewhere in this Volume (pp. 285–328) so only the main points will be considered here. It is concerned with an experimental observation made about 10 years ago which focussed attention upon a comparable but much older clinical observation.

There have been sporadic reports, mainly emanating from Warren (1927) and LeCompte (1958), that some children dying in the early acute stages of diabetes exhibit 'insulitis', a lesion characterized by infiltration of the islets of Langerhans with small round cells. Though these authors considered such lymphocytic infiltration of the islets rare, Gepts (1965) found it in 15 of 22 young diabetic patients dying within 6 months of the onset of their disease; no such lesions appeared in 32 young diabetics dying after more than one year. Similar lesions have been found in cattle given repeated injections of bovine or porcine insulins in Freund's adjuvant. In these animals LeCompte et al. (1966) reported lymphocytic infiltration, fibrosis and distortion of the islets, variable reduction in number but some individual enlargement of the beta cells, and complete absence of evidence of necrosis. Similar lesions were found in some sheep given repeated injections of insulin (Federlin, 1971) but in neither of these species of injected animals did hyperglycemia appear. By contrast, Grodsky et al. (1966) induced hyperglycemia which was usually transient in rabbits and within a few weeks of receiving their first injection of insulin in Freund's adjuvant they showed round cell infiltration of the pancreatic islets (Toreson et al., 1968).

These experimental lesions and the 'insulitis' found in juvenile diabetics resemble one another so closely that they have renewed practical interest in the possibility that the human disease could be the result of an auto-immune process. This hypothesis will no doubt be discussed in detail elsewhere but one point should be made here about the experimental observations. The experimental lesions were not induced by hormonal preparations which contained only insulin. Until very recently the insulin preparations used for clinical and experimental purposes contained not only insulin and derivatives or precursors of similar molecular weight, but also an unidentified mixture of components of much higher molecular weight. This latter 'A' component of extracted insulin, as shown originally by Steiner and Oyer (1967), elutes first from gel filtration (Sephadex) columns, well in advance of proinsulin ('B' component) and insulin ('C' component). In a recent study of the immunogenic properties of these 3 fractions, Schlichtkrull et al. (1972) found that the 'A' component of bovine insulin was more immunogenic in rabbits than the hormone itself, the 'C' component. We were unable to confirm this when we carried out similar experiments in guinea pigs but we did find that after about 4 months the animals which had originally been immunized with bovine 'A' component showed fibrotic changes in their islets; half of the 8 survivors originally immunized with 'A' component but none of the 11 originally immunized with insulin ('C' component) showed significant islet fibrosis (Fig. 1). In a second but very limited study of guinea pigs given the same bovine 'A' component in Freund's adjuvant, we have found focal areas of round cell infiltration along pancreatic ducts, round and in islets, and in the interstitial spaces of the acinar tissue after only 14 to 28 days (Fig. 2). Similar lesions appeared in guinea pigs given injections of rat islet homogenates in Freund's adjuvant (Fig. 3). Such lesions, it should be emphasized, were not numerous but they were not found in control animals given Freund's adjuvant alone or killed after no treatment at all. In mentioning these isolated and preliminary observations, my intention is to emphasize that insulin itself may not be the antigen responsible for experimental 'insulitis'; some other component of extracted insulin or of the islets themselves could be inducing the lesions.

If, and this is by no means agreed, juvenile diabetes is the results of an auto-immune process, its initiation would require the release of islet cell constituents. Craighead (1966) reported that the M-variant of the encephalomyocarditis virus causes necrotic lesions in the islets of infected mice and can induce temporary or permanent signs of diabetes (Craighead, 1968; Craighead and Steinke, 1971). The Coxsackievirus also induces pancreatitis in mice, and viral crystals of the B_1 strain have been observed in beta cells of the islets (Tsui et al., 1972). These observations do suggest that viral infections could cause progressive destruction of islet tissue and might initiate an immune response by release of islet constituents. These possibilities warrant further investigation in the experimental field; the possibility that Coxsackievirus B_4 could be responsible in man is already being considered (Gamble and Taylor, 1969).

THE FATE OF INSULIN IN INSULIN-IMMUNIZED ANIMALS

When radio-iodinated insulin is injected intravenously into insulin-treated diabetic patients it disappears from the blood at an abnormally slow rate (Berson et al., 1956; Welsh et al., 1956). Nothing is known, however, of the ultimate fate of such injected insulin or of how that fate may differ from that of insulin injected into a normal subject. There is little doubt that in both animals (Rabkin and Colwell, 1969) and man (Rabkin et al., 1970) the kidneys remove a large proportion of the insulin which they receive in arterial

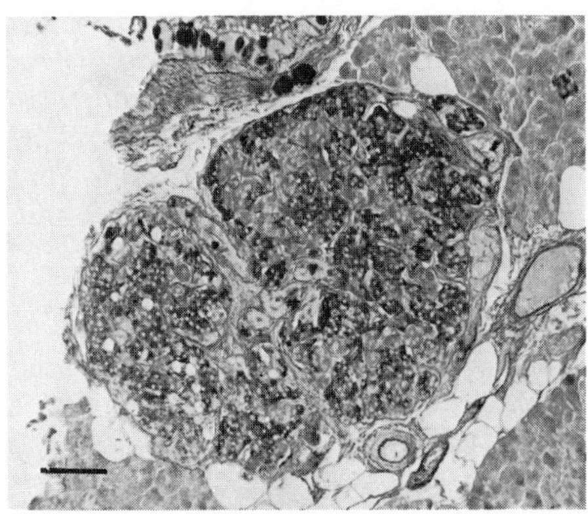

FIG. 1. Fibrosed islet of a guinea pig killed 135 days after initial (Day 0) and one subsequent (Day 63) subcutaneous injection of bovine 'A' component in Freund's adjuvant (aldehyde-fuchsin; black bar represents 100 μ).

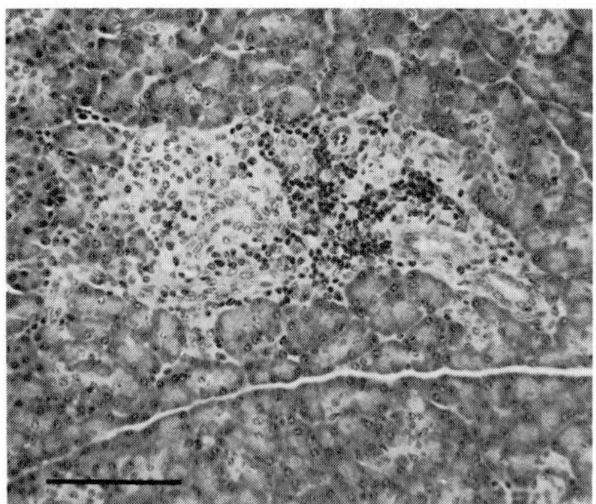

FIG. 2. Lymphocytic infiltration around ducts, small blood vessels and a small islet in a guinea pig killed 15 days after a single subcutaneous injection of bovine 'A' component in Freund's adjuvant (hematoxylin and eosin; black bar represents 100 μ).

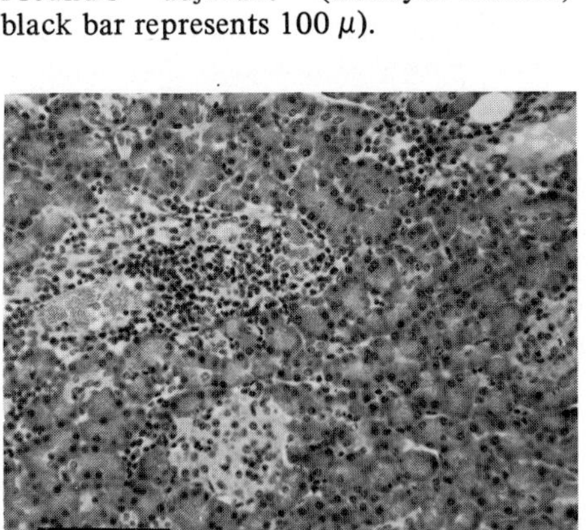

FIG. 3. Lymphocytic infiltration in or around ducts, small blood vessels and islets of a guinea pig killed 59 days after an initial (Day 0) and 2 subsequent (Days 22 and 46) subcutaneous injections of homogenates of isolated rat islets in Freund's adjuvant (hematoxylin and eosin; black bar represents 100 μ).

blood. It is also thought that the liver plays a major, possibly the major, role in endogenous insulin metabolism but the evidence is mainly indirect (Field, 1972). This normal pattern in the experimental animal is affected by the presence of insulin antibodies.

When insulin is allowed to react with guinea pig anti-insulin serum in vitro and is then injected into normal mice (Beck et al., 1966), dogs (Zaharko et al., 1966), rats or guinea pigs (Frikke et al., 1973), the insulin-antibody complexes do not accumulate in the kidneys but concentrate in the liver and spleen. If the hormone itself is injected into insulin-immunized guinea pigs, it disappears slowly from the blood (Horino et al., 1966) and concentrates mainly in the liver (Fig. 4). Preformed complexes are seen to be taken up by reticuloendothelial cells but this could not be demonstrated after injection of the hormone itself into insulin-immunized guinea pigs (Frikke et al., 1973). Thus the presence of antibodies does affect the metabolism of insulin in animals and could do so in the insulin-treated diabetic.

Abnormal metabolism of insulin in man could result in abnormalities in its metabolic action. Berson and Yalow (1958) first suggested that antibodies to insulin probably have an 'insulin transporting' action in most diabetics; they take up the insulin as it enters the blood from the injected depot and release it again to the tissues which require it. At the other extreme, in patients who may require very large doses for adequate control of their disease, Berson and Yalow (1964) suggested that there may be a very high rate of insulin turnover, the insulin-antibody complexes formed in the blood being degraded without the hormone itself ever reaching the tissues which require it. This change in the fate of the injected hormone could be due to a change in the nature rather than in the amount of circulating antibodies. In fact, Kerp et al. (1968) have shown that diabetic patients with antibodies having high affinity for the hormone require more insulin than those whose circulating antibodies have low affinity for insulin. Also, Dixon et al. (1972) have claimed that the presence of moderate amounts of antibodies with low affinity for insulin is needed for stability of control with insulin; they buffer and smooth action of the injected hormone. In their absence, or when avid antibodies are present, such buffering is reduced and the diabetic becomes 'labile'.

DIABETIC COMPLICATIONS

The cause or causes of debilitating and sometimes fatal complications of diabetes mellitus are not known but there are 2 contrasting theories which have clinical implications. According to one, the lesions develop under conditions in which the diabetic syndrome is

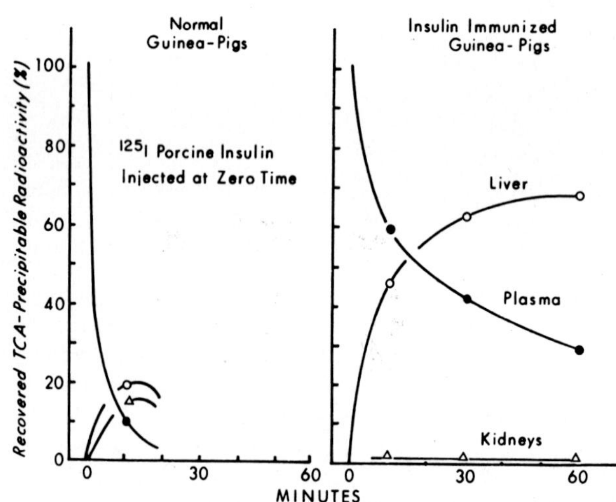

FIG. 4. Recovery of TCA-precipitable radioactivity from the plasma, liver and kidneys of normal and insulin-immunized guinea pigs injected (intracardiac) at zero time with mixtures of ^{125}I-labeled (ca 10 μc; 123 μc/μg) and unlabeled (200 mU) porcine insulin in normal guinea pig serum (0.5 ml). Each point represents the mean of observations in 5 to 7 animals.

poorly controlled and could be prevented by strict attention to good therapeutic control. The second theory implies that microvascular lesions result from the deposition in the walls of small blood vessels of insulin-antibody complexes and are therefore iatrogenic. Both theories have their advocates but neither has been adequately substantiated.

In spite of all the experimental work which has been done over the last 50 years with chronically diabetic animals, few vascular or renal lesions similar to those seen in the human diabetic have been reported. Ricketts et al. (1959), for example, were unable to find any in pancreatectomized dogs which they had maintained for about 10 years. Bloodworth et al. (1969), on the other hand, reported 'moderately severe' diffuse diabetic glomerulosclerosis in dogs made diabetic with growth hormone or alloxan and maintained in poor metabolic control for 5 years; some of these animals also exhibited retinal lesions (Engerman and Bloodworth, 1965). In addition to such conflicting reports, the most consistent lesion found in persistently hyperglycemic animals is cataract; this is frequently seen and easily induced in alloxan-diabetic rats (Lukens, 1948). Impaired neural function which can be partially corrected with insulin has also been observed in streptozotocin-diabetic rats (see Gabbay, 1973). These 2 lesions have been attributed to the accumulation in these tissues of sorbitol which is produced from glucose under hyperglycemic conditions by way of the sorbitol pathway, which has been recently reviewed by Gabbay (1973). By direct study of human tissue, Spiro and his co-workers (Spiro, 1963; Beisswinger and Spiro, 1970) have suggested that thickened basement membranes contain deposits of abnormal glycoproteins which are formed under conditions of insulin deficiency. Thus there is some experimental evidence to support the hypothesis that abnormal lesions can develop under conditions of hyperglycemia but the evidence is still poor in the cases of microangiopathies which have yet to be induced consistently in experimental animals.

The second hypothesis is commonly attributed to Blumenthal et al. (1962) who were among the first to note the similarity between renal lesions found in diabetics and those induced with antigens such as albumin in experimental animals. In support of this hypothesis have been scattered reports of renal lesions in normal and diabetic animals treated with insulin. Grieble (1960) and Mohos et al. (1963) reported them in rabbits and Zampa and Mancini (1965) and Andreev et al. (1970) found them in guinea pigs given repeated injections of insulin. In each case the lesions were said to resemble those found in human diabetics and in some it was claimed that they bound fluoresceinated insulin. Others, such as Federlin (1971) who studied insulin-immunized guinea pigs, failed to find any such lesions so this hypothesis also lacks consistent experimental support.

CONCLUSIONS

To those who are concerned with the management of patients, an experimental model is only useful if it mimics some aspect of the human condition and can be used to aid in diagnosis, treatment or basic understanding of the condition itself. For many years the only models available for the study of human diabetes were the insulin deficiency syndromes produced by the methods outlined above. They served their purpose and have contributed greatly to our understanding of the actions of insulin. In recent years, as I hope that I have shown, other aspects of the human disease have been studied experimentally. Thus, for example, some of the lesions seen in the pancreas of young diabetics have been induced in animals and their causes are being actively investigated. It is suggested that insulin itself or some other components of extracted insulin or of the islet tissue could be responsible for the disease itself or for the complications which appear in later life in the diabetic. Old arguments about the relationship of control of the metabolic disorder to the incidence of complications are being reviewed and submitted to experimental study. Explanations are being sought for the lability and resistance of diabetic patients to treatment with insulin. In fact, those who are studying diabetes now, whether in the clinic or the laboratory, are no longer obsessed with glucose concentration in the blood. They are now studying patients and experimental models with a view towards finding the cause of the disease and its development, and hope that they can do something in the future which will improve its treatment or, far better, prevent it.

ACKNOWLEDGEMENTS

The author wishes to thank Dr. Paul E. Lacy, St. Louis, Missouri, in whose Department the preliminary studies of experimental insulitis were carried out, and Drs. Ronald A. Chance and William Bromer of Eli Lilly and Company, Indianapolis, Indiana, who provided the bovine insulin preparations.

REFERENCES

ANDERSON, J. W., KILBOURN, K. G., ROBINSON, J. and WRIGHT, P. H. (1963): Diabetic acidosis in rats treated with anti-insulin serum. *Clin. Sci., 24,* 417.

ANDREEV, D., DITZOV, S. and DASHEV, G. (1970): Diabetes-like vascular lesions in the kidneys of guinea pigs immunized with insulin-adjuvant mixtures. *Acta diabet. lat., 7,* 243.

ARISON, R. N., CIACCIO, E. I., GLITZER, M. S., CASSARO, J. A. and PRUSS, M. P. (1967): Light and electron microscopy of lesions in rats rendered diabetic with streptozotocin. *Diabetes, 16,* 51.

ARMIN, J., GRANT, R. T. and WRIGHT, P. H. (1960): Experimental diabetes in rats produced by parenteral administration of anti-insulin serum. *J. Physiol., 153,* 146.

BECK, L. V., ZAHARKO, D. S., ROBERTS, N. and KING, C. (1966): On insulin-I^{131} metabolism in mice. Modifying effects of anti-insulin serum and of total insulin dosage. *Diabetes, 15,* 336.

BEISSWINGER, P. J. and SPIRO, R. G. (1970): Human glomerular basement membrane; chemical alteration in diabetes mellitus. *Science, 168,* 596.

BERSON, S. A. and YALOW, R. S. (1958): Insulin antagonists, insulin antibodies and insulin resistance. *Amer. J. Med., 25,* 155.

BERSON, S. A. and YALOW, R. S. (1964): The present status of insulin antagonists in plasma. *Diabetes, 13,* 247.

BERSON, S. A., YALOW, R. S., BAUMAN, A., ROTHSCHILD, M. A. and NEWERLY, K. (1956): Insulin-I^{131} metabolism in human subjects; demonstration of insulin binding globulin in the circulation of insulin treated subjects. *J. clin. Invest., 35,* 170.

BLACKARD, W. G., GARCIA, A. R. and BROWN, C. L. (1970): Effect of streptozotocin on qualitative aspects of plasma insulin in a patient with a malignant islet cell tumor. *J. clin. Endocr., 31,* 215.

BLOODWORTH, J. M. B., ENGERMAN, R. L. and POWERS, K. L. (1969): Experimental diabetic microangiopathy. 1. Basement membrane statistics in the dog. *Diabetes, 18,* 455.

BLUMENTHAL, H. T., BERNS, A. W., OWENS, C. T. and HIRATA, Y. (1962): The pathogenesis of diabetic glomerulosclerosis. 1. The significance of various histopathological components of the disease. *Diabetes, 11,* 296.

BRODSKY, G. and LOGOTHETOPOULOS, J. (1966): Streptozotocin diabetes in the mouse and guinea pig. *Diabetes, 18,* 606.

BROWN, E. E. (1956): Infectious origin of juvenile diabetes. *Arch. Pediat., 73,* 191.

CRAIGHEAD, J. E. (1966): Pathogenicity of the M and E variants of the encephalomyocarditis (EMC) virus. II. Lesions of the pancreas, parotid and lachrymal glands. *Amer. J. Pathol., 48,* 375.

CRAIGHEAD, J. E. (1968): Virus induction of diabetes mellitus in mice. *Amer. J. Pathol., 52,* 56a.

CRAIGHEAD, J. E. and STEINKE, J. (1971): Diabetes mellitus-like syndrome in mice infected with encephalomyocarditis virus. *Amer. J. Pathol., 63,* 119.

DANOWSKI, T. S. (1957): *Diabetes Mellitus – With Emphasis on Children and Young Adults.* Williams and Wilkins, Baltimore.

DIXON, K., EXON, P. D. and HUGHES, H. R. (1972): Insulin antibodies in aetiology of labile diabetes. *Lancet, i,* 343.

DUFF, G. L. (1945): The pathology of the pancreas in experimental diabetes mellitus. *Amer. J. med. Scis, 210,* 381.

ENGERMAN, R. L. and BLOODWORTH, J. M. B. (1965): Experimental diabetic retinopathy in dogs. *Arch. Ophthal., 73,* 205.

FEDERLIN, K. (1971): *Immunopathology of Insulin; Clinical and Experimental Studies.* Springer Verlag, New York.

FIELD, J. B. (1972): Insulin extraction by the liver. In: *Handbook of Physiology, Section 7, Endocrinology, Volume 1, Endocrine pancreas, Chapter 32,* pp. 505–513. Editors: R. O. Greep and E. B. Astwood. American Physiological Society, Washington, D.C.

FRIKKE, M. J., GINGERICH, R. L., STRANAHAN, P. D., CARTER, G., BAUMAN, A. K., GREIDER, M. H., WRIGHT, P. H. and LACY, P. E. (1973): Distribution of insulin and insulin-antibody complexes in normal and insulin-immunized animals. *Diabetologia,* submitted for publication.

GABBAY, K. H. (1973): The sorbitol pathway and the complications of diabetes. *New Engl. J. Med., 288,* 831.

GAMBLE, D. R. and TAYLOR, K. W. (1969): Seasonal incidence of diabetes mellitus. *Brit. med. J., 3,* 631.

GEPTS, W. (1965): Pathologic anatomy of the pancreas in juvenile diabetes mellitus. *Diabetes, 14,* 619.

GILLMAN, T., HATHORN, M. and LAMONT, N. McE. (1957): Alloxan as a possible therapeutic agent for primary carcinoma of the liver. *Lancet, i,* 80.

GRIEBLE, H. G. (1960): Renal lesions induced with heterologous insulin: an example of foreign protein nephritis. *J. lab. clin. Med., 56,* 819.

GRODSKY, G. M., FELDMAN, R., TORESON, W. E. and LEE, J. C. (1966): Diabetes mellitus in rabbits immunized with insulin. *Diabetes, 15,* 579.

HORINO, M., YU, S. Y. and BLUMENTHAL, H. T. (1966): Studies on experimental insulin immunity. I. Dynamics of insulin immunity in the guinea pig. *Diabetes, 15,* 812.

JUNOD, A., LAMBERT, A. E., ORCI, L., PICTET, R., GONET, A. E. and RENOLD, A. E. (1967): Studies of the diabetogenic action of streptozotocin. *Proc. Soc. exp. Biol. Med. (N.Y.), 126,* 201.

JUNOD, A., LAMBERT, A. E., STAUFFACHER, W. and RENOLD, A. E. (1969): Diabetogenic action of streptozotocin; relationship of dose to metabolic response. *J. clin. Invest., 48,* 2129.

KERP, L., KASEMIR, H. and KIELING, F. (1968): Insulinbindende Antikörper und Insulinbedarf bei Diabetikern. *Klin. Wschr., 46,* 376.

KREMER, H. U. (1947): Juvenile diabetes as a sequal to mumps. *Amer. J. Med., 3,* 257.

LeCOMPTE, P. M. (1958): 'Insulitis' in early diabetes. *Arch. Pathol., 66,* 450.

LeCOMPTE, P. M., STEINKE, J., SOELDNER, J. S. and RENOLD, A. E. (1966): Changes in the islets of Langerhans of cows injected with heterologous and homologous insulin. *Diabetes, 15,* 586.

LUKENS, F. D. W. (1948): Alloxan diabetes. *Physiol. Rev., 28,* 304.

VON MERING, J. and MINKOWSKI, O. (1889–90): Diabetes mellitus nach Pankreasexstirpation. *Arch. exp. Pathol. Pharmakol., 26,* 371.

MOHOS, S. C., HENNIGAR, G. R. and FOGELMAN, J. A. (1963): Insulin induced glomerulosclerosis in the rabbit. *J. exp. Med., 118,* 667.

MOLONEY, P. J. and COVAL, M. (1955): Antigenicity of insulin; diabetes induced by specific antibodies. *Biochem. J., 59,* 179.

MULLER, W. A., FALOONA, G. R. and UNGER, R. H. (1971): The effect of experimental insulin deficiency on glucagon secretion. *J. clin. Invest., 50,* 1992.

MULLER, W. A., FALOONA, G. R. and UNGER, R. H. (1973): Hyperglucagonemia in diabetic ketoacidosis. Its prevalence and significance. *Amer. J. Med., 54,* 52.

MURRAY-LYON, I. M., EDDLESTON, A. L. W. F., WILLIAMS, R., BROWN, M., HOGBIN, B. M., BENNETT, A., EDWARDS, J. C. and TAYLOR, K. W. (1968): Treatment of multiple-hormone-producing malignant islet-cell tumour with streptozotocin. *Lancet, ii,* 895.

NEEL, J. V., FAJANS, S. S., CONN, J. W. and DAVIDSON, R. T. (1965): Diabetes Mellitus. In: *Genetics and the Epidemiology of Chronic Diseases,* pp. 105–132. Editors: J. V. Neel, M. W. Shaw and W. J. Schull. U. S. Public Health Service Publication No. 1163.

PAVY, F. W. (1885): Introductory address to the discussion on the clinical aspect of glycosuria. *Lancet, ii,* 1033.

RABKIN, R. and COLWELL, J. A. (1969): The renal uptake and excretion of insulin in the dog. *J. lab. clin. Med., 73,* 893.

RABKIN, R., SIMON, N. M., STEINER, S. and COLWELL, J. A. (1970): Effect of renal disease on renal uptake and excretion of insulin in man. *New Engl. J. Med., 282,* 182.

RICKETTS, H. T., TEST, C. E., PETERSON, E. S., LINTS, H., TUPIKOVA, N. and STEINER, P. E. (1959): Degenerative lesions in dogs with experimental diabetes. *Diabetes, 8,* 298.

SCHLICHTKRULL, J., CHRISTIANSEN, A. H., HEDING, L. G., JORGENSEN, K. H. and VOLUND, A. (1972): Clinical aspects of insulin-antigenicity. *Diabetes, 21,* 649.

SCOW, R. O. (1957): 'Total' pancreatectomy in the rat; operation, effects and postoperative care. *Endocrinology, 60,* 359.

SPIRO, R. G. (1963): Glycoproteins; structure, metabolism and biology. *New Engl. J. Med., 269,* 566 and 616.

STEINER, D. F. and OYER, P. E. (1967): The biosynthesis of insulin and a probable precursor of insulin by a human islet cell adenoma. *Proc. nat. Acad. Sci. U.S.A., 57,* 473.

STEINKE, J., CAMERINI-DAVALOS, R., MARBLE, A. and RENOLD, A. E. (1961): Elevated levels of serum insulin-like activity (ILA) as measured with adipose tissue in early untreated diabetes and prediabetes. *Metabolism, 10,* 707.

THOROGOOD, E. and ZIMMERMANN, B. (1945): The effects of pancreatectomy on glycosuria and ketosis in dogs made diabetic with alloxan. *Endocrinology, 37,* 191.

TORESON, W. E., LEE, J. C. and GRODSKY, G. M. (1968): The histopathology of immune diabetes in the rabbit. *Amer. J. Pathol., 52,* 1099.

TSUI, C. Y., BURCH, C. E. and HARB, J. M. (1972): Pancreatitis in mice infected with Coxsackievirus B_1. *Arch. Pathol., 93,* 379.

UNGER, R. H. (1971): Glucagon physiology and pathophysiology. *New Engl. J. Med., 285,* 443.

WARREN, S. (1927): The pathology of diabetes in children. *J. Amer. med. Ass., 88,* 99.

WELSH, G. W., HENLEY, F. H., WILLIAMS, R. H. and COX, R. W. (1956): Insulin-I^{131} metabolism in man. *Amer. J. Med., 21,* 324.

WHITE, P. (1959): Diabetic children and their later lives. In: *Treatment of Diabetes Mellitus, 10th Edition, Chapter 27,* pp. 655–689. Editors: E. P. Joslin, H. F. Root, P. White and A. Marble. Lea and Febinger, Philadelphia, Pa.

WRIGHT, P. H. (1965): Experimental diabetes induced with insulin antibodies. In: *On the Nature and Treatment of Diabetes, Chapter 24,* pp. 354–360. Editors: G. A. Wrenshall and B. S. Leibel. Excerpta Medica, Amsterdam.

ZAHARKO, D. S., BECK, L. V. and BLANKENBAKER, R. (1966): Role of the kidney in the disposal of radioiodinated and non-radioiodinated insulin in dogs. *Diabetes, 15,* 680.

ZAMPA, G. A. and MANCINI, A. M. (1965): Kimmelstiel-Wilson-like nephropathology. *Lancet, ii,* 300.

JUVENILE DIABETES

R. L. JACKSON

Department of Pediatrics, University of Missouri School of Medicine,
Columbia, Mo., U.S.A.

Diabetes in children and young adults is so different from diabetes in the middle-aged or elderly patient that it requires special consideration. The term 'insulin deficient' or 'insulin dependent' often is applied to the juvenile type of diabetes because the availability of endogenous insulin is decreased or absent. Juvenile diabetes also is referred to as growth-onset diabetes because the onset of the symptoms and signs frequently occurs at the time of prepubertal growth spurt.

An ever increasing number of younger diabetics are finding themselves handicapped by serious vascular disease in early adult life. The difficulties encountered in the long-term treatment of juvenile diabetes indicate that, too often, the disease is managed inadequately.

The relationship of genetic factors to the development of diabetes or to variations in metabolic processes which may contribute to the development of vascular complications of diabetes are poorly understood. Diabetes mellitus has been the subject of many genetic studies. Despite this, the mode of genetic transmission remains obscure. To date, the carrier state can only be assumed rather than biochemically defined.

Prior to the availability of accurate techniques for the determination of the concentration of insulin in blood, all forms of diabetes mellitus were considered to have an absolute insulin deficiency. The development and application of immunoassay methods led to results which necessitated a rethinking of the relationship between circulating insulin and the development of diabetes.

In the early stages of *chemical* diabetes in children, an increased insulin response to an oral glucose load has been found with only minor changes in the blood sugar values. The more typical serum insulin response is a delayed response with elevated values at 3 hours. As the disease progresses to late chemical diabetes, there is a progressive decrease in insulin response and overt diabetes develops. At some point the insulinogenic reserve of the islets is exceeded and 'overt diabetes' develops. Definite deficiency of insulin release occurs in association with the development of juvenile diabetes. Figure 1 demonstrates the serial oral glucose tolerance test (OGTT) of a 12-year-old white boy (A.I.) whose 5-year-old sister had overt diabetes. Figure 2 demonstrates the progressive decrease in his insulin response to oral glucose tolerance tests over a 9-month period of time. Figure 3 demonstrates patient A.I.'s decreasing insulin response to the rapid infusion of glucose and glucose with glucagon over a 10-week period of time. There also is essentially no response of serum insulin to tolbutamide at the same dates. In spite of the decreased insulin response, the child remained aglycosuric except during glucose tolerance tests. He

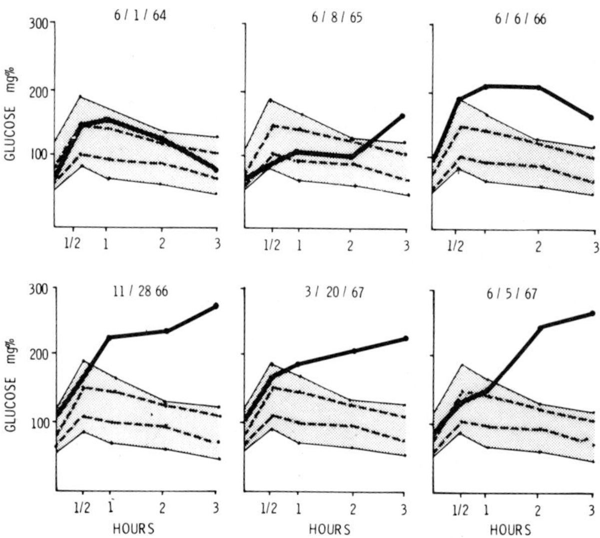

FIG. 1. Progressive changes in a serial standard oral glucose tolerance test of patient A.I. from 9 to 12 years of age.

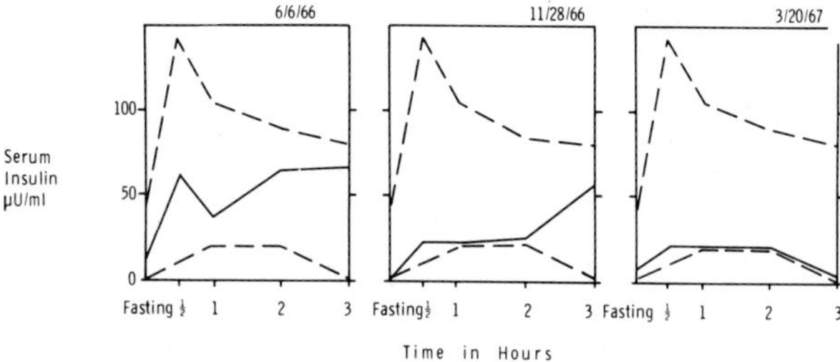

FIG. 2. Serum insulin response during standard oral glucose tolerance tests in patient A.I. Broken lines enclose the normal range. Solid line is the response of this patient.

was given insulin before he developed symptoms or signs of diabetes. His exogenous insulin requirement, to maintain excellent control of his diabetes, has been only 0.5 U/kg/day, which is about half the amount required by boys of his age with overt diabetes. Figure 4 demonstrates serial OGTT's over a 4-month period of time, of patient D.O., a 7-year-old girl who was found to have transient glycosuria and an abnormal OGTT by her family doctor. This child had mild transient glycosuria. Figure 4 also demonstrates a decreasing insulin response to repeated OGTT's. Figure 5 demonstrates a decreasing insulin response of the same child to a rapid i.v. infusion of glucose and to a rapid infusion of glucose with glucagon. Impaired glucose clearance (K) also was observed during this time. She was also given insulin and has required only 0.1–0.2 U of insulin/kg body weight/day to maintain an excellent degree of control of her diabetes which is less than one third of the maintenance amount required by most children with overt diabetes.

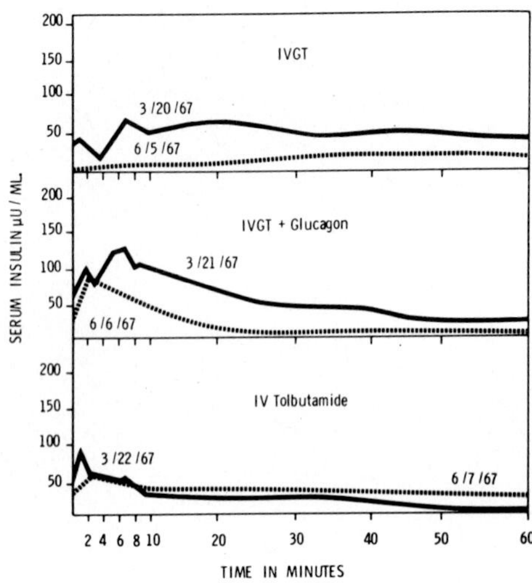

FIG. 3. Progressive decrease in serum insulin response during i.v. tolerance tests in patient A.I.

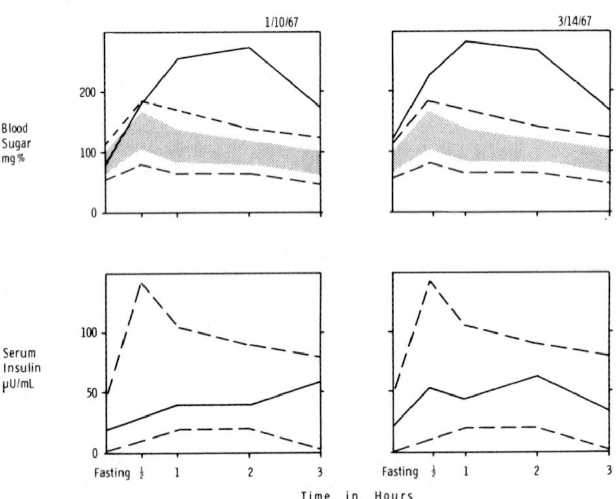

FIG. 4. Serum insulin response during standard oral glucose tolerance tests in a 7-year-old girl (patient D.O.). Broken lines enclose the normal range. Solid line is the response of this patient.

The child with overt juvenile diabetes has low basal insulin levels with little or no insulin release after islet cell stimulation. In the juvenile diabetic, the pancreatic structure varies from a picture of hypertrophic islets with a gross reduction of beta cells to one of complete hyalinization of islets. With the passage of time, only a few atrophic islets can be found.

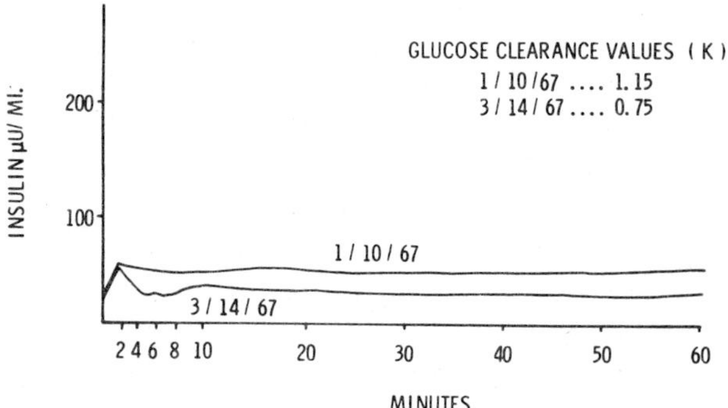

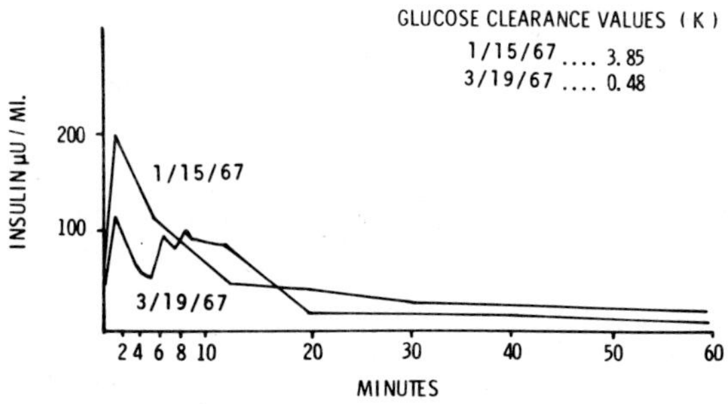

FIG. 5. Progressive decrease in insulin response during i.v. tests in patient D.O.

The biochemical alterations characterizing the child with diabetes result from insulin deficiency. Marked insulin deficiency produces a metabolic state similar to that of starvation. *Without insulin, food cannot be stored effectively for future use.* There is: (1) inhibition of peripheral glucose uptake, (2) decreased synthesis of glycogen, protein, and lipid, (3) reversal of the glycolytic pathway with active hepatic production of glucose from amino acids despite the presence of hyperglycemia, (4) active mobilization of fats from adipose tissue, leading to marked elevations in the concentration of total lipids, cholesterol, triglycerides, and free fatty acid in plasma, and (5) development of ketoacidosis.

Insulin-deficiency diabetes produces an extreme catabolic state. When overt diabetes mellitus occurs in childhood, the signs and symptoms of insulin deficiency are usually severe and appear abruptly, especially if the child has an acute infection. The child or parents usually can recall the week or even the day when symptoms were first noticed. For a few weeks or months after the onset of the clinical disease, the increased intake of food and liquids compensates for the urinary losses, and mild ketosis may be tolerated, even though increased catabolism and defective protein synthesis interferes with normal growth. Ketonemia gradually increases, finally causing anorexia and vomiting, after which ketoacidosis develops rapidly.

There is a growing body of evidence that the glucose tolerance test may be abnormal for a long time (years) before the onset of clinical or overt diabetes. The pattern of development and the terms used are delineated in Table 1. Figure 6 demonstrates the normal range of blood sugars and serum insulin values during an OGTT (Jackson et al., 1967).

The progressive decrease in insulin response to the children with chemical diabetes and the excellent results of early insulin therapy in children with early diagnosis of overt diabetes suggest that substitution insulin therapy may be indicated even prior to the onset of the overt form of the disease.

Every child with overt diabetes should receive insulin therapy as soon as the diagnosis is confirmed. The exogenous insulin requirement varies depending on how early the diagnosis is made and how soon insulin is given. The earlier the diagnosis is made, the lower the insulin needed and the easier it will be to attain and maintain a high degree of control with little risk of hypoglycemia.

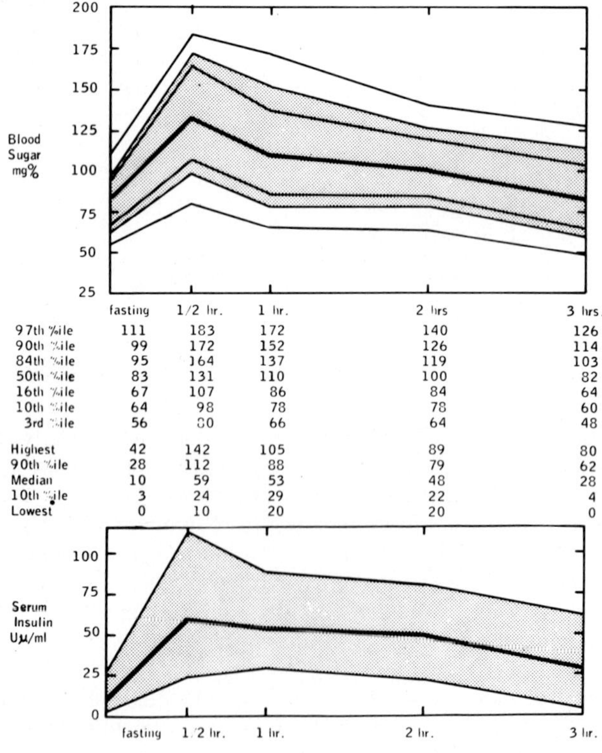

	fasting	1/2 hr.	1 hr.	2 hrs	3 hrs.
97th %ile	111	183	172	140	126
90th %ile	99	172	152	126	114
84th %ile	95	164	137	119	103
50th %ile	83	131	110	100	82
16th %ile	67	107	86	84	64
10th %ile	64	98	78	78	60
3rd %ile	56	80	66	64	48
Highest	42	142	105	89	80
90th %ile	28	112	88	79	62
Median	10	59	53	48	28
10th %ile	3	24	29	22	4
Lowest	0	10	20	20	0

FIG. 6. Blood sugar and serum insulin during the standard oral glucose tolerance test in children.

TABLE 1
The pattern of development of diabetes

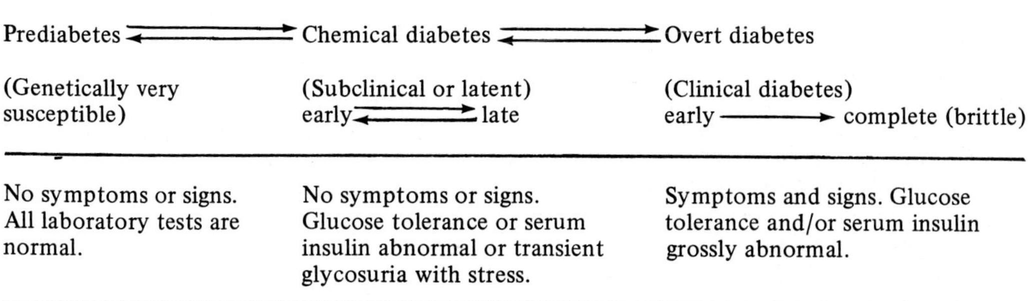

Prediabetes ⇄	Chemical diabetes ⇄	Overt diabetes
(Genetically very susceptible)	(Subclinical or latent) early ⇄ late	(Clinical diabetes) early → complete (brittle)
No symptoms or signs. All laboratory tests are normal.	No symptoms or signs. Glucose tolerance or serum insulin abnormal or transient glycosuria with stress.	Symptoms and signs. Glucose tolerance and/or serum insulin grossly abnormal.

In our opinion, too many children receive inadequate treatment at the time of onset of overt diabetes. Most often they are given a single daily dose of an intermediate type of insulin with some modifications of food intake. A few are also given an ineffective therapeutic trial with an oral hypoglycemic agent. During the early weeks or even months after onset of the disease, most children will have a good response to only a single dose of exogenous insulin as they are still producing some endogenous insulin. However, *with suboptimal therapy the insulin deficiency progresses* and, consequently, the morning dose of insulin is increased in an attempt to control the polyuria and glycosuria which develops during the night. The child then begins to experience hypoglycemic episodes of varying intensities, usually during the later morning or early afternoon, and is then considered to have *brittle* diabetes with the added possibility of a convulsive disorder. It is not until this time, when the child has total diabetes, that he is referred to a diabetic clinic in a medical center.

Children with complete or total (brittle) diabetes have an advanced stage of the disease. In order for them to maintain a good to fair degree of control, they need to receive at least twice daily injections of insulin and proper meal planning which includes 3 meals and 3 snacks. In contrast to the children with recent onset of diabetes they will not have a recovery period. Their daily insulin requirement will be about 0.6 to 1.0 U/kg/day.

At the University of Missouri Medical Center 63 children with recent onset of overt diabetes have been studied, to compare differences in responses of children with early diagnosis and prompt insulin treatment with children with delayed diagnosis and insulin treatment. It is well known that the exogenous insulin requirement of most children with recent onset of diabetes decreases rapidly to a relatively low level for a variable period. This state of partial remission is known as the 'honeymoon period'. During this time, glycosuria can be controlled completely without any symptoms or signs of an insulin reaction. It is usually possible to attain and maintain complete regulation (without insulin reactions) and with a relatively low dosage of insulin (0.02 to 0.12 U/kg/day) during the early months after onset of overt diabetes. In this so-called 'honeymoon period', the child's pancreas is still producing some endogenous insulin.

In 23 children with early diagnosis and treatment, the insulin requirement was very low (0.05 to 0.10 U/kg/day) and the period of partial remission was as long as 4 years. In

12 children admitted with severe ketoacidosis who had delayed diagnosis and delayed insulin treatment, the period of hospitalization was longer, the insulin requirement was 0.5 to 0.8 U/kg/day and the period of partial remission as short as 2 months.

As previously stated, at least a 2 dose insulin program is needed for the treatment of juvenile diabetes. In our clinic, a mixture of NPH insulin and regular insulin is given half an hour before breakfast, and NPH insulin is given one hour before the evening meal. The insulin mixture for the morning injection consists of 2 parts of NPH insulin to one part of regular insulin. The insulins are mixed by injecting them into a sterile bottle in an amount not to exceed a 2 weeks' supply. This method is convenient and provides much greater accuracy in measurement than mixing the insulins in a syringe. Two-thirds of the total daily dosage is given as the mixture of regular and NPH before breakfast, and the other one third is given as NPH insulin one hour before the evening meal. Regular insulin is given with the morning dose of NPH insulin so that the breakfast can be eaten within 30 minutes after the morning insulin injection; the intermediate insulin in the mixture will be reaching its peak activity for the noon meal. The usual dietary distribution used with this insulin regimen is one in which 4/18 of the caloric intake is given at breakfast, followed by a mid-morning snack approximately 2 hours after breakfast, consisting of 2/18 of the diet; the noon meal is 5/18 of the daily allowance with a mid-afternoon snack about 3 hours later of 1/18; 5/18 is given as the evening meal; and a bedtime snack of the remaining 1/18 of the caloric intake is given about 3 hours after the evening meal. Most young patients *with total or so-called brittle diabetes* will make a good response to this plan of treatment which provides insulin throughout the day (24 hours) with sufficient insulin available at the approximate times so that the child can have meals and snacks in keeping with the usual food pattern of non-diabetic children (Fig. 7). Some patients with total diabetes will have a better response to more frequent injections of regular insulin given 20 to 30 minutes prior to individual meals. *I have often stated that it is not the total diabetes that is brittle; it is the doctors that are brittle and unwilling or reluctant to modify their therapy to meet the needs of the patients with total diabetes.*

One of the major differences in the management of children with diabetes in our clinic as compared to most other children's clinics is that insulin is given as often as necessary to keep the urine as sugar-free as practicable.

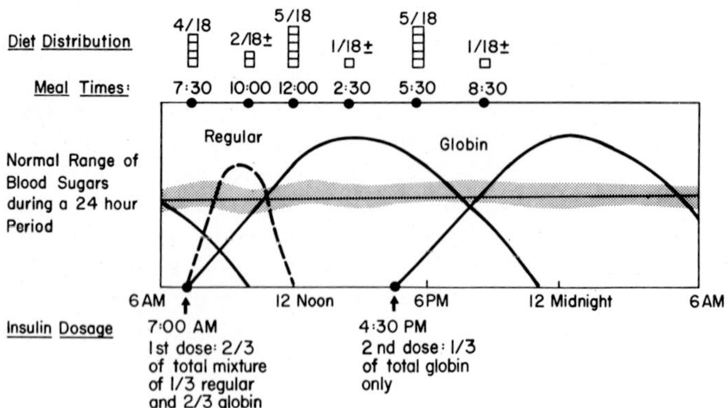

FIG. 7. Insulin action over a 24-hour period. Two-dose regimen.

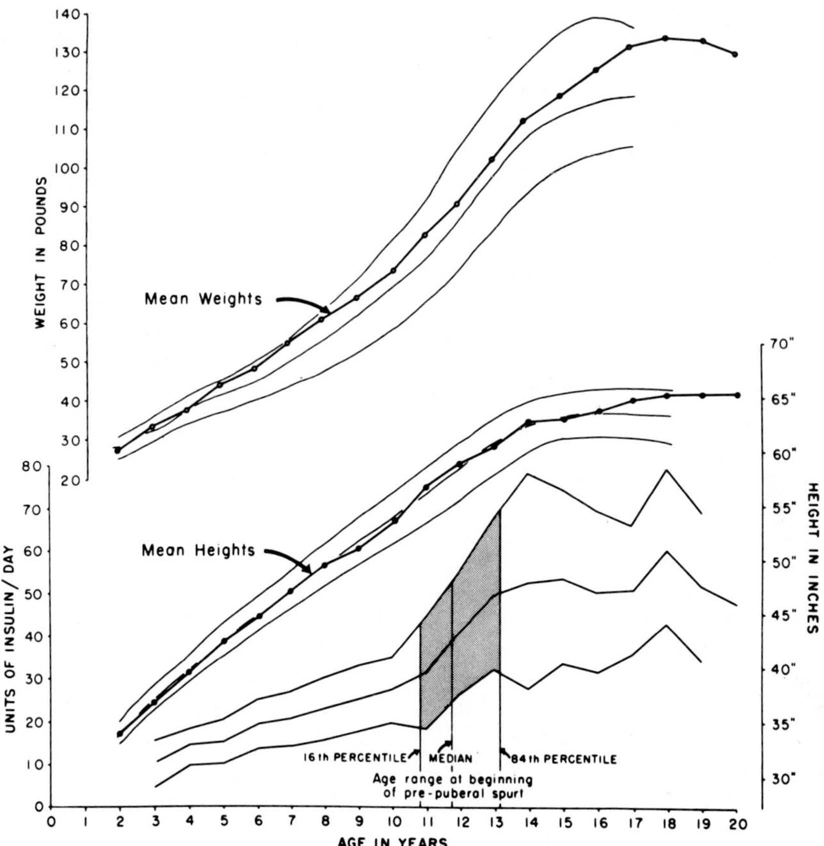

FIG. 8. Mean body weight and height and range of insulin requirements in a group of well-controlled diabetic girls.

It is important to know and be able to predict future insulin requirements of a given child. *There is a close interrelationship between the changing insulin requirement and physical growth, as indicated in Figures 8 and 9.* The insulin requirement gradually rises in the prepubertal child as a result of increase in body weight, but the ratio of insulin dosage to ideal body weight increases only slightly. With the prepubertal growth spurt, there is a sharper rise in insulin requirement, and control is more difficult to maintain. After puberty, the insulin requirement will decrease to a lower level and remain relatively constant during adulthood. The age of onset of the disease does not significantly influence the insulin requirement per unit of body weight. As adulthood is reached, it is important that insulin dosage and caloric intake be reduced gradually to the person's adult requirement. The adolescent girl is especially prone to become obese if her insulin dosage and caloric intake are not adjusted to a lower requirement in keeping with her age. It is much easier to prevent than to treat obesity.

A knowledge of insulin requirements and growth at varying age periods of well-con-

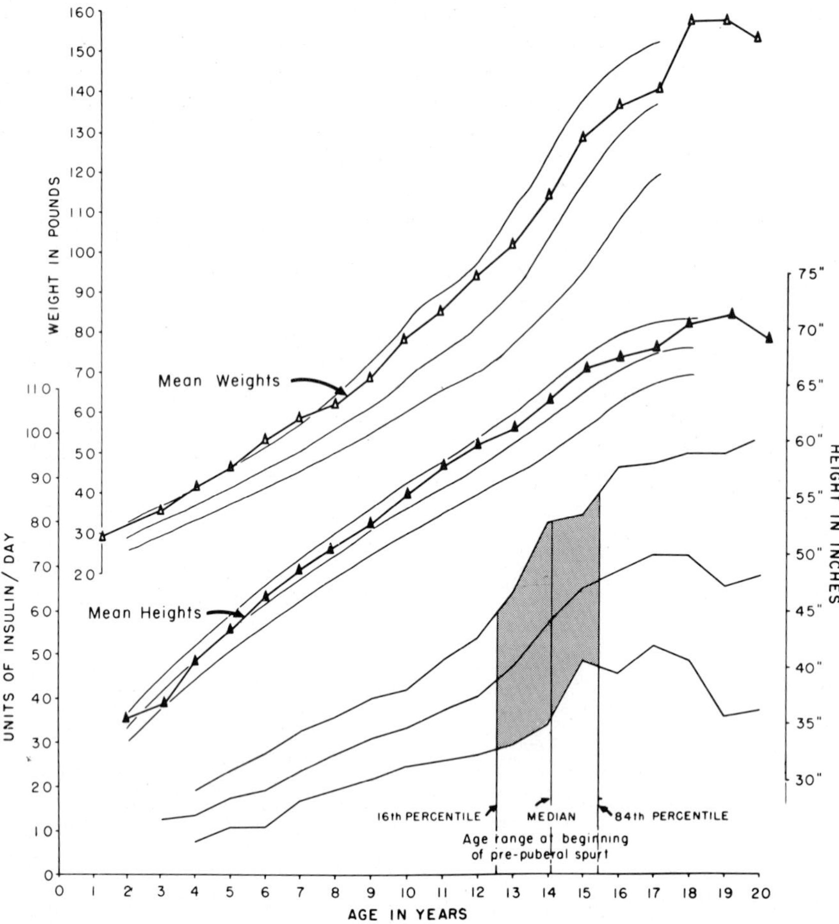

FIG. 9. Mean body weight and height and range of insulin requirements in a group of well-controlled diabetic boys.

trolled diabetic patients helps in the prediction of insulin and nutritional requirements and for maintaining good control of the disease and a normal growth pattern (Kelly et al., 1955). Figures 8 and 9 indicate the average and standard deviation of insulin requirements of girls and boys from infancy to adulthood. Also plotted on this chart are mean heights and weights of a group of well-controlled diabetic patients in relation to the standard Iowa Growth Charts. On these 2 charts, the 'zones of rapid growth' are marked to indicate the relation of insulin requirements to periods of rapid growth. Up to 10 years, the growth patterns of boys and girls are quite similar, in contrast to the great difference after 10 years. The insulin requirements reflect the periods of similarity and differences in the sexes and clearly show a relationship of insulin requirement to growth. The insulin requirement of girls increases rapidly after the age of 10 years, concomitantly with their prepubertal growth spurt, and decreases after the period of rapid growth. The insulin requirement for boys increases rapidly after 12 years, concomitantly with their prepubertal growth spurt, and both decrease gradually as adulthood is reached. As the child's insulin requirements increase with growth, many parents may fear that the disease is becoming more severe unless they have been informed that this is to be expected.

During a febrile illness the insulin requirement usually increases provided the child continues to ingest and absorb his food. In addition to needing somewhat larger doses of insulin in the morning and evening, the child also may require a supplementary dose of regular insulin at noon and late in the evening.

It has been well established that drugs such as tolbutamide and phenformin are not effective for the treatment of the insulin-deficient overt juvenile diabetic. We are doing a controlled longitudinal study to determine if tolbutamide may be useful for treating selected children with early chemical diabetes.

The maintenance diet of the child with diabetes should be essentially the same as for normal children. In the initial instruction of the parents and the child, it is most important to teach them how to use high quality common foods in preparing simple menus.

The only differences in the diabetic child's dietary program as compared to that of the non-diabetic child is that the diet is planned as a predictable caloric intake and is given in the proper relationship to the type and amount of insulin that has been administered to avoid glycosuria and insulin reactions. The daily caloric intake needs to be varied according to the physical activity pattern of the child.

The well diabetic child may be as active as any child with whom he plays. It is not necessary to limit his physical activity; it is, however, necessary to understand his need to have more or less food depending on whether exercise is increased or decreased (Jackson and Kelly, 1948).

When juvenile diabetes is not well controlled, serious consequences such as retardation of growth, progression of the disease itself, and degenerative vascular changes such as diabetic retinitis and arteriosclerosis have been found to develop. Observations by Hardin et al. (1956) at the University of Iowa on a group of 140 juvenile diabetic patients with a duration of the disease ranging from 10 to 29 years have indicated that duration of the disease is not the deciding factor in the development of retinopathy. The degree of control of the diabetes was the only identifiable factor bearing a constantly significant relationship to the incidence and severity of this complication. New knowledge has become available recently regarding the relationship of vascular disease in diabetics to the carbohydrate intolerance and diabetic control. Winegrad et al. have studied the polyol pathway of glucose metabolism (Morrison and Winegrad, 1971; Rasio et al., 1972). They have shown this pathway to be operative in the lens of the eye, the aorta and most recently in capillary tissue. In the lens, hyperglycemia results in the shunting of glucose into the polyol pathway with an accumulation of sorbitol and fructose. These compounds in turn increase the osmotic pressure in the lens with an increase in water content and disruption of the fibers of the lens. The accumulation of sorbitol, fructose and water results in thickening of the vascular tissue with a decrease in the diffusion of oxygen and a resulting hypoxic damage to the vascular tissue.

Convincing data in the controversy about the relationship of diabetic control to the development of vascular disease comes from the work of Spiro who has studied extensively the metabolism of glycoproteins (Spiro, 1969; Beisswenger and Spiro, 1973). The capillary basement membrane is a glycoprotein made up primarily of lysine molecules. These chains of lysine molecules are tightly bound to each other forming a compact membrane. Periodically the lysine molecules become hydroxylated and substituted with galactose and glucose units. At these points the bonds between the chains of lysine are broken and the membrane is thickened. In the non-diabetic individual these substitutions are infrequent and the chains closely packed. In the diabetic the substitutions are very frequent, as often as every third lysine molecule in long-standing poorly controlled diabetics. Spiro has recently identified the enzymes, transferases, responsible for the transfer of the galactose, glucose units to the lysine molecules (Spiro and Spiro, 1971). He has shown that the action of these enzymes is suppressed by insulin. Thus hyperglycemia increases the substrate for the basement membrane reaction and a low tissue insulin level allows the enzymes responsible for transfer of glucose to lysine to become activated. Whether the hyperglycemia or hypoinsulinism is the most important factor is under investigation. Both, however, occur concurrently.

Cahill (1971) has presented evidence that there must be detectable serum insulin levels during the entire 24-hour period in order to prevent the reactions Spiro has described and thus prevent capillary basement membrane thickening (CBMT). *Clinically, anatomically and biochemically the evidence is accumulating that the vascular disease of diabetes is related to abnormal blood glucose and serum insulin levels, i.e., the degree of control of the diabetes.*

Electron microscopic measurements of the capillary basement membrane (CBM) obtained by muscle biopsy in our clinic are in keeping with the findings of Kilo et al. (1972): CBMT does not precede the onset of carbohydrate intolerance but is related to the duration and degree of control of the diabetes. Data to date indicates that CBMT is not seen in children with chemical diabetes or in children with newly diagnosed overt diabetes. CBMT develops in less than 5 years in children with poorly controlled diabetes but may not develop even after 17 years in well controlled diabetics. The CBM's in children with well controlled diabetes of more than 15 years' duration were thinner than CBM's of children with poorly controlled diabetes of less than 5 years' duration (Guthrie, unpublished observations).

Until more knowledge concerning the pathologic physiology of vascular disease in diabetics is available, good control offers the best means of delaying or averting degenerative changes. Recent advances in diabetes research have been encouraging. We are looking forward to the day when we will know the cause of the disease and how to prevent it. The doctor should retain an optimistic outlook in caring for children with diabetes.

REFERENCES

ARLANS, L., ROSENBLOOM, M. D., DRASH, A. and GUTHRIE, R. A. (1970): *Chemical Diabetes Mellitus in Childhood.* Proceedings of a conference held at Ponte Vedra Beach, Florida, December, 1970, Vol. XXII. *Metabolism,* 1973.

BEISSWENGER, P. J. and SPIRO, R. G. (1973): Studies on the human glomerular basement membranes. Composition, nation of the carbohydrate units and chemical changes in diabetes mellitus. *Diabetes, 22,* 180.

CAHILL, G. F. (1971): Physiology of insulin in man. The Banting Memorial Lecture. *Diabetes, 20,* 785.

HARDIN, R. C., JACKSON, R. L., JOHNSTON, R. L. and KELLY, H. G. (1956): The development of diabetic retinopathy. Effects of duration and control of diabetes. *Diabetes, 5,* 397.

JACKSON, R. L., GUTHRIE, R. A., MURTHY, D. Y. N., WOMACK, W. N. and McCANN, M. L. (1967): Diabetes and pre-diabetes in children. In: *Supplement to the Proceedings of the sixth Congress of the International Diabetes Federation, Stockholm, 1967,* pp. 79–102. Editor: J. Östman. International Congress Series No. 172S, Excerpta Medica, Amsterdam.

JACKSON, R. L. and KELLY, H. G. (1948): A study of physical activity in juvenile diabetic patients. *J. Pediat., 33,* 155.

KELLY, H. G., RAO, T. R. and JACKSON, R. L. (1955): Insulin requirements of children with diabetes mellitus maintained in good control. *Amer. J. Dis. Child., 89,* 31.

KILO, C., VOGLER, N. and WILLIAMSON, J. R. (1972): Muscle capillary basement membrane changes related to aging and diabetes mellitus. *Diabetes, 21,* 881.

MORRISON, A. D. and WINEGRAD, A. I. (1971): Regulation of polyol pathway activity in aorta. *Diabetes, 20,* 329.

RASIO, E. A., MORRISON, A. D. and WINEGRAD, A. I. (1972): Demonstration of polyol pathway activity in an isolated capillary preparation. *Diabetes, 21,* 330.

SPIRO, R. G. (1969): Glycoproteins: their biochemistry, biology, and role in human disease. *New Engl. J. Med., 281,* 991, 1043.

SPIRO, R. G. and SPIRO, M. J. (1971): Effect of diabetes on the biosynthesis of the renal glomerular basement membrane. Studies on the glucosyl transferase. *Diabetes, 20,* 641.

CONTINUOUS BLOOD GLUCOSE MONITORING IN BRITTLE DIABETES

J. MIROUZE and F. COLLARD

Clinique des Maladies Métaboliques et Endocriniennes,
Hôpital Saint Eloi, Montpellier, France

Continuous blood glucose monitoring, accepted by some groups as a regular method of investigation in diabetes, has provided important information, especially in relation to brittle diabetes in which most authors believe a total lack of insulin to be present. This paper attempts to put together the information obtained over the past 11 years.

METHOD OF INVESTIGATION

The classical method of oxidoreduction of ferricyanide to ferrocyanide allows the determination of blood glucose; it seemed more reliable than the peroxidase reaction because of the rapid alteration of enzymatic reagents in prolonged glycemic recordings.

The technical appliance and its different steps have been described elsewhere (Mirouze et al., 1963a, 1972). Monitoring of insulin-treated diabetics is particularly interesting if prolonged over at least 24 hours. It requires the withdrawal of blood at a rate of 3.32 ml/min. or 460 ml/24 hour, although it can be less, i.e. 6 ml/hour (Mayo clinic). Because of the dangers of strong heparinization associated with continuous blood glucose monitoring, patients with severe hemorrhagic retinopathy and those suffering from diffuse vascular diseases were excluded.

CONTINUOUS BLOOD GLUCOSE MONITORING IN INSULIN-TREATED BRITTLE DIABETES

Figure 1 shows a continuous record of 2 insulin-treated diabetics, one brittle (solid line), the other stable (dotted line): glycemic fluctuations are obvious, especially in the brittle form of the disease.

We noticed *3 or 6 glycemic depressions* in the 24-hour cycle, which are related to the frequency of the various meals. The duration of the depression is variable: sometimes there is a very transient episodic minimum, sometimes there is a longer lasting lower plateau interrupted by the next food intake. The lowest level of the depression is sometimes normoglycemic, sometimes hyperglycemic and sometimes hypoglycemic. *A clinically obvious hypoglycemia* is clearly indicated by this technique and therefore allows better education of the patient. Thus, when hypoglycemia is nearly asymptomatic, a search must be made for neglected slight symptoms that have so far not been recognized,

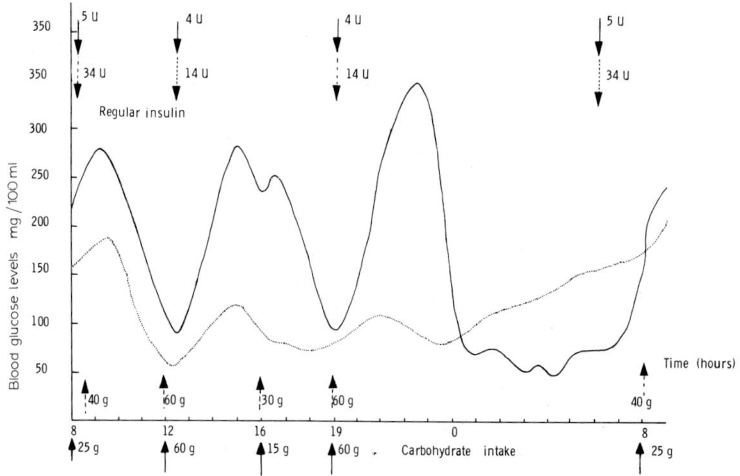

FIG. 1. Continuous blood glucose monitoring: brittle diabetes (———), stable diabetes (-----).

but could help the patient to identify hypoglycemia. Sometimes, despite this search, hypoglycemia episodes remain absolutely latent, but it is essential to know their incidence because they have to be avoided, either by additional food intake or by adjustment of insulin dosage. The depression of blood sugar shows the *duration of effect of previously injected insulin,* the action of which stops at the very moment the depression ceases. Thus, in the examples given in Figure 1, regular insulin had an effective duration of 12 hours in cases of brittle diabetes and of only 6 hours in cases of stable diabetes. Experience shows that the duration of a given insulin preparation may differ greatly from one subject to another. In some individuals, the duration differs from the mean by several hours. However, the means do not markedly differ between stable and brittle cases as shown in Table 1. Finally, *identification of previously unexplained clinical symptoms* becomes easy when they occur during the recording.

Hyperglycemic peaks as opposed to falls in blood glucose are obvious when insulin is lacking, but are always evident, particularly in the most severe cases of brittle diabetes

TABLE 1

Comparison between stable and brittle diabetes in relation to the duration of administration of different insulin preparations

	Long-acting insulin	Semi-lente insulin	Regular insulin
Stable diabetes	19.38 hr ± 26 min.	7.29 hr ± 54 min.	6.44 hr ± 46 min.
Brittle diabetes	17.06 hr ± 27 min.	7.43 hr ± 37 min.	5.35 hr ± 30 min.

(Fig. 1). There seems to be no correlation between the rise of the peak and the carbohydrate intake. The peak generally appears as a transient projecting point. The slopes of the peaks are influenced by insulin treatment in brittle diabetes, and therefore it is most important to know their sharpness.

Falls in blood sugar occur in the period following complete food absorption and depend on whether or not the patient is treated with insulin. Without insulin, glycemic decreases are very slow and irregular. Under the effect of insulin, however, the blood glucose curve falls even more abruptly than in non-diabetic patients and a secondary rise in the slope is seldom seen. Indeed this can be detected in normal individuals and in those with chemical diabetes. The more brittle the diabetes, the more abrupt the fall in blood sugar.

Postprandial blood glucose rises are very rapid and acute in all forms of diabetes mellitus, but especially in the brittle form. Insulin treatment only moderately reduces the sharpness of the rise.

Spontaneous nightly blood glucose rises occur during sleep. The start of a spontaneous blood glucose rise indicates that the hypoglycemic treatment is coming to an end and allows a precise estimation of the duration of the hypoglycemic effect of previously injected insulin. Knowing that time of action it is possible to decide whether the patient has to be treated by 1, 2 or 3 injections of insulin per day. The rate of the spontaneous rise in blood glucose seems proportional to the severity of the diabetes. The nightly rise in blood glucose is almost always sensitive even to a small injection of insulin, as is shown in Figure 2.

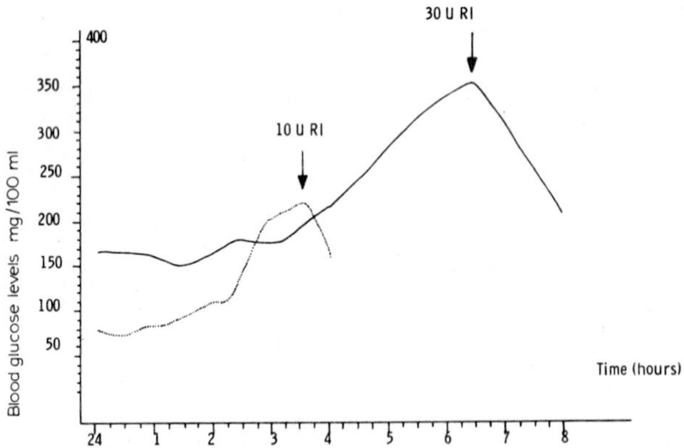

FIG. 2. Insulin effect upon nightly spontaneous 'rate of blood glucose rise' (RBGR) in 2 patients. ----- = 10 U of regular insulin, ——— = 30 U of regular insulin.

The course of the nightly rise in blood glucose can be evaluated by prolonging the morning fast until lunch and by delaying the hour of morning insulin injection (see Fig. 3). Sometimes the rise in blood sugar is followed by ketoacidosis which can become severe if no further insulin is given. Sometimes stabilization of blood glucose occurs at abnormally high levels.

Other cases, after an initial nocturnal reascension following the loss of insulin effect, show in the morning a spontaneous reduction in blood glucose levels until stability is attained; these levels either remain pathological or tend to approach normoglycemia.

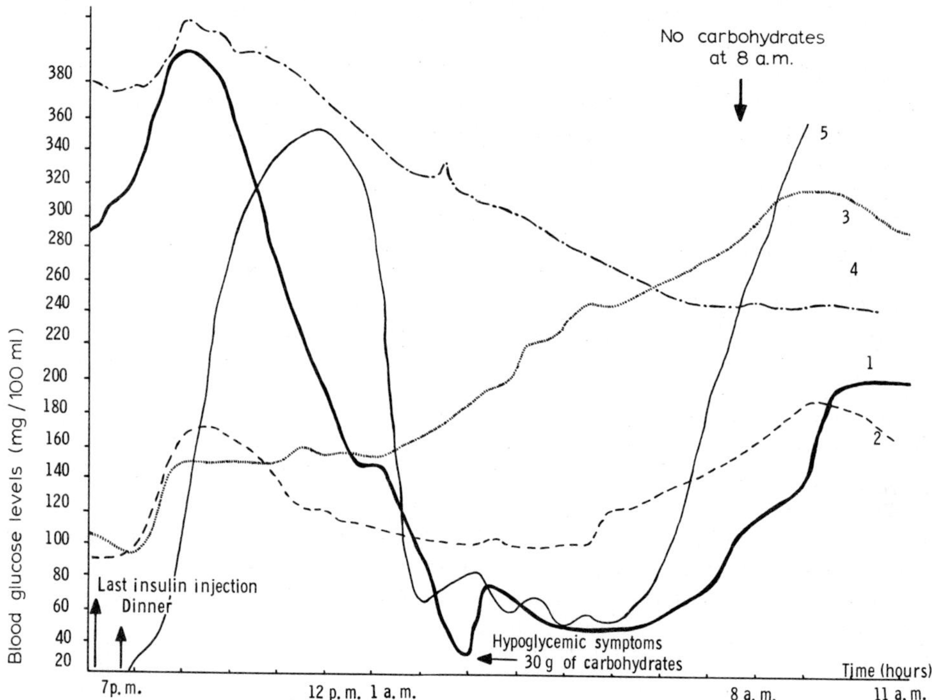

FIG. 3. Five continuous blood glucose recordings with prolongation of morning fast and without insulin therapy.

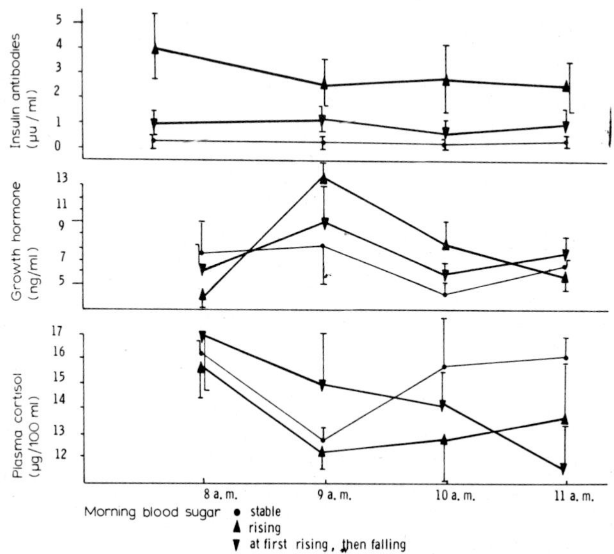

FIG. 4. Plasma cortisol, growth hormone and insulin antibodies in the same conditions as in Figure 3.

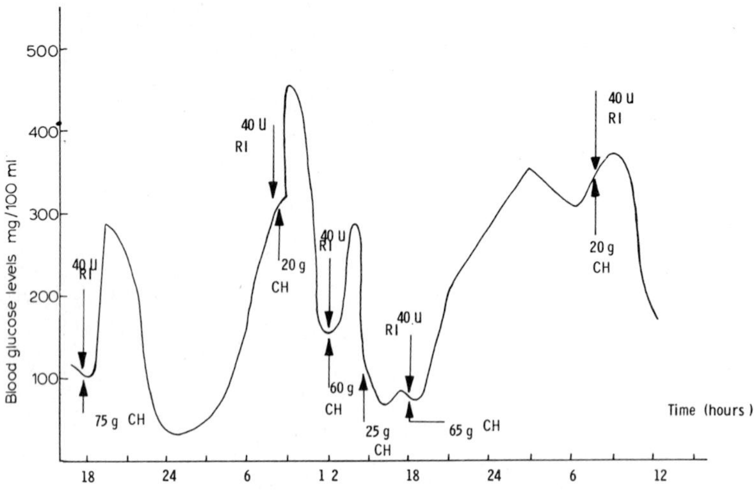

FIG. 5. Continuous blood glucose monitoring over 48 hours in a case of very brittle diabetes showing on the first day a spontaneous nightly hyperglycemic rise beginning between 3 and 4 a.m. and on the second day a nightly hyperglycemia followed by preprandial hypoglycemia without postprandial hypoglycemia, indicating a Somogyi effect. RI = regular insulin, CH = carbohydrate intake.

Repeated testing of growth hormone and cortisol in the morning is not helpful. The levels of anti-insulin antibodies are always higher in those patients with rapid and continuous rises in blood sugar (Fig. 4).

Day-to-day reproducibility of recordings is not constantly observed and this irregularity provides further information. Figure 5 shows a blood glucose monitoring prolonged over 48 hours. The dinner on the first day was followed by a hyperglycemic rise and by a secondary hypoglycemia. The dinner on the following day, however, although containing slightly less carbohydrate and preceded by exactly the same dose of insulin, was followed by a continuous hyperglycemic rise lasting till early in the morning. The first day the dinner was ingested while the blood glucose was at a normal level, the second day it was taken while hypoglycemic. This curve seems to be an obvious demonstration of a Somogyi effect: that hyperglycemia following hypoglycemia impedes further hypoglycemia after food absorption. Thus, continuous blood glucose recording gives very important information for the control of difficult cases. It helps to detect the very *frequent latent hypoglycemic episodes* and permits their prevention. The *duration of insulin efficiency* may be measured quite precisely; thus, the choice of insulin and the number of injections per day can be accurately monitored in each individual patient. The *existence of a spontaneous nightly rise in blood glucose* without food intake indicates a severe form of diabetes which must be carefully controlled.

Rapid rises in blood sugar, with or without insulin, and abrupt falls in blood sugar after insulin are the best signs of the severity and the lability of diabetes. Continuous monitoring of such diabetics shows that there is no phase of blood sugar stability.

TABLE 2

Studies in stable and brittle diabetics divided according to the number and type of insulin injections

	Group 1 (1 insulin injection per day)		Group 2 (2 insulin injections per day)		Group 3 (3 insulin injections per day)	
	Brittle diabetes	Stable diabetes	Brittle diabetes	Stable diabetes	Brittle diabetes	Stable diabetes
Number	60	61	30	11	27	11
Sex: Male	34	42	20	10	14	5
Female	26	19	10	1	13	6
Age (years)	32.1 ± 1.9	34.2 ± 2.1	37.4 ± 2.3	37.5 ± 4.5	36.0 ± 2.4	31.3 ± 4.8
Weight (kg)	56.9 ± 1.5	61.7 ± 1.3	62.7 ± 2.6	61.2 ± 2.3	60.4 ± 1.7	54.7 ± 2.7
Height (cm)	164.2 ± 1.5	167.5 ± 1.2	167.5 ± 1.7	169.5 ± 2.4	164.9 ± 1.8	163.5 ± 2.6
Duration of diabetes (years)	5.2 ± 0.8	7.2 ± 0.7	10.6 ± 1.5	9.5 ± 2.9	11.1 ± 1.8	7.2 ± 1.7
Insulin dosage (U)	54.7 ± 3	45.9 ± 2.6	46.1 ± 2.8	48.1 ± 7.1	55.3 ± 5.2	46.5 ± 4.3

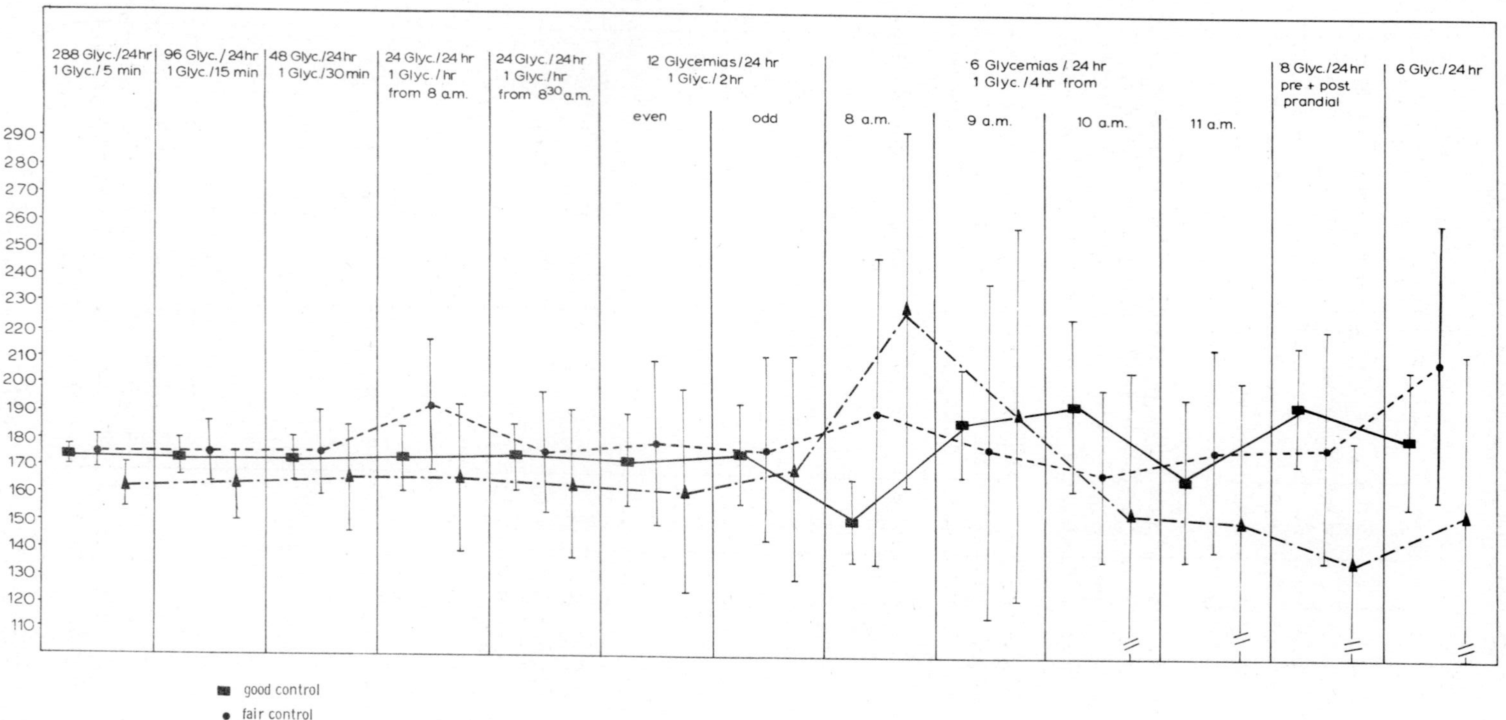

FIG. 6. Mean blood glucose (MBG) of cases 1, 2 and 3.

OBSERVATIONS ON INSULIN-TREATED DIABETICS, SEPARATE OR GROUPED

In order to evaluate previous methods of investigation by continuous blood glucose monitoring, let us consider 3 insulin-treated diabetics: one with a good control (case 1), one with a fair control (case 2) and one with a poor control (case 3). Similar studies were carried out in stable and brittle diabetics divided according to the number and type of insulin injections: one injection of long-acting insulin (group 1), 2 injections of insulin with intermediate effect (group 2), and 3 injections with regular insulin (group 3) (see Table 2).

Mean blood glucose (MBG) proposed by Molnar et al. (1968) corresponds to the mean values recorded every 5th minute over 48 hours. These authors indicated rates of 78, 80, and 83 mg/100 ml in 3 normal subjects; in 3 stable diabetics rates of 110, 111 and 115 mg/100 ml, and in 6 brittle diabetics rates of 146, 149, 170, 196, 208, and 244 mg/100 ml were observed.

We have tried to establish whether in the brittle form mean blood glucose could provide an accurate profile of diabetes and we determined the minimum number of blood sugar values necessary to give a valid MBG. Figure 6 shows the results of the 3 previously mentioned observations.

Obviously MBG obtained by just testing for hypoglycemia or hyperglycemia is not

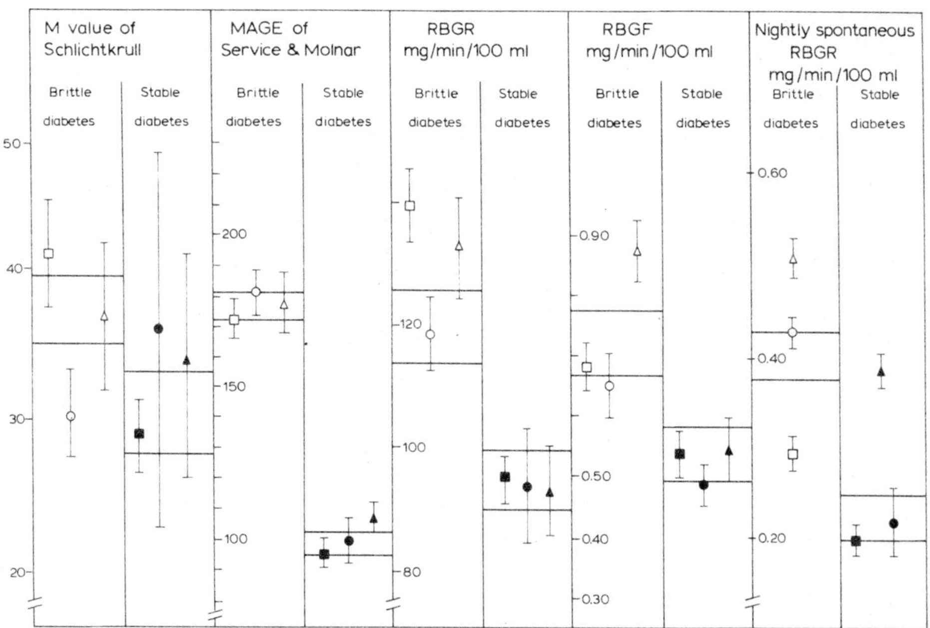

FIG. 7. Summary of all data calculated in cases with brittle or stable diabetes belonging to group 1 (with one injection of long-acting insulin, □ brittle, ■ stable diabetes), group 2 (2 injections of insulin with intermediate duration, ○ brittle, ● stable diabetes), and group 3 (3 injections of regular insulin, △ brittle, ▲ stable diabetes).

very reliable; with a sufficient number of blood glucose values, however, MBG becomes very precise. Determining blood sugar every other hour, no matter whether even or odd hours are chosen, is as good as testing blood sugar every hour, every half hour, every quarter of an hour or even every 5 minutes. MBG appears to be inadequate to distinguish between stable or brittle diabetes or give the incidence of the daily hypoglycemic episodes (see Fig. 7).

The coefficient of insulin efficiency or M-value of Schlichtkrull et al. (1961) considers the level of blood sugar and of glucosuria, the presence of urinary ketone bodies, and the appearance of hypoglycemic episodes. The reference blood sugar is arbitrarily fixed at 120 mg/ml and the M value is defined by the following formula:

$$M = 10\,(\log \cdot \frac{\text{glycemia}}{120})^3$$

whereas Service et al. (1970) define it:

$$M = 10\,(\log \frac{\text{glycemia}}{80})^3$$

In Schlichtkrull's coefficient the mean M value is established by measuring 7 glucose values each day over a 6 to 8 day period. We showed that by the technique of continuous blood glucose monitoring it was possible to obtain a much larger number of blood glucose values, so that it was no longer possible to take glycosuria, hypoglycemia and ketonuria into account. It is only necessary to establish a mean M value from the blood sugar/hour/day by adding up the M value so determined and dividing by the chosen number of blood sugar measurements, i.e. 24. The diabetic control is considered very good if the value is less than 18, fair if it is less than 31 and poor if it is above 31.

An obvious disadvantage of the proposed method is the fact that it only covers periods of 24–72 hours. Between Schlichtkrull's technique, covering periods of 6 to 8 days, and our own method the extreme differences proved to be only of the order of 17–19% and it was therefore considered unnecessary to continue the procedure for longer than 72 hours. By continuous blood glucose recording it is now possible to code the fluctuations in Schlichtkrull's coefficient according to the number of daily samples and to the hours of sampling, as shown in Figure 8. With a sufficient number of blood glucose values, i.e. more than 6 per 24 hours, or with 6 or 8 pre- and postprandial readings, the coefficient is stable; it affords an excellent means for estimating diabetic control, but does not distinguish between stable and brittle diabetes. The study of M value in our grouped patients (Table 2) shows that all the patients submitted to continuous blood glucose monitoring could have their balance improved (see Fig. 7).

Mean amplitude of glycemic excursions (MAGE) (Service et al., 1970) also indicates the extreme variability of glycemia, but different from Schlichtkrull's M value and from mean blood glucose. This index is obtained by measuring the rate difference between peak blood sugar and succeeding minimum blood sugar, or vice versa, considering only fluctuations exceeding standard error of MBG; the mean of the fluctuations thus defined corresponds to MAGE. Service et al. give the following rates: in 3 normal subjects, MAGE is equivalent to 60, 40, and 21 mg/100 ml respectively; in 3 stable diabetics to 67, 82 and 79 mg/100 ml; and in 6 brittle diabetics to 119, 154, 169, 184 and 200 mg/100 ml.

Figure 10 shows MAGE for the 3 patients studied for comparison: 102, 450 and 260 mg/100 ml respectively. In brittle diabetes our MAGE rates correspond to those of

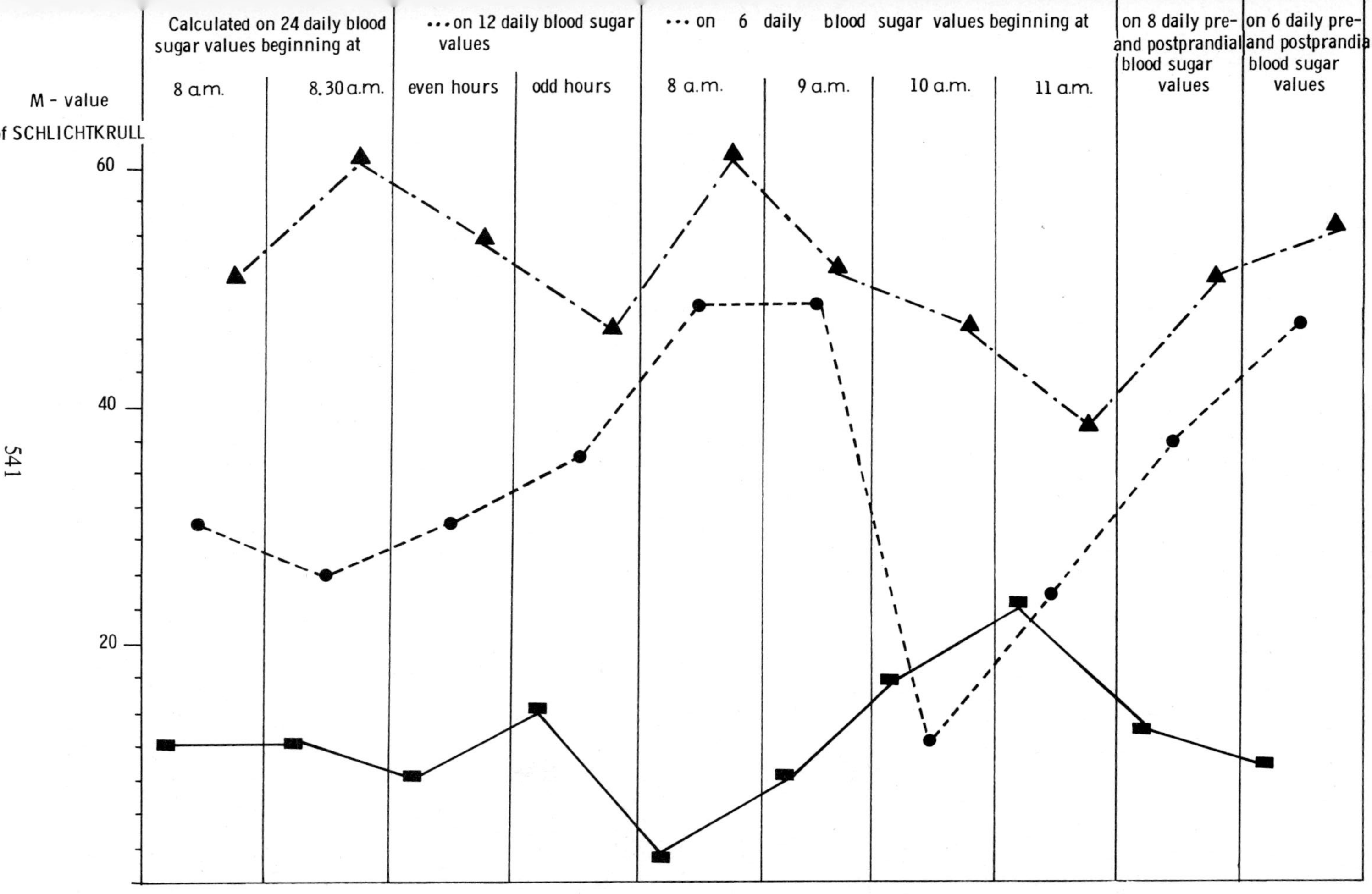

FIG. 8. M value of Schlichtkrull: example of calculation in cases 1, 2 and 3. Case 1 (■) good control; Case 2 (●) fair control; Case 3 (▲) poor control.

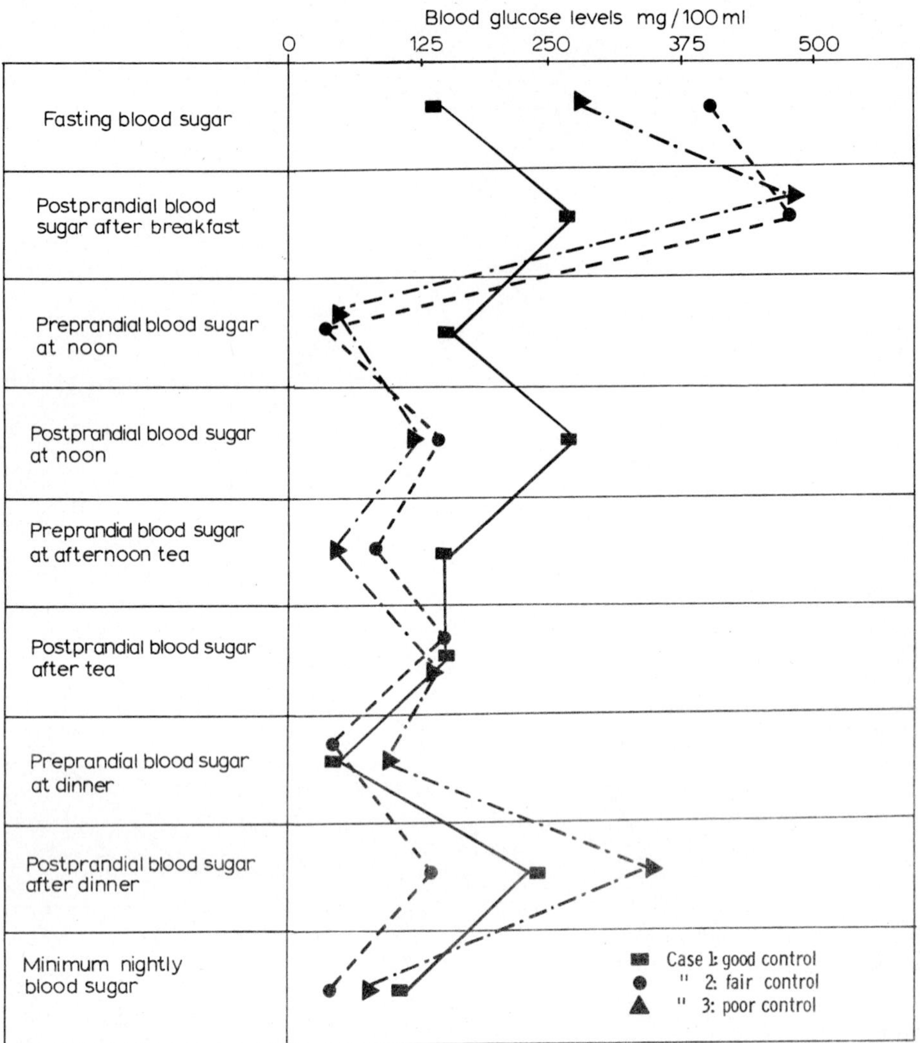

FIG. 9. Blood glucose key values obtained in cases 1, 2 and 3.

Service et al. and they do not seem to be corrected by improved insulin therapy. MAGE may recognize the stable or brittle pattern of diabetes but gives no estimate of diabetic control, as clearly illustrated in Figure 7.

Detection of glycemic key values corresponding to highest and lowest blood glucose levels (i.e. slope changes) is only practicable through continuous blood glucose monitoring. Thus it is possible to define postprandial blood glucose peaks after breakfast, lunch, afternoon tea and dinner, as well as day and night minimum blood glucose levels long after food absorption as shown in Figure 9.

Rates of mean rise in blood glucose and of mean fall in blood glucose, whatever the

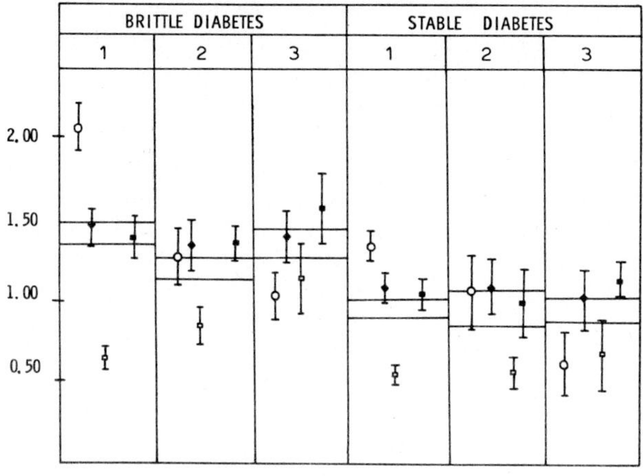

FIG. 10. Rate of blood glucose rise (RBGR) (mg/min./100 ml) in groups of treatment 1, 2 and 3 of cases with stable or brittle diabetes (same definitions as in Fig. 7).

blood glucose baseline values and postprandial blood glucose peaks might be, indicate the magnitude and speed of glucose fluctuations.

The rate of blood glucose rise (RBGR) is expressed in mg/min./100 ml of blood:

$$\text{RBGR} = \frac{\text{Peak blood glucose-baseline blood glucose (mg/100 ml)}}{\text{Time at peak blood glucose-time at baseline blood glucose (min.)}}$$

The rate of blood glucose fall (RGBF):

$$\text{RBGF} = \frac{\text{Peak blood glucose-return blood glucose (mg/100 ml)}}{\text{Time at lowest blood glucose level-time at peak blood glucose (min.)}}$$

In physiological conditions:

RBGR = 1.1 ± 0.1 mg/min./100 ml of blood
RBGF = 0.6 ± 0.1 mg/min./100 ml of blood

The advantage of RBGR lies in the fact that it can be calculated even without continuous monitoring of blood glucose but with 2 or 3 early postprandial blood glucose determinations, since the rise in blood glucose is linear. *The risk of error is important in determination of RGBF* without continuous blood glucose monitoring because there is no certainty about all the blood glucose samples having been chosen on the falling curve.

In observations 1, 2 and 3 mean RGBR are, respectively, 0.91 ± 0.48, 1.16 ± 0.22, 2.01 ± 0.79, and mean RBGF 0.51 ± 0.20, 1.20 ± 0.57, 1.37 ± 0.37. In stable cases we notice that the rates are reduced and subnormal; in brittle cases, however, rapid rises are uncontrolled by insulin and rapid falls demonstrate an abnormally high sensitivity to insulin.

RBGR of brittle diabetes are constantly faster than in stable cases (Figs 7 and 10), especially after the main meals (lunch and supper). In the presence of long-acting insulin (group 1) RBGR after breakfast demonstrates a spontaneous rise almost without insulin effect and is about twice as fast in brittle diabetes. The rate following the afternoon tea is always slight due to the moderate carbohydrate intake. In the same way, RBGF are faster in brittle diabetics than in stable diabetics (Figs 7 and 11) and in normal subjects after all

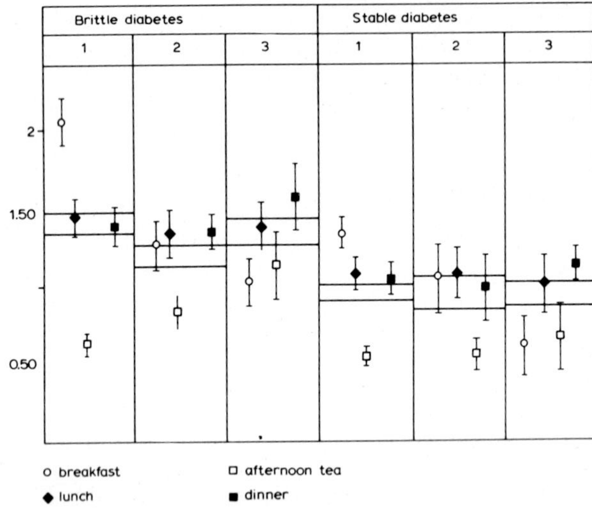

FIG. 11. Rate of blood glucose fall (RBGF) (mg/min./100 ml) in groups 1, 2 and 3 of cases with stable or brittle diabetes.

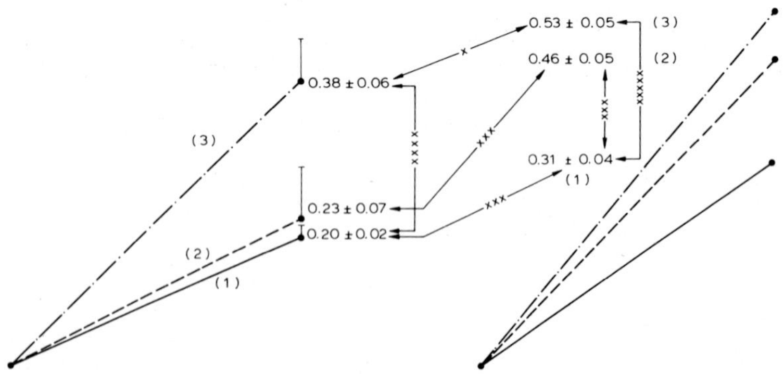

FIG. 12. Nightly spontaneous rate of blood glucose rise in groups of treatment 1, 2 and 3 of cases with stable or brittle diabetes (same definitions as in Fig. 7). X: P<0.05; XXX: P<0.01.

meals except the afternoon tea; the difference is more evident in patients treated by 3 daily injections.

Nightly RBGF are constantly faster in all cases of brittle diabetes treated by 1, 2 or 3 daily injections (Fig. 12), the difference being always significant.

CONCLUSIONS

This study shows that diabetics can be systematically studied, monitored and controlled by continuous blood glucose monitoring. The determination of maximum and minimum blood sugar levels or circadian key values and their precise incidence in time are very important.

M value of Schlichtkrull evaluates diabetic control; *MAGE and RBGR* indicate the brittle character of diabetes; *RBGF* indicates the sensitivity to antidiabetic therapy; *Nightly RBGR* will give a warning against ketosis.

In these conditions criteria of brittle diabetes are evident:
constant lack of glycemic stability;
abnormally fast postprandial blood glucose rise;
abnormally fast postprandial blood glucose fall showing an excessive sensitivity to insulin;
rapid spontaneous nightly blood glucose rise becoming dangerous when the effect of insulin therapy ceases.

REFERENCES

MIROUZE, J., COLLARD, F. and TEISSEIRE, J. P. (1972): Intérêt de l'enregistrement glycémique continu dans l'analyse du diabète sucré insuliné. In: *Journées de Diabétologie Hôtel Dieu,* p. 285. Flammarion, Paris.

MIROUZE, J., JAFFIOL, C. and SANY, C. (1962): Enregistrement glycémique nycthéméral continu dans le diabète instabile. *Rev. Franç. Endocr., III,* 337.

MIROUZE, J., JAFFIOL, C. and SANY, C. (1963a): Enregistrement glycémique nycthéméral continu dans le diabète sucré. *Pathol.-Biol., II,* 553.

MIROUZE, J., SATINGHER, A., SANY, C. and JAFFIOL, C. (1963b): Coefficient d'efficacité insulinique. Coefficient M de Schlichtkrull corrigé et simplifié par la technique de l'enregistrement glycémique continu. *Diabète, 6,* 267.

MOLNAR, G. D., ACKERMAN, E. and ROSEVEAR, J. W. (1968): Continuous blood glucose analysis in ambulatory fed subjects. I. General methodology. *Mayo Clin. Proc., 43,* 833.

SCHLICHTKRULL, S., MUNCK, O. and JERSILD, M. (1961): The M value, an index of blood sugar control in diabetics. *Acta med. scand., 177,* 95.

SERVICE, J. F., MOLNAR, G. D., ROSEVEAR, W., ACKERMAN, E., GATEWOOD, L. C. and TAYLOR, W. F. (1970): Mean amplitude of glycemic excursions, a measure of diabetic instability. *Diabetes, 19,* 644.

UNSTABLE DIABETES: CONCEPTS OF ITS NATURE AND TREATMENT BASED ON CONTINUOUS BLOOD GLUCOSE MONITORING STUDIES

GEORGE D. MOLNAR

Mayo Clinic and Mayo Foundation, Rochester, Minn., U.S.A.

After 50 years of clinical experience with insulin therapy, we still have difficulties in treating diabetics with insulin. Variability of response to consistent therapy is generally called 'unstable diabetes'. Extreme variability is brittle (hyperlabile) diabetes.

This operational definition, of course, excludes conditions that may make stable diabetes appear unstable or unstable diabetes appear even more unstable. The conditions to be excluded are other health problems coexisting with the diabetes and errors of testing, dieting, or injecting insulin (Molnar, 1964).

The studies by Colwell (1953), Izzo and Crump (1950), Somogyi (1959), and our group (Molnar et al., 1965) in this country and by Schlichtkrull et al. (1965) in Europe helped to define unstable diabetes as a clinical entity. The advent of the technique of continuous blood glucose monitoring provided the means for complete documentation of blood glucose behavior. Following early studies by Weller et al. (1960), Mirouze et al. (1962) (in France) first applied continuous blood glucose monitoring to the study of unstable diabetes.

In our own work, my colleagues and I combined continuous blood glucose monitoring, as an intensive means of scientific scrutiny, with optimal conditions for diabetes regulation (Molnar et al., 1968; Rosevear et al., 1969; Service et al., 1969) to seek answers to the following questions:

Can blood glucose stability or instability be consistently identified and quantified in diabetes?

Is it possible to transform an unstable diabetic into a stable diabetic?

Can the blood glucose patterns of diabetics be made to conform to the patterns of non-diabetics?

What causes blood glucose instability or stability in diabetes?

METHODS

In all of our studies, we compared unstable and stable diabetics and normal (non-diabetic) subjects. Because we had previously found prolonged investigations necessary for decisive results, we combined long-term study methods (Molnar et al., 1965) with continuous blood glucose monitoring of 48 hours' duration (Molnar et al., 1968; Rosevear et al., 1969; Service et al., 1969). Also, because of the importance of exercise-related phenomena in unstable diabetics, we included standardized but realistic exercise as a part of our experimental conditions. To permit freedom of movement, the intravenously placed catheter connecting the patient to the automated analytical equipment was 10 feet long (Molnar et al., 1968; Rosevear et al., 1969).

To aid in the analysis of prolonged studies under ambulatory-fed conditions, we added shorter dynamic tests under resting-fasting conditions (Fatourechi et al., 1969; Cremer et al., 1971; Molnar et al., 1974). During these tests, a single stimulus usually was applied. Where appropriate, mathematical models and simulation techniques were used to interpret those results (Gatewood et al., 1970; Yipintsoi et al., 1973).

Figure 1 illustrates our experimental design. A prolonged preparation period of several weeks served 3 major purposes: (1) achievement of clinically optimal therapy with diet, exercise, and insulin or oral antidiabetic agents; (2) performance of the resting-fasting single stimulus tests; and (3) training the patients to follow a consistent schedule of activities. Throughout the studies, complete urine collections were made for multiple analyses. A 6-day nitrogen balance period followed the preparation period. The 48-hour continuous blood glucose monitoring was done in the middle of this 6-day period.

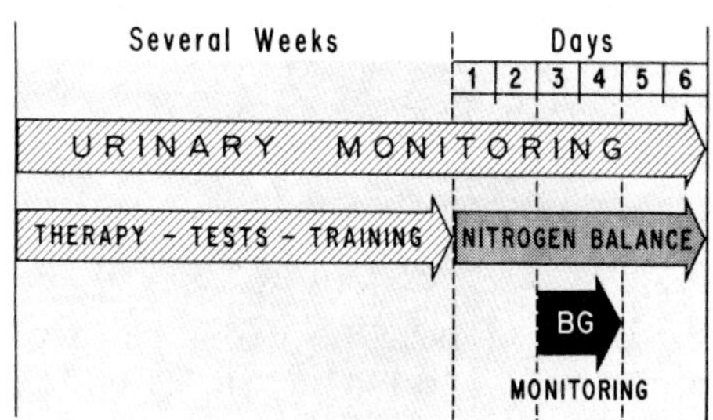

FIG. 1. Diagram of experimental design to clarify time relationships of measurements and activities. For details, see Tables 1 and 2 as well as text.

Table 1 lists the urine glucose, ketone body, and nitrogen measurements made throughout all studies. The measurements in feces and blood added during the nitrogen balance and continuous blood glucose monitoring are also listed.

Table 2 enumerates the activities during the segments of each study. Once a patient was ready for the nitrogen balance period, we kept the therapy as constant as feasible. During the continuous blood glucose monitoring, we sampled blood hourly, or more frequently, for the additional measurements listed.

We repeated the studies both with and without intentional changes. As shown in Figure 2, diabetics were studied on 2 regimens of therapy: with 4 daily injections of short-acting insulin and with 1 or 2 daily injections of (primarily) intermediate-acting insulin. The resting-fasting tests were done while the diabetics were on the short-acting insulin regimen. The training usually took place during the initial investigative session.

RESULTS AND COMMENTS

Figure 3 shows the daily schedule of activities and the averaged 48-hour blood glucose patterns of 3 unstable diabetics, 3 stable diabetics, and 3 normal subjects. The patients

TABLE 1
Measurements made during experimental periods

A. Throughout all studies
   1. Urinary glucose
      a. Quantitatively from meal to meal
      b. Semiquantitatively 60 and 30 minutes before meals
   2. Urinary ketone bodies
      Quantitatively from meal to meal
   3. Urinary total nitrogen
      Quantitatively per 24 hours
B. During nitrogen balance studies
   Above plus fecal nitrogen
C. During continuous monitoring studies
   Above plus: 1. Continuous BG
   2. Hourly hGH, IRI, FFA, ketone bodies

ate breakfast, lunch, dinner, and supper at 5-hour intervals. These meals provided equal calories and were of equal composition. There was also a half-size snack at mid-afternoon (Molnar et al., 1968). Exercise was an hour's standardized walk during the third post-prandial hour. During these studies, diabetics received insulin once daily before breakfast. The glucose fluctuations were greater and more variable in diabetics, especially in unstable diabetics. Only the normals had prolonged baseline levels.

TABLE 2
Activities during experimental periods

A. Preparation period
   1. Complete urine collections
   2. Development of individualized clinically optimal therapy
   3. Training for standard schedule of activities
   4. Tests (resting-fasting) with arginine, insulin, glucose, tolbutamide, etc.
B. Nitrogen balance period
   1. Stool collections added
   2. Therapy kept as constant as feasible
C. Continuous BG monitoring
   1. Collections, activities, and therapy continued and kept constant
   2. Hourly blood sampling (for hGH, IRI, FFA, and ketone bodies)
   3. Continuous blood sampling (for glucose)

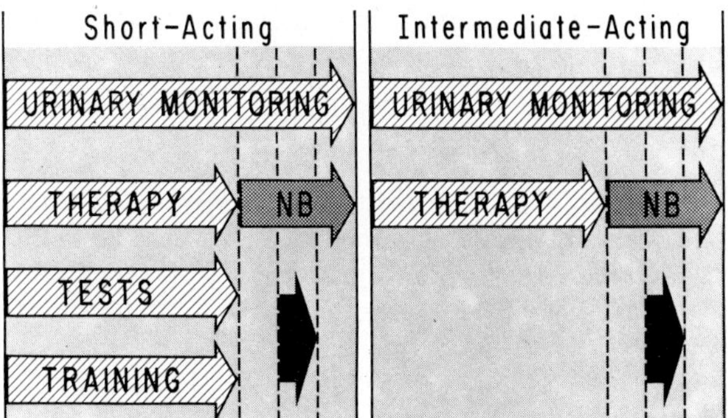

FIG. 2. Diagram of experimental design to clarify time relationships of measurements and activities during 2 insulin regimens. Symbols: NB = nitrogen balance; solid black arrow = continuous blood glucose monitoring. For details, see Tables 1 and 2 as well as text.

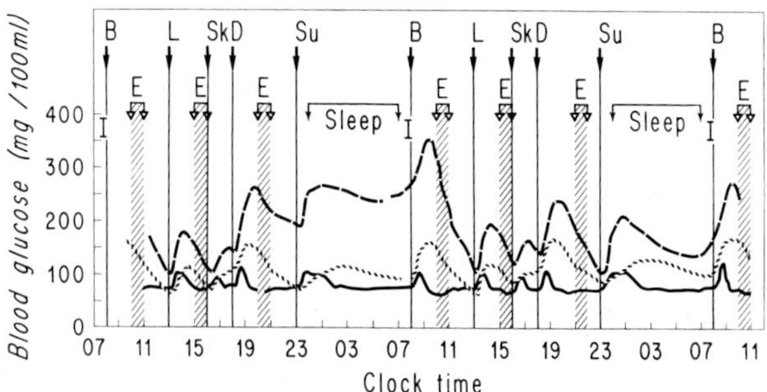

FIG. 3. Averaged BG patterns of 3 unstable (D2, 4, 8; interrupted line), 3 stable diabetics (D9, 10, 11; dotted line), and 3 normal subjects (N1, 2, 3; solid line) studied under matching conditions. Time scale is in 24-hour clock time. Symbols: B = breakfast; L = lunch; Sk = snack; D = dinner; Su = supper; E = walking exercise; I = insulin injection (in diabetics). Vertical lines indicate start of meals; shaded areas indicate exercise periods.

The vertical lines in Figure 3 indicate the start of meals. The major blood glucose increases occurred only after meals. The minor blood glucose increases before breakfast in unstable diabetics have been shown to be associated with a decrease in plasma immunoreactive insulin (Molnar et al., 1972b). The vertical shaded areas in Figure 3 indicate the exercise periods. Blood glucose decreases accelerated in diabetics during the periods of exercise.

Our results bear out the findings of Klachko et al. (1972) who, in their continuous blood glucose studies, have best defined the effect of exercise on blood glucose changes. They found that both the blood glucose concentration at the time the exercise is started and the intensity of exercise affect the magnitude of blood glucose decreases. Because unstable diabetics are often hyperglycemic, it is no wonder that they have extensive blood glucose decreases during intensive and prolonged exercise.

In contrast to the meals, exercise, and insulin therapy in Figure 3, Figure 4 shows a 4-hour study without food, exercise, or insulin administration. Diabetics had had no long-acting insulin preparations for at least 48 hours prior to this study. The last dose of short-acting insulin was given 9 hours prior to this test. This study examined the conditions under which all of the resting-fasting tests were done. Under these conditions, as Möllerström (1943) had observed more than 3 decades ago, unstable diabetics have a gradual blood glucose increase. Some stable diabetics may have a blood glucose decrease. Normal subjects tend to maintain their blood glucose level. Contrary to the widespread notion that unstable diabetics have extensive glucose fluctuations without known cause, we did not see major glucose fluctuations during these tests. Unidirectional changes did occur, but large, sequentially bidirectional fluctuations did not. Similarly, during the ambulatory-fed studies we have not seen major blood glucose fluctuations unless related to food intake, exercise, or insulin therapy (Molnar et al., 1968, 1972b).

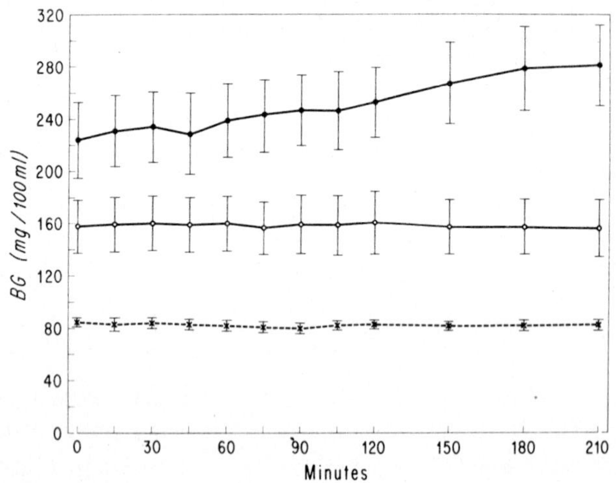

FIG. 4. Blood glucose patterns during infusion of 0.45% saline in 9 unstable diabetics (solid circles), 10 stable diabetics (open circles), and 8 normal subjects (x). Values shown are means ± 1 S.E.M.

To summarize quantitative aspects of ambulatory-fed studies, Figure 5 shows more averaged blood glucose results in 3 normal subjects, 3 stable diabetics, and 6 unstable diabetics on both the short-acting and the intermediate-acting insulin regimen. The 48-hour mean blood glucose concentration was determined by averaging 576 values at 5-minute intervals, from the continuous record. A line transecting each panel shows the mean blood glucose value for the group. The 48-hour mean amplitude of glycemic excursions (MAGE) for each group of subjects is shown bracketed between interrupted lines. This is a measure of the within-day glucose variability (Service et al., 1970). The mean of (each group of subjects') daily differences (MODD) of paired blood glucose values on successive days is shown as the shaded area. This absolute difference between 2 successive days' glucose curves is a measure of the day-to-day glucose variability (Molnar et al., 1972a).

With short-acting insulin therapy, the mean glucose level of unstable diabetics was significantly decreased (Service et al., 1970). However, neither the mean amplitude of

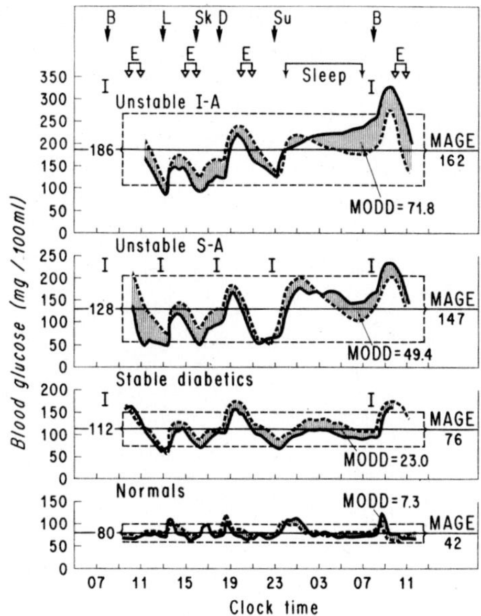

FIG. 5. Averaged blood glucose curves of 3 normal subjects, 3 stable diabetics, and 6 unstable diabetics. The unstable diabetics are shown during therapy with short-acting insulin injections (S-A) 4 times daily as well as with intermediate-acting insulin (I-A) once (or twice) daily. First 24 hours (solid line) and second 24 hours (interrupted line) are superimposed. The absolute difference between the first and second 24 hours is the mean of daily differences of paired blood glucose values (MODD: hatched area). The mean amplitude of glycemic excursions (MAGE) averaged for each group is shown bracketing the averaged mean blood glucose. The average of the individual 48-hour mean blood glucose values (MBG) is indicated by the line transecting each panel and by the value at the left. The values shown for MAGE and MODD are also averages of the individual 48-hour values.

glycemic excursions nor the mean of daily glucose differences was significantly decreased (Service et al., 1970; Molnar et al., 1972a). Intensified therapy with short-acting insulin merely transposed the essentially same glucose pattern downward.

Figure 5 contains answers to some of the questions we had posed. It was possible to identify and quantify the blood glucose stability or instability consistently (Service et al., 1970; Molnar et al., 1972a). It was not possible to make the blood glucose patterns of unstable diabetics conform to those of stable diabetics. Neither was it possible to conform the blood glucose patterns of stable diabetics to those of normal subjects.

In searching for causes of diabetic instability, it seemed reasonable to postulate that growth hormone might have a pathogenetic role (Molnar et al., 1968). Growth hormone levels increase during hypoglycemia and exercise, especially in lean persons (Glick et al., 1965). Unstable diabetics have hypoglycemic episodes, they are sensitive to the effects of muscular exercise, and they tend to be lean.

The experimental findings are illustrated in Figure 6 by the superimposed hourly growth hormone and continuous blood glucose patterns of 3 men: a normal, a stable diabetic, and an unstable diabetic. The higher growth hormone increases in the unstable diabetic are striking. On analyzing our data we found that hypoglycemic episodes, exercise, and sleep all contributed to the higher growth hormone levels in unstable diabetics (Molnar et al., 1968, 1972c). Yet none of these events accounted for the observed differences, in that unstable diabetics have higher mean hourly and higher peak growth hormone levels. We did not see a significant change in growth hormone levels in unstable diabetics during intensified therapy with 4 daily injections of short-acting insulin (Molnar et al., 1972c).

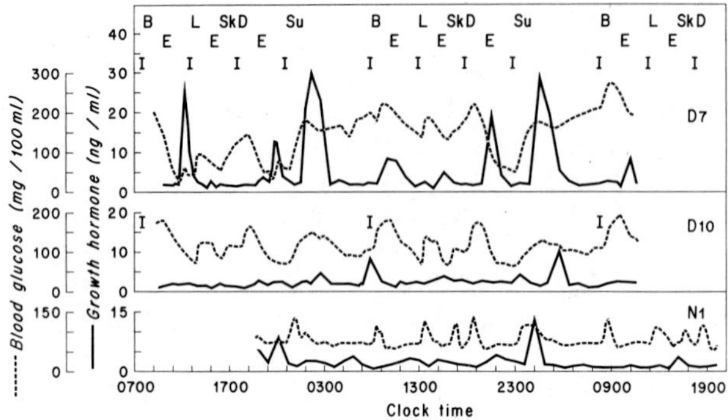

FIG. 6. Growth hormone (solid line) and blood glucose (broken line) values during 48 hours in 3 men. N1 = normal; D10 = stable diabetic; D7 = unstable diabetic (From Molnar et al., 1972c, by permission of J. B. Lippincott Co.).

Johansen and Hansen (1971) have confirmed our observations concerning diurnal growth hormone levels. Moreover, in one of his groups of juvenile diabetics, Hansen (1971) was able to achieve greater relative normalization of blood glucose patterns than we did. His success may have been due to the fact that his subjects were recently discovered diabetics. Intensive antidiabetic treatment during spontaneous partial remission may explain his excellent blood glucose results. What is even more interesting is that, with improved blood glucose levels in this one group of diabetics, the growth hormone hyperresponse to exercise was also improved.

The hyperresponse of growth hormone to exercise was also Hansen's (1970) observation. He found that diabetic young men have a lower exercise threshold for growth hormone increase than do non-diabetic young men. During exercise of sufficiently low intensity so that normals (non-diabetics) have no growth hormone increases, unstable diabetics consistently have growth hormone increases.

In contrast to the apparently consistent effect of exercise, growth hormone increases do not always occur during hypoglycemic episodes. Among 46 inadvertent hypoglycemic episodes which we completely documented in our ambulatory-fed studies in unstable diabetics, no growth hormone increases occurred in 12 episodes (Molnar et al., 1971). The rate of blood glucose decrease and the concentration at the nadir were similar whether or not growth hormone increase occurred. Moreover, 17 of the 46 episodes were asymptomatic. The occurrence of growth hormone increases was most consistently related to the symptomatic stress of hypoglycemia (Molnar et al., 1971). Growth hormone increases were lower in hypoglycemic unstable diabetics when they were ambulatory and fed than when they were resting and fasting (Fatourechi et al., 1969; Molnar et al., 1971).

Whether or not growth hormone increase occurred during hypoglycemic episodes, there was no apparent effect on subsequent blood glucose changes and levels (Molnar et al., 1971). Similarly, we could not detect any difference in urinary ketone body levels whether or not the hypoglycemia was associated with growth hormone increase (Molnar et al., 1971).

With the role of growth hormone in the pathogenesis of unstable diabetes remaining equivocal, we examined whether insulin patterns in plasma could account for the abnormal blood glucose patterns of unstable diabetes.

Because therapy with insulin generates endogenous antibodies (Berson et al., 1956), immunoreactive insulin measurements had not previously been examined systematically in chronically insulin-treated subjects. We determined the validity of radioimmunoprecipitation assays in plasma containing antibodies to beef and pork insulin (Cremer et al., 1971; Moxness et al., 1971; Molnar et al., 1974). During our studies (Moxness et al., 1971; Molnar et al., 1974) we found the following:

1. Precision was only moderately impaired with low degrees of insulin binding by antibodies.

2. The species specificity of our antisera discriminated only bovine insulin among bovine, porcine, and human insulins.

3. The effect of endogenous antibodies was an exaggeration of immunoreactive insulin concentrations. This occurred in proportion to the antibody's ability to bind tracer amounts of radioactive insulin. Recovery of insulin was excessive only with higher degrees of insulin binding. But even then it was linearly related to the actual insulin measurements.

4. During in vivo tests, other variables (glucose, free fatty acids, ketone bodies) measured simultaneously showed the expected biologic effects of insulin consistent with the measured changes in immunoreactive insulin concentrations (Cremer et al., 1971; Molnar et al., 1974; Yipintsoi et al., 1973).

5. The disappearance of intravenously injected insulin was delayed in proportion to the degree of insulin binding by antibodies (Palumbo et al., 1972).

6. Insulinogenic reserve (tested with the stimuli listed in Table 2) was absent in unstable diabetics. It was preserved in stable diabetics but decreased in comparison with normals (Cremer et al., 1971; Molnar et al., 1974).

7. Differences in insulin-glucose relationships between normals, stable diabetics, and unstable diabetics during acute tests could be ascribed in our model studies primarily to differences in ability to secrete insulin (Gatewood et al., 1970; Yipintsoi et al., 1973).

Figure 7 compares averaged 48-hour immunoreactive insulin and blood glucose curves of 3 normals, 3 stable diabetics, and 3 unstable diabetics (on the 2 regimens of insulin therapy). From below upward the curves are less regular and more variable and there is progressively less of the normal synchrony between insulin and glucose maxima and minima.

Simultaneously measured immunoreactive insulin and blood glucose levels in normals showed a positive trend: higher insulin and glucose concentrations coincided. In unstable diabetics, the insulin-glucose relationship showed a negative trend: higher insulin and lower glucose concentrations coincided. Stable diabetics had an intermediate trend (Molnar et al., 1972b). With short-acting insulin treatment of unstable diabetics, the insulin-glucose relationship was always less negative than with intermediate-acting insulin (Molnar et al., 1972b). This less negative relationship may account, in part, for the

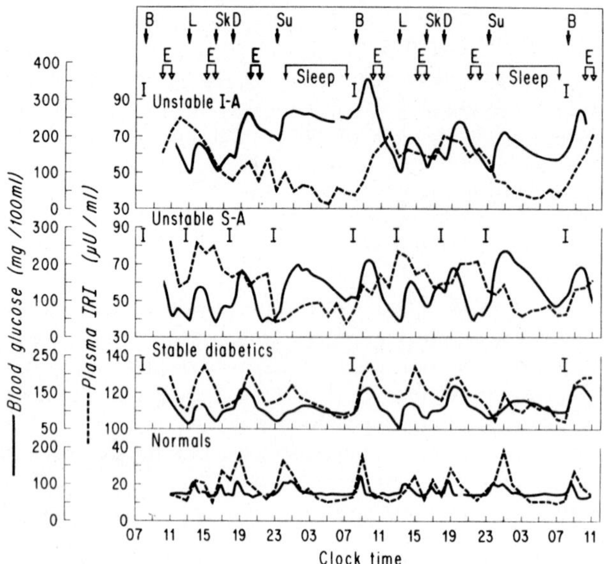

FIG. 7. Averaged simultaneous continuous blood glucose (solid line) and hourly immunoreactive insulin (IRI) (interrupted lines) patterns in 3 normal subjects, 3 stable diabetics, and 3 unstable diabetics. Both short-acting (S-A) and intermediate-acting (I-A) insulin regimens are shown for the unstable diabetics.

improved but still unphysiologic blood glucose patterns of unstable diabetics on 4 daily injections of short-acting insulin (Service et al., 1970; Molnar et al., 1972a, b).

We noted several associations between insulin and glucose changes (Molnar et al., 1972b). The wider the amplitude of glycemic excursions, the lower was the frequency of insulin increases and the greater was the delay in attaining insulin maxima and minima. In unstable diabetics, both the diminished frequency of insulin increases and the delayed attainment of insulin maxima and minima may have contributed to the amplitude of glycemic excursions being wider. This is also in accord with predictions based on our model studies (Gatewood et al., 1970; Yipintsoi et al., 1973).

The greater the day-to-day glucose variability, the greater also was the day-to-day insulin variability (Molnar et al , 1972b). In unstable diabetics, greater day-to-day insulin variability may have contributed to the greater day-to-day glucose variability.

We interpret the immunoreactive insulin findings as follows. Rapid and adequate plasma immunoreactive insulin increases and decreases, well synchronized with blood glucose increases and decreases, characterize normal persons. Delayed and inadequate immunoreactive insulin changes relative to glucose changes characterize the results of insulin therapy in unstable diabetics. These inadequacies in unstable diabetics reflect the shortcomings of therapy with exogenous insulin (Molnar et al., 1972b).

In stable diabetics, the findings of Rubenstein's group (Block et al., 1972a, b) support our impression that continuing secretion of endogenous insulin permits the degree of stability noted in these patients (Molnar et al., 1972b). Even during therapy with exogenous insulin, stable diabetics apparently release endogenous insulin early after glucose administration (Block et al., 1972a, b) or meals (Molnar et al., 1972b). Their blood glucose increases are therefore moderate. Late after glucose or meals, with the stimuli to insulin release abated, endogenous insulin release diminishes. Insulin therapy acts therefore as a supplement, compensating for a partial deficiency. Autoregulation of insulin secretion persists and, with judicious therapy, both insulin deficiencies and excesses are easily avoided. This hypothesis explains why consistently good therapeutic results may easily be achieved in stable diabetics.

Endogenous antibodies to insulin contribute to the delays with which the immunoreactive insulin maxima and minima are reached (Molnar et al., 1972b). Therefore, antibodies impede synchronization of immunoreactive insulin and blood glucose changes. This affects stable and unstable diabetics alike. Palumbo et al. (1969) found that the degree of insulin binding by endogenous antibodies in vitro was similar in stable and unstable diabetics. More recent findings (Palumbo et al., 1972) in vivo, concerning the delaying effects of antibodies on the intravascular persistence of injected insulin, confirm this lack of difference between stable and unstable diabetics.

Dixon et al. (1972) have recently suggested, however, that stable diabetics may possess greater buffering capacity through their endogenous insulin antibodies. They demonstrated in a few patients that, for a given total increment of injected insulin, a smaller free insulin increment resulted in stable than in unstable diabetics. If this is confirmed, the behavior of insulin antibodies could account in part for the varying degrees of instability which unstable diabetic patients display despite their similar lack of insulinogenic reserve.

Turning to the possible role of glucagon, Unger et al. (1970, 1971) have demonstrated that patients with apparently total beta cell failure continue to secrete pancreatic glucagon. We are in the process of confirming their observations in patients whose insulinogenic reserve has been tested (Reynolds et al., 1973). Just as with growth hormone, hyperglycemia poorly suppresses glucagon in diabetics. However, both stable and unstable diabetics have hyperglucagonemia relative to their hyperglycemia (Reynolds et al., 1973). The first direct relevance of alpha cell dysfunction to diabetic instability is the failure of plasma glucagon levels to increase during insulin-induced hypoglycemia in unstable diabetics, in contrast to stable diabetics and normals (Reynolds et al., 1973).

The essence of our concept of unstable diabetes may now be outlined as group differences among unstable and stable diabetics and normal (non-diabetic) subjects.

Under ambulatory-fed conditions only the within-day (MAGE) and between-day (MODD) blood glucose variability measurements differentiate all 3 groups of subjects. Unstable diabetics also differ from stable diabetics and normals by having higher diurnal plasma growth hormone levels and higher and more variable urinary glucose excretion. Although withdrawal from insulin therapy provokes greater fasting ketogenesis (Cremer et al., 1971) and negative nitrogen balance (Izzo et al., 1955) in unstable diabetics, nitrogen balance and urinary ketone body excretion are not significantly different in the 3 groups during intensive therapy of fed diabetics (Thomas et al., 1974).

Under resting-fasting conditions, only the ability to release endogenous insulin differentiates among all 3 groups of subjects. In addition, the unstable diabetics differ from the stable diabetics and normals during withdrawal from insulin by having greater increases in blood glucose and serum ketone body concentrations (Cremer et al., 1971). Unstable diabetics also show greater lability of their growth hormone release mechanism, both at rest (Cremer et al., 1974) and during exercise (Hansen, 1970). In all diabetics, hyperglycemia fails to inhibit growth hormone (Fatourechi et al., 1969; Molnar et al. 1971, 1972c; Cremer et al., 1974) and glucagon release (Unger et al., 1970, 1971;

Reynolds et al., 1973). Other tests we have used* failed to distinguish any of the groups (Gatewood et al., 1970; Yipintsoi et al., 1973; Cremer et al., 1974).

No discussion of the nature of unstable diabetes is complete without mention of the Somogyi phenomenon (Somogyi, 1959; Mintz et al., 1968; Bloom et al., 1969) and the role of the emotions. The design of our studies precluded decisive studies and critical analyses of the Somogyi phenomenon and of emotional effects on blood glucose patterns. This occurred because our subjects were cooperative, trained, research volunteers who lived by the clock on regimens of rhythmic feedings and controlled activities. By design, we avoided overinsulinization and promptly treated inadvertent hypoglycemic episodes when recognized. Mirouze et al. (1972), using a looser experimental design, found examples of Somogyi phenomena during continuous blood glucose monitoring.

We therefore cannot confirm or deny that posthypoglycemic hyperglycemia occurs. With sufficiently deep and prolonged hypoglycemia, counter-regulatory surges of insulin-antagonistic hormones occur (Somogyi, 1959; Mintz et al., 1968). Among these, the catecholamines antagonize and glucagon enhances endogenous insulin release. Catecholamines, corticosteroids, and growth hormone all impair responsiveness to endogenous or exogenous insulin. In combination with glycogenolytic and gluconeogenetic and other effects of the counter-regulatory hormones, impaired availability or effectiveness of insulin may increase circulating glucose and ketone body concentrations.

By overinsulinization, stable diabetics could be made unstable through insulin-induced hypoglycemic episodes (Somogyi, 1959). By suppression of their endogenous insulin-releasing capabilities, stable diabetics could be made to lose their best defense against excessive blood glucose fluctuations. But our data do not support the hypothesis that totally insulin-deficient, inherently unstable diabetics, can be conformed to the blood glucose patterns of stable diabetics merely by avoiding hypoglycemic episodes or by less intensive therapy.

It is worth emphasizing that both hypoglycemia and emotional states may alter eating and exercise habits and schedules and may exert some of their effects through altering the rhythmic patterns of behavior in diabetics. Such alterations of pattern are deleterious to good therapeutic results.

The 2 known principal abnormalities of unstable diabetics are the reasons for their need for careful regulation of the timing and supply of insulin, food, and exercise. These abnormalities are lack of endogenous insulin (Cremer et al., 1971) and inability to regulate the supply of insulin to tissues (Molnar et al., 1972b). Probably some other abnormalities of unstable diabetics (relative to ketosis proneness and to having high diurnal growth hormone levels) are caused by unphysiologic therapy consequent to the lack of insulin autoregulation (Molnar et al., 1972b).

Additional causes of unstable blood glucose regulation are likely to be discovered, possibly through studies of the gut hormones and of insulin-receptor interactions to explain the gaps in our present knowledge. It seems likely, even with our present concepts (Ackerman et al., 1968), that a continuous spectrum of blood glucose regulatory stability exists from the normal through the stable to the brittle diabetics.

* Tests of growth hormone release with insulin, arginine, glucagon, epinephrine, and tolbutamide intravenously and glucose orally.

SUMMARY

Varying degrees of blood glucose stability can best be identified and measured by continuous blood glucose monitoring under standardized ambulatory-fed conditions. Excessive within-day and between-day blood glucose variability, high diurnal growth hormone levels, and negative correlation of immunoreactive insulin with blood glucose levels characterize unstable diabetes under ambulatory-fed conditions. In the resting-fasting state, inability to release endogenous insulin and higher growth hormone, blood glucose, and ketone body increases on insulin withdrawal characterize unstable diabetes. Unstable diabetics also have a low threshold for growth hormone release during exercise.

The ability to release endogenous insulin is probably essential to stable blood glucose regulation. The difference between supplementing or totally supplying an individual's needs with exogenous insulin may account for most of the ease or difficulty of treating diabetes mellitus.

REFERENCES

ACKERMAN, E., GATEWOOD, L. C., MOLNAR, G. D., ROSEVEAR, J. W. and SERVICE, F. J. (1968): Quantitative measures of instability of blood glucose regulation (abstract). *Federation Proceedings; Federation of American Societies for Experimental Biology, 27,* 565.

BERSON, S. A., YALOW, R. S., BAUMAN, A., ROTHSCHILD, A. and NEWERLY, K. (1956): Insulin-I^{131} metabolism in human subjects: demonstration of insulin binding globulin in the circulation of insulin treated subjects. *J. clin. Invest., 35,* 170.

BLOCK, M. B., MAKO, M. E., STEINER, D. F. and RUBENSTEIN, A. H. (1972a): Circulating C-peptide immunoreactivity: studies in normals and diabetic patients. *Diabetes, 21,* 1013.

BLOCK, M. B., MAKO, M. E., STEINER, D. F. and RUBENSTEIN, A. H. (1972b): Diabetic ketoacidosis: evidence for C-peptide and proinsulin secretion following recovery. *J. clin. Endocr., 35,* 402.

BLOOM, M. E., MINTZ, D. H. and FIELD, J. B. (1969): Insulin-induced posthypoglycemic hyperglycemia as a cause of 'brittle' diabetes: clinical clues and therapeutic implications. *Amer. J. Med., 47,* 891.

COLWELL, A. R. (1953): Treatment of diabetes: selection of technic according to severity. *Diabetes, 2,* 262.

CREMER, G. M., MOLNAR, G. D., TAYLOR, W. F., MOXNESS, K. E., SERVICE, F. J., GATEWOOD, L. C., ACKERMAN, E. and ROSEVEAR, J. W. (1971): Studies of diabetic instability. II. Tests of insulinogenic reserve with infusions of arginine, glucagon, epinephrine, and saline. *Metabolism, 20,* 1083.

CREMER, G. M., MOLNAR, G. D., TAYLOR, W. F., ROSEVEAR, J. W. and ACKERMAN, E. (1974): Growth hormone release in unstable diabetes: tests with saline, arginine, glucagon, and epinephrine. *Acta diabet. lat.,* in press.

DIXON, K., EXON, P. D. and HUGHES, H. R. (1972): Insulin antibodies in aetiology of labile diabetes. *Lancet, 1,* 343.

FATOURECHI, V., MOLNAR, G. D., SERVICE, F. J., ACKERMAN, E., ROSEVEAR, J. W., MOXNESS, K. E. and TAYLOR, W. F. (1969): Growth hormone and glucose interrelationships in diabetes: studies with insulin infusion during continuous blood glucose analysis. *J. clin. Endocr., 29,* 319.

GATEWOOD, L. C., ACKERMAN, E., ROSEVEAR, J. W. and MOLNAR, G. D. (1970): Modeling blood glucose dynamics. *Behav. Sci., 15,* 72.

GLICK, S. M., ROTH, J., YALOW, R. S. and BERSON, S. A. (1965): The regulation of growth hormone secretion. *Rec. Progr. Hormone Res., 21,* 241.

HANSEN, A. P. (1970): Abnormal serum growth hormone response to exercise in juvenile diabetics. *J. clin. Invest., 49,* 1467.

HANSEN, A. P. (1971): Normalization of growth hormone hyperresponse to exercise in juvenile diabetics after 'normalization' of blood sugar. *J. clin. Invest., 50,* 1806.

IZZO, J. L. and CRUMP, S. L. (1950): A clinical comparison of modified insulins. *J. clin. Invest., 29,* 1514.

IZZO, J. L., HOFFMASTER, J. and SUSKIE, A. G. (1955): The interrelationships of exogenous insulin and the metabolism of carbohydrate and protein: studies in cases of stable and unstable diabetes mellitus. *Diabetes, 4,* 113.

JOHANSEN, K. and HANSEN, A. P. (1971): Diurnal serum growth hormone levels in poorly and well-controlled juvenile diabetics. *Diabetes, 20,* 239.

KLACHKO, D. M., LIE, T. H., CUNNINGHAM, E. J., CHASE, G. R. and BURNS, T. W. (1972): Blood glucose levels during walking in normal and diabetic subjects. *Diabetes, 21,* 89.

MINTZ, D. H., FINSTER, J. L., TAYLOR, A. L. and FEFAR, A. (1968): Hormonal genesis of glucose intolerance following hypoglycemia. *Amer. J. Med., 45,* 187.

MIROUZE, J., COLLARD, F. and TEISSIERE, J. P. (1972): Intérêt de l'enregistrement glycémique continu dans l'analyse du diabète sucré insuliné. In: *Journées Annuelles de Diabetologie de l'Hôtel-Dieu,* pp. 285–301. Flammarion, Paris.

MIROUZE, J., JAFFIOL, C. and SANY, C. (1962): Enregistrement glycémique nycthéméral continu dans le diabète instable. *Rev. franç. Endocr., 3,* 337.

MÖLLERSTRÖM, J. (1943): Das Diabetesproblem: die rhythmischen Stoffwechselvorgänge. *Acta med. scand., Suppl. 147,* 1.

MOLNAR, G. D. (1964): Observations on the etiology and therapy of 'brittle' diabetes. *Canad. med. Ass. J., 90,* 953.

MOLNAR, G. D., ACKERMAN, E., ROSEVEAR, J. W., GATEWOOD, L. C. and MOXNESS, K. E. (1968): Continuous blood glucose analysis in ambulatory fed subjects. I. General methodology. *Mayo Clin. Proc., 43,* 833.

MOLNAR, G. D., CREMER, G. M., MOXNESS, K. E., SERVICE, F. J., ROSEVEAR, J. W. and ACKERMAN, E. (1974): Insulinogenic reserve in diabetics and normal subjects. In: *Endocrines and Enzymes in Anesthesiology.* Editors: C. M. Ballinger and V. Brechner. Charles C. Thomas, Springfield, Ill., in press.

MOLNAR, G. D., FATOURECHI, V., ACKERMAN, E., TAYLOR, W. F., ROSEVEAR, J. W., GATEWOOD, L. C., SERVICE, F. J. and MOXNESS, K. E. (1971): Growth hormone and glucose interrelationships in diabetes: studies of inadvertent hypoglycemic episodes during continuous blood glucose analysis. *J. clin. Endocr., 32,* 426.

MOLNAR, G. D., GASTINEAU, C. F., ROSEVEAR, J. W. and MOXNESS, K. E. (1965): Quantitative aspects of labile diabetes. *Diabetes, 14,* 279.

MOLNAR, G. D., TAYLOR, W. F. and HO, M. M. (1972a): Day-to-day variation of continuously monitored glycaemia: a further measure of diabetic instability. *Diabetologia, 8,* 342.

MOLNAR, G. D., TAYLOR, W. F. and LANGWORTHY, A. L. (1972b): Plasma immunoreactive insulin patterns in insulin-treated diabetics: studies during continuous blood glucose monitoring. *Mayo Clin. Proc., 47,* 709.

MOLNAR, G. D., TAYLOR, W. F., LANGWORTHY, A. and FATOURECHI, V. (1972c): Diurnal growth hormone and glucose abnormalities in unstable diabetics: studies of ambulatory-fed subjects during continuous blood glucose analysis. *J. clin. Endocr., 34,* 837.

MOXNESS, K. E., MOLNAR, G. D., TAYLOR, W. F., OWEN Jr., C. A., ACKERMAN, E. and ROSEVEAR, J. W. (1971): Studies of diabetic instability. I. Immunoassay of human insulin in plasma containing antibodies to pork and beef insulin. *Metabolism, 20,* 1074.

PALUMBO, P. J., MOLNAR, G. D., TAYLOR, W. F., MOXNESS, K. E. and TAUXE,

W. N. (1969): Insulin antibody binding in diabetes mellitus and factitious hypoglycemia. *Mayo Clin. Proc., 44,* 725.

PALUMBO, P. J., TAYLOR, W. F., MOLNAR, G. D. and TAUXE, W. N. (1972): Disappearance of bovine insulin from plasma in diabetic and normal subjects. *Metabolism, 21,* 787.

REYNOLDS, C., MOLNAR, G. D., JIANG, N.-S., JONES, J. D. and TAYLOR, W. F. (1973): Abnormal glucagon response to hypoglycemia in unstable diabetics (abstract). *Diabetes, 22/Suppl. 1,* 327.

ROSEVEAR, J. W., PFAFF, K. J., SERVICE, F. J., MOLNAR, G. D. and ACKERMAN, E. (1969): Glucose oxidase method for continuous automated blood glucose determination. *Clin. Chem., 15,* 680.

SCHLICHTKRULL, J., MUNCK, O. and JERSILD, M. (1965): The M-value, an index of blood sugar control in diabetics. *Acta med. scand., 177,* 95.

SERVICE, F. J., MOLNAR, G. D., ROSEVEAR, J. W., ACKERMAN, E., TAYLOR, W. F., CREMER, G. M. and MOXNESS, K. E. (1969): Continuous blood glucose analysis in ambulatory fed subjects. II. Effects of anticoagulation with heparin. *Mayo Clin. Proc., 44,* 466.

SERVICE, F. J., MOLNAR, G. D., ROSEVEAR, J. W., ACKERMAN, E., GATEWOOD, L. C. and TAYLOR, W. F. (1970): Mean amplitude of glycemic excursions, a measure of diabetic instability. *Diabetes, 19,* 644.

SOMOGYI, M. (1959): Exacerbation of diabetes by excess insulin action. *Amer. J. Med., 26,* 169.

THOMAS, S. K., TAYLOR, W. F. and MOLNAR, G. D. (1974): Continuous blood glucose analysis in ambulatory fed subjects. III. Nitrogen balance and urinary ketone bodies related to other measurements in the characterization of unstable diabetes. *Mayo Clin. Proc., 49,* 28.

UNGER, R. H. (1971): Seminars in medicine of the Beth Israel Hospital, Boston: glucagon physiology and pathophysiology. *New Engl. J. Med., 285,* 443.

UNGER, R. H., AGUILAR-PARADA, E., MÜLLER, W. A. and EISENTRAUT, A. M. (1970): Studies of pancreatic alpha cell function in normal and diabetic subjects. *J. clin. Invest., 49,* 837.

WELLER, C., LINDER, M., MACAULAY, A., FERRARI, A. and KESSLER, G. (1960): Continuous in vivo determination of blood glucose in human subjects. *Ann. N.Y. Acad. Sci., 87,* 658.

YIPINTSOI, T., GATEWOOD, L. C., ACKERMAN, E., SPIVAK, P. L., MOLNAR, G. D., ROSEVEAR, J. W. and SERVICE, F. J. (1973): Mathematical analysis of blood glucose and plasma insulin responses to insulin infusion in healthy and diabetic subjects. *Computers in Biology and Medicine, 3,* 71.

SHORT- AND LONG-TERM EFFECTS OF ORAL HYPOGLYCEMIC AGENTS

SULFONYLUREAS: NEWER ASPECTS OF PHARMACOLOGY AND CLINICAL EFFICACY*

ERNST F. PFEIFFER

Department of Endocrinology and Metabolism, Center of Internal Medicine and Pediatrics, University of Ulm, Federal Republic of Germany

The area of the new sulfonylureas of the ‘second generation’, as we called it elsewhere (Pfeiffer, 1971; Raptis and Pfeiffer, 1971) has been opened by the extremely potent hypoglycemic agent glibenclamide (Schwarz et al., 1968) (Fig. 1). Extended substitution

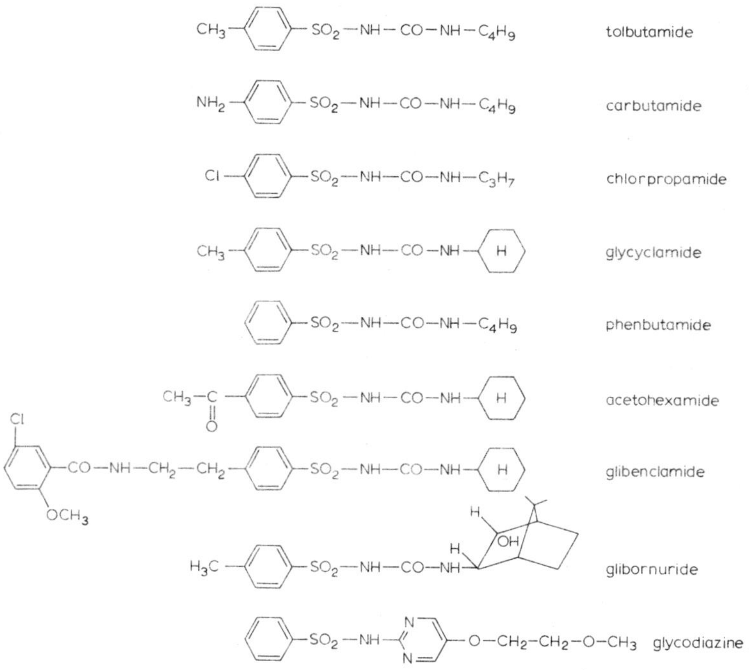

CH_3–⟨⟩–SO_2–NH–CO–NH–C_4H_9 tolbutamide

NH_2–⟨⟩–SO_2–NH–CO–NH–C_4H_9 carbutamide

Cl–⟨⟩–SO_2–NH–CO–NH–C_3H_7 chlorpropamide

CH_3–⟨⟩–SO_2–NH–CO–NH–⟨H⟩ glycyclamide

⟨⟩–SO_2–NH–CO–NH–C_4H_9 phenbutamide

CH_3–C(=O)–⟨⟩–SO_2–NH–CO–NH–⟨H⟩ acetohexamide

Cl, OCH_3 ⟨⟩–CO–NH–CH_2–CH_2–⟨⟩–SO_2–NH–CO–NH–⟨H⟩ glibenclamide

H_3C–⟨⟩–SO_2–NH–CO–NH– (H, H, OH) glibornuride

⟨⟩–SO_2–NH–(N, N)–O–CH_2–CH_2–O–CH_3 glycodiazine

FIG. 1. Chemical configuration of various sulfonylureas of the first and second generation.

* Supported by grants from the Deutsche Forschungsgemeinschaft, Bad Godesberg.

of the radical on the left side of the benzene ring of the sulfonylurea nucleus distinguishes that compound from its precursors.

Five lines of evidence have accumulated to suggest a new and, at least partially, different mechanism of action:

1. In the isolated perfused rat pancreas in vitro, in the presence of high, i.e. 200 mg%, glucose, tolbutamide – after effecting its rapidly appearing peak of insulin secretion in the interval between the 2 glucose-induced phases of insulin release – blocks any further enhancement of insulin release, both while it is infused and after its withdrawal (Fig. 2). Glibenclamide, on the other hand, is acting synergistically with the glucose-effected stimulation of insulin release, both during and after withdrawal of the perfusion (Fussgänger et al., 1969).

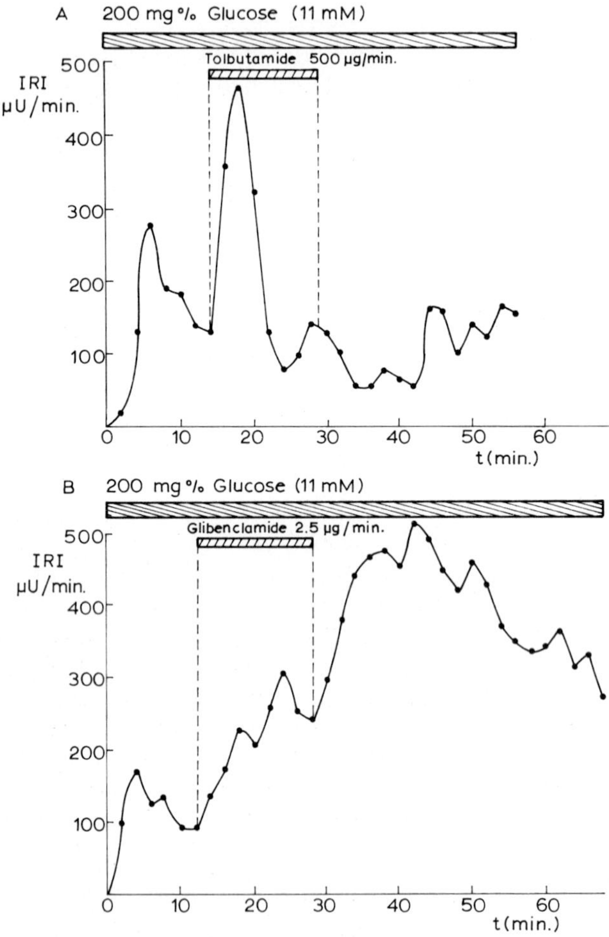

FIG. 2. Dynamics of insulin secretion of the perfused rat pancreas in response to 200 mg% glucose and tolbutamide and glibenclamide, respectively (From Fussgänger et al., 1969, by courtesy).

2. In the healthy human subject the rapid release of insulin exerted by i.v. tolbutamide is contrasted by a much slower and lower increment of longer duration following i.v. glibenclamide, resulting in a more pronounced blood sugar decrease. According to the kinetics of the insulin responses, all further sulfonylurea preparations might be profitably classified as belonging either to the tolbutamide- or to the glibenclamide-type (Fig. 3) (Raptis et al., 1971).

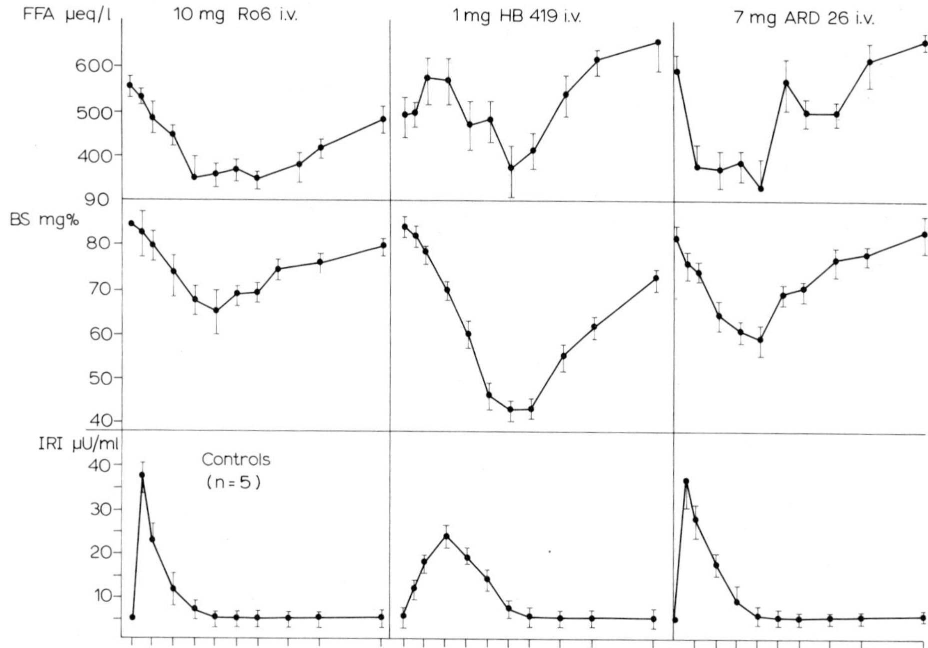

FIG. 3. Tolbutamide- and glibenclamide-type of insulin secretion in response to various sulfonylurea preparations in man. BS = blood sugar.

3. Addition of a phosphodiesterase inhibitor to i.v. tolbutamide changes neither the insulin nor the blood glucose response; considerably higher and steeper insulin rises, however, follow the combined glibenclamide-inhibitor action (Raptis et al., 1973).

4. (*a*) Similar and even more pronounced variations in the character of the insulin curve following glibenclamide occur in human subjects when glucose is injected concomitantly, whereas the tolbutamide-induced insulin releases are not influenced in the same way (Fig. 4). A supra-additive if not potentiating action might be ascribed either to glucose in the presence of glibenclamide or to the sulfonylurea compound, adding its effect to the glucose action (Raptis et al., 1969). (*b*) Clinically, this specific capacity of glibenclamide might become decisive. In secondary failures of tolbutamide therapy the addition of glucose changes neither the insulin nor the blood sugar responses to tolbutamide; however, the combined glibenclamide-glucose injection is followed by a marked rise in insulin and a normalization of the key value of glucose assimilation (Fig. 5). In the more severe maturity-onset diabetics, and also in some early juvenile-onset diabetics, glibenclamide is not exceeded in efficacy by any of the newer sulfonylurea preparations.

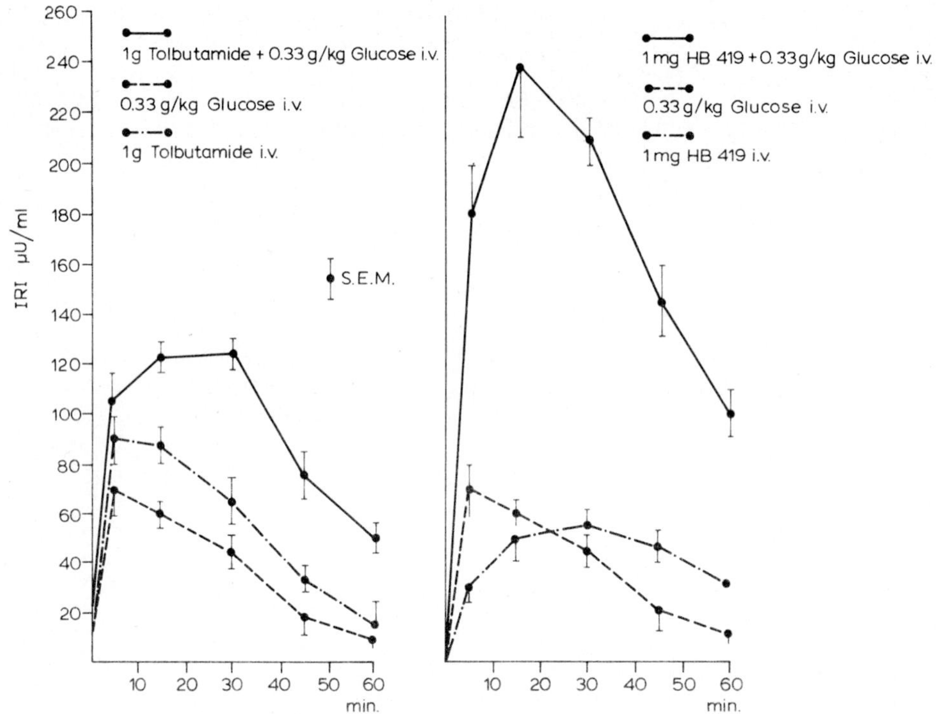

FIG. 4. Potentiation of glucose-induced insulin secretion by concomitant glibenclamide injection or simple addition of actions by combined glucose-tolbutamide action. N = 15 normal subjects. (From Raptis et al., 1969, by courtesy).

5. As described before (Pfeiffer et al., 1960, 1961; Pfeiffer, 1967), in severe maturity-onset diabetics repeated application of tolbutamide 4 hours after the first injection is not followed by a new rise in serum insulin and a new fall in blood sugar. Glibenclamide, on the other hand, is acting again already after that interval (Raptis et al., 1969), suggesting the administration of the drug in 2 doses per day is feasible, if necessary.

The potentiating action of glibenclamide on the defective glucose and also tolbutamide-mediated insulin secretion is utilized profitably for predicting the outcome of long-term sulfonylurea therapy (Pfeiffer and Raptis, 1972). In 11 out of 40 maturity-onset diabetics, insulin-dependent up to more than 100 U of a long-acting insulin daily, a mean increase of insulin of more than 500% above the initial value was associated with successful long-term treatment with glibenclamide. Smaller increases recorded in the other 29 cases were correlated with failures (Fig. 6). The responses to i.v. tolbutamide and glucose combined in those groups were not superior to the action of glucose alone. We demonstrated this combined i.v. glibenclamide-glucose response test 2 years ago.

The disadvantage associated with prior removal of antibodies from serum in the formerly insulin-treated cases is obvious. We therefore tried to base the test solely on blood glucose determinations. As seen in Figure 6 also, in the positive responders the blood sugar, 3 hours after injection, decreased to less than the initial values indicated as 100%.

The continued response test was applied to 225 elderly diabetics, having an average

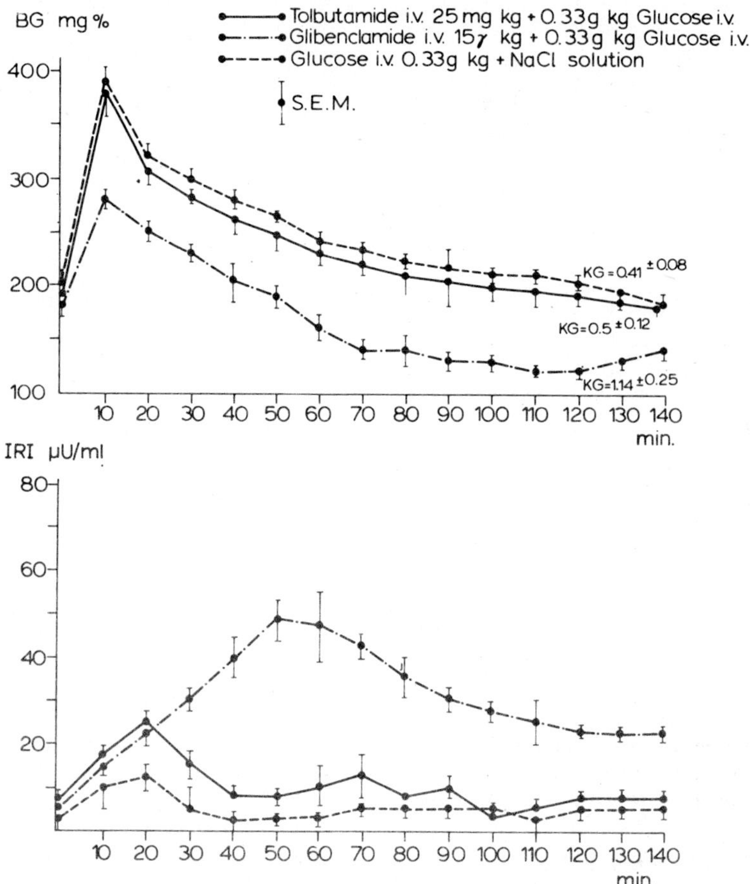

FIG. 5. Glucose and insulin concentrations in serum of patients after secondary failure of tolbutamide therapy following glucose, tolbutamide + glucose, and glibenclamide + glucose, respectively. (From Raptis and Pfeiffer, 1971, by courtesy).

duration of diabetes of 10 years, out of which 139 were on insulin and 86 were secondary failures of other sulfonylurea preparations (Pfeiffer et al., 1973). In 130 cases where the 3-hour blood glucose concentration was at least 20 mg% below the average initial value of 200 mg% of the fasting blood sugar concentration, the long-term treatment was successful; in the remaining 95 cases with 3-hour blood glucose above the initial value of about 250 mg% glibenclamide therapy failed (Fig. 7). Similarly, though not identical individually, was the correlation between the result of the oral therapy and the blood glucose response recorded as percent changes. Hence, evaluation of the absolute and relative blood sugar decreases resulted in 82.49 and 88.52% of correct prediction for the combined response test, respectively, which percentage was further improved up to 93.87% if the absolute and the relative changes in serum insulin were also included.

A higher rate of *hypoglycemic attacks* than was encountered following other sulfonylurea preparations is the tribute we have to pay for that 'controlled extension of oral antidiabetic therapy on former insulin-dependent diabetics' (Pfeiffer and Raptis, 1972).

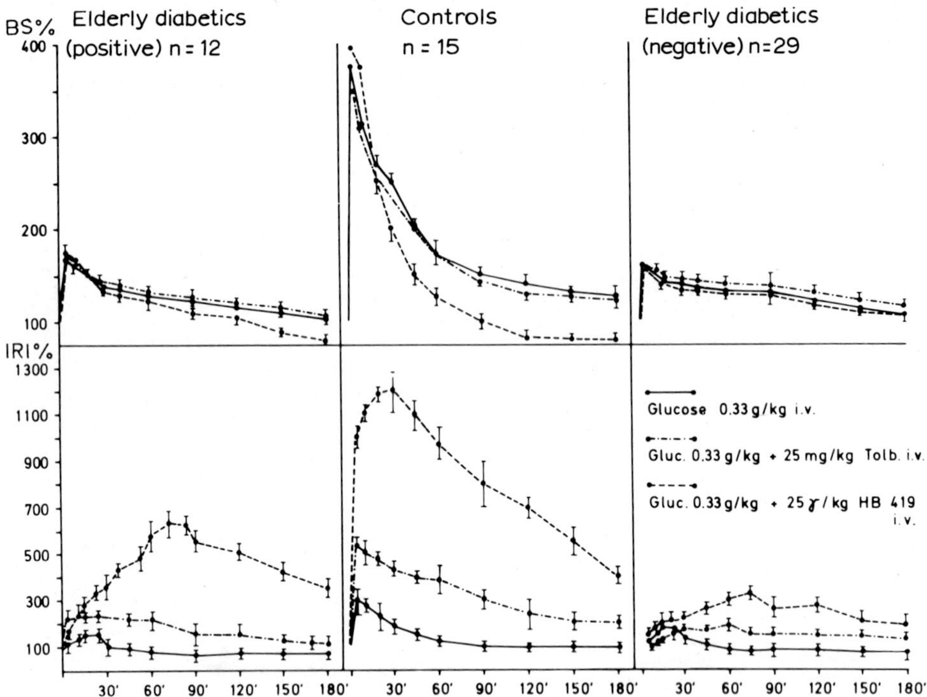

FIG. 6. Glucose and insulin (% changes from initial) responses to glucose, glucose + tolbutamide, and glucose + glibenclamide i.v. combined, in 40 apparently insulin-dependent elderly diabetics not responding to tolbutamide, and 15 normal controls. Note the more than 500% increase in serum insulin, the more than 20% decrease in blood glucose at 1.5 and 3 hours, respectively, following glucose + glibenclamide in elderly diabetics afterwards maintained successfully on glibenclamide (left part of Figure), and absence of significant changes in the failures of maintenance treatment (right part of Figure). (From Pfeiffer and Raptis, 1972, by courtesy).

Strangely enough, glibenclamide-associated hypoglycemias were experienced 1–4 weeks after commencement of the tablet therapy, and usually in the afternoon hours.

There is no need to speculate on some major extrapancreatic hypoglycemic actions (Beyer et al., 1973). As emphasized on several occasions (Pfeiffer et al., 1958, 1959; White and Dupré, 1968; Berger et al., 1973) measurement of serum insulin in the portal rather than in the cubital venous blood, via catheterization of the umbilical vein, is revealing remarkable rises after *oral* administration of various sulfonylurea preparations, HB 419 included, in both normal and diabetic individuals (Fig. 8).

The hypoglycemia in the afternoon, on the other hand, might be convincingly ascribed to the different dynamics of insulin secretion effected by glibenclamide in relation to food, i.e. carbohydrate intake. Whereas tolbutamide administered orally at 7 a.m. exhibited the maximal insulin increases and blood sugar decreases at 11 a.m., glibenclamide effected, exactly in accord with the observations of the group of Boshell (cf. Chandalia et al., 1969) and of Quabbe and Kliems (1969), the highest insulin and the lowest blood

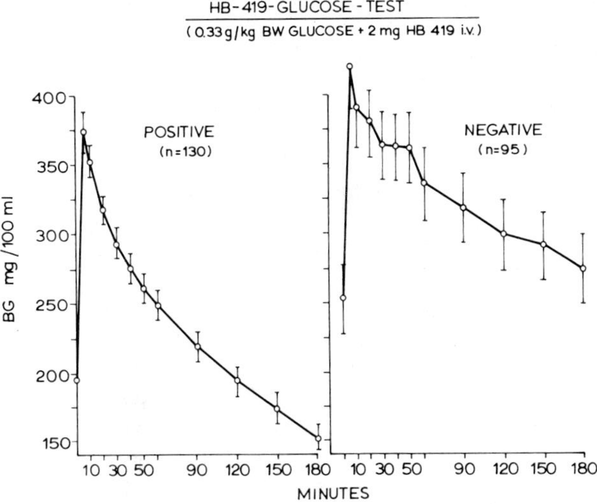

FIG. 7. Significant differences between blood glucose changes in positive and negative responders to glibenclamide maintenance therapy induced by glucose and glibenclamide i.v. combined as a method of predicting the outcome of chronic treatment. For details see text. (From Pfeiffer et al., 1973, by courtesy).

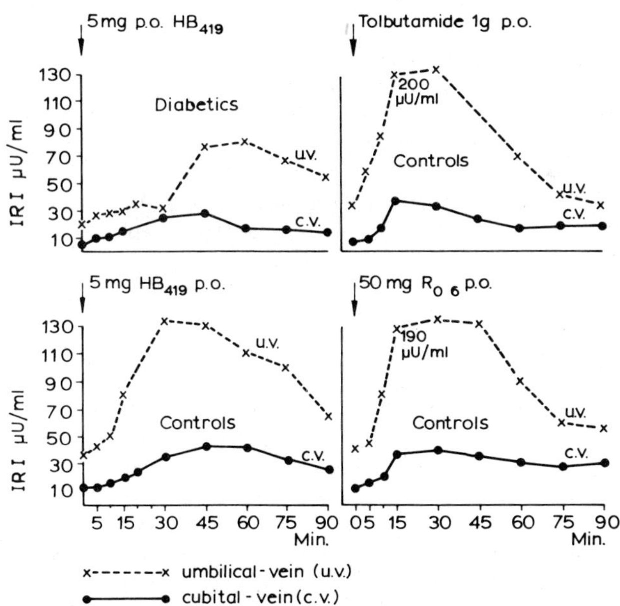

FIG. 8. Serum insulin in peripheral and portal circulation (provided by umbilical vein catheterization) in normal and diabetic subjects following various sulfonylurea preparations given orally. (From Raptis, 1972, by courtesy).

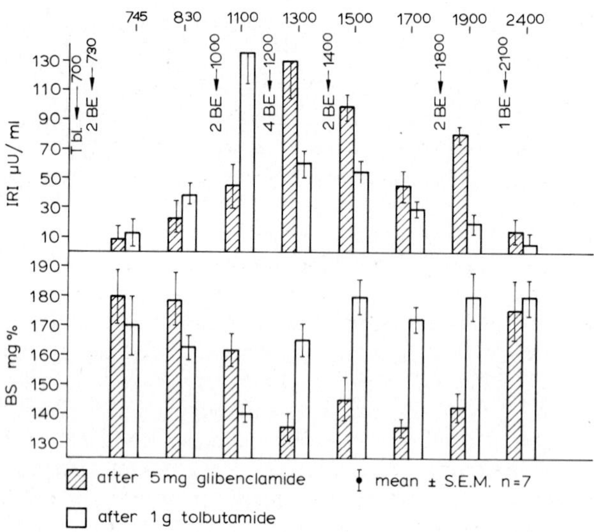

FIG. 9. Glucose and insulin concentrations in blood of 7 diabetics maintained on tolbutamide and glibenclamide, respectively, from 7 a.m. to 12 p.m. Highest increase in serum insulin and lowest blood glucose concentrations recorded under tolbutamide in the morning hours, under glibenclamide in the afternoon. 1 BE = 12.5 g carbohydrates. (From Rothenbuchner et al., 1971, by courtesy).

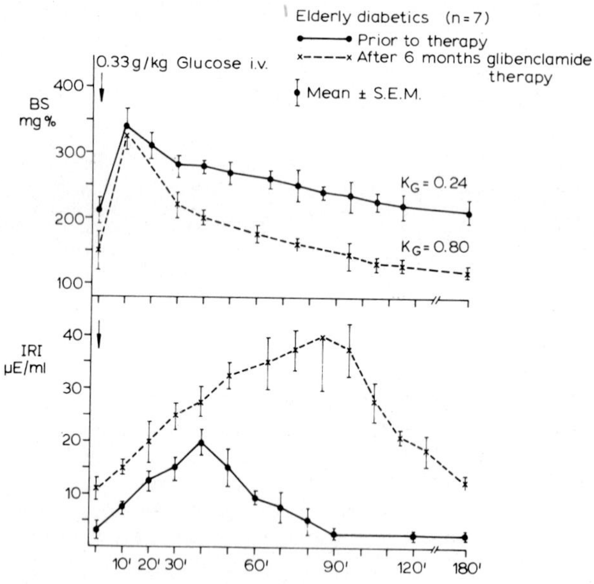

FIG. 10. Blood glucose and insulin following i.v. glucose in 7 maturity-onset diabetics maintained successfully for 6 months on glibenclamide therapy. (From Raptis et al., 1971, by courtesy).

glucose levels between 1 and 4 p.m., i.e. after lunch and after the highest carbohydrate intake (Rothenbuchner et al., 1971) (Fig. 9). This finding strongly reminds us of the former observation of Chu Ping-Chi et al. (1968) that in long-term treatment with tablets, chlorpropamide too did not increase serum insulin in the fasting state but did so only following the physiological stimulus of food ingestion. Incidentally, in our mind chlorpropamide is likely to be registered as one of the 'classical' sulfonylureas for, though weaker quantitatively, it is qualitatively closest to those of the second generation.

There is not the slightest indication of a lasting improvement in the response of the beta cell to glucose effected by glibenclamide. Intravenous injection of glucose after some months of therapy resulted in a remarkable increase in reactive insulin which, however, was only observed as long as the glibenclamide therapy was applied (Fig. 10); immediately upon withdrawal of the drug the former, unsatisfactory and diabetic, response returned (Raptis et al., 1971). Hence, we might reasonably assume re-sensitization of the defective glucose sensor of the diabetic beta cell (Maier and Pfeiffer, 1971) by purely pharmacochemical action. Whether this effect remains through the course of the long-term treatment proper remains to be elucidated. The minute per minute blood sugar determinations performed by continuous blood sugar monitoring (Molnar et al., 1972) constantly exhibited much smoother blood glucose and also, if measured, insulin concentrations in the group of patients suitable for oral therapy in general than in the juvenile insulin-deficient diabetics.

As far as the action of glibenclamide and other sulfonylureas on the biosynthesis and conversion of pro-insulin to insulin is concerned, Schatz et al. (1972) did not observe potentiation of glucose action. Incorporation of ^{3}H-leucine did not show any differences, in contrast to former observations (Tanese et al., 1970), even in the presence of high glucose inhibitions. Only very recently and at variance to tolbutamide, non-interference of glibenclamide with the release of newly synthesized insulin has been suggested (Schatz and Pfeiffer, 1973). For the time being, the influence of the new compound on the second phase of insulin secretion, even after the first hour of application, appears to be the most likely explanation for its action.

In essence, these newer drugs are affecting sites of the diabetic beta cells which are different from both the glucose and the tolbutamide receptors, and by doing so they are permitting oral treatment of the more severe type of diabetes formerly regarded as non-responsive to tablet treatment.

REFERENCES

BERGER, W., GÖSCHKE, H., MOPPERT, J. and KÜNZLI, H. (1973): Insulin concentrations in portal venous and peripheral venous blood in man following administration of glucose, galactose, xylitol and tolbutamide. *Hormone metabol. Res., 5,* 4.

BEYER, J., HAUPT, E., CORDES, U., KUTSCHERA, J. and SCHÖFFLING, K. (1973): Different amounts of insulin secretion following an equal total decrease of blood glucose as an indication of possible extrapancreatic activities of different sulfonylurea drugs. *Hormone metabol. Res., 5,* 9.

CHANDALIA, H. B., HOLLOBAUGH, S. L., PENNINGTON, L. F. and BOSHELL, B. R. (1969): Use of glybenzcyclamide in maturity-onset diabetes. Effect of the drug on serum insulin levels. *Hormone metabol. Res., 1/Suppl. 1,* 73.

CHU-PING-CHI, CONWAY, M. J., KROUSE, H. A. and GOODNER, C. J. (1968): The pattern of response of plasma insulin and glucose to meals and fasting during chlorpropamide therapy. *Ann. int. Med., 68,* 757.

FUSSGÄNGER, R. D., GOBERNA, R., HINZ, M., JAROS, P., KARSTEN, C. and PFEIFFER, E. F. (1969): Comparative studies on the dynamics of insulin secretion following HB 419 and tolbutamide on the perfused isolated rat pancreas and the perifused isolated islets of Langerhans. *Hormone metabol. Res., 1/Suppl. 1,* 34.

MAIER, V. and PFEIFFER, E. F. (1971): Influence of δ-neuraminidase treatment on biosynthesis and secretion of insulin from isolated mouse islets of Langerhans. *Hoppe-Seyler's Z. physiol. Chem., 352,* 1733.

MOLNAR, G. D., TAYLOR, W. F. and HO, M. M. (1972): Day-to-day variation of continuously monitored glycaemia: A further measure of diabetic instability. *Diabetologia, 8,* 342.

PFEIFFER, E. F. (1967): Dynamics of insulin secretion in normal, obese and diabetic subjects following beta-cell stimulation. In: *Tolbutamide ..... After ten years, Proceedings of the Brook Lodge Symposium, Augusta, Mich., 1967,* pp. 127–139. Editors: W. J. H. Butterfield and W. Van Westering. International Congress Series No. 149, Excerpta Medica, Amsterdam.

PFEIFFER, E. F. (1971): Fortschritte der Diabetologie. *Therapiewoche, 21,* 553.

PFEIFFER, E. F., DITSCHUNEIT, H. and ZIEGLER, R. (1960): Untersuchungen zur Pathogenese des menschlichen Altersdiabetes: Die Dynamik der Insulinsekretion des Stoffwechselgesunden und des Altersdiabetikers nach wiederholter Belastung mit Glukose, Sulfonylharnstoffen und menschlichem Wachstumshormon. In: *VII. Symposium der Deutschen Gesellschaft für Endokrinologie, Homburg (Saar), 1960,* p. 206. Springer Verlag, Berlin.

PFEIFFER, E. F., DITSCHUNEIT, H. and ZIEGLER, R. (1961): Über die Bestimmung von Insulin im Blut am epididymalen Fettanhang der Ratte mit Hilfe markierter Glukose. IV. Die Dynamik der Insulinsekretion des Stoffwechselgesunden und des Altersdiabetikers nach wiederholter Belastung mit Glukose, Sulfonylharnstoffen und menschlichem Wachstumshormon, ein Beitrag zur Pathogenese des menschlichen Altersdiabetes. *Klin. Wschr., 39,* 415.

PFEIFFER, E. F., PFEIFFER, M., DITSCHUNEIT, H. and CHANG-SU-AHN (1959): Über die Bestimmung von Insulin im Blut am epididymalen Fettanhang der Ratte mit Hilfe markierter Glukose. II. Experimentelle und klinische Erfahrungen. *Klin. Wschr., 37,* 1238.

PFEIFFER, E. F. and RAPTIS, S. (1972): Controlled extension of oral antidiabetic therapy on former insulin dependent diabetics by means of the combined i.v. glibenclamide-glucose-response-test. *Diabetologia, 8,* 41.

PFEIFFER, E. F., RAPTIS, S. and SCHRÖDER, K. E. (1973): Die Bedeutung der einmaligen kombinierten i.v. Glibenclamid-Glukose-Belastung für Auswahl, Indikationsstellung und Prognose der oralen Dauertherapie des sogenannten 'insulinbedürftigen' Tolbutamid-resistenten Erwachsenendiabetes. In preparation.

PFEIFFER, E. F., RENOLD, A. E., MARTIN, D. B., DAGENAIS, Y., MEAKIN, J. W., NELSON, D. H., SHOEMAKER, G. and THORN, G. W. (1958): Untersuchungen über die Rolle des Pankreas im Wirkungsmechanismus blutzuckersenkender Sulfonylharnstoffe. In: *Diabetes mellitus, III Congress of the International Diabetes Federation, Düsseldorf, 1958,* pp. 298–303. Editors: K. Oberdisse and K. Jahnke. Georg Thieme Verlag, Stuttgart.

QUABBE, H.-J. and KLIEMS, G. (1969): Verhalten von Plasma-Insulin, Blutzucker und freien Fettsäuren nach Gabe von Tolbutamid und HB 419 bei Stoffwechselgesunden und Diabetikern. In: *Tegernsee-Konferenz über das Neue Orale Antidiabetikum HB 419, 1969.* Farbwerke Hoechst A.G. – Boehringer Mannheim GmbH.

RAPTIS, S. and PFEIFFER, E. F. (1971): Sulfonylharnstoffe als orale Antidiabetika der 1. und 2. Generation. *Therapiewoche, 21,* 578.

RAPTIS, S., DOLLINGER, H., CHRISSIKU, M., ROTHENBUCHNER, G. and PFEIFFER, E. F. (1973): The effect of the β-receptor blockade (propranolol) on the endocrine and exocrine pancreatic function in man after the administration of intestinal hormones (secretin and cholecystokinin-pancreozymin). *Europ. J. clin. Invest., 3,* 163.

RAPTIS, S., RAU, R. M., SCHRODER, K. E., FAULHABER, J. D. and PFEIFFER, E. F. (1969): Comparative study of insulin secretion following repeated administration of glucose, tolbutamide and glibenclamide (HB 419) in diabetic and non-diabetic human subjects. *Hormone metabol. Res., 1/Suppl. 1,* 65.

RAPTIS, S., THUM, C., SCHRÖDER, K. E., ROTHENBUCHNER, G., KLÖR, U., RAU, R. M. and PFEIFFER, E. F. (1971): Die Insulinsekretion nach der einfachen und wiederholten Injektion von RO_6-4563/8, Glibenclamid (HB 419), Tolbutamid oder Chlorpropamid ohne und mit gleichzeitiger Gabe von Glukose bei Stoffwechselgesunden und Altersdiabetikern. In: *Diabetes mellitus, Vol. 1,* p. 347. Editors: I. Magyar and A. Beringer. Verlag der Wiener Medizinischen Akademie, Wien.

ROTHENBUCHNER, G., RAPTIS, S. and PFEIFFER, E. F. (1971): Insulin oder orale Antidiabetika aus der Sicht von Forschung und Klinik. *Heilkunst, 84,* 215.

SCHATZ, H. and PFEIFFER, E. F. (1973): Regulation der Insulinbiosynthese. In: *3. Internationales Donau-Symposium über Diabetes mellitus, Salzburg, 1973,* pp. 67–72. Editor: A. Beringer. Verlag Wilhelm Maudrich, Wien, München, Bern.

SCHATZ, H., MAIER, V., HINZ, M., NIERLE, C. and PFEIFFER, E. F. (1972): The effect of tolbutamide and glibenclamide on the incorporation of ^{3}H-leucine and on the conversion of proinsulin to insulin in isolated pancreatic islets. *FEBS Letters, 26,* 237.

SCHWARZ, H., AMMON, J., YEBOAH, J. E., HILDEBRANDT, H. E. and PFEIFFER, E. F. (1968): Förderung der Insulinsekretion in vitro durch ein neues, hochwirksames Antidiabeticum. *Diabetologia, 4,* 10.

TANESE, T., LAZARUS, N. R., DEVRIM, S. and RECANT, L. (1970): Synthesis and release of proinsulin and insulin by isolated rat islets of Langerhans. *J. clin. Invest., 49,* 1394.

WHITE, J. J. and DUPRE, J. (1968): Regulation of insulin secretion by the intestinal hormone secretin: studies in man via transumbilical portal vein catheterization. *Surgery, 64,* 204.

ORAL HYPOGLYCEMIC DRUG PROPHYLAXIS IN ASYMPTOMATIC DIABETES*

ROBERT FELDMAN,† DEREK CRAWFORD,‡ ROBERT ELASHOFF§
and ALVIN GLASS‡

Since 1965, in the Kaiser-Permanente Medical Centers in Oakland and San Francisco, we have been testing the hypothesis that the carbohydrate tolerance of patients with asymptomatic (chemical) diabetes may be improved by the prophylactic administration of oral hypoglycemic drugs, and that such improvement would prevent or postpone overt diabetes (Feldman and Fitterer, 1967; Feldman and Crawford, 1970; Feldman et al., 1973). Two drugs have been used in this prospective double-blind study: tolbutamide was selected because sulfonylurea drugs had been shown in animals to be beta cell cytotropic, and treatment with tolbutamide had been reported to improve glucose tolerance in patients with mild diabetes (Fajans and Conn, 1960). Phenformin was used because it had been widely employed in diabetic therapy, and had been reported to reduce excessive insulin response in obese patients and to increase peripheral glucose utilization. The present paper extends summarization of our experience to September, 1972.

MATERIAL AND METHODS

Three hundred and fifty subjects have been admitted to the study on the prophylactic use of oral hypoglycemic drugs in asymptomatic diabetes conducted in the Diabetic Research Laboratory, Kaiser-Permanente Medical Center, Oakland, California. The methods by which the subjects were selected, their demographic characteristics, the methods of testing for diabetes, and the therapy used have been described (Feldman et al., 1973). Salient points are that the subjects are members of the prepaid Kaiser Foundation Health Plan, residing in the San Francisco-Oakland area; that they entered the study voluntarily after having been informed of its purpose and risks, and of the general patterns of activity that would be incumbent upon them. The first subject was admitted to the study during

* This work was supported by USPHS Grants CD 00051 and HS 00267; The Permanente Medical Group and the Kaiser Foundation Research Institute, Oakland, California; and in part by the Automated Multiphasic Screening Program, USPHS Grant CD 00142.
† Invited speaker; Kaiser-Permanente Medical Center, Oakland, Calif.
‡ Kaiser-Permanente Medical Center, San Francisco, Calif.
§ Instruction and Research Division, Information Systems, Computer Center, and Department of Biostatistics, University of California, San Francisco, Calif., U.S.A.

the closing weeks of 1964; the goal of 350 admissions was reached early in 1969. The subjects were 15 to 59 years of age with a mean age of 44.7 years; 28% were younger than 40 years, 62% were male, 73% white, 12% black. A total of 23% were more than 20% above their ideal weight; the average deviation from ideal weight for the entire study group was +11%. All patients were free of other significant disease. None was taking a drug known to affect glucose tolerance, and none had received hypoglycemic therapy.

In all cases, the presence of chemical diabetes was newly discovered. Because of the known variability of carbohydrate tolerance in early diabetes, abnormal responses to 3 testings were required before any patient was admitted to the study:

1. Of the subjects, 75% were referred to the study from the Automated Multiphasic Health Check clinic, to which members of the Health Plan may voluntarily present themselves for multiphasic health examination. The examination includes a screening test for glucose tolerance 1 and 2 hours after a glucose load. The remaining 25% of the study group had been investigated for diabetes in the Oakland or San Francisco clinic of The Permanente Medical Group because of a family or obstetrical history suggesting diabetes.

2. For confirmation of those results, a glucose tolerance test was conducted in a routine clinical laboratory. Only patients who showed a positive response were considered further for entry into the study.

3. A third set of tests was performed in the Diabetic Research Laboratory before the patient was admitted to the study. The subject was prepared by the addition of 150 g carbohydrate daily to his regular diet for 3 days, then by overnight fast. After the oral administration of 100 g glucose, glucose in whole venous blood was measured by the glucose oxidase method, plasma insulin by the immunoassay method of Grodsky and Forsham, and plasma free fatty acid by Trout's modification of Dole's method. When the criteria of Fajans and Conn (1960) were applied to these results, 280 subjects with chemical diabetes and 70 with probable diabetes were admitted to the study. For this analysis, the findings of these 2 subgroups are combined.

The asymptomatic nature of the diabetes in the study population is emphasized by the mean fasting blood sugar of the total group: 105 mg/100 ml; and of three-fourths of the total group: less than 110 mg/100 ml. The glucose tolerance curve for the entire group was well above normal (Fig. 1). While insulin response varied widely among subjects, the mean curve was typical of mild maturity-onset diabetes (hyperinsulin response to the glucose load, with peak values at 2 hours). Individual free fatty acid values also varied widely, but the mean exceeded that of normal controls at 30, 60, and 90 minutes after the glucose load.

Patients were randomly assigned to 3 treatment groups. The success of randomization was apparent in the absence of significant differences among the 3 groups with respect to entry age, sex, race, weight, and curves for mean values of glucose, insulin, and free fatty acid (Fig. 1).

Of the subjects, 50% (174 patients) were given tolbutamide, 1 g daily as 0.5 g with breakfast and dinner. The preponderant number of patients was assigned to this group because of the reported beta cell cytotropism of tolbutamide. One quarter (91) of the patients received phenformin, 100 mg daily as 50 mg with breakfast and dinner, in timed-release capsules. One quarter (85) of the patients received a placebo and were considered as controls. The drugs were dispensed in double-blind fashion, in containers of 130 capsules given to the patient every 2 months. Unused capsules were returned to the Diabetic Research Laboratory and tabulated as an indication of adherence to schedule. To test for improved beta cell function, research drugs were discontinued 3 days before

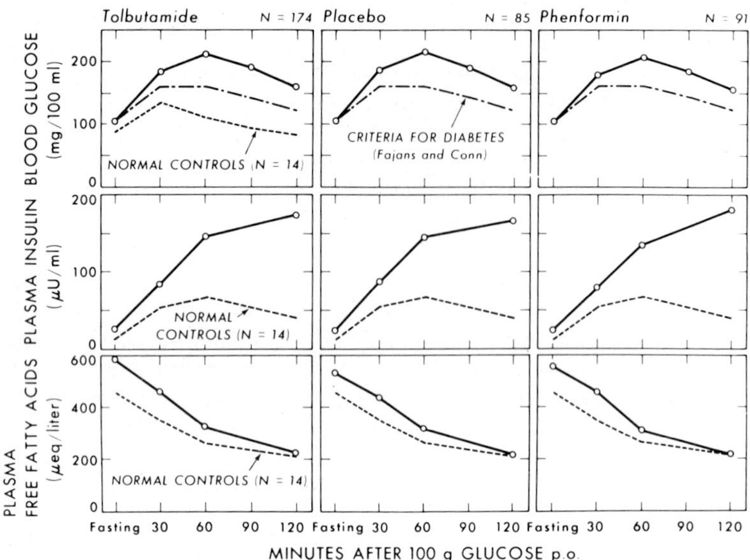

FIG. 1. Mean values for all subjects in each drug group upon entry to study, compared with criteria of Fajans and Conn (1960) for diabetes, employed in the study, and with mean curves for 14 normal controls examined in our laboratory. (Reproduced by permission from Feldman et al., 1973.)

follow-up glucose tolerance testing, which was repeated every 4 months during the first year and every 6 months thereafter.

Diabetic diets were prescribed to all patients. In addition, reduction diets were prescribed to those who were 10% or more above their ideal weight.

To assess the long-term effects of treatment on some neurovascular aspects of diabetes, beginning early in 1968 after somewhat more than half of the patients were under treatment, peripheral nerve function was evaluated annually. Standard techniques for measuring the conduction velocity of both motor and sensory nerves were used; these techniques had shown decreased nerve function in diabetic patients having no clinical evidence of peripheral neuropathy (Downie and Newell, 1961; Lawrence and Locke, 1961).

Arterial pulse wave velocity was also measured annually, as an early indicator of peripheral arteriosclerosis. Simultaneous tracings from the right carotid and right radial arteries were made by the method of Woolam et al., which had been reported by a number of authors to show significantly higher velocity in diabetic and prediabetic subjects than in normal controls (Woolam et al., 1962; Gunn et al., 1965; Katz et al., 1970).

In view of the success of randomization previously demonstrated by other parameters, it was assumed that nerve conduction and pulse wave velocity were also comparable in the 3 groups at entry.

The frequencies of deaths and of fatal and non-fatal cardiovascular events were reviewed.

The research subjects underwent an annual health examination.

RESULTS AND DISCUSSION

Considered in this progress report are 7 categories of change in patients undergoing the regimens described, over the study period to September, 1972: (1) chemical changes (glucose, insulin, free fatty acids) noted in the Diabetic Research Laboratory, (2) changes in weight, (3) changes on annual health examination, (4) changes in nerve conduction velocity, (5) changes in arterial pulse wave velocity, (6) removals from the study and deaths, and (7) fatal and non-fatal cardiovascular events.

Chemical changes

The sums of the results from glucose tolerance testing (Fig. 2) and the mean 2-hour glucose levels (Fig. 3) determined in the Diabetic Research Laboratory were directly

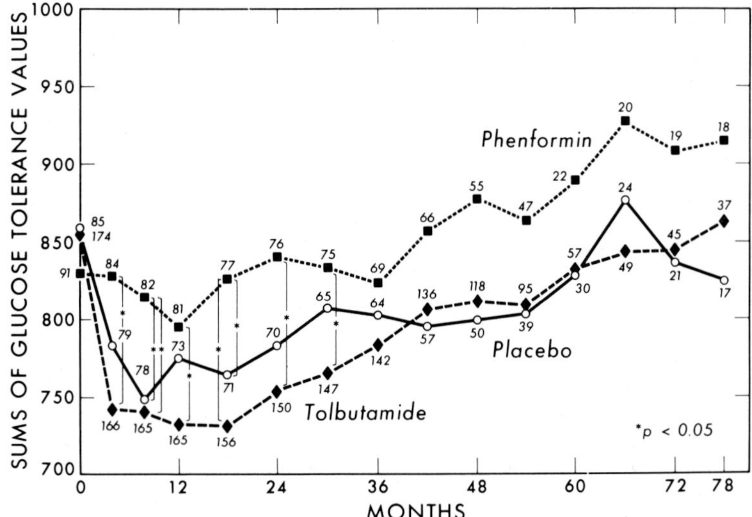

FIG. 2. Sums of glucose tolerance values in the 3 drug groups for the first 78 months of the study.

comparable throughout the first 78 months of therapy, and are considered together here. It is to be noted that these tests were made after the drug had been withdrawn for 3 days.

During the entire 78 months, glucose tolerance was more impaired and 2-hour glucose levels were higher in the phenformin group than in the placebo or tolbutamide group. At 9 and 18 months, both values were significantly ($P < 0.05$) higher in the phenformin than in the control group. During the first 36 months the glucose tolerance sums on 6 occasions, and the 2-hour glucose means on 4 occasions, were significantly ($P < 0.05$) higher in the phenformin group than in the tolbutamide group. Tolbutamide group values, while lower than those of the control group during the first 36 months, did not show a statistically significant difference from them.

After 30 months, glucose tolerance impairment and 2-hour glucose values gradually increased in all groups. At 78 months, the tolbutamide and placebo group values were near baseline, while the phenformin-associated levels continued to rise. When these results

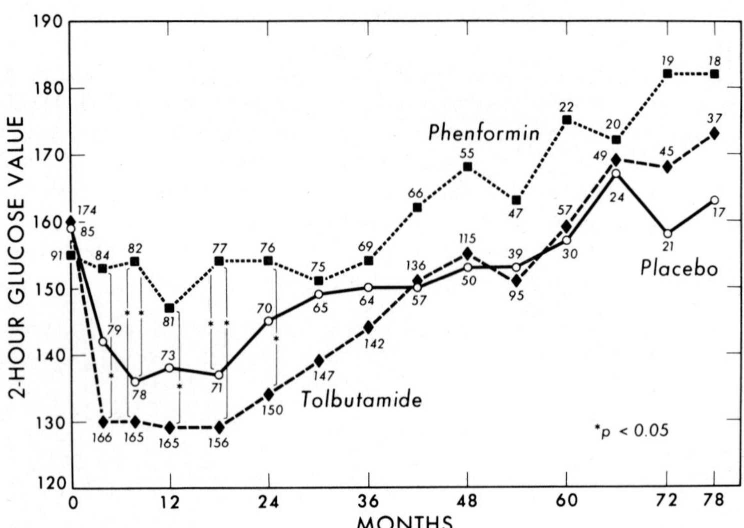

FIG. 3. Sums of 2-hour blood glucose values in the 3 drug groups for the first 78 months of the study.

were plotted as percentage changes from baseline, a similar pattern emerged: at 78 months, the tolbutamide group means had returned to baseline, while those for the phenformin group were 10% above the initial levels.

The sums of insulin values before therapy and up to 60 months of therapy appear in Figure 4. Although statistical significance was not achieved because of the large standard

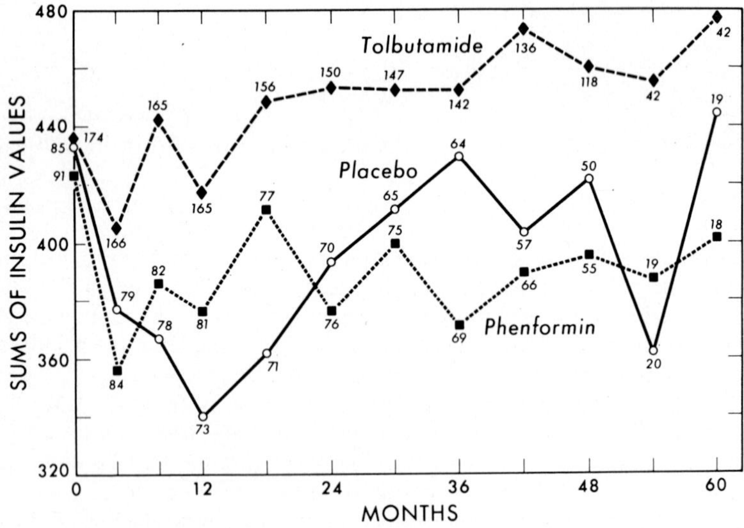

FIG. 4. Sums of insulin values for the 3 drug groups for the first 78 months of the study.

deviations, the trends are evident: starting 24 months after the beginning of therapy, the values for the phenformin group were for the most part slightly lower than for controls; values for the tolbutamide group were consistently higher than for controls. Calculations of percentage changes in sums of insulin values from the baselines gave a similar pattern. On several occasions, the 30-minute and 60-minute insulin values for patients receiving phenformin were significantly ($P < 0.05$) lower than those of the tolbutamide group.

Thus, the initial improvement in glucose tolerance that was observed with tolbutamide was associated with increased plasma insulin during the glucose tolerance studies, whereas in the phenformin group no change in insulin levels was seen despite gradual deterioration of glucose tolerance. In the controls, insulin values varied widely but showed no consistent trend. Free fatty acids did not change significantly with any form of therapy.

Changes in weight

Percent changes from ideal weight are shown in Figure 5. Starting from means of about

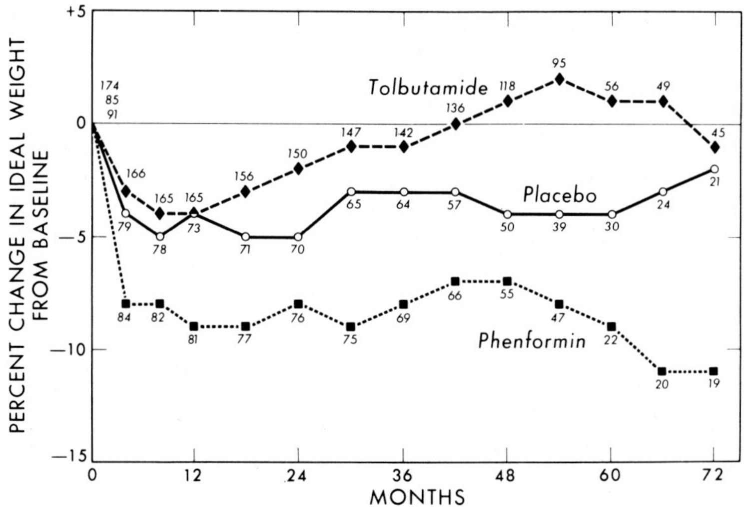

FIG. 5. Percent changes from ideal weight: means for the 3 drug groups.

11% above ideal weight at entry for each of the 3 treatment groups, the mean for the patients receiving phenformin declined persistently throughout the study period. The mean weight of the tolbutamide group decreased initially, then rose gradually above baseline. The percentage changes from ideal weight of each treatment group did not differ significantly from those of controls.

Changes in annual health examination data

Selected mean values from the annual health examination data during the first 6 years of the study are shown in Figure 6. These serum glucose measurements were made while the patient was following his diabetic research drug regimen; the blood samples were taken at various times of day. While certain trends are of interest, none reached statistical

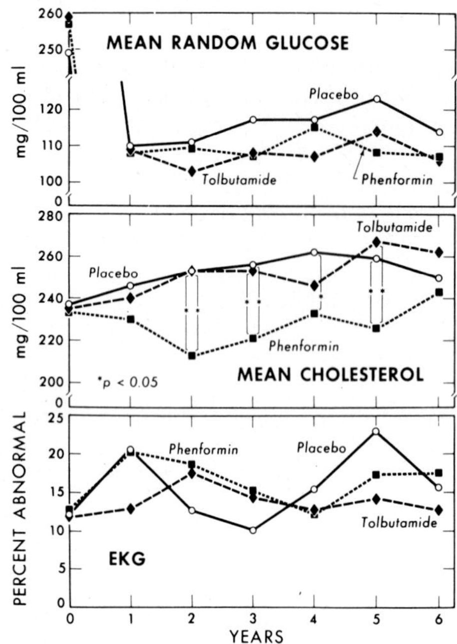

FIG. 6. Annual health examination data: mean random glucose levels and serum cholesterol levels, and mean percentages of subjects within each drug group showing an abnormality on the electrocardiogram during the first 6 years.

significance: in the fourth year, the mean level for the tolbutamide group was lower than for both the placebo and the phenformin groups; by the end of the sixth year, the means for both drug groups were lower than for controls.

In each of the 3 treatment groups, the mean serum cholesterol level at entry was 235 mg/100 ml. From years 2 through 5, the mean level for the phenformin group was significantly lower than for controls. The curve of mean cholesterol values of the tolbutamide group was close to that for controls during all but one of the 6 years: at the fourth checkpoint, it was nonsignificantly lower than the control mean. At 6 years, the mean tolbutamide group level was higher than control, and the phenformin group mean was lower than control; neither of these differences was statistically significant.

The percentages of patients showing a deviation from normal on the electrocardiogram fluctuated in each treatment group throughout the 6 years. The total percentages rose slightly over the entire period, but no significant differences emerged.

Nerve conduction velocities

Motor nerves Nerve conduction velocities are compared as means for each treatment group, and as differences in velocities in individual subjects, at annual intervals over 4 years, in Table 1. Conduction velocity in all of the 3 motor nerves tested was comparable in the 3 treatment groups and within the normal range throughout the 4 years. Paired differences demonstrated no significant difference between the effect of either drug and

TABLE 1
Motor nerve conduction velocities

Treatment group		Test*				Paired differences		
		1	2	3	4	2nd–1st	3rd–1st	4th–1st
Median nerve								
Tolbutamide	N	115	127	107	39	101	81	27
	Mean (meters/sec.)	55.6	55.0	55.2	55.1	−1.00	0.53	−1.64
	S.D.	4.2	3.8	5.1	4.0	4.6	6.3	4.2
Placebo	N	57	59	47	17	45	35	13
	Mean (meters/sec.)	55.4	54.4	55.5	55.1	−1.22	−1.03	−0.25
	S.D.	4.4	4.3	3.8	4.2	5.0	4.0	4.4
Phenformin	N	61	63	52	23	50	41	18
	Mean (meters/sec).	55.0	54.9	54.9	54.8	−0.31	−0.62	−0.74
	S.D.	4.5	4.2	4.6	3.1	5.0	4.8	5.3
Ulnar nerve								
Tolbutamide	N	99	105	103	37	72	70	20
	Mean (meters/sec.)	56.8	56.1	57.6	57.1	−0.29	1.15	1.12
	S.D.	5.2	4.9	5.6	3.0	5.3	5.9	4.9
Placebo	N	48	48	45	15	34	27	9
	Mean (meters/sec.)	55.5	55.8	57.4	56.7	−0.39	0.62	−0.30
	S.D.	5.4	5.6	6.8	6.3	6.4	7.3	4.2
Phenformin	N	55	57	48	22	38	35	17
	Mean (meters/sec.)	55.4	57.1	58.4	57.9	0.06	1.96	3.96
	S.D.	10.4	5.4	6.4	4.5	5.1	11.1	12.9
Peroneal nerve								
Tolbutamide	N	100	118	103	39	83	69	22
	Mean (meters/sec.)	47.3	47.2	47.4	45.6	0.19	0.66	−3.99
	S.D.	5.0	4.2	5.6	4.2	4.5	5.2	4.8
Placebo	N	49	55	45	16	37	29	9
	Mean (meters/sec.)	46.9	46.1	46.5	45.8	−0.41	−0.88	−3.02
	S.D.	3.8	5.3	4.0	4.9	4.3	4.3	3.7
Phenformin	N	56	62	50	22	44	33	13
	Mean (meters/sec.)	46.5	47.1	47.7	47.3	0.68	0.86	1.42**
	S.D.	4.2	3.3	4.1	3.8	4.4	5.1	4.9

* The interval between tests was approximately one year.
** Phenformin significantly different from tolbutamide and placebo $P < 0.05$.

that of the placebo on median nerve conduction velocity; in general, velocities were slightly lower on the second and subsequent examinations than on the first. Mean conduction velocity improved in the ulnar nerve in the phenformin group at all time points, and was apparent in the paired differences, especially at the fourth testing. In the peroneal nerve, the improvement with phenformin seen in the paired differences was sufficient to make a statistically significant ($P < 0.05$) difference from the individuals receiving tolbutamide or placebo.

Sensory nerves Sensory latency (orthodromic distal) nerve conduction studies in the median and ulnar nerves (Table 2) showed no significant difference between the control group and either group receiving an oral hypoglycemic drug.

TABLE 2
*Sensory latency (orthodromic distal) nerve conduction velocities**

Treatment group		Test				Paired differences		
		1	2	3	4	2nd–1st	3rd–1st	4th–1st
Median nerve								
Tolbutamide	N	120	128	108	39	107	89	28
	Mean (meters/sec.)	3.5	3.5	3.1	3.1	0.04	–0.31	–0.26
	S.D.	0.3	0.4	0.2	0.1	0.51	0.42	0.32
Placebo	N	65	60	47	17	53	41	14
	Mean (meters/sec.)	3.4	3.5	3.1	3.1	0.03	–0.36	–0.39
	S.D.	0.4	0.3	0.2	0.1	0.53	0.42	0.39
Phenformin	N	68	66	52	21	57	44	20
	Mean (meters/sec.)	3.3	3.5	3.2	3.1	0.10	–0.14	–0.36
	S.D.	0.4	0.3	0.2	0.1	0.51	0.43	0.51
Ulnar nerve								
Tolbutamide	N	120	128	107	39	107	89	28
	Mean (meters/sec.)	3.3	3.3	3.0	3.0	0.08	–0.19	–0.07
	S.D.	0.6	0.4	0.2	0.1	0.60	0.57	0.37
Placebo	N	60	60	47	17	48	38	12
	Mean (meters/sec.)	3.3	3.3	3.0	3.0	0.05	–0.12	0.20
	S.D.	0.4	0.3	0.2	0.1	0.52	0.46	0.26
Phenformin	N	65	66	50	22	54	40	19
	Mean (meters/sec.)	3.1	3.3	3.1	3.0	0.20	–0.03	–0.04
	S.D.	0.4	0.3	0.2	0.1	0.47	0.44	0.36

* The interval between testing was approximately one year.

Arterial pulse wave changes

Arterial pulse wave velocity increases with the rigidity of the arterial wall, and is thus presumably an indicator of the degree of arteriosclerosis. Arterial pulse wave changes were observed at approximately annual intervals for 4 years in these subjects. The means for each treatment group at these intervals are shown in Table 3, together with paired differences for individual subjects. The mean velocity increased with time in all treatment

TABLE 3
*Arterial pulse wave velocity**

Treatment group		Test 1	Test 2	Test 3	Test 4	Paired differences 2nd–1st	3rd–1st	4th–1st
Tolbutamide	N	139	99	79	33	93	75	31
	Mean (meters/sec.)	9.1	9.4	10.0	10.4	0.23	0.75	1.71
	S.D.	1.4	1.7	2.0	2.1	2.11	2.42	2.13
Placebo	N	65	47	34	16	42	31	14
	Mean (meters/sec.)	9.0	9.4	9.1	10.2	0.20	0.25	1.36
	S.D.	1.8	1.6	1.5	1.5	2.73	1.48	1.47
Phenformin	N	71	41	33	11	39	31	9
	Mean (meters/sec.)	9.2	9.0	9.8	10.6	−0.39	0.60	0.62
	S.D.	1.6	1.6	1.7	1.9	1.99	1.53	2.28

* The interval between tests was approximately one year.

groups and in paired determinations, without significant difference between either drug and the placebo group. Among the paired differences, the least increase in velocity was in the patient treated with phenformin; indeed, uniquely among all comparisons, this patient's velocity actually slowed between the first and second studies, indicating an improvement in this parameter.

Removals and deaths

By September 1972, 110 (32%) of the 350 subjects had been removed from the program or had died (Table 4). The largest number of removals occurred because the subjects failed to cooperate, had moved from the area, or had left the Health Plan. Eleven patients (3%) were removed because they incurred overt diabetes. Five of the 11 had received tolbutamide, 6 the placebo; none had received phenformin. Although these numbers are small, the difference between the frequency of overt diabetes in the phenformin and control groups is statistically significant at the 5% level. This is in surprising contrast to the glucose tolerance and 2-hour blood sugar determinations after the drugs had been withdrawn for 3 days; there, the performance of phenformin was the poorest of the 3 forms of treatment.

Toxicity was a rare cause of removal from the program; its incidence did not differ among the treatment groups.

Of particular interest, in view of the adverse effects of tolbutamide and phenformin reported by the University Group Diabetes Program (1970) and Knatterud et al. (1971), are the data respecting deaths and non-fatal cardiovascular events during the study period. Only 4 deaths occurred (Table 5). Three, which resulted from carcinoma, were in patients taking tolbutamide.

TABLE 4
Reasons for removal of subjects from the diabetic research study during the first 8 years

	Tolbutamide N = 174		Placebo N = 85		Phenformin N = 91		All drug groups N = 350	
	No.	%	No.	%	No.	%	No.	%
Expired	3	1.7	1	1	0		4	1
Overt	5	2.9	6	8 ←*→	0		11	3
Toxicity	2	1	1	1	1	1	4	1
Moved/off plan	21	12	8	9	11	12	40	11
Lack of cooperation	18	10	17	20	16	17	51	14
Total	49	28	33	39	28	31	110	32

* $P < 0.05$.

TABLE 5
*Deaths during the first 8 years of treatment**

Treatment group	Age at entry	Length of treatment prior to death	Cause of death
	Years	Months	
Placebo**	47	24	Myocardial infarction
Tolbutamide	58	47	Carcinoma – hepatobiliary
Tolbutamide	50	57	Carcinoma – colon
Tolbutamide	56	78	Carcinoma – liver

* All of these 4 subjects were male. Not included is one 44-year-old man, treated with tolbutamide for 3 months, who died of complications of renal transplant, 45 months after leaving the program.
** This patient's electrocardiogram was normal; serum cholesterol 235 mg/100 ml; blood pressure 143/80 on entry.

Fatal and non-fatal cardiovascular events

In this study population, which contained no patients with clinical evidence of cardiovascular disease at entry, there were 9 cardiovascular events. One of the 4 deaths (Table 6) was due to myocardial infarction. It occurred in a patient on placebo, whose

TABLE 6
Non-fatal cardiovascular events during the first 8 years of treatment

Cardiovascular event	Treatment group	Age at entry	Sex	Length of treatment prior to cardiovascular event	Risk factors		
					EKG	Cholesterol mg/100 ml	Blood pressure mm Hg
		Years		Months			
Myocardial infarction							
	Tolbutamide	48	M	12 months	Normal	230	136/72
	Tolbutamide	47	M	25 months	Normal	232	130/86
	Placebo	39	M	60 months	Normal	225	140/70
Angina pectoris							
	Phenformin	50	M	67 months	Borderline	241	120/80
	Phenformin	50	M	27 months	Normal	227	120/80
	Phenformin	57	M	44 months	Normal	227	120/80
	Placebo	54	F	21 months	Normal	238	150/90
Cerebral and peripheral arteriosclerosis							
	Tolbutamide	55	M	46 months	Normal	345	132/73

electrocardiogram, serum cholesterol, and blood pressure were within the normal range at entry into the study.

Among the 8 patients who suffered a non-fatal cardiovascular event, 3 were taking tolbutamide, 3 phenformin, and 2 placebo. Six had values within the normal range for the recognized cardiovascular risk factors. Of the 2 who had abnormal values, the patient who showed evidence of both cerebral and peripheral arteriosclerosis while taking tolbutamide had a cholesterol level of 345 mg/100 ml of serum; and one of the patients with angina pectoris had a blood pressure of 150/90. Again, it should be noted that half of the study population was receiving tolbutamide, and one quarter each were on placebo or phenformin.

SUMMARY

During nearly 8 years of prophylactic treatment of asymptomatic diabetes with tolbutamide, phenformin, or placebo, there was suggestive – although not conclusive – evidence that phenformin may be of practical benefit to patients in this phase of the disease. Trends suggesting long-term improvement with phenformin were seen in reduction toward ideal weight, lowered mean cholesterol values, and prevention of deterioration in motor nerve conduction velocity and pulse wave velocity. In a few instances, differences between the phenformin group and controls in these factors were statistically significant. Importantly, in the phenformin group there was no death, myocardial infarction, or overt diabetes during the study period.

Although tolbutamide showed early promise of improving glucose tolerance, this effect did not persist. Phenformin showed no beneficial effect on this factor.

The frequency of death or a cardiovascular event was not greater in either group taking a hypoglycemic drug than in the control group.

REFERENCES

DOWNIE, A. W. and NEWELL, D. J. (1961): Sensory nerve conduction in patients with diabetes mellitus and controls. *Neurology, 11,* 876.

FAJANS, S. S. and CONN, J. W. (1960): Tolbutamide-induced improvement in carbohydrate tolerance of young people with mild diabetes mellitus. *Diabetes, 9,* 83.

FELDMAN, R. and CRAWFORD, D. (1970): Prophylactic use of oral hypoglycemic drugs in asymptomatic diabetes. In: *Early Diabetes,* pp. 443–448. Editors: R. Camerini-Dávalos and H. S. Cole. Academic Press, New York, N.Y.

FELDMAN, R. and FITTERER, D. (1967): Prophylactic use of oral hypoglycemic drugs in asymptomatic diabetes. In: *Tolbutamide – After 10 Years,* pp. 243–254. Editors: W. J. H. Butterfield and W. Van Westering. International Congress Series No. 149, Excerpta Medica, Amsterdam.

FELDMAN, R., CRAWFORD, D., ELASHOFF, R. and GLASS, A (1973): Progress report on the prophylactic use of oral hypoglycemic drugs in asymptomatic diabetes: neurovascular studies. In: *Vascular and Neurological Changes in Early Diabetes,* pp. 557–567. Editors: R. A. Camerini-Dávalos and H. S. Cole. Academic Press, New York and London.

GUNN. G. C., DOBSON, H. L., GRAY, T., GEDDES, L. A. and VALLBONA, C. (1965): Studies of pulse wave velocity in potentially diabetic subjects. *Diabetes, 14,* 489.

KATZ, H. P., CHEITLIN, M. D., WASSER, A. H. and FLAIR R. C. (1970): Observations on the pulse wave velocity and tissue biopsy in children with diabetes mellitus. *Johns Hopkins Med. J., 127,* 336.

KNATTERUD, G. L., MEINERT, C. L., KLINT, C. R., OSBORNE, R. K. and MARTIN, D. B. (1971): Effects of hypoglycemic agents on vascular complications in patients with adult-onset diabetes. IV. A preliminary report on phenformin results. *J. Amer. med. Ass., 217,* 777.

LAWRENCE, D. G. and LOCKE, S. (1961): Motor nerve conduction velocity in diabetes. *Arch. Neurol., 5,* 483.

UNIVERSITY GROUP DIABETES PROGRAM (1970): A study of the effects of hypoglycemic agents on vascular complications in patients with adult-onset diabetes. *J. Amer. Diabetes Ass., 19/Suppl. 2,* 747.

WOOLAM, G. L., SCHNUR, P. L., VALLBONA, C. and HOFF, H. E. (1962): The pulse wave velocity as an early indicator of atherosclerosis in diabetic subjects. *Circulation, 25,* 533.

TOLBUTAMIDE AND ARTERIAL DISEASE IN BORDERLINE DIABETICS

H. KEEN, R. J. JARRETT and J. H. FULLER

Unit for Metabolic Medicine, Department of Medicine, Guy's Hospital Medical School, London, United Kingdom

The evidence relating to the effects of tolbutamide on the vascular accompaniments of diabetes in man is conflicting. On the one hand, there is the assertion of the University Group Diabetes Program (U.G.D.P.) that the risk of cardiovascular death may be increased in adult, asymptomatic maturity-onset diabetics treated with the agent (U.G.D.P., 1970). On the other is our own earlier finding, in a somewhat different setting, that the manifestations of arterial disease may be lessened by the administration of tolbutamide (Keen et al., 1968; Keen and Jarrett, 1970). Many of the other contributions to this controversy are difficult to interpret, since they are based on retrospective observations made in diabetic patients assigned to one or other form of treatment, not randomly, but because of some characteristic of their disease. In such cases it is not possible to distinguish the effects of treatment from the forms of the disease for which the treatment was given. There are, however, 3 other long-term studies in which people have been randomly assigned to different treatments, including tolbutamide (Paasikivi, 1970; Feldman et al., 1973; Carlstrom et al., 1971). In general the results of these studies have been more comparable to ours than to the U.G.D.P.

We have made analyses of our data on 2 occasions since our study started in April 1962, one after 5 and the other after 7 years of treatment (Keen et al., 1968; Keen and Jarrett, 1970). On both occasions there was a lower rate of arterial events in the group receiving tolbutamide than in the placebo-treated group. In neither case was there any excess of total or of cardiovascular mortality in tolbutamide-treated subjects. This comparison has been repeated at 8½ years up to 1st January 1971, and forms the substance of the present communication. This 8½ year analysis is presented in 2 forms. The first is similar to our first analysis, that is to say it compares (using the chi-square test of significance) the accumulated number of individuals affected by arterial events in the group of subjects assigned to tolbutamide with that of those assigned to placebo. It further seeks systematically to locate any particular group of individuals in whom a difference between these 'treatments' may be concentrated; and it groups individuals by the type (and combinations of types) of arterial event sustained to see if any particular form (or combination of forms) of arterial disease is more or less susceptible to treatment.

A second, considerably more rigorous analytical approach uses the Logrank test procedure (Peto and Pike, 1973), which is a form of life-table analysis in which cumulative comparisons of event rates can be made for the various treatment groups. The Logrank test can be shown to be the best available test of significance for this type of data and is suitable for the comparative analysis in clinical trials of various 'treatments' of time to death or time to other non-fatal events. Among its advantages are that 'censored' data can be dealt with easily, that is, the method can allow for subjects dropping out of the trial at various time points through death, default or for any other reason. Also, no distributional assumptions are necessary with this method.

MATERIALS AND METHODS

The derivation of the study population has been described in previous communications. In brief, it consists of 248 borderline diabetics, 228 of whom were identified in a large-scale population screening programme for diabetics in 1962 (Sharp et al., 1964) and 20 of whom were recruited by comparable techniques over the subsequent 15 months from participants in a glaucoma screening survey in Bedford in the course of a study of the prevalence of glaucoma in the same community (Wright, 1966). After exclusion of previously known diabetics and persons with metabolic disorders, the sole defining criterion for recruitment to the trial was a capillary blood sugar exceeding 119 mg/dl and less than 200 mg/dl, 2 hours after a 50 g oral glucose load. The subjects were recruited to a long-term double blind therapeutic trial of tolbutamide (half with and half without accompanying dietary carbohydrate restriction) 0.5 g twice daily, versus placebo (with or without carbohydrate restriction) 1 tablet twice daily, each placebo tablet containing 0.003 g tolbutamide.

Efforts have been made to review each subject at 6-monthly intervals. At each review a series of pre-arranged standardized examinations was conducted. Those examinations concerning the cardiovascular system, from which the present analysis stems, are tabulated in Table 1, together with the various 'event combinations' used in the analysis. The W.H.O. cardiovascular questionnaire (Rose and Blackburn, 1968) was used to identify symptomatic arterial disease. Resting electrocardiograms were read independently by 2 'Minnesota coders', conflicts being reconciled by a third observer. Failure of a subject to attend for follow up examination was exhaustively investigated. When the reason was illness or death, hospital records and/or death certificates were obtained. Major illnesses reported between periodic visits were also investigated by correspondence with hospital and/or general practitioner. All interrogations and examinations were conducted in ignorance of the nature of the treatment which the subject was receiving.

SUBGROUPINGS

In the present analysis subjects have been grouped by (1) age (those under 60 years of age at entry into trial; those aged 60 years or more at entry), (2) sex, (3) tertile of 'diagnostic' blood sugar level (the diagnostic blood sugar was taken as the arithmetic mean of the 2 hour blood sugar measured at the survey and that measured at the first follow up clinic visit before treatment had been initiated), and (4) tertile of ponderal index (height/weight $^{-1/3}$) measured at the survey. The cutting points which separate the distributions of blood sugar and ponderal index into 3 numerically equal segments (tertiles) are shown in Table 2. The number of subjects in the placebo/tolbutamide comparisons and their baseline characteristics, subdivided into age and sex groups and ponderal index tertiles, is

TABLE 1
Cardiovascular events and event combinations used as end-points in the placebo/tolbutamide comparisons

Cardiovascular death (Cv. Dth)	Death attributed primarily to a cardiovascular cause using hospital records and/or death certificates
Coronary death (Cor. Dth)	Myocardial infarction, coronary thrombosis or sudden death
ECG event (ECG)	Development of Q/qs changes, depression of S-T segments or T wave changes (Minnesota code) compared with baseline ECG
Angina Infarct Claudication Stroke	Onset assessed by standard questionnaire
Ang/Inf	Onset of angina *or* infarct
Ang/Inf/ECG	Onset of ang/inf *or* ECG event
Ang/Inf/Cor. Dth	Onset of ang/inf *or* coronary death
Ang/Inf/Cor. Dth/ECG	Onset of ang/inf/Cor. Dth *or* ECG event
Cv. event/Cv. Dth	Onset of angina *or* infarct *or* claudication *or* stroke *or* cardiovascular death
Cv. event/Cv. Dth/ECG	Onset of Cv. event/Cv. Dth *or* ECG event

TABLE 2
Definition of blood sugar and ponderal index tertiles

Blood sugar (mg/dl)		Male	Female
	BST 1	<125	<123
	BST 2	125–147	123–149
	BST 3	$\geqslant 148$	$\geqslant 150$
Ponderal index			
	PIT 1	<11.95	<11.43
	PIT 2	11.95–12.39	11.43–12.09
	PIT 3	$\geqslant 12.40$	$\geqslant 12.10$

TABLE 3*

Baseline characteristics by age, sex, ponderal index tertiles and treatment groups

	Age				Sex				Ponderal index tertile							
	Age < 60 yr		Age ⩾ 60 yr		Male		Female		PIT 1		PIT 2		PIT 3		Total	
	(n=61) Plac	(n=74) Tolb	(n=64) Plac	(n=49) Tolb	(n=68) Plac	(n=61) Tolb	(n=57) Plac	(n=62) Tolb	(n=38) Plac	(n=43) Tolb	(n=45) Plac	(n=36) Tolb	(n=42) Plac	(n=42) Tolb	(n=125) Plac	(n=123) Tolb
Mean entry age (yr)	45.7	46.6	70.8	68.6	56.4	54.1	61.1	56.6	60.8	57.9	56.6	55.6	58.6	52.0	58.5	55.4
(± S.E.)	(± 1.27)	(± 1.16)	(± 0.88)	(± 0.90)	(± 1.82)	(± 1.71)	(± 2.01)	(± 1.82)	(± 2.34)	(± 1.52)	(± 2.17)	(± 2.30)	(± 2.55)	(± 2.55)	(± 1.36)	(± 1.25)
Mean entry blood sugar (mg/dl)	134.9	136.0	146.4	143.4	141.9	138.7	139.5	139.2	144.4	139.8	143.7	137.0	134.4	139.2	140.8	139.0
(± S.E.)	(± 2.83)	(± 3.28)	(± 3.31)	(± 3.18)	(± 3.15)	(± 3.29)	(± 3.18)	(± 3.40)	(± 4.39)	(± 3.95)	(± 3.71)	(± 4.32)	(± 3.48)	(± 4.22)	(± 2.24)	(± 2.36)
Mean entry ponderal index	12.06	12.06	11.97	11.92	12.27	12.14	11.71	11.88	11.30	11.25	11.98	11.99	12.71	12.79	12.02	12.00
(± S.E.)	(± 0.08)	(±0.08)	(± 0.09)	(± 0.13)	(± 0.08)	(± 0.08)	(± 0.07)	(± 0.11)	(± 0.05)	(± 0.06)	(± 0.04)	(± 0.05)	(± 0.08)	(± 0.07)	(± 0.06)	(± 0.07)
% smoking ⩾ 15 cigarettes per day @ entry	13.1	13.5	7.8	4.1	14.7	18.0	5.3	1.6	7.9	9.3	11.1	11.1	11.9	9.5	10.4	9.8
% Arterial disease @ entry	6.6	6.8	17.2	20.4	11.8	14.8	12.3	9.7	13.2	7.0	11.1	16.7	11.9	11.9	12.0	12.2
% Hypertension @ entry	13.1	13.5	23.4	40.8	11.8	11.5	26.3	37.1	13.2	30.2	26.7	22.2	14.3	21.4	18.4	24.4
% Females	36.1	45.9	54.7	57.1	–	–	–	–	50.0	46.5	48.9	47.2	38.1	59.5	45.6	50.4

* The numbers and mean values shown differ from our previously published figures because of an earlier incorrect treatment group coding of 2 subjects which came to light during checking procedures for this analysis.

TABLE 4

Baseline characteristics by age, blood sugar tertiles and treatment

	Age < 60 yr						Age ⩾ 60 yr						All ages					
	BST 1		BST 2		BST 3		BST 1		BST 2		BST 3		BST 1		BST 2		BST 3	
	Plac (n=23)	Tolb (n=37)	Plac (n=21)	Tolb (n=17)	Plac (n=17)	Tolb (n=20)	Plac (n=13)	Tolb (n=11)	Plac (n=25)	Tolb (n=19)	Plac (n=26)	Tolb (n=19)	Plac (n=36)	Tolb (n=48)	Plac (n=46)	Tolb (n=36)	Plac (n=43)	Tolb (n=39)
Mean entry age (yr)	44.5	44.7	46.0	45.8	47.0	50.9	69.2	66.8	70.0	69.5	72.2	68.7	53.4	49.8	59.1	58.3	62.3	59.6
(± S.E.)	(± 1.73)	(± 1.67)	(± 2.33)	(± 2.64)	(± 2.76)	(± 1.74)	(± 1.81)	(± 1.68)	(± 1.54)	(± 1.34)	(± 1.29)	(± 1.64)	(± 2.37)	(± 1.90)	(± 2.23)	(± 2.45)	(± 2.32)	(± 1.87)
Mean entry blood sugar (mg/dl)	114.0	114.1	135.2	137.4	162.8	175.4	112.0	115.0	137.2	138.1	172.5	165.1	113.3	114.3	136.3	137.8	168.7	170.4
(± S.E.)	(± 1.83)	(± 1.07)	(± 1.58)	(± 1.74)	(± 3.50)	(± 4.24)	(± 2.68)	(± 2.01)	(± 1.60)	(± 1.76)	(± 3.15)	(± 3.43)	(± 1.50)	(± 0.94)	(± 1.12)	(± 1.22)	(± 2.44)	(± 2.84)
Mean entry ponderal index	12.11	12.12	12.00	12.16	12.09	11.85	12.08	11.92	11.94	11.91	11.94	11.93	12.10	12.07	11.97	12.03	12.00	11.89
(± S.E.)	(± 0.11)	(± 0.12)	(± 0.14)	(± 0.16)	(± 0.24)	(± 0.15)	(± 0.18)	(± 0.23)	(± 0.16)	(± 0.24)	(± 0.15)	(± 0.19)	(± 0.09)	(± 0.10)	(± 0.11)	(± 0.15)	(± 0.11)	(± 0.12)
% Smoking ⩾ 15 cigarettes per day @ entry	17.4	8.1	9.5	17.6	11.8	20.0	23.1	18.2	4.0	0.0	3.8	0.0	19.4	10.4	6.5	8.3	7.0	10.3
% Arterial disease @ entry	0.0	5.4	14.3	11.8	5.9	5.0	0.0	45.5	24.0	26.3	19.2	0.0	0.0	14.6	19.6	19.4	14.0	2.6
% Hypertension @ entry	21.7	5.4	0.0	17.6	17.6	25.0	23.1	54.5	24.0	26.3	23.1	47.4	22.2	16.7	13.0	22.2	20.9	35.9
% Females	47.8	48.7	28.6	41.2	29.4	45.0	53.8	45.5	60.0	57.9	50.0	63.2	50.0	47.9	45.7	50.0	41.7	53.8

shown in Table 3. Table 4 similarly shows the baseline characteristics for the subjects subdivided into age groups and blood sugar tertiles. In all the comparisons made, the numbers, frequencies and percentages refer to affected individuals and not to events; when combinations of events are used, they group those individuals sustaining one or another element of the combination as their first event. Thus, an individual developing angina pectoris will be assigned to the angina event class and will remain there, though he may later sustain a myocardial infarct, show electrocardiographic abnormality or die suddenly. In any event, an individual figures only once as a contributor to the tally of 'arterial disease' in any treatment group. In the results which follow, the dietary treatment subdivision has been ignored. Preliminary study of results suggested that it had no obvious effect in its own right nor was there any clear indication of interaction between diet and tolbutamide in respect of arterial events.

RESULTS

Simple comparison of event rates in tolbutamide and placebo groups

Comparability of tolbutamide and placebo subgroups at baseline Many variables, often termed 'risk-factors' are known to influence the chance of an arterial event (e.g. age, sex, blood pressure, degree of glucose intolerance, obesity, etc.). In simple comparisons of treatment groups therefore, one needs to ensure that differences apparently due to treatment are not in fact due to dissimilarity in the representation of such variables. Tables 3 and 4 enable comparisons to be made of the representation of the major risk factors recorded in the variety of groups and subgroups considered in the analyses.

Cardiovascular events in tolbutamide/placebo subgroups Table 5 shows the 8½ year incidence of deaths and cardiovascular events per 100 subjects at risk for the placebo- and tolbutamide-treated groups. In this Table the subjects are subdivided into age and sex groups and tertiles of ponderal index distribution. For the event combination angina *or* infarct *or* ECG event in the younger age group, 41% of 61 placebo-treated subjects were affected compared with 23% of 74 tolbutamide-treated subjects ($\chi^2 = 5.06$, $P < 0.05$). When correction for continuity is applied, the value for chi-square becomes 4.25 ($P < 0.05$). This difference was not due to age differences since the mean entry age for the tolbutamide-treated subjects in this subgroup was higher (46.6) than that for the placebo-treated group (45.7). That it was probably those younger subjects in the highest tertile of blood sugar distribution who contributed most to this difference is shown in Table 6, where the incidence of cardiovascular events per 100 subjects at risk is shown subdivided into age groups and blood sugar tertiles.

As is shown in Table 6, those tolbutamide-treated subjects in the youngest age group and highest blood sugar tertile had lower event rates than their placebo-treated counterparts in the following event combinations:

(i) Angina *or* infarct *or* ECG event ($\chi^2 = 9.74$, $P < 0.01$; continuity corrected $\chi^2 = 7.79$, $P < 0.01$);

(ii) Angina *or* infarct *or* coronary death *or* ECG event ($\chi^2 = 7.94$, $P < 0.01$; continuity corrected $\chi^2 = 6.19$, $P < 0.05$);

(iii) Cardiovascular event *or* cardiovascular death *or* ECG event ($\chi^2 = 4.98$, $P < 0.05$; continuity corrected $\chi^2 = 3.60$, N.S.).

TABLE 5

Incidence of cardiovascular events and combinations in placebo and tolbutamide groups by age, sex, ponderal index tertiles (PIT)
(Figures show percentage affected)

Cardiovascular events	Age				Sex				Ponderal index tertile							
	Age < 60 yr		Age ≥ 60 yr		Male		Female		PIT 1		PIT 2		PIT 3		Total	
	Plac (n=61)	Tolb (n=74)	Plac (n=64)	Tolb (n=49)	Plac (n=68)	Tolb (n=61)	Plac (n=57)	Tolb (n=62)	Plac (n=38)	Tolb (n=43)	Plac (n=45)	Tolb (n=36)	Plac (n=42)	Tolb (n=42)	Plac (n=125)	Tolb (n=123)
Death (all causes)	6.6	8.1	35.9	38.8	20.6	18.0	22.8	22.6	21.0	20.9	20.0	16.7	23.8	21.4	21.6	20.3
Cardiovascular death (Cv. Dth)	3.3	6.8	26.6	26.5	16.2	14.8	14.0	14.5	15.8	16.3	13.3	11.1	16.7	14.3	15.2	14.6
Coronary death (Cor. Dth)	0.0	5.4	14.1	12.2	7.4	9.8	7.0	6.4	5.3	11.6	8.9	2.8	7.1	9.5	7.2	8.1
ECG event (ECG)	26.2	17.6	17.2	20.4	23.5	24.6	19.3	12.9	15.8	25.6	26.7	11.1	21.4	16.7	21.6	18.7
Angina (Ang)	18.0	8.1	17.2	16.3	14.7	13.1	21.1	9.7	31.6	20.9	8.9	8.3	14.3	4.8	17.6	11.4
Infarct (Inf)	4.9	1.4	1.6	12.2	2.9	4.9	3.5	6.5	2.6	9.3	2.2	8.3	4.8	0.0	3.2	5.7
Claudication	0.0	9.5	4.7	4.1	1.5	8.2	3.5	6.5	2.6	11.6	2.2	5.6	2.4	4.8	2.4	7.3
Stroke	6.6	0.0	7.8	4.1	4.4	3.3	10.5	0.0	10.5	0.0	8.9	2.8	2.4	2.4	7.2	16.3
Ang/Inf	21.3	9.4	17.2	22.4	16.2	14.8	22.8	14.5	31.6	23.2	11.1	16.7	16.7	4.8	19.2	14.6
Ang/Inf/ECG	41.0	23.0*	28.1	34.7	32.4	27.9	36.8	27.4	39.5	39.5	33.3	22.2	31.0	19.0	34.4	27.6
Ang/Inf/Cor. Dth	21.3	13.5	31.2	34.7	23.5	23.0	29.8	21.0	36.8	34.9	20.0	19.4	23.8	11.9	26.4	22.0
Ang/Inf/Cor. Dth/ECG	41.0	25.7	42.2	44.9	39.7	36.1	43.8	30.6	44.7	46.5	42.2	25.0	38.1	26.2	41.6	33.3
Cv. event/ Cv. Dth	27.9	17.6	51.6	53.1	33.8	32.8	47.4	30.6	57.9	41.9	31.1	30.6	33.3	21.4	40.0	31.7
Cv. event/Cv. Dth/ ECG	45.9	29.7	59.4	63.3	48.5	45.9	57.9	40.3	63.2	53.5	48.9	36.1	47.6	35.7	52.8	43.1

* $P < 0.05$ for chi-square test with one degree of freedom.

TABLE 6

Incidence of cardiovascular events and combinations in placebo and tolbutamide groups by blood sugar tertiles (BST) within age groups (Figures show percentage affected)

Cardiovascular events	Age < 60 yr						Age ≥ 60 yr						All ages					
	BST 1		BST 2		BST 3		BST 1		BST 2		BST 3		BST 1		BST 2		BST 3	
	Plac (n=23)	Tolb (n=37)	Plac (n=21)	Tolb (n=17)	Plac (n=17)	Tolb (n=25)	Plac (n=13)	Tolb (n=11)	Plac (n=25)	Tolb (n=19)	Plac (n=26)	Tolb (n=19)	Plac (n=36)	Tolb (n=48)	Plac (n=46)	Tolb (n=36)	Plac (n=43)	Tolb (n=39)
Death (all causes)	8.7	0.0	9.5	11.8	0.0	20.0	27.3	27.3	32.0	47.4	46.2	36.8	13.9	6.2	21.7	30.6	27.9	28.2
Cardiovascular death (Cv. Dth)	4.3	0.0	4.8	11.8	0.0	15.0	15.4	27.3	28.0	31.6	30.8	21.1	8.3	6.2	17.4	22.2	18.6	17.9
Coronary death (Cor. Dth)	0.0	0.0	0.0	11.8	0.0	10.0	7.7	18.2	16.0	15.8	15.4	5.3	2.8	4.2	8.7	13.9	9.3	7.7
ECG event (ECG)	8.7	18.9	33.3	17.6	41.2	15.0	15.4	27.3	12.0	21.1	23.1	15.8	11.1	20.8	21.7	19.4	30.2	15.4
Angina (Ang)	13.0	2.7	9.5	17.6	35.3	10.0	23.1	9.1	20.0	15.8	11.5	21.1	16.7	4.2	15.2	16.7	20.9	15.4
Infarct (Inf)	0.0	0.0	9.5	5.9	5.9	0.0	7.7	18.2	0.0	5.3	0.0	15.8	2.8	4.2	4.3	5.6	2.3	7.7
Claudication	0.0	0.0	0.0	23.5	0.0	15.0	0.0	9.1	8.0	5.3	3.8	0.0	0.0	2.1	4.3	13.9	2.3	7.7
Stroke	4.3	0.0	9.5	0.0	5.9	0.0	0.0	9.1	4.0	0.0	15.4	5.3	2.8	2.1	6.5	0.0	11.6	2.6
Ang/Inf	13.0	2.7	19.0	23.5	35.3	10.0	23.1	27.3	20.0	15.8	11.5	26.3	16.7	8.3	19.6	19.4	20.9	17.9
Ang/Inf/ECG	17.4	21.6	38.1	23.5	76.5	25.0**	30.8	45.5	24.0	31.6	30.8	31.6	22.2	27.1	30.4	27.8	48.8	28.2
Ang/Inf/Cor. Dth	13.0	2.7	19.0	29.4	35.3	20.0	30.8	45.5	36.0	31.6	26.9	31.6	19.4	12.5	28.3	30.6	30.2	25.6
Ang/Inf/Cor. Dth/ ECG	17.4	21.6	38.1	29.4	76.5	30.0**	38.5	63.6	40.0	42.1	46.2	36.8	25.0	31.2	39.1	36.1	58.1	33.3*
Cv. event/Cv. Dth	21.7	2.7*	28.6	35.3	35.3	30.0	38.5	72.7	56.0	52.6	53.8	42.1	27.8	18.8	43.5	44.4	46.5	35.9
Cv. event/Cv. Dth/ ECG	26.1	21.6	42.8	35.3	76.5	40.0*	46.2	90.9*	60.0	63.2	65.4	47.4	33.3	37.5	52.2	50.0	69.8	43.6*

* $P < 0.05$
** $P < 0.01$ for chi-square test with one degree of freedom.

TABLE 7
Numbers of subjects excluded from the trial by age group, treatment category and reason for exclusion

	Age < 60 yr		Age ⩾ 60 yr		Total	
Reason for exclusion	Plac (n=61)	Tolb (n=74)	Plac (n=64)	Tolb (n=49)	Plac (n=125)	Tolb (n=123)
1. Became diabetic*	5 (8.2%)	6 (8.1%)	5 (7.8%)	5 (10.2%)	10 (8.0%)	11 (8.9%)
2. Emigrated	2 (3.3%)	3 (4.1%)	2 (3.1%)	0 (0.0%)	4 (3.2%)	3 (2.4%)
3. Uncooperative	0 (0.0%)	4 (5.4%)	1 (1.6%)	1 (2.0%)	1 (0.8%)	5 (4.1%)

* Criteria used in assigning a subject to the 'diabetic' category:
(1) 2-hour blood sugar ⩾ 200 mg/dl on 2 consecutive visits;
(2) 2-hour blood sugar ⩾ 200 mg/dl on 3 non-consecutive visits;
(3) 2-hour blood sugar ⩾ 200 mg/dl on one visit plus clear clinical signs or symptoms of diabetes (e.g. diabetic ketoacidosis).

For the latter 2 event combinations, (ii) and (iii), the tolbutamide-treated group still retained an advantage compared to the placebo group when all ages were considered in the upper blood sugar tertile ($P < 0.05$ for the uncorrected and for the continuity-corrected chi-square test). For the younger subjects in the lowest blood sugar tertile, Table 6 also shows an advantage for the tolbutamide-treated group for the event combination cardiovascular event *or* cardiovascular death ($\chi^2 = 5.71$, $P < 0.05$, continuity corrected $\chi^2 = 3.79$, N.S.).

The only comparison which shows a significant advantage for the placebo-treated group is for the event combination cardiovascular event *or* cardiovascular death *or* ECG event for the older age group with the lowest blood sugar tertile (Table 6) ($\chi^2 = 5.73$, $P < 0.05$; continuity corrected $\chi^2 = 3.56$, N.S.). However, from Table 2 it can be seen that the tolbutamide-treated subjects in this subgrouping had a much higher prevalence of arterial disease and hypertension at baseline than their placebo-treated counterparts.

Analysis using Logrank test procedure Using the Logrank test procedure, a cumulative comparison between the placebo- and tolbutamide-treated groups has been made using as end-points the various events and event combinations described above for the single time-point chi-square analysis. With this procedure, subjects become excluded from the cumulative comparison once they suffer the particular event or combination being considered, as soon as they 'become diabetic' or from the time that they default from follow-up (Table 7). This method of dealing with 'censored' data causes rapid reductions in the numbers 'at risk' as time advances and is the reason why the Logrank method is much more rigorous than the single time-point method of chi-square comparison, which retains the full number of 'starters'.

TABLE 8

Logrank analysis of placebo/tolbutamide comparisons for cardiovascular events and combinations by age, sex, ponderal index tertile and blood sugar tertile

		Age		Sex		Ponderal index tertile			Blood sugar tertile			χ^2 for treatment effect	Total
		$<$ 60 yr	$\geqslant$ 60 yr	Male	Female	1	2	3	1	2	3		
ardiovascular	O/E (Tolb)	1.28	1.01	0.87	1.11	1.08	0.91	0.88	0.89	1.17	0.97	1.02	0.99
ath	χ^2	0.52	0.00	0.29	0.20	0.08	0.07	0.16	0.10	0.30	0.02	0.01	0.01
v. Dth)	χ^2 (corr)	0.10	0.02	0.09	0.04	0.00	0.00	0.01	0.01	0.07	0.02	0.00	0.01
oronary	O/E (Tolb)	1.90	0.96	1.03	1.11	1.53	0.45	1.03	1.18	1.32	0.89	1.10	1.07
ath	χ^2	2.71	0.01	0.01	0.10	2.03	1.18	0.01	0.13	0.56	0.08	0.17	0.09
or. Dth)	χ^2 (corr)	1.14	0.02	0.05	0.00	1.03	0.40	0.11	0.05	0.13	0.01	0.03	0.00
	O/E (Tolb)	0.69	1.10	0.98	0.76	0.82	1.26	0.46	0.71	1.13	0.81	0.92	0.86
ng/Inf	χ^2	2.05	0.17	0.01	1.24	0.88	0.49	2.41	1.06	0.18	0.54	0.22	0.78
	χ^2 (corr)	1.45	0.03	0.02	0.79	0.51	0.13	1.48	0.50	0.03	0.22	0.09	0.52
	O/E (Tolb)	0.82	1.12	0.96	0.90	1.01	0.83	0.77	1.11	1.11	0.68	0.97	0.93
ng/Inf	χ^2	1.60	0.40	0.06	0.43	0.01	0.48	1.14	0.37	0.19	3.77	0.05	0.43
CG	χ^2 (corr)	1.20	0.20	0.01	0.23	0.01	0.20	0.70	0.14	0.04	3.02	0.01	0.29
	O/E (Tolb)	0.86	1.05	1.00	0.85	0.97	0.97	0.69	0.82	1.20	0.84	0.98	0.92
g/Inf	χ^2	0.51	0.06	0.00	0.70	0.02	0.01	1.37	0.53	0.63	0.60	0.02	0.33
r. Dth	χ^2 (corr)	0.25	0.00	0.03	0.42	0.00	0.03	0.83	0.20	0.33	0.31	0.00	0.20
	O/E (Tolb)	0.87	1.05	0.98	0.88	1.06	0.75	0.83	1.12	1.12	0.68	0.97	0.93
g/Inf	χ^2	0.82	0.08	0.03	0.64	0.17	1.32	0.85	0.49	0.31	4.48*	0.06	0.47
r. Dth/ECG	χ^2 (corr)	0.55	0.02	0.00	0.40	0.05	0.87	0.52	0.24	0.13	3.74	0.02	0.33
	O/E (Tolb)	0.84	1.01	0.99	0.81	0.81	1.03	0.81	0.84	1.11	0.82	0.96	0.90
. Ev. Dth	χ^2	0.82	0.00	0.00	1.83	1.88	0.01	0.78	0.68	0.34	1.09	0.13	0.94
	χ^2 (corr)	0.52	0.01	0.01	1.43	1.45	0.00	0.45	0.35	0.17	0.74	0.06	0.74
	O/E (Tolb)	0.87	1.03	0.99	0.85	0.92	0.86	0.89	1.07	1.11	0.70	0.97	0.92
. Ev. Dth	χ^2	0.94	0.06	0.00	1.51	0.44	0.59	1.54	0.22	0.35	4.93*	0.10	0.83
CG	χ^2 (corr)	0.66	0.01	0.01	1.18	0.25	0.33	1.30	0.08	0.18	4.24*	0.05	0.66

E (Tolb) = ratio of observed to expected events in tolbutamide group;
= overall chi-square (one degree of freedom);
(corr) = chi-square corrected for continuity;
ndicates values of chi-square for which $P < 0.05$.
e chi-square for treatment effect makes an adjustment for the effects of age, sex and
eline blood sugar.

Table 8 shows the values of chi-square (for one degree of freedom) for the various event combinations comparing placebo- with tolbutamide-treated subjects using the Logrank procedure. As before, subanalyses have been performed within age, sex, blood sugar and ponderal index groupings. For subjects in the upper blood sugar tertile, there appears to be a significant advantage for the tolbutamide-treated group when we consider the event combination cardiovascular event *or* cardiovascular death *or* ECG event ($\chi^2 = 4.93$, $P < 0.05$) and the combination angina/infarct/coronary death/ECG change ($\chi^2 = 4.48$, $P < 0.05$). Only the first of these comparisons retains the 5% level of significance when correction for continuity is made.

We have also evaluated the various event combinations in age, sex and baseline blood sugar categories using the 'chi-square test for treatment effect' (Table 8). Conventional levels of significance are not reached, but 75% of the observed/expected ratios show an advantage to tolbutamide.

DISCUSSION

The findings of this most recent analysis of the Bedford data are compatible with our conclusions drawn from previous analyses. Simple chi-square analysis, made at a fixed point in time, gives stronger support to the hypothesis that tolbutamide exerts some protective action against arterial events than the more rigorous Logrank procedure. However, even this latter approach provides some evidence for the hypothesis and none against it.

In assessing the validity of the previous evidence several objections must be considered. We have, as in previous analyses, pooled a number of different manifestations of vascular disease, ranging from codable ECG items on the one hand, to death, certified as cardiovascular, on the other. We accept that there are differences in degree amounting almost to differences in kind between these 'events', but consider that the underlying process leading to them is similar and gives some sanction to the pooling process. There are many studies which confirm the grave prognostic import of ECG changes of even lesser degree. Our analysis of the individual component events has ruled out the theoretical possibility that, although 2 groups might be similar in number of total events, in one group they might consist predominantly of deaths and in the other of symptomless ECG changes. Further sanction for the use of 'soft' end-points like symptoms or ECG changes can be derived from the double-blind nature of the trial which denies the observer the opportunity for bias in his judgement of the event. The use of validated questionnaires also confers increased objectivity in the record of subjective complaints.

The availability of many end-points provides an opportunity for selective presentation of those combinations favouring the hypothesis (and, per contra, suppression of those which refute it). We have tried to meet this objection by listing all the groupings we have tested, without selection. A further objection to this form of 'multiple analysis' is that, if enough comparisons are made, simply by chance some of them would achieve technical significance at the 1 in 20 level. The likelihood that a difference is 'real' rather than generated by 'chance' can only be assessed by exercising non-statistical judgements and these must be to some extent dependent upon prior experience and 'common sense'. No great security can be drawn from the fact that several comparisons showed differences which achieved statistical significance, for most of the comparisons were not independent one of the other and contained common elements.

TABLE 9
Deaths in tolbutamide- and placebo-treated subjects (to January 1st, 1971)

	Placebo			Tolbutamide		
	Male	Female	Total	Male	Female	Total
Number at risk of death	68	57	125	61	62	123
Cardiovascular causes						
Myocardial infarction	5	4	9	6	4	10
Sudden death	0	0	0	0	0	0
Other heart disease	2	2	4	2	2	4
Extracardiac vascular disease	4	2	6	1	3	4
All cardiovascular causes	11	8	19	9	9	18
Noncardiovascular causes						
Cancer	2	2	4	1	2	3
Other causes	1	3	4	1	3	4
All causes	14	13	27	11	14	25
Percent dead from:						
Cardiovascular	16.2	14.0	15.2	14.8	14.5	14.6
All causes	20.6	22.8	21.6	18.0	22.6	20.3

Since serious assertions have been made about an increased rate of cardiovascular mortality in tolbutamide- compared with placebo-treated diabetics (U.G.D.P., 1970), we have paid special attention to this single end-point. Table 9 shows the mortality experience of the 2 Bedford treatment groups analysed and laid out in a manner as like that of the U.G.D.P. presentation as possible. Cumulative mortality comparisons have been published elsewhere (Keen et al., 1973). Neither give any indication of differences between groups in respect of mortality. No support for a lethal influence of oral antidiabetic drugs comes from the more indirect evidence derived from a cohort of Birmingham diabetics (Fitzgerald and Malins, 1973). The standardised mortality ratio of these diabetics, computed from the regional non-diabetic population, has shown a progressive fall over the successive quinquennia from 1946. The British national mortality data, quoted by Reid and Grimley Evans (1970), show a rise in mortality from diabetes in certain age groups. However, as Warren and Corfield (1973) have suggested, a rise in deaths from diagnosed myocardial infarction among diabetics would actually lead to a *fall* in deaths classified to diabetes. The rise in death rates attributed to diabetes could thus be presented as evidence of a *diminished* susceptibility to coronary death! National mortality statistics, however, are of doubtful validity. Diabetes is often not mmentioned on the death certificate (Lancaster and Maddox, 1958) and the data need to be interpreted in conjunction with diabetes incidence rates, which are never known with any accuracy.

Our study has not demonstrated a beneficial effect of tolbutamide upon mortality. Apart from the immediate and unquestioned effect of the substance on certain diabetic symptoms, its putative benefits may therefore be upon cardiovascular morbidity. Other studies give some support to this view, notably those of Carlstrom et al. (1971, 1973) in Lund, Sweden, those of Feldman et al. (1973) in San Francisco and even those of the U.G.D.P. The study of Carlstrom et al. is similar to the Bedford study, though with some differences in design and in numbers. The subjects in the continuing trial of Feldman et al. were also derived from screening a normal population group. Table 13 of the U.G.D.P. publication on tolbutamide (1970) indicates a lower frequency of ECG changes in tolbutamide- compared with placebo-treated diabetics, though more detailed data have not yet been published.

What several of these studies have in common is that they took as their experimental subjects individuals with lesser degrees of glucose intolerance ('borderline' or 'chemical' diabetics), usually asymptomatic and often coming to light (as in the case of the Bedford group) as a result of a screening programme. It is possible that the response to tolbutamide may be different in subjects with slighter (or earlier) degrees of abnormality by comparison with diabetics with more usual clinical onset and probably with more severe (or longer lasting) disturbance of metabolism. Indeed, the experimental studies of Reaven and co-workers (Reaven and Miller, 1968; Reaven and Farquhar, 1969) and others (Chiles and Tzagournis, 1970; Seltzer et al., 1967) have suggested that the kinetics of the glucose-insulin relationship are quite different in these 2 classes. This may account for the different findings of Paasikivi (1970). The subjects of his study were found to be carbohydrate intolerant only by systematic testing and are therefore more like the Bedford/Lund/San Francisco type of population. The possibility must also be considered that the fundamental nature of the disturbance in 'borderline' diabetics differs in kind rather than degree from that in the maturity-onset diabetic subjected to clinical trial in the U.G.D.P.

Much further analytical work remains to be done with our Bedford group. Explanations for differences between the treatment groups will be sought in detail in the differential behaviour of blood sugar, body weight, blood pressure etc. during the course of the trial. A detailed analysis of this nature at the 10-year time point is in preparation and will be published elsewhere.

CONCLUSION

The influence of tolbutamide on arterial disease in a group of borderline diabetics had been made after 8½ years of treatment. Two methods of analysis, one a simple chi-square analysis of event rates at a given point in time, the other a Logrank procedure which gives a cumulative comparison of the experience of unaffected members of the groups with time, have been used. For both types of analysis, treatment effects have been sought in specified subsets of the experimental subjects and against various elements and combinations of elements of arterial disease.

Neither form of analysis indicated the existence of a statistically significant, untoward influence of tolbutamide. In certain subgroupings, a beneficent influence of tolbutamide in respect of arterial disease events was suggested. Subsidiary analysis showed that this apparently protective effect, shown principally in those aged less than 60 at recruitment to the trial and falling into the upper third of the distribution of diagnostic blood sugars, could not be attributed to maldistribution of other 'risk' factors such as age, blood pressure or smoking habits, between groups. No obvious explanation was forthcoming to explain the differences in the apparent effects of tolbutamide between our Bedford Group and the U.G.D.P., though this may be due to differences in the populations studied, to the different drug dosage employed or simply to chance.

ACKNOWLEDGEMENTS

We remain indebted to many helpers at Bedford and, of course, to the subjects of the follow-up study who have cooperated so willingly. Mr. R. Peto, Dr. M. Pike and Mrs. D. Bull have advised us on the use of the Logrank analysis and have kindly allowed us to use their computer program. The Borderline Diabetes Project is supported by a grant from the Department of Health and Social Security, London, United Kingdom.

REFERENCES

CARLSTROM, S., LUNDQUIST, A., LUNDQUIST, I., NORDEN, A., SCHERSTEN, B. and WOLLMARK, G. (1971): Studies in subjects with positive postprandial Clinistix test. *Acta med. scand., 189,* 415.

CHILES, R. and TZAGOURNIS, M. (1970): Excessive serum insulin response to oral glucose in obesity and mild diabetes. Study of 501 patients. *Diabetes, 19,* 458.

FELDMAN, R., CRAWFORD, C., ELASHOFF, R. and GLASS, A. (1973): In: *Vascular and Neurological Changes in Early Diabetes,* p. 557. Editors: R. A. Camerini-Davalos and H. S. Cole. Academic Press, New York – London.

FITZGERALD, M. G. and MALINS, J. M. (1973): Paper presented at: The Spring Meeting of the Medical and Scientific Section of the British Diabetic Association.

KEEN, H. and JARRETT, R. J. (1970): In: Atherosclerosis. Proceedings, II Symposium, p. 435. Editor: R. H. Jones. Springer-Verlag, New York N.Y.

KEEN, H., JARRETT, R. J., CHLOUVERAKIS, C. and BOYNS, D. R. (1968): The effect of treatment of moderate hyperglycaemia on the incidence of arterial disease. *Postgrad. med. J., 44,* 960.

KEEN, H., JARRETT, R. J., WARD, J. D. and FULLER, J. H. (1973): In: *Early Diabetes,* p. 571. Editors: R. A. Camerini-Davalos and H. S. Cole. Academic Press, New York – London.

LANCASTER, H. O. and MADDOX, J. K. (1958): *Aust. Ann. Med., 7,* 145.

PAASIKIVI, J. (1970): Long-term tolbutamide treatment after myocardial infarction. *Acta med. scand., Suppl. 507.*

PETO, R. and PIKE, M. C. (1973): Conservatism of the approximation $\Sigma(O\text{-}E)^2/E$ in the logrank test for survival data or tumor incidence data. *Biometrics, 29,* 579.

REAVEN, G. M. and FARQUHAR, J. W. (1969): Steady state plasma insulin response to continuous glucose infusion in normal and diabetic subjects. *Diabetes, 18,* 273.

REAVEN, G. M. and MILLER, R. (1968): Study of the relationship between glucose and insulin responses to an oral glucose load in man. *Diabetes, 17,* 560.

REID, D. D. and GRIMLEY EVANS, J. (1970): New drugs and changing mortality from non-infectious disease in England and Wales. *Brit. med. Bull., 26,* 191.

ROSE, G. A. and BLACKBURN, H. (1968): *Cardiovascular Survey Methods.* World Health Organization, Geneva.

8. Phase of recovery.

The relevant problems in biguanide research and in the clinical use of these drugs can be summarized as follows:

a. Three biguanide derivatives are in use as oral antidiabetics. Is there a prevalence for one of the three preparations?

b. Three theories about the mechanism of action of the blood sugar lowering effect by the biguanides are currently under discussion. Which one is the most convincing?

c. There are three possible indications for the clinical use of biguanides. When should biguanides preferentially be prescribed?

Although it is neither possible nor necessary to give here a complete discussion on the theory and practice of biguanide therapy, the above-mentioned questions should be considered.

PHENFORMIN – BUFORMIN – METFORMIN

Little can be said about the prevalence of the different biguanide preparations. From the literature (Beckmann, 1971), and from our own experience with all 3 biguanides (Mehnert, 1969) we can generally assume that phenformin, buformin and metformin, in spite of their different pharmacokinetics, do not present any significant differences regarding their blood sugar lowering effect and the underlying mechanism of action. The 3 biguanide preparations have a different potency but the same efficacy. Similar doses therefore cause a different blood sugar lowering effect which will be equalized by the fact that the stronger acting substances will only be tolerated in a smaller dose. The other biguanides may be tolerated in a larger dose without gastrointestinal side effects but the larger dose again is necessary for adequate lowering of the blood sugar. On the basis of an equal dose, tolerance of the drugs increases in the following sequence: phenformin – buformin –metformin. However, the blood sugar lowering effect diminishes in the same order. In the standard preparations the advantages and disadvantages offset each other and it has been impossible to prove without doubt that one preparation is superior to another. It is only certain that the introduction of long-acting preparations has improved the tolerance of these drugs, compared with the previous standard preparations.

Formerly, biguanides were often not prescribed because there were frequent gastrointestinal side effects. A change occurred through the restrictive recommendations of drug manufacturers. Thus low dosage was often prescribed which, although reducing the frequency of side effects, also impairs the therapeutical success. The individual tolerance of biguanide preparations is so different that a firm dosage scheme cannot be generally accepted. In rare cases 300 mg of phenethylbiguanide or 600 mg of butylbiguanide (or even higher doses) can be tolerated without any problems and will also be necessary for the desired effect (Mehnert, 1970). A trial of the biguanides should therefore not be curtailed too soon and the tolerance limit approached by slowly increasing the dose of the drug.

INVESTIGATIONS ON THE MECHANISM OF ACTION OF BIGUANIDES

The mode of action of the biguanides still remains unresolved. It is clear that the biguanides have an extra-pancreatic action and do not lower blood sugar by stimulating the secretion of endogenous insulin. There is no doubt that the biguanides lower the blood sugar in diabetics; but, as a rule it is not possible to produce hypoglycemia in a healthy person. Counterregulatory mechanisms which compensate for the blood sugar lowering effect could be the cause of this in normal subjects. Even in diabetics, there are no hypoglycemic reactions with biguanide treatment alone.

The following theories have been postulated for their mechanism of action: (1) inhibition of intestinal absorption, (2) increased peripheral utilisation of glucose, and (3) inhibition of hepatic glucose production (Beckmann, 1971; Mehnert, 1970; Mehnert and Haese, 1971). Studies in our own group (Dietze et al., 1973) were concerned with biguanide inhibition of hepatic gluconeogenesis in man. Studies with the isolated perfused rat liver indicate that biguanides may inhibit hepatic glucose synthesis (Beckmann, 1971; Söling, 1969), but there is no support that this is true for the human liver. Tranquada et al. (1960), who determined the liver blood flow and the arteriohepatic venous glucose differences, could not show any significant change in hepatic glucose output. The data of Searle et al. (1969) and Kreisberg et al. (1970) indicate that gluconeogenesis might even be stimulated under the influence of the biguanides. It seemed therefore important to reinvestigate this problem with an improved catheterization technique, which allows for simultaneous measurements of total liver blood flow and splanchnic substrate differences.

After pretreatment with 150 mg of phenformin per day for 5 days and a fasting period of 15 hours, 5 healthy volunteers underwent right hepatic vein catheterization. In addition a Cournand needle was inserted into the left femoral artery. Arterial and hepatic venous blood was sampled in 10-minute intervals during a control period and under the influence of lactate (0.03 mmoles/kg/min.). During each period the liver blood flow was calculated with a ^{133}Xenon inhalation technique developed in our laboratory. Five control subjects without phenformin medication underwent the same procedure.

Figure 2 summarizes our results and shows the hepatic glucose production of the controls and of the biguanide-treated subjects during a control period from 0 to 30

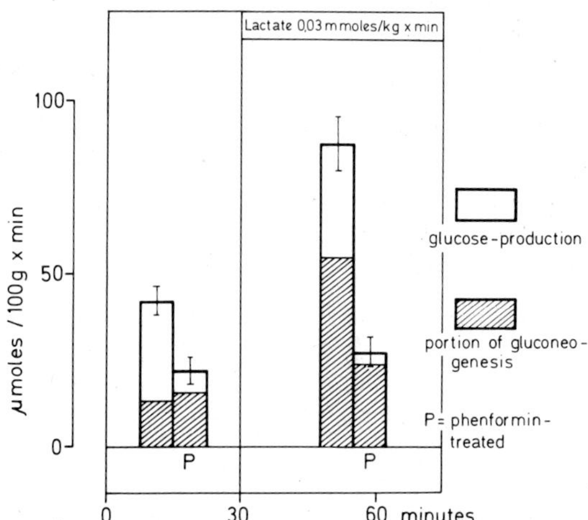

FIG. 2. Glucose production and estimated portions of glycogenolysis and gluconeogenesis during a basal period and lactate infusion in control and phenformin-treated healthy volunteers.

tion but is initiated on the basis of clinical criteria. Figure 4 shows our results. In contrast to Meinert and Schwartz, an initial reduction in body weight was only seen in 2 groups of patients: those on diet alone and those on biguanides. However, in the prospective study,

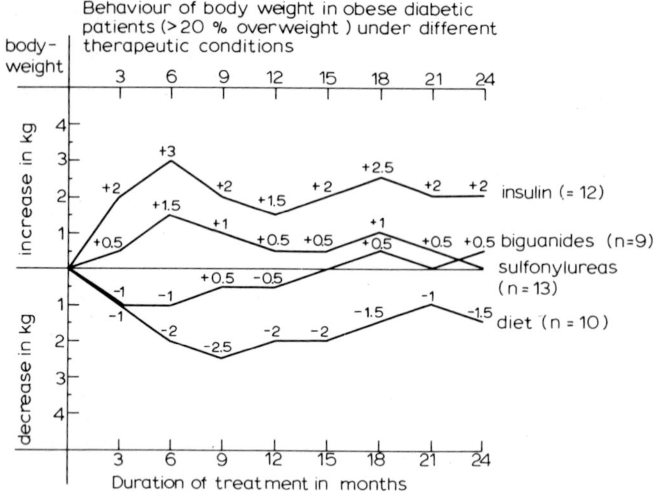

FIG. 4. Behaviour of body weight in obese diabetics (overweight > 20%) under different therapeutic conditions.

patients on insulin and sulfonylureas also lost weight. This difference can be easily explained: our overweight patients on insulin received insulin because they did not keep to their diet and could not be managed on oral drugs alone. Under insulin these, from a diet standpoint uncooperative patients, showed an increase in their body weight. Similar observations were made in patients treated with sulfonylureas, who should have been treated by diet alone, had they been fully cooperative. The diabetics on biguanides had been so treated also because of lack of cooperation, and the anorexigenic effect of these substances. Those patients who were on diet alone were the most successful because they were the most cooperative and therefore did not need any additional medications. It should be noted that these patients exhibit a small but constant rate of weight reduction over the whole period of observation, corresponding to the results of Meinert and Schwartz. The weight-reducing effect of the biguanides decreases with time, and towards the end of the test period the 2 treated groups are no longer different.

These observations surely indicate that the problem of weight reduction in overweight diabetics cannot be permanently solved by biguanide therapy.

Combined treatment of insulin and biguanides is still controversial. It is well to remember that many cases chosen for combined therapy are so unstable that they can hardly ever be stabilized whatever is done subsequently. Usually the biguanides are underdosed and are therefore not effective (Mehnert, 1970). Table 1 shows that 24-hour urine sugar in 10 insulin-treated unstable diabetics without change in insulin dosage is significantly reduced after additional therapy with 300–500 mg butylbiguanide. It is interesting to know that in the second control period, after the termination of biguanide therapy, there is still a better metabolic situation compared with the first control period.

The third form of biguanide treatment, the combination of biguanides and sulfon-

TABLE 1

24 hr urine glucose in 10 insulin-treated diabetics before, during and after additional therapy with 300–500 mg butylbiguanide without change in insulin dosage

	Mean urine glucose (g/24 hr) during 10-day periods		
Patient No.	Control period I	Test period	Control period II
1	33	15	30
2	72	12	10
3	17	20	21
4	64	43	52
5	55	7	18
6	15	10	28
7	50	43	32
8	27	5	10
9	31	17	18
10	19	11	21
Mean ± S.E.M.	38.3 ± 6.5	18.3 ± 4.3	24.0 ± 3.9
Difference, P	<0.02		>0.1

amides, which we described in 1958 (Mehnert and Seitz, 1958), should be the most widely used form of treatment with guanidine derivatives. Because of the different mechanism of action of the 2 compounds, combined oral therapy has a good theoretical basis and has been found useful for maturity-onset diabetes. There are no incompatibilities known among the 2 groups of compounds, and it is often possible to reduce the gastrointestinal side effects of biguanides with sulfonylureas since the biguanide dose can be reduced. Quite often it is the other way round: the sulfonylureas alone are not enough but the addition of biguanides brings about a further and often satisfactory lowering of the blood sugar.

SUMMARY

Phenformin, buformin and metformin have a different potency but the same efficacy. Also, regarding the mechanism of action, there are no known significant differences. Three theories are under discussion: (1) inhibition of intestinal absorption, (2) improved peripheral glucose utilisation, and (3) inhibition of gluconeogenesis. Our own studies in healthy volunteers showed that with usual doses of phenformin a significant reduction in gluconeogenesis can be found in the postabsorptive state, when an additional precursor such as lactate is infused.

Of all 3 indications for biguanide treatment, i.e., monotherapy, combination with insulin, and combination with sulfonylureas, the combined oral therapy is the most widely used and the one which has the best theoretical basis.

ADVERSE EFFECTS OF THE ORAL HYPOGLYCEMIC DRUGS

THADDEUS E. PROUT

Department of Medicine, Johns Hopkins Hospital, and Department of Medicine,
Greater Baltimore Medical Center, Baltimore, Md., U.S.A.

A serious look at clinical information available in 1959 failed to reveal any evidence based on controlled studies to demonstrate either that insulin or the oral agents were preventing long-term complications in diabetic patients. Stetten (1957), among others, had previously noted the developing widespread use of the sulfonylureas and had given a note of caution since the exact mode of action and the long-term effects of these drugs were not known. There was an obvious need to initiate a study in non-insulin dependent diabetics in which both insulin and oral agents could be tested against treatment with diet alone. For such a study to be useful, patients with non-insulin dependent diabetes of similar duration and severity had to be randomly allocated to various treatment groups to determine the degree to which we were truly influencing the prognosis and the development of complications in our diabetic patients. Thus began the long-term prospective controlled clinical trial on the efficacy of various methods of treatment of the diabetic that was called the University Group Diabetes Program (UGDP, 1970).

Much emphasis has been placed on the results of the UGDP relating to the evidence of adverse effects of both tolbutamide, as a representative of the sulfonylurea drugs, and of phenformin, as a representative of the biguanide drugs, but too little emphasis has been placed on the comparative effects of various degrees of control of diabetes on the development of complications. Observations on the effects of control on complications will continue in the UGDP at least through 1975, and additional data on this most important question will be forthcoming at a later time.

In looking at the long-term effects of the oral agents, based in part on the UGDP, it is essential to emphasize clinically important facts that should now be used in determining the use for these drugs in the long-term treatment of patients. Because many clinicians outside of the United States have not had an opportunity to discuss these facts in an open meeting with one of the members of the UGDP, I should like to anticipate some of the important clinical questions that have led clinicians to believe that the results of the UGDP were not applicable to their own patients and to answer them briefly. I hope that this will then bring us to a common understanding of the importance of the UGDP to clinical practice.

First, it has been asked whether patients in the UGDP had less severe diabetes than that for which use of oral agents are generally recommended. In answer to this, it is well to recall first that oral agents have been proposed for the treatment of minor abnormalities of glucose tolerance in order to prevent further deterioration of this disorder. Although the studies of the UGDP do not bear directly on this question, it may be stated inferentially that there is no evidence thus far that treatment of chemical diabetes or prediabetes is justified. Important studies have also been initiated on patients with borderline diabetes in the hope that the development of vascular complications in such patients might be prevented or postponed (Keen et al., 1968). These patients too are generally less severe than those studied in the UGDP. In addition, worldwide records of use of the oral agent make it abundantly clear that these medications are being given in a completely uncritical manner to a spectrum of patients that stretches from those with trivial blood glucose abnormalities to those clearly unresponsive to oral agents. In the middle of this spectrum, and quite closely identified with the group of patients for which these agents are commonly recommended, are to be found the patients of the UGDP.

The values for the sum of the fasting, 1-, 2-, and 3-hour blood glucose (SUM GTT) are shown in Table 1 and are compared with conventional glucose tolerance curves. Two-thirds of the patients had an average blood glucose value during the 3-hour glucose tolerance test of over 200 mg%. All but 6% of the patients had an average blood glucose above 170 mg%. The 6% of the patients below this level were equally distributed among the treatment groups, and their presence made it more difficult to show differences because of the dampening effect of this small group, but did not alter the conclusions of the study in any way. We may safely conclude that the UGDP studied a spectrum of patients most important to the practising clinician (Table 1).

TABLE 1

Baseline glucose tolerance test results for patients in the UGDP

SUM GTT	Representative glucose levels	% Patients
500	90–170–150–90	6
500–574	110–195–160–110	19
575–650	130–220–170–130	14
650	130–220–170–130	61

The sum of the fasting, 1-, 2-, and 3-hour postchallenge whole blood glucose level in mg/100 ml (SUM GTT) after an oral test utilizing 30 g of glucose/m^2 of body surface has been contrasted with representative blood glucose values for the 4 specimens. The percentage of patients in each SUM GTT group is shown (Berndt et al., 1970).

Second, it has been stated that only patients from the lowest economic strata were admitted to the study and that these results are therefore not applicable to the patients seen in private practice. In fact, there was a wide geographic representation of rural and urban people. Ethnic divisions included descendants from pioneer stock in the northwest United States, descendants of Scandinavia and Northern Europe in Minnesota and the midwest, a proportion of Jewish patients from the large cities, particularly New York, a virtually pure Anglo-Saxon strain from Appalachia as well as southern Negroes and Puerto

TABLE 2

Percent of patients with the first occurrence of a specified non-fatal event identified at a follow-up examination (denominators given in parentheses)

	PLBO	TOLB	ISTD	IVAR
Heart examination				
Significant ECG abnormality*	14.1 (198)	8.2 (196)	8.2 (195)	7.9 (190)
New use of digitalis	4.7 (190)	8.9 (180)	6.8 (190)	5.4 (184)
Hospitalized for heart disease	6.2 (194)	5.8 (190)	2.1 (190)	3.2 (187)
Hypertension†	36.8 (125)	44.4 (135)	41.3 (138)	44.3 (140)
Eye examination				
Visual acuity ⩽ 20/200 (either eye)	6.7 (179)	9.4 (181)	5.6 (179)	5.7 (175)
Opacity (vitreous, lens or corneal, either eye)	5.4 (149)	8.4 (155)	4.1 (146)	9.6 (146)
Fundus photo abnormalities excluding exudates**	38.9 (126)	40.0 (120)	43.5 (115)	37.3 (118)
Kidney examination				
Urine protein ⩾ 1 g/liter	0.5 (204)	2.5 (204)	0.0 (204)	2.0 (198)
Serum creatinine ⩾ 1.5 mg/100 ml	6.5 (184)	5.9 (188)	3.6 (192)	5.4 (186)
Peripheral vascular examination				
Amputation of all or part of either limb	1.0 (202)	0.0 (202)	0.0 (209)	0.0 (204)
Arterial calcification***	11.3 (168)	14.8 (155)	16.8 (161)	17.2 (157)
New intermittent claudication	8.2 (182)	14.8 (182)	11.1 (190)	10.0 (180)

* Major or minor Q-waves (codes 1-1-1 through 1-2-7), S-T depression (code 4-1), T-wave inversion (code 5-1), complete heart block (code 6-1), left bundle branch block (code 7-1), or ventricular tachycardia (code 8-1). All ECG's evaluated using the Minnesota Code (Chu et al., 1968).

** Readings of right central fundus photographs for one or more of the following abnormalities: retinal hemorrhages and microaneurysms, preretinal and vitreous hemorrhages, venous pathology, arterial pathology or proliferative changes and neovascularization.

*** Evidence of arterial calcification noted in both of 2 independent readings of the same set of soft-tissue X-rays of the right lower limb.

† Systolic blood pressure ⩾ 160 mm Hg and/or diastolic blood pressure ⩾ 95 mm Hg.

may be considered relatively small. It seems unlikely, however, that a commercial insurance company would survive if it consistently extracted a penalty of 1% per annum over those of other insurance policies without giving additional benefits. The participants of the UGDP, therefore, concluded that when a hypoglycemic agent is indicated in addition to diet, preference must be given to insulin because it provides equal benefits at a smaller risk.

Equally important to the neglect of long-term clinical trials and the application of the

TABLE 3

Mortality results of the UGDP group comparisons

	All deaths	Cardiovascular deaths
A*		
Tolbutamide versus placebo	0.17	0.005
Tolbutamide versus insulin standard	0.11	0.02
Tolbutamide versus variable insulin	0.07	0.02
(p values based on chi-square tests of significance)*		
B**		
Phenformin versus placebo	0.36	0.08
Phenformin versus insulin	0.02	0.02
Phenformin versus insulin plus placebo	0.02	0.08
(p values based on Fisher exact test)**		

A* See Berndt et al. (1970) for discussion of these results.
B** See Brod (1959) for discussion of these results.

TABLE 4

*The percentage of deaths due to cardiovascular causes in each of the treatment groups, in the absence of specific known cardiovascular risk factors**

	PLBO	TOLB	ISTD	IVAR
No hypertension	3.9	11.5	4.2	0.7
No history of digitalis	3.6	10.9	5.1	4.7
No history of angina	3.6	11.8	5.2	5.7
No major ECG abnormalities	3.6	10.9	5.6	4.7
Cholesterol 300 mg/100 ml	5.0	12.4	4.6	4.0
None of above	2.0	9.0	2.0	0.0

* As defined in Berndt et al. (1970).
An increase in cardiovascular mortality was noted in TOLB in patients without risk factors. TOLB exceeds all other treatment groups in all categories shown.

results of these trials to clinical practice has been the failure to be aware of the many other actions of these complex chemicals that cannot be related to their usefulness as hypoglycemic drugs. Stetten (1957), in his discussion of the need for caution in the use of these drugs, concluded that the mode of action of the sulfonylureas was apparently

TABLE 6
*Some drugs that interact with sulfonylureas**

Alcohol	Barbiturates
Coumadins	MO inhibitors
Phenylbutazone	Analgesics
Diphenylhydantoin	Vasopressin
Hydralazine	Oxytocin
Diazoxide	Sulfonamides
Thiazides	Catecholamines

* See text for discussion.

biguanides have been discovered (Schafer, 1969), demonstrating once again that the complexity of their biologic effects is well documented and far exceeds their use in the control of simple hyperglycemia. It is mandatory that we review the benefits of these agents in relation to their possible risk before embarking on their long-term use in our diabetic patients (Table 7).

TABLE 7
*Metabolic effects of biguanides**

Anaerobic glycolysis	Increased blood pressure
Increased glucose to lactate	Heart rate
Decreased glyconeogenesis	Need for digitalis
Lactic acidosis	
Decreased glucose absorption	Other actions
Anorexia	Anti-infection

* See text for discussion.

It is popular in a panel such as this to decry the widespread use of these agents on the one hand but to heartily endorse the continuation of this practice on the other despite evidence that they are of limited benefit and frequently cause unnecessary harm. The widespread use of drugs in the treatment of diabetes is a phenomenon which has burgeoned during the past decade. The usefulness of mortality statistics in relation to existing medical practices as described by Reid and Evans (1970) has already been noted. It is disturbing that there has been a striking increase in annual death rate for diabetes during this same period of time (Table 8). This is a virtually universal phenomenon and has been documented for the continents of Asia, Africa, and Australia as well as Europe and America (Marks, 1971). It is by no means clear that a deterioration in death rate on a worldwide basis can be attributed solely to the wide use of the oral agents. But this cannot be dismissed as a methodologic phenomenon related to data retrieval. This is a fact that is occurring in the real world. For this reason, I should like to close with a rhetorical question:

What changes in therapy have been initiated in the past 15 years on a global basis which could possibly account for the fact that we are doing less well in 1973 than we were doing in 1953 as regards mortality for diabetes?

Or perhaps stated more positively: What changes in therapy should we recommend in 1973 which will reverse this disastrous trend?

TABLE 8
Percentage change in annual death rate for diabetes, 1951–1967

Country	1951–53	1961–63	1965–67
United States	16.3	16.8	17.5
Belgium	17.8	22.0	32.0
France	10.9	14.0	17.3
German Federal Republic	10.6	14.5	17.1
The Netherlands	11.3	14.4	16.5
England	7.8	8.2	8.8
Sweden	11.1	14.5	17.3

From: Joslin's *Diabetes Mellitus, 17,* p. 248.

ACKNOWLEDGEMENTS

It is only possible to refer here to the original report in order to acknowledge all of the participants of the University Group Diabetes Program whose work has been liberally quoted (Berndt et al., 1970; Brod, 1959). The editorial comments as regards the implications of the University Group Diabetes Program are the responsibility of the author. In the event of any inadvertent discrepancy between figures or percentages quoted here and those of previous reports, the previous reports are to be accepted as final.

REFERENCES

ASHMORE, J., CAHILL, G. F. and HASTINGS, A. B. (1956): Inhibition of glucose 6-phosphatase by hypoglycemia sulfonylureas. *Metabolism, 5,* 774.

BERNDT, W. O., MILLER, M. and KETTYLE, W. M. (1970): Potentiation of the anti-diuretic effect of vasopressin by chlorpropamide. *Endocrinology, 86,* 1028.

BLOODWORTH Jr., J. M. B. (1963): Morphologic changes associated with sulfonylurea therapy. *Metabolism, 12,* 287.

BORSTEIN, J. (1957): Inhibition of alanine transaminase by the hypoglycaemic sulfonylurea derivatives. *Nature (Lond.), 179,* 534.

BREIDAHL, H. D., ENNIS, G. C. and MARTIN, F. L. (1972): I. Physiological and clinical pharmacological aspects. *Drugs, 3,* 79.

WHAT TO AIM AT IN THE TREATMENT OF DIABETES?

TABLE 1

Comparison of basement membrane thickness in diabetic patients and normals (From Siperstein, 1972, by courtesy.)

	Basement Membrane Thickness	
	Å + S.E.	% Abnormal
Diabetic (120)	2404 ± 68	91
Normal	1082 ± 24	2

whose parents have diabetes, have thickened basement membranes in the absence of abnormal glucose tolerance (Table 2). Although such a finding might indicate dissociation between thickening of the basement membrane and the carbohydrate abnormality, it may be pertinent that the mean age of this group was 11 years higher than that of the controls. Kilo et al. (1972) have reported a relationship between basement membrane thickness and age. Furthermore, the mean thickness for the prediabetic group, although significantly greater than that of the control group, is considerably less than that found in the 120 patients with overt diabetes. This difference could indicate that deterioration of carbohydrate metabolism exerts a further deleterious effect on basement membrane thickness. Siperstein provides additional evidence that thickening of the muscle capillary basement membrane is characteristic of genetic diabetes unrelated to aberrations in blood sugar control since only 1 of 13 patients with hyperglycemia associated with pancreatitis had such thickening. Hyperglycemia in these patients was frequently present for more than 10 years. Furthermore, 8 of 13 patients with retinopathy, suggestive of diabetic retinopathy but with reportedly normal glucose tolerance tests, had muscle capillary basement membrane thicknesses greater than 1600 Å. However, scrutiny of the glucose tolerance tests in these 8 patients indicates that at least 5 of them had abnormal 2-hour post-glucose blood sugars indicative of diabetes mellitus. Even if thickening of the muscle capillary basement membrane is an independent characteristic of genetic diabetes, this

TABLE 2

Comparison of average basement membrane thickness in normals and prediabetic patients (From Siperstein et al., 1968, by courtesy.)

	Average Basement Membrane Thickness	
	Å ± S.E.	Average Age
Normal (50)	1080 ± 27	32
Pre-diabetic (30)	1373 ± 44	43

does not necessarily or unequivocally establish that the vascular degenerative complications are unrelated to some metabolic abnormality of the disease. Siperstein, himself, has not excluded this possibility and states in his recent article in *Advances in Internal Medicine:* 'Whereas thickening of muscle capillary basement membrane is an early and sensitive indication of diabetes mellitus, it is unlikely that the capillary basement membrane width in muscle will provide an accurate indication of this lesion in tissues such as the kidney or eyes, where basement membrane thickness is probably related to duration of overt diabetes'. If the muscle capillary basement membrane thickening is unrelated to the microangiopathy in the kidneys and eyes, it would still be an important finding but is somewhat irrelevant to our primary concern – the degenerative complications of diabetes mellitus.

In addition, Dr. Siperstein's hypothesis concerning the independence of muscle capillary basement membrane thickening from the metabolic abnormality of diabetes has been questioned as a consequence of several other studies. Williamson's group (Kilo et al., 1972), in contrast to Siperstein, found that the minimal muscle capillary basement thickness siginificantly increases from 650 Å at one year of age to 1050 Å at age 70 (Fig. 1).

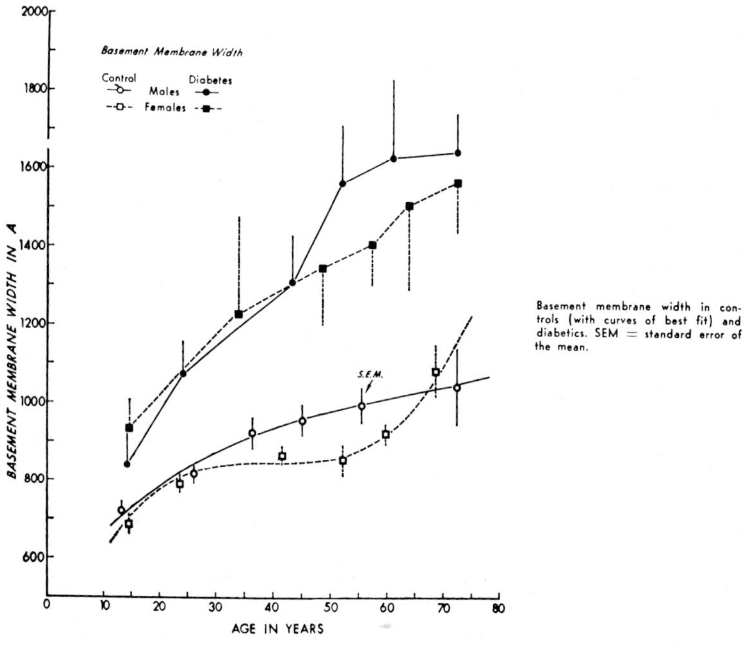

FIG. 1. Basement membrane width in controls and diabetics as a function of age and sex. (From Kilo et al., 1972, by courtesy.)

This effect of age is different for males and females and might account for some of the differences between these 2 laboratories. Dr. Siperstein calculates the average basement membrane thickness utilizing a grid with 20 equidistant lines, while Dr. Williamson computes the minimal basement membrane thickness from the average of 2 measurements of each muscle capillary. Williamson feels this parameter is less likely to be influenced by

TABLE 4

Comparison of basement membrane measurements obtained by the methods of Williamson et al. and Siperstein et al. on 28 normal males and 40 male diabetics†
(From Kilo et al., 1972, by courtesy)

	Williamson method	Siperstein method
Mean BMW ± SD in Å		
Controls	859 ± 148	1.533 ± 314
Diabetics	1.499 ± 615	2.927 ± 1.331
Correlation coefficient of BMW and age		
Controls	0.51|| (9.7)††	0.64§ (42.5)
Diabetics	0.35** (18.6)	0.38** (42.5)
Incidence of BMT‡‡		
Controls	1 of 28	2 of 28
Diabetics	24 of 40	24 of 40

* Twenty-eight normal male subjects were age matched and equal in number to those in the series of Siperstein et al.
† In forty male diabetics between ages twenty and seventy-eight, the diagnosis was verified by the criteria of Siperstein et al., e.g. two fasting plasma sugar levels of 140 mg./100 ml. or greater.
§ $P < 0.001$.
|| $P < 0.01$.
** $P < 0.05$.
†† Regression coefficient in parentheses as angstroms per year.
‡‡ Basement membrane thickening is defned as BMW exceeding mean BMW + 1.703 (SD) of controls (e.g. 95 per cent confidence limits).

in diabetics of 5 years and longer compared to patients whose disease was less than 5 years in duration. Thickening of the basement membrane correlated with retinopathy since only one patient with normal fundi had a measurement outside the normal range. Correlations with other clinical parameters were lacking although renal disease was not considered. The results obtained and the analysis of variance were essentially the same, whether the method of Siperstein or that of Williamson was used. Pardo et al. concluded that discrete changes in capillary basement membrane thickness are not sufficient to establish the presence of early diabetic microangiopathy and that identifiable vessel involvement is a late event appearing only after a prolonged period of disturbed carbohydrate metabolism. Dr. Lundbaek will comment further on this extremely important subject (this Volume, pp. 657–666).

The discrepancies between the various studies might preclude an unambiguous statement concerning the relationship between thickening of the muscle capillary basement membrane, the degenerative complications of diabetes and the carbohydrate abnormality. Nonetheless, at the current time, I think it is more constructive to consider that development of diabetic complications is related to the duration of the disease and somehow reflects the metabolic abnormality which the diabetic has. Is there other evidence that *control of the metabolic disorder will prevent or delay the degenerative complication?* In a recent review, Bondy and Felig (1971) delineated the difficulties in interpretation of most of the previously published studies. However, I would like to review the study of Johnsson (1960) which supports the argument that control of the metabolic abnormality exerts a beneficial effect on the degenerative complications. He studied all diabetic patients diagnosed in Malmö, Sweden, between 1922 and 1945 and who were less than 40 years old at the age of onset. Series I comprised 54 patients diagnosed between 1922 and 1935 while Series II consisted of 105 patients diagnosed from 1936 to 1945. Nineteen Series I patients died of late complications of diabetes – 11 from cardiac disease after an average of 21 years' duration (range 15–30 years) and 8 from nephropathy after 22 years (range 17–29). The remaining 35 patients were examined. Five Series II patients had died – 4 of nephropathy after a mean duration of 16 years and 1 of cardiac disease. Ninety-nine of the remaining 100 were examined. Nephropathy, defined as proteinuria in more than ½ of all urine samples examined during the prior year, was more common in Series II than in Series I although the latter had their diabetes for an average of 8.6 years longer (Table 5). Comparing patients with diabetes for at least 15 years, 9% in Series I and 61%

TABLE 5
Incidence of nephropathy in the 2 series of diabetic patients diagnosed in Malmö, Sweden, from 1922 to 1935 and 1936 to 1945
(From Johnsson, 1960, by courtesy)

	Series I	Series II
Duration of diabetes in years	19–35 (24.5)	10–21 (15.9)
Number of patients	56	104
Patients with nephropathy	18 (32%)	56 (54%)

The frequency of nephropathy was lower in Series I (32 per cent against 54 per cent) though the patients in Series I had had diabetes for 8.6 years longer than those in Series II. The difference is statistically significant ($P < 0.001$).

in Series II had nephropathy. Retinopathy, especially severe involvement, was also more common in Series II despite diabetes for an average of 10.5 years less than the patients in Series I (Table 6). To what can we attribute this apparent reduced incidence of complications in patients in Series I despite a significantly longer duration of diabetes? Series I patients were initially treated with strict diet control and multiple injections of regular insulin per day, while Series II received a freer diet and long-acting insulin was available when their diabetes was diagnosed. I want to emphasize the use of multiple injections of regular insulin for the control of diabetes in relation to the complications of the disease. This area will be more thoroughly discussed by Dr. Tchobroutsky (this Volume, pp. 667–682). Eighteen of the 35 patients in Series I always had at least 2 injections of insulin per day while only 26% of the patients in Series II had received only multiple insulin

TABLE 6
Incidence of retinopathy in the 2 series of diabetic patients diagnosed in Malmö, Sweden, from 1922 to 1935 and 1936 to 1945 (From Johnsson, 1960, by courtesy)

	Series I	Series II
Duration of diabetes in years	21–35 (26.5)	10–21 (15.9)
Number of patients	33	97
Normal ocular fundi	14 (42%)	49 (51%)
Retinopathy degree I	13 (40%)	16 (16%)
II	5 (15%)	14 (14%)
III	– } (3%)	9 } (19%)
IV	1 }	9 }

injections. Series I patients received only one injection of insulin for an average of 10% of their cumulative diabetic history, while the Series II patients received a single daily injection 45% of their cumulative diabetic history. Johnsson did not analyze the incidence of diabetic complications based on the number of insulin injections per day. Excellent control of diabetes includes normal blood sugar values at least some time during the day. Attempts at such excellent control will be associated with frequent hypoglycemia. However, this in itself may not be entirely deleterious, espicially if it indicates that normoglycemia exists some time during the day. This is consistent with Johnsson's finding that Series I patients had more hypoglycemia and insulin coma than Series II patients, reflecting attempts to achieve normoglycemia and the use of multiple insulin injections per day. The 8 patients in Series I with more than 20 episodes of insulin coma had no proteinuria and 4 had no retinal changes. The retinopathy in the other 4 was mild. Can one interpret this study to indicate that strict control of diabetes probably necessitates multiple daily injections of insulin, including regular insulin? Attainment of normal blood sugar values at some time during the day will probably be accompanied by increased hypoglycemia. If we can establish, as I believe, that such treatment will prevent or delay the complications of diabetes, I strongly endorse it and accept the hypoglycemia as the lesser of two evils.

The case for multiple injections of regular insulin in the treatment of diabetes and prevention of its complications was impressively summarized by Dr. Francis Lukens in his Joslin Lecture (1965). He reviewed 3 series of patients with diabetes of 30–40 years' duration who were treated with multiple injections of regular insulin. A surprisingly high percentage of the patients were free of serious diabetic complications. Lukens cited a patient who took 2 injections of regular insulin per day for 32 years. Despite what was defined as poor diabetic control, the patient was apparently free from complications. One must be extremely cautious about drawing conclusions from such anecdotal experiences and the one of Dr. Shepherd (1971), but perhaps these are not isolated incidents, but are applicable to all diabetic patients. Dr. Shepherd, whose diabetes began in 1925 when he was 6 years old, had only a few perivascular microaneurysms, mild proteinuria of about 200–250 mg per day and some decrease in vibration sensation after 43 years of diabetes. He used regular insulin 3 times a day but after 27 years he omitted his pre-lunch insulin because of mid-afternoon hypoglycemia. He frequently had early morning ketonuria without glycosuria which suggests nocturnal hypoglycemia (Bloom et al., 1969). He also mentioned 3 other patients with diabetes of 40 years' duration without significant complications and also using regular insulin several times per day. The frequent hypoglycemia reported by such patients provides further evidence for the serious attempt to achieve normal blood sugar values at some time during the day. Subsequently we will consider pancreatic and islet cell transplants and artificial β-cell devices as more efficient methods of achieving normoglycemia without hypoglycemia.

Recent studies support the concept that strict control may prevent or delay development of diabetic neuropathy. Ward et al. (1971) found that nerve conduction time was significantly impaired in diabetics at the onset of their diabetes. After 6 months of treatment, significant improvement was apparent even though the values were still less than normal. Terkildsen and Christenson (1971) also noted beneficial effects of strict diabetic control measuring changes in vibratory sensation threshold induced during ischemia. Normalization of the response probably represents remyelination of the nerves since the basic pathologic defect in diabetic neuropathy is segmental demyelination. A recent editorial in *Lancet* (1972) summarizes data indicating beneficial effects of control of hyperglycemia on diabetic neuropathy. A similar salutary effect of strict control of diabetes on retinopathy is also suggested by the prospective study of Kohner cited by Lundbaek (1972). During a 2-year period retinopathy progressed more slowly in those patients having good diabetic control. Additional support for the benefit of good diabetic control on the development of retinopathy has been presented by Pirart et al. (1973).

The important recent studies from Dr. Spiro's laboratory have provided a basis for the effectiveness of strict control of the diabetes and will be presented in greater detail elsewhere in this Volume (pp. 387–430). Beisswenger and Spiro (1970) reported that diabetic glomeruli contain increased amounts of basement membrane which had a significant

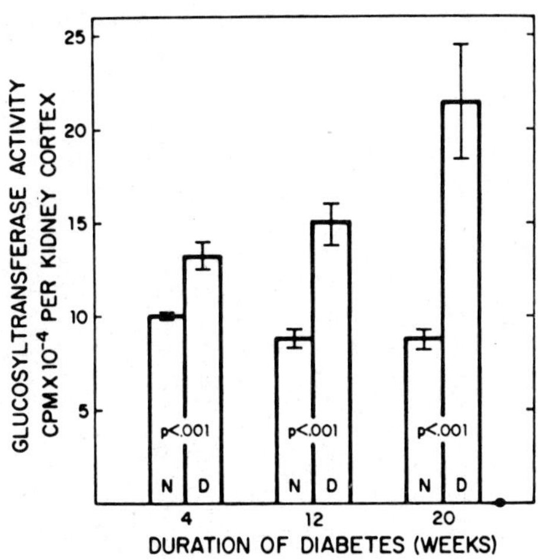

FIG. 3. Effect of diabetes on the total glucosyltransferase activity of rat kidney cortex at various times after the administration of alloxan. The diabetic animals (D) are compared to age-matched controls (N). (From Spiro and Spiro, 1971.)

decrease in lysine concentration with an equivalent increase in hydroxylysine and hydroxylysine-linked disaccharide units. Spiro and Spiro (1971) found that a glucosyltransferase involved in synthesis of disaccharide units is increased in the renal cortex of alloxan diabetic rats (Fig. 3). Furthermore, the increase was more marked as the duration of the diabetes increased. After one week of alloxan diabetes, treatment of the rats for 3 weeks with insulin significantly returned glucosyltransferase activity back toward normal (Fig. 4). The importance of the early, vigorous treatment of diabetes was suggested, since if the 3-week treatment was delayed until the animals had been diabetic for 9 weeks, insulin was less efficacious. Alloxan diabetes did not increase glucosyltransferase activity in other tissues nor did it increase the activity of UDP galactose-N-acetylglucosamine. This enzyme is important in glycoprotein synthesis but not in the synthesis of basement membrane. Galactosyltransferase, which attaches galactose to the hydroxylysine of the basement membrane, is also increased in the diabetic rat (Spiro and Spiro, 1971). Thus, if activities of these enzymes accurately reflect synthesis of the abnormal basement membrane in diabetes, the beneficial effect of insulin supports the importance of strict control of the diabetes in relationship to the microangiopathic complications. In addition, strict control of the blood sugar should diminish the formation of sorbitol and other products of the polyol pathway.

For a moment I would like to consider some aspects of the *definition of good control.* This has usually included freedom from both marked hyperglycemia and glycosuria on the one hand and hypoglycemia on the other. A diabetic could be considered well-controlled within such a context and yet never actually have normal blood sugar values.

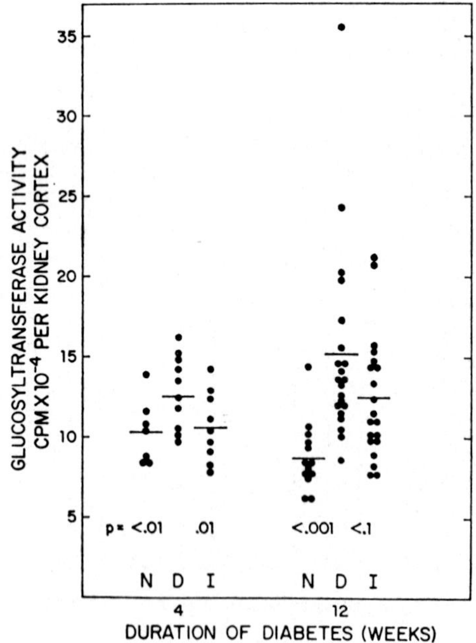

FIG. 4. Effect of insulin treatment on the glucosyltransferase activity of the kidney cortex of diabetic rats. (From Spiro and Spiro, 1971.)

From the data I have cited, several periods of true normoglycemia each day may be more important to prevent complications even though moderate to marked hyperglycemia and glycosuria exist at other times. Today, this may be accomplished only by multiple insulin injections and the appropriate use of rapid acting insulins. The frequent hypoglycemic reactions, rather than indicating poor diabetic control, provide evidence that normoglycemia was achieved. This approach to the degenerative complications has never been tested in a long-term prospective study.

If strict control of the blood sugar provides the best chance of preventing diabetic complications, how can it be attained? Dr. Krall and Dr. Jackson will discuss dietary management, a necessary but insufficient approach for insulin-requiring diabetics (this Volume, pp. 645–656 and 639–644). Dr. Tchobroutsky will discuss his important studies utilizing regular insulin and the exciting new possiblilities of artificial β-cell devices (pp. 667–682).

Another hopeful approach is pancreatic transplants, either whole organ or isolated islets. Successful transplantation would permit insulin secretion to be regulated by normal physiologic factors avoiding both hyperglycemia and hypoglycemia. Presently the major problem of transplantation is the immunologic one. The observation that tissues grown in culture lose their antigenicity when transplanted could provide a solution to the immunologic problem involved in isolated islet transplants (Summerlin et al., 1973). Ballinger and Lacy (1972) and Leonard et al. (1973) successfully controlled hyperglycemia in experimental animals with isolated islet transplants. Dr. Frederick Goetz (personal communication) of the University of Minnesota has kindly summarized their results with pancreatic transplants for me. Ten diabetic, uremic patients received both a kidney and a pancreas transplant, except for one patient who received only a pancreas. Under favorable circumstances, such pancreas transplant immediately reverses the metabolic effects of insulin deficiency and the patients no longer require insulin injections. Glucose tolerance and fasting blood glucose may be normal for at least 6 months, especially considering the large doses of steroids the patients receive for immunosuppression. However, only one patient survived beyond 6 months, and he died one year after transplantation, still not requiring insulin injections. At autopsy, the pancreas appeared relatively intact in almost the entire group of patients. Since Dr. Goetz felt that the total burden of such double transplants was unacceptably great, 3 patients without uremia, but with severe retinopathy, received only a pancreas transplant. The transplant functioned well for only 1 to 5 weeks. One had clearcut histologic evidence of rejection while the other 2 had multiple venous thromboses. These results suggest that uremia facilitates the acceptance of the transplant, but the additional problems associated with renal failure cannot be minimized. However, preliminary results of Gliedman et al. (1973), presented at the recent meeting of the American Diabetes Association, suggest that the asynchronous transplantation of the pancreas and kidney provides better function of both organs than when they are simultaneously transplanted. One can be confident that in time we will possess both the knowledge and the techniques to provide better metabolic control for the diabetic and the prevention of the degenerative complications of the disease.

REFERENCES

BALLINGER, W. F. and LACY, P. E. (1972): Transplantation of intact pancreatic islets in rats. *Surgery, 72,* 175.

BEISSWENGER, P. J. and SPIRO, R. G. (1970): Human glomerular basement membrane: Chemical alteration in diabetes mellitus. *Science, 168,* 596.

BLOOM, M., MINTZ, D. H. and FIELD, J. B. (1969): Insulin-induced post-hypoglycemic hyperglycemia as a cause of 'Brittle' diabetes: Clinical clues and therapeutic implications. *Amer. J. Med., 47,* 891.

BONDY, P. K. and FELIG, P. (1971): Relation of diabetic control to development of vascular complications. *Med. Clin. N. Amer., 55,* 888.

DANOWSKI, T. S., FISHER, E. R., KHURANA, R. C., NOLAN, S. and STEPHAN, T. (1972): Muscle capillary basement membrane in juvenile diabetes mellitus. *Metabolism, 21,* 1125.

EDITORIAL (1972): Diabetic neuropathy: A preventable complication. *Lancet, 2,* 583.

GLIEDMAN, M. C., RIFKIN, H., ROSS, H., SOTERMAN, R., ZARDEY, Z., TELLIS, V., FREED, S. and VEITH, F. J. (1973): Clinical segmental pancreatic transplantation with ureter to pancreatic duct anastomosis for exocrine drainage. *Diabetes, 22/Suppl. 1,* 295.

JOHNSSON, S. (1960): Retinopathy and nephropathy in diabetes mellitus: Comparison of the effects of two forms of treatment. *Diabetes, 9,* 1.

KILO, C., VOGLER, N. and WILLIAMSON, J. R. (1972): Muscle capillary basement membrane changes related to aging and to diabetes mellitus. *Diabetes, 21,* 881.

LEONARD, R. J., LAZAROW, A. and HEGRE, O. D. (1973): Pancreatic islet transplantation in the rat. *Diabetes, 22,* 413.

LUKENS, F. D. (1965): The rediscovery of regular insulin. *New Engl. J. Med., 272,* 130.

LUNDBAEK, K. (1972): Recent contributions to the study of diabetic angiopathy and neuropathy. In: *Advances in Metabolic Disorders, Vol. 6,* Chapter 4, pp. 99–129. Editors: R. Levine and R. Luft. Academic Press, New York, N.Y.

PARDO, V., PEREZ-STABLE, E., ALZAMORA, D. B. and CLEVELAND, W. W. (1972): Incidence and significance of muscle capillary basal lamina thickness in juvenile diabetes. *Amer. J. Pathol., 68,* 67.

PIRART, J., LAUVAUX, J. P. and VASSART, G. (1973): Development and evolution of nervous and vascular complications in the course of diabetes: a prospective study. II. Diabetic retinopathy: relation to sex, age, severity of diabetes and degree of control. In: *Abstracts, VIII Congress of the International Diabetes Federation, Brussels, 1973,* p. 185. International Congress Series No. 280, Excerpta Medica, Amsterdam.

SHEPHERD, G. R. (1971): Diabetes mellitus of juvenile onset with 40 years' survival and no gross damage. In-depth study of and by a 50-year-old physician. *Arch. int. Med., 128,* 284.

SIPERSTEIN, M. D. (1972): Capillary basement membranes and diabetic microangiopathy. In: *Advances in Internal Medicine, Vol. 18,* Chapter 15, pp. 325–344. Editor: G. Stollerman. Year Book Medical Publishers, Inc., Chicago, Ill.

SPIRO, R. G. and SPIRO, M. J. (1971): Effect of diabetes on the biosynthesis of the renal glomerular basement membrane. Studies on the glucosyltransferase. *Diabetes, 20,* 641.

SUMMERLIN, W. T., MILLER, G. E. and GOOD, R. A. (1973): Successful tissue and organ allotransplantation without immunosuppression. *Program 65th Annual Meeting of The American Society for Clinical Investigation.*

TERKILDSEN, A. B. and CHRISTENSON, N. J. (1971): Reversible nervous abnormalities in juvenile diabetics with recently diagnosed diabetes. *Diabetologia, 7,* 113.

WARD, J. D., BARNES, C. G., FISHER, D. J., JESSOP, J. D. and BAKER, R. W. R. (1971): Improvement in nerve conduction following treatment in newly diagnosed diabetics. *Lancet, 1,* 428.

DIAGNOSIS AND DIETARY MANAGEMENT OF MILD, OBESE AND BORDERLINE DIABETICS

W. P. U. JACKSON

Endocrine Research Group, Department of Medicine, University of Cape Town and Groote Schuur Hospital, Observatory, Cape, South Africa

I want to discuss the mild, asymptomatic, chemical diabetic, but must first of all consider his diagnosis. One could compose a treatise on 'when is hyperglycemia diabetes?' and also, more simply, on 'when is hyperglycemia?'. I am not here concerned with differences in methods or interpretations of blood glucose levels and glucose tolerance tests, or with the influence of age or time of day, but more with differences in the variability of individuals and between individuals. Unless hyperglycemia is associated with symptoms, or with vascular or other complications, can we call it diabetes? In the course of a population study among Bantu Africans in the Transvaal we found completely asymptomatic people whose blood sugars rose to 800 mg/100 ml after a carbohydrate load and I believe similar levels have been seen among the Pima Indians. Locally I have observed people with blood sugars in the 300s, refusing treatment and being seemingly none the worse 2 or 3 years later. Hyperglycemia after a glucose load is so common in the elderly that it may almost be considered a normal state. We have already given our reasons for believing that while much of this elderly hyperglycemia indicates diabetes, a good deal does not (Jackson and Vinik, 1970).

The variability of blood glucose levels in single individuals was clearly shown by McDonald et al. (1965) who analyzed the results of oral glucose tolerance tests repeated 6 times at 2-monthly intervals in all of 334 male prisoners being kept under constant conditions of diet and exercise. The individual variability even in these comparatively young men was remarkable in some instances. For example the 1-hour post-glucose level in one subject varied between 86 and 215 mg/100 ml. The authors say 'with variations of this magnitude ..... it is difficult to interpret ..... single glucose tolerance tests that show abnormalities which are not extreme'. Thus 30 of their subjects recorded 64 total 'diabetic' tests as judged by Fajans and Conn criteria. We have found the same sort of thing in our population studies, as exemplified by one overweight man aged 37 who produced a 2-hour post-glucose screening test level of 70 mg/100 ml, then in succession a grossly diabetic glucose tolerance test, a normal glucose tolerance test and an intermediate or 'borderline' test (Jackson et al., 1970).

This difficulty in diagnosing diabetes from a single glucose tolerance test is found also in juveniles. In Table 1 are the figures of 4 youngsters who gave abnormal screening values *and* diabetic initial glucose tolerance curves. However, 3 were normal when retested a year later without any treatment (Jackson and Kalk, 1972). Had they been on sulphonylureas during this period we might have been inclined to ascribe such 'improvement' to the drug. To get around these difficulties Butterfield (1964) has suggested that diabetes

TABLE 1
Discovered diabetics under 20 years, on no therapy

Age	Sex	Initially obese	Weight change*	Family history	Screening level	1st GTT Fasting	1st GTT 1 hr	1st GTT 2 hr	2nd GTT Fasting	2nd GTT 1 hr	2nd GTT 2 hr	Designation
17	M	Yes	No	0	162	141	205	109	82	118	69	Normal
17	M	No	No	0	171	128	226	185	84	136	86	Normal
11	M	No	No	0	188	165	200	144	102	120	111	Normal
14	M	No	No	+	164	100	219	140	88	192	188	Diabetic

* Apart from that commensurate with 1 year's growth.

should be diagnosed only when the 2-hour level is over 200 mg/100 ml, lower levels being doubtful or borderline. Generally speaking our criteria are considerably less stringent than this, but O'Sullivan and Williams (1966) estimated that different reported criteria applied to their own data from Sudbury would vary the prevalence rate of 'discovered diabetics' between 1.2 and 13.4%.

DIETARY CONTROL

Following a population study we made in 1970 (Michael et al., 1971) all those who were diagnosed as new diabetics over the age of 20 were instructed to modify their diet; all were told to restrict carbohydrates and eschew sugar entirely; in addition overweight subjects were instructed to reduce calorie intake. Thirty-eight of these asymptomatic 'diabetics' were retested one year later. At this time they could be divided into 3 groups: those who had dieted and lost weight; those who had made some effort to diet but had lost no weight; and those who had not changed their eating habits at all (Jackson and Kalk, 1972). We found a significant improvement in mean glucose tolerance in those so-called 'diabetics' who lost weight and no change in those who did not diet or lose weight. The intermediate group who dieted without loss of weight were also improved, to an intermediate degree. Of the original 15 diabetics who lost weight 9 could be classified as normal by glucose tolerance test. The mean plasma insulin (IRI) levels in this group showed a significant fall from previous levels, presumably indicating a reduction in insulin resistance rather than any improvement in beta cell function.

The small amount or even absence of weight loss consistent with improvement in carbohydrate tolerance suggests that the operative factor is reduction in dietary carbohydrate (especially sugar) rather than actual weight loss.

The Kings College Hospital group (Wall et al., 1973) have recently confirmed this belief on a larger scale, achieving satisfactory metabolic control in 159 of 200 fat diabetics by carbohydrate restriction, with little mean weight loss (5.7%). Actually 18 of these 159 gained weight. They conclude that control by diet is usually independent of weight loss. This clinical observation can be matched by recent elegant demonstrations that carbohydrate restriction rather than weight change is responsible for reduction in insulin output in obese (Grey and Kipnis, 1971) and non-obese (Muller et al., 1971) subjects. The clinically important corollary is that carbohydrate restriction can be as effective in normal-weight maturity-onset diabetics as in obese diabetics.

Pavel and Pieptea (1970) in Rumania have used similar dietary and other simple prophylactic advice for over 25 years in normal subjects with diabetic relatives. They found that the proportion of 'hereditary' (i.e., positive family history) diabetes fell by 50% over a 20-year period, whereas logically it would have been expected to rise.

On the other hand, Brunzell et al. (1971) argue in favour of *high* carbohydrate feeding in mild diabetics leading to improved glucose tolerance and reduced insulin output. Their period of observation on this diet was only 10 days, which does not seem to me to constitute a valid argument, since we all know that *short-term* high carbohydrate intake is essential for proper preparation for the glucose tolerance test whatever long-term regimen may be in use.

IN PREGNANCY

I now want to turn to gestational or mild maturity-onset diabetes in pregnancy. I believe the same principles apply and have seen only good results from the use of strict 600 or 800 calorie diets. Pregnant women are rather liable to ketosis and indeed diabetic keto-acidosis is highly toxic for the fetus. Certainly some ketonuria may appear during a restricted carbohydrate regimen in pregnancy but we have never found any systemic ketosis by plasma acetest reaction, and believe that this is a safe situation. Occasionally in fact ketosis may be abolished by restricted diet as in the following example (Fig. 1). This 36-year-old, overweight, coloured woman had been put on insulin after the diagnosis of diabetes in the third trimester, but, as is so often the case, proved rather insulin-resistant and was poorly controlled on around 80 units a day, with acetone in the urine. On proper

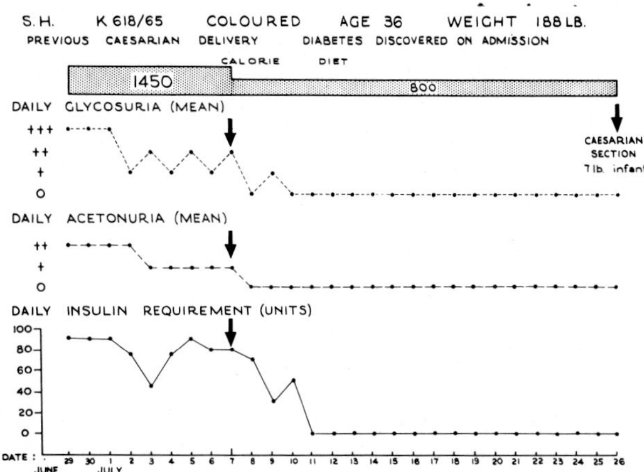

FIG. 1. Reduction in caloric intake leading to rapid abolition of glycosuria, acetonuria and insulin requirement in an obese pregnant woman.

dietary restriction she stopped gaining weight, totally lost glycosuria and ketonuria, and needed no more insulin.

We have recently started a trial of the effects of dietary restriction in pregnancy and I should like to show some early results. Our 3 groups of pregnant subjects comprised: (1) normal weight for height; (2) obese diabetics; and (3) obese non-diabetics. Oral glucose tolerance tests were performed with proper preparation at around 20 weeks and again after 6–10 weeks on a 800-calorie diet in the two obese groups. At this later stage in pregnancy the mean glucose tolerance test of the control group was significantly worse, while that of the dieted, obese diabetics had significantly improved. There was slight improvement in the obese non-diabetics. There was a similar, and in general satisfactory, fall in the day to day urine and blood sugar levels. Changes in plasma insulin are difficult to interpret and more data are needed.

Mean weight changes were: normal non-diabetics gained 4.5 kg, obese diabetics lost 1.8 kg and obese non-diabetics gained 1.35 kg, but the dieting of the latter group could not be supervised in hospital, and was certainly less strictly imposed than in the diabetics.

The babies were all satisfactory, none appeared typically 'diabetic' in type and the low mean birth weight of the obese diabetics' infants (3 kg) probably shows the effect of diet, since the mean weight of their previous 25 infants had been 3.64 kg.

SPECIAL CASES: AGEING, CHRONIC PANCREATITIS

The next special case I want to consider is old age. If I develop diabetes at the age of 70 or 75 I should not be too worried about *further* damage to my blood vessels, and provided I had no symptoms I should not worry much about my blood sugar. I should not like to be fat, though. I used to think it rather unfair to try to restrict the caloric enjoyment of elderly people, but as I get older myself I believe more and more in maintaining correct weight at any age. The difficulty lies in *losing* weight in the elderly, but I have on occasions been most gratified in the improvement when weight loss has been achieved.

Another special case in which we are not worried about vascular disease is that of chronic pancreatitis (Joffe et al., 1968). The danger here is more likely to be hypoglycemia, which may be severe and intractable, for reasons not entirely clear, though probably related in part to a concomitant deficiency of glucagon. Here again, then, we do not treat the high blood sugar itself.

'TRUE AIMS'

To return to our true aims in treating the ordinary mild, asymptomatic diabetic, naturally we will try to avoid symptoms developing later, and this alone is a good argument for reasonable control of the blood glucose level. Secondly we should like to prevent complications. We are not really sure about retinopathy; certainly the most severe grades can occur with minimal hyperglycemia. Nevertheless there is fairly good evidence that on the whole those with lower blood sugars do best.

Much recent work has tied together hyperglycemia, hyperinsulinemia and ischemic heart disease (Weaver et al., 1970) so that any factors we believe help to prevent heart disease in general should apply *a fortiori* to diabetics and should logically apply from an early age.

Reaven et al. (1972) found that the blood glucose levels of glucose tolerance (or chemical) diabetics were no higher than those of normal subjects when estimated after a standard American-type meal. Plasma insulin levels, however, were significantly higher in the chemical diabetics both after oral glucose and after the standard meal. They therefore suggest that hyperinsulinemia is more characteristic than hyperglycemia in the day to day life of the patients with chemical diabetes, and that it is this hyperinsulinemia that needs to be controlled. Correspondingly we (Jackson et al., 1972) found that the more potentially diabetic a group became the higher the mean insulin response to glucose, whether this potentiality was indicated by overweight, borderline glucose tolerance tests or diabetic parentage.

Therefore I think we can recommend that we should aim to reduce the obese and re-activate the physically lazy, since these objectives will help to control the diabetes and the coronary vessels together. In particular we can recommend the abolition of sugar from the diet, which will materially reduce calorie intake and insulin levels. Other risk factors include the blood pressure and the serum lipids, and these may be helped by dietary and by chemical means. One most important risk factor over which we have no control is our inheritance – but no one can choose his parents.

Now what about those who are doubtfully diabetic, according to whatever definition we wish to apply? Surely since these peoples' coronary vessels are also at risk they should be dealt with in the same manner. Going further, the same principles regarding the maintenance of correct weight, reducing sugar intake and saturated fat intake and exercising must apply to others at risk such as relatives of diabetics, any overweight person, anyone else who does not want to develop diabetes, obesity, or heart disease, and so by logical extension to you and me.

REFERENCES

BRUNZELL, J. D., LERNER, R. L., HAZZARD, W. R., PORTE, D. and BIERMAN, E. (1971): Improved glucose tolerance with high carbohydrate feeding in mild diabetes. *New Engl. J. Med., 284,* 521.

BUTTERFIELD, W. J. H. (1964): Summary of results of the Bedford Diabetes Survey. *Proc. Roy. Soc. Med., 57,* 196.

GREY, N. and KIPNIS, D. M. (1971): Effect of diet composition on the hyperinsulinemia of obesity. *New Engl. J. Med., 285,* 827.

JACKSON, W. P. U. and KALK, J. (1972): Glucose intolerance retested. *S. Afr. med. J., 46,* 2065.

JACKSON, W. P. U., VAN MIEGHEM, W. and KELLER, P. (1972): Insulin excess as the initial lesion in diabetes. *Lancet, I,* 1040.

JACKSON, W. P. U. and VINIK, A. I. (1970): Hyperglycaemia and diabetes in the elderly. In: *Diabetes Mellitus: Theory and Practice,* p. 526. Editors: M. Ellenberg and H. Rifkin. McGraw-Hill, New York, N.Y.

JACKSON, W. P. U., VINIK, A. I., JOFFE, B. I., SACKS, A. and EDELSTEIN, I. (1970): Vicissitudes encountered in a diabetes population study. *S. Afr. med. J., 44,* 1283.

JOFFE, B. I., BANK, S. and MARKS, I. N. (1968): Hypoglycaemia in pancreatitis. *Lancet, 2,* 269.

McDONALD, G. W., FISHER, G. F. and BURNHAM, C. (1965): Reproducibility of the oral glucose tolerance test. *Diabetes, 8,* 473.

MICHAEL, C., EDELSTEIN, I., WHISSON, A., MacCULLUM, M., O'REILLY, I., HARDCASTLE, A., TOYER, M. G. and JACKSON, W. P. U. (1971): Prevalence of diabetes, glycosuria and related variables among a Cape coloured population. *S. Afr. med. J., 45,* 795.

MULLER, W. A., FALOONA, G. R. and UNGER, R. H. (1971): Influence of antecedent diet upon glucagon and insulin secretion. *New Engl. J. Med., 285,* 1450.

O'SULLIVAN, J. B. and WILLIAMS, R. F. (1966): Early diabetes mellitus in perspective. *J. Amer. med. Ass., 198,* 579.

PAVEL, I. and PIEPTEA, R. (1971): Prevention of diabetes in the prediabetic stage: Results after 25 years. In: *Proceedings of the VII Congress of the International Diabetes Federation, Buenos Aires, 1970,* p. 421. Editor: R. R. Rodriguez. International Congress Series No. 231, Excerpta Medica, Amsterdam.

REAVEN, G. M., OLEFSKY, J. and FARQUHAR, J. W. (1972): Does hyperglycaemia or hyperinsulinaemia characterise the patient with chemical diabetes? *Lancet, I,* 1247.

WALL, J. R., PYKE, D. A. and OAKLEY, W. G. (1973): Effect of carbohydrate restriction in obese diabetics: Relationship of control to weight loss. *Brit. med. J., 1,* 577.

WEAVER, J. A., BHATIA, S. K., BOYLE, D., HADDEN, D. R. and MONTGOMERY, D. A. D. (1970): Cardiovascular state of newly discovered diabetic women. *Brit. med. J., 1,* 783.

GOALS OF TREATMENT AND WHY THEY ARE NOT ACHIEVED

LEO P. KRALL

Joslin Clinic and New England Deaconess Hospital, Education Division, Joslin Diabetes Foundation, Harvard Medical School, Boston, Mass., U.S.A.

It is a strange paradox that, more than 100 years after Langerhans and 50 years after the development of insulin, there should even be a discussion concerning the treatment of diabetes. Moreover, 50-odd years after the discovery of the 'cure' for diabetes, the confusion is compounded by the fact that there is no universally accepted definition of what diabetes is! In 1922, Elliott P. Joslin was quoted as saying: 'Now there is no excuse for any diabetic to ever be sick again and no reason for a diabetic to miss any time from his work because of diabetes'. Indeed, in a bitter-sweet way, there has been remarkable progress for the diabetic, who, prior to the development of insulin, often died shortly after the onset of his diabetes, generally of acidosis, acute infection, or both. Now the diabetic survives long enough to succumb to cancer, cerebrovascular accident or cardiovascular disease just like the rest of the population. That is progress!

This Panel will not settle in 2 hours those problems which have accumulated for the past half-century. It might, however, make a contribution if it not only expresses pleasure at the progress that has been made, but also mirrors the frustration of almost all those who try to treat diabetes because of those gaps in knowledge still present, and if it further makes clear the faults and inadequacies of the tools given us to treat the diabetics of today.

As for a definition of diabetes, with today's knowledge, it might be best stated as an insufficiency of adequate or effective available insulin. This is true whether the cause be (a) insufficient insulin production; (b) improper type or quality of insulin; (c) no production at all; (d) harassment by the anterior pituitary, thyroid, adrenal or by glucagon; (e) binding of insulin; (f) antibody production; (g) destruction by known or unknown enzymes; (h) destruction by known or unknown viruses; (i) improper enzyme activity; or (j) any other reason for defective physiology. In any event, the result is always the same. Other body dysfunctions may be involved but at this point in our knowledge, while it is possible that elevated blood glucose may exist without diabetes, clinical diabetes as we know it does not exist without elevated blood glucose.

Our present-day treatment is directed at insulin use in every instance: (a) diet permits the diabetic to use his own insulin, which is presumably superior to that of the sheep, cow or pig; (b) the sulfonylureas may help to produce or release more insulin; (c) biguanides in some fashion make what insulin is available more effective; (d) exogenous insulin itself is a replacement of insufficient endogenous insulin, whether this be by the use of slow, intermediate or rapid insulin or a combination of these. The very plethora of treatment methods shows that there is no single perfect road to physiological normalcy.

It would be a futile exercise to sit here and air our own therapeutic prejudices or to regurgitate those data which we all know and which at this time do not lead to a firm single conclusion but which are often used to reinforce the beliefs which we individually cherish. In the spectrum of world diabetologists, possibly one-third believe in strict regulation of diabetes while 10% are therapeutic nihilists who feel that such efforts are useless and absolve themselves by asking the rhetorical question 'who knows what diabetes is anyway?' Meanwhile, the majority of practising physicians daily face problems that demand answers. They feel insecure with hyperglycemic promiscuity and would like to treat their diabetics with greater effectiveness but are not certain how to achieve that goal. Researchers can afford the luxury of doubt but those who treat patients must do so daily to the best of their ability while being prepared to change their views when the evidence warrants.

Since there can be no really definitive answers and since each panel member already knows most of the data known to the others, it would be best to (a) define therapeutic goals; (b) determine why they have not or cannot be achieved; (c) ascertain what can be done more effectively with the knowledge we have; and (d) project the improvements of the future.

GOALS OF TREATMENT

These vary with each physician and each treatment center. No conscientious physician is really happy about accepting 'abnormality' as desirable. Physicians have been trained to strive for normal body function and laboratory results and quite naturally bridle at the thought of accepting any abnormal body chemical measurements as not only satisfactory, but also desirable. Would not everyone prefer the normalcy of all blood chemistry *including glucose* if it were possible to achieve this easily? Under these circumstances, would any physician deliberately attempt to achieve hyperglycemia? The fact is that chemical normalcy is very difficult and sometimes impossible to achieve in the diabetic. Furthermore, the penalty for deviation from normal may well be delayed long enough so that the unregulated diabetic patient may succumb from some other medical problem anyway.

The oft-repeated platitude that 'the diabetic should be able to live a normal life' is nonsense. This is because of the tools for treatment at our disposal today. If a person must think continually about diet, blood and urine sugar testing, oral hypoglycemic agents or insulin with adjustment of doses for activity and diet, this is no longer a 'normal' life.

The goals of treatment should be: (1) To keep the patient functioning as normally as possible now and in the future. (2) To keep body physiology and chemistry, including blood glucose, urine glucose, cholesterol, triglyceride, possibly the mucoproteins, the polyol pathway, and a host of other measurements known and unknown, within normal limits, avoiding distressing side effects.

To achieve this *physiologically normal* state, it may be necessary to attenuate or re-adjust the patient's habits and life style.

For the diabetic, *short-term benefits* include a smoother course, ideal weight, normal strength, freedom from severe reactions, from acidosis and possible avoidance of infections. *Long-term benefits* are more debatable but the goal still is to attempt to avoid circulatory or cardiovascular deficiencies, nephropathy, neuropathy and retinopathy, or at least to ameliorate them. While it may be argued that *good control* as practised today may not prevent these complications, certainly no one has ever demonstrated that *poor control* (either purposely or by default) ever prevented or improved these complications.

What is meant by 'good control'? In the ideal sense, good control simply means 'normal'. It might be argued that this is nearly impossible to achieve, that it has never been accomplished in any large series of cases, or that it must be modified by the realities and circumstances of modern life. This, however, is another question. The inability to achieve an ideal does not necessarily dilute the ideal. Fajans has been quoted as saying that all other things considered, it is still 'appropriate to strive to achieve the best hormonal and biochemical control feasible and practical in any given patient with the methods available today and at the earliest time possible that an abnormality can be identified' (see Table 1).

TABLE 1

Criteria for control (Marble-Camerini). Maximal venous blood glucose levels ('true sugar'). Blood sugar levels in mg/100 ml. At least 70% of all blood sugar levels must be at or below a given standard in order that the degree of control may be designated

Time	Good	Fair	Poor
Fasting	110	130	
1 hour p.c.	150	180	All
2 hours p.c.	130	150	others
3 hours p.c.	110	130	

RELATIONSHIP OF COMPLICATIONS TO DEGREE OF CONTROL

This topic may cause a difference of opinion and simply citing the available evidence could fuel endless discussion. Part of the problem lies in the fact that many statements in the literature which are questionable may be used out of context and are repeated until they are accepted as dogma although they may have been used in a contemplative or rhetorical manner in the first place. For example, consider the statement of Bondy and Felig (1971): 'Under normal circumstances, the normal human being keeps his blood glucose concentration between approximately 50 and 150 mg/100 ml'. In the first 15,000 blood sugar determinations during the course of the Oxford diabetes studies, which were started back in 1946 by Wilkerson and Krall (1947), the blood glucose levels of non-diabetics one or more hours after a meal rarely approached the Folin Wu level of 140 mg/100 ml. In the small group whose blood sugar levels were more elevated were those persons subsequently identified as diabetic at a rate 10 times that of the truly 'normal' population.

Another statement, this time of Gabbay (1973), notes that '. . . it is quite clear that the clinical expression and development of the various complications are a function of the duration of diabetes'. This is not without challenge since many diabetics have survived 25 to 50 years without serious complications while, on the other hand, short-term diabetics sometimes have been shown to have complications. Another often-heard statement is that complications develop in diabetic patients despite 'good control'. While this is not completely erroneous, it is misleading because if 'control' means constant normalization of blood glucose levels, there simply have not been any sizable groups of long-term patients who have been well controlled. Bondy and Felig (1971) very succinctly make this clear with the statement: 'Moreover, most authors . . . have concluded that the relationship between control of the metabolic disorder and the incidence and progression of . . . complications is difficult, if not impossible, to demonstrate'. The classic statement by Priscilla White (1956) that, after 20 years of diabetes, over 82% of juvenile-onset diabetics had retinopathy, has been interpreted to suggest that even patients as well controlled as hers had severe complications, etc. The fact is that while many juvenile-onset diabetics do have some vascular changes, sometimes after many years, in many instances they are not severe. The number of those who actually become blind or have very severe visual loss may be statistically small. Moreover, Priscilla White has never claimed to have a large series of constantly and superbly regulated diabetics with perfectly normal blood sugar levels, simply because most of the patients in her series are juvenile-onset diabetics who are notoriously difficult to regulate, even under hospital conditions. Krall and Podolsky (1971) reported that even after the onset of retinopathy, a significant number of patients may improve or have no further visual regression. The classic work of Siperstein et al. (1968) has been cited as proof that attempted 'control' is useless. Danowski et al. (1971) point out other possibilities with thickening of the basement membrane and state that glucose intolerance present in persons with myopathy or neuromyopathy appears to be 'an entity distinct from diabetes mellitus'. Moreover, Soeldner et al. (1967) have shown that glucose tolerance tests can be negative many times even in those persons with a strong hereditary tendency to diabetes, but after numerous repeated test, occasional evidence of carbohydrate defect is found in many of these.

There are many who feel strongly that there is a definite correlation between degree of control and incidence of complications of diabetes. Marble's (1967) excellent review cites many of these and concludes: 'At the very least, one must concede that the primacy of the vascular abnormality is far from proven and with present knowledge it is unwarranted to assume that vascular disease in its origin is unrelated to the metabolic defect'. Lundbaek (1953) found a significant difference in the frequency of retinopathy in those with 'good' and those with 'poor' control. Bloodworth et al. (1970) found a definite increase in the basement membrane width of the muscle, kidney and retinal capillaries of the diabetic dog. Camerini-Dávalos et al. (1973) reported that basement membrane thickening was greater in insufficiently-treated diabetics. Among other adherents of good control, Constam (1972) also vigorously supports careful regulation of diabetes, starting early in its course.

It is obvious that at this time there are no final answers and those who advocate good control admit reluctantly that, while the point is hard to prove, they do feel strongly that such control is beneficial. On the other hand, those who feel that attempts at good control make no difference are handicapped by the fact that there is no sizable group of patients with poor control who have survived any length of time, to say nothing of having avoided complications. Bondy and Felig (1971) summarize their discussion thus: 'Under the circumstances, it appears appropriate to strive to achieve the best biochemical control practical with the methods available, always keeping in mind the fact that the biochemistry in question is occurring in a patient, and that the patient's comfort, safety and ability to lead a rewarding life may force compromises in the objectives of treatment'. This is a very fair and objective statement which is not inconsistent with the goals of therapy cited earlier.

If there is any new evidence which might point to prolonged hyperglycemia as a potential culprit, it is the recent data which suggests that in cases of insulin insufficiency the reverse of some of the usual metabolic pathways may take place. The polyol pathway, which may result in excess deposition of sorbitol (Gabbay and O'Sullivan, 1968; Gabbay, 1973), takes place when hyperglycemia apparently influences an increased accumulation of glucose within the Schwann cell with decreased use of the usual metabolic pathway, common glycolysis. The glucose then becomes an alcohol sugar called sorbitol because of increased activity of the enzyme, aldose reductase. This accumulation and swelling may damage the sheath of the Schwann cell and conduction down the peripheral nerves is impaired. This probably takes place in other tissues as well. Some of the work by Spiro (1973) strongly suggests that the basement membrane lesions are the sequelae of insulin deficiency and that careful hormonal replacement therapy can prevent or mitigate their development. Other pathways include the glycoprotein pathway where, in the presence of insulin deficiency, glycoprotein is increased in the diabetic basement membrane, and the glucuronic acid pathway in which glucose again finds itself going through an alternate pathway resulting in increased amounts of glucose converted into two substances called xylulose and xylitol, which may be incorporated into mucopolysaccharides, said to be the ground substance in tissue. If none of these bits of evidence are conclusive, they are at least highly suggestive at this point.

Differences in complications of insulin-dependent and insulin-independent diabetics

It is difficult to generalize on differences in the fates of the insulin-dependent and insulin-independent diabetics. Classifications and categories are a snare and a delusion because the 'juvenile-onset diabetic' whose diabetes starts at an early age sometimes has the adult type of course, while diabetics in their fifth and sixth decades may have a very unstable, juvenile-like course. Indeed, hospital and diabetes centers are quite accustomed to the admission of elderly diabetics who were 'insulin-independent' and 'acidosis-resistant' until they developed an infection of some type which ultimately resulted in ketoacidosis. Table 2 shows what is happening to the diabetic population. Diabetic coma, which was the cause of death in 47.7% of all diabetic deaths prior to the development of insulin, has now decreased to about 1%. Infections and tuberculosis deaths have dropped considerably, due largely to better care with the use of insulin and antibiotics. While gangrene of the extremities has not disappeared, it has diminished to one-tenth of its previous total as a cause of death. On the other hand, because diabetics are living longer, their chances to die of cardiovascular, cerebrovascular and renal causes as well as of cancer are greatly increased. One way to distinguish between 'insulin-dependent' and 'insulin-independent diabetics' is to identify the categories of juvenile- and adult-onset diabetes.

In observing these data, some facts are immediately apparent. Coma is still a possible cause of death in either adults or juveniles. Interestingly enough, among insulin-dependent adults, there are a significant number who die of coma because of other complications such as myocardial infarction. Both adult- and juvenile-onset diabetics may die of myocardial infarction, probably at an earlier age and sometimes with fewer obvious

TABLE 2
Trends in causes of death (percentage of total deaths; Joslin Clinic)
25,489 patients

All causes	1898–1922 (1162)	1923–1949 (11,877)	1950–1964 (12,450)
		Percent of Total	
Diabetic Coma	47.7	4.5	1.0
Vascular	22.6	63.6	77.0
Cardiac	---	36.1	53.3
Renal	---	5.1	9.0
Nephropathy	---	---	5.5
Cerebral	---	10.1	12.5
Gangrene	---	10.4	1.3
Infections	11.2	9.4	5.8
Tuberculosis	4.9	2.2	0.3
Cancer	3.2	9.2	10.1

symptoms than non-diabetics.

In the most classical of 'insulin-dependent' patients, the juvenile-onset diabetics, evidence of arterial calcification appeared between the ages of 10 and 19 years in 6.5% of the group of 1,072 patients who were living 20 years or more following the time of diagnosis of the disease according to White and Graham (1971). The first lesions to appear were in the foot and leg, then in the pelvic arteries, including the uterine vessels, still later in the abdominal aorta and finally in the thoracic aorta. Among 478 patients with juvenile-onset diabetes who in 1960 had survived 30 or more years, while gangrene of the foot or leg had occurred in only 3%, coronary involvement was more common with 19% having had myocardial infarctions.

Retinopathy, considered the bane of young-onset diabetics, is not necessarily peculiar to them. While malignant retinopathy may be found in this group, some of those who did best in a 15-year observation series reported by Krall and Podolsky (1971) were those whose onset of diabetes was at an early age.

Nephropathy is a most important complication from the viewpoint of morbidity and eventual mortality in juvenile-onset diabetes. In general, these diabetics more often succumb to nephropathy and kidney failure while the adult-onset diabetic succumbs to cardiac disease. In is difficult to completely equate adult insulin-dependent and non-insulin-requiring diabetics in long series of observations because many adults who should be treated with insulin are not, while others, who are treated with insulin, might do as well with diet alone.

THE TOOLS OF TREATMENT

It has been estimated that the world diabetic population may be somewhere between 20 and 30 million persons. Since there is definite evidence that at least the short-term, acute complications of diabetes can be avoided, and suggestive evidence that some of the long-term complications may be ameliorated, why are there so few really well controlled or regulated diabetics? This question is increasingly important now when hospital costs are under scrutiny everywhere in the world and people are more and more aware of the high cost of diabetic morbidity.

There are more reasons for this.

1. Lack of awareness on the part of the physician. Over many decades it has become habitual to look for diabetes with the classical triad of polyuria, polydipsia and polyphagia. These symptoms really represent a breakdown of the insulin delivery system. It is as logical to wait to start treatment of diabetes at this level of symptomatology as it is to start treating cardiac disease when there is pulmonary edema. These classical signs of diabetes indicate a gross pancreatic beta cell decompensation. The physician who prides himself on the detection and treatment of other diseases at an early stage should be aware that a positive family history, obesity and hyperglycemia are among the forerunners of diabetes. Very often treatment is started late. Treatment does not necessarily mean large doses of insulin or even the use of oral hypoglycemic agents. If a person's weight is reduced sufficiently so that he is able to survive with his own endogenous insulin, the finest possible treatment has been started.

2. In a world which is rapidly developing increased prosperity for more people, the tendency toward a hedonistic society mitigates against the discipline needed to follow a diet. There are cultural and ethnic habit patterns which often lead to the equating of obesity with prosperity. The onset of diabetes in a large segment of the population comes at an age when many of the other pleasures are no longer available and the necessity of a diet takes away one of the last remaining joys. While some of the more educated portions of the world population are increasingly diet-conscious, there still remain sizable groups to whom any form of diet is anathema.

3. Insulin in its present form has not been changed or improved greatly for at least 30 years and in spite of its basic life-saving properties, it is a difficult tool to use in the treatment of severe or unstable diabetes.

At the present time, the clinician is forced to choose an insulin dose 24 hours in advance, estimating the patient's diet, activity, emotional state, chance of incipient infection and other factors which might change the insulin requirement. Once insulin is injected, the patient must then pattern his living according to this insulin dose.

Exogenous insulin itself is a complex group of amino acids from a foreign species. Too large a dose results in hypoglycemia. Insufficient doses may result in acidosis. There is always the possibility of insulin allergy, resistance or local complications in the form of dystrophies. Possibly the best method for administering present-day insulin would be the use of regular (crystalline, rapid) insulin 3 or 4 times daily, simulating the insulin-releasing activity of the normal pancreas. This would be unacceptable to most people.

If diabetic patients are difficult to treat, it is not always the fault of the physician or the patient. Sometimes it is due to the awkwardness of the therapeutic tools themselves.

What could be achieved if the ideal diabetic patient were found early enough and would wholeheartedly cooperate? There is such a group of patients previously reported in the literature by Krall (1970a, b). These are airline jet pilots, who are as a group becoming older, many of them now reaching the fifth and the sixth decades. An increasing number of pilots are entering those decades of life when diabetes is more likely to occur. The problem is further underscored by the fact that in that same airline, the causes of pilot grounding were (1) cardiovascular disease, (2) psychiatric reasons, (3) diabetes mellitus, (4) central nervous system disorders, (5) ear, nose and throat problems, and (6) malignancies, in that order. This incidence of diabetes poses a great threat to the pilots because they are likely to be grounded at the height of their careers. If it is necessary to treat them with either insulin or oral hypoglycemic agents, their flying status is terminated with a subsequent loss of skilled personnel to the airlines and a substantial livelihood to the pilots.

Although these pilots are usually not much overweight, they are superb subjects for diet therapy because they are intelligent, cooperative and, of course, extremely well motivated. The series of pilots who over the past 15 years have been closely observed numbers 20. Of the 20, one failed completely with diet therapy, two continued for 5 and 7 years respectively, while the rest have been able to show normal postprandial blood glucose levels with none of the clinical or laboratory abnormalities found with diabetes. The problem with these pilot patients is exactly the opposite of what one would expect with the usual population. The pilots tend to eat *less* than the diets allowed them. In general, they are given a moderate-carbohydrate, high-protein, moderate-fat diet, relatively modest in calories and with frequent smaller feedings distributed throughout the waking hours. Thus, at no time is there a challenge to the pancreatic function.

Case #PA-A-1 was age 48, height 68 inches, weight 198 pounds, with a history of diabetes in his family. His symptoms were polyuria, polydipsia and polyphagia as well as tiredness. Some years earlier he had been told that he had an 'elevated blood sugar' which was 'not diabetic'. At the time of his arrival at the Clinic, his oral glucose tolerance test was unquestionably diabetic (Fig. 1). He was hospitalized and first treated with a 1000 calorie diet. This did not lower his blood glucose level. The diet was reduced to 900 calories with the true blood sugar results (mg/100 ml) shown in Table 3.

The patient was discharged with an exercise program and a 730 calorie diet. Blood sugar levels continued normal even postprandially. There were no longer symptoms. The diet was later raised to 1166 calories daily and finally to 1584 calories. The weight decreased slowly and blood glucose levels were consistently within normal limits month after month, whether fasting or postprandially. In May, 1973, the patient's weight had been

TABLE 3
Recovery of patient PA-A-I

Hospital day	Fasting (venous)	11.00 a.m. (capillary)	15.00 p.m. (capillary)
		(Diet: 1000 calories)	
6	170	145	165
7	140	135	120
	(Diet was then reduced to 900 calories daily)		
8	150	125	140
9	155	160	136
10	130	150	123

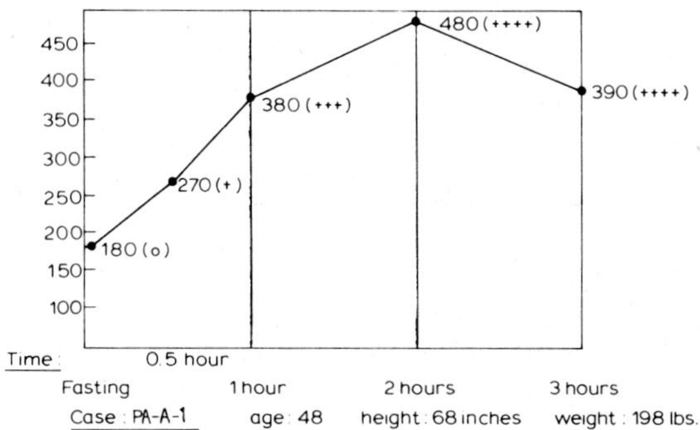

FIG. 1. 100 gram glucose tolerance test (October, 1972). Numbers indicate blood glucose in mg/100 ml true sugar. Numbers in brackets indicate amount of glucose in urine.

reduced from the original 198 pounds to 167 pounds. A blood glucose one hour postprandially at that time was 123 mg/100 ml and he returned to flying status with normal health and ability.

Case #E-rw-1 was more complex. He was found to have glycosuria in October, 1970, during a routine physical examination. Although he was slender, with a height of 72 inches and a weight of 186 pounds, it was noted that he once weighed 230 pounds and had a history of diabetes in his family. The glucose tolerance test results of fasting 103 (urine sugar 0), 1-hour 149 (urine 0), 2-hour 129 (urine 0) and 3-hour 82 mg% (urine 0) were considered 'abnormal'. He had consistently normal blood glucose levels during the next 2 years. In May, 1972, he developed diabetes symptoms and was found to have a blood glucose level of 278 mg% 2 hours p.c. with a urine glucose of 3.9% and 3+ acetonuria. He was hospitalized but treatment with an 800 calorie diet was ineffective. The blood glucose was 211 mg% fasting, 320 mg% at 11.00 a.m. and 270 mg% at 15.00 p.m. He was treated with insulin, and after 8 days his blood sugar levels returned to normal. He was discharged to a work program at his farm with a 1630 calorie diet and 26 units of insulin daily. He was given careful instructions to adjust the insulin as needed to keep him on the verge of hypoglycemic reaction or in a state of frequent mild reactions. These were to be treated promptly with just enough oral glucose to keep him out of hypoglycemia. During a 2-month period, his blood sugar levels continued normal and the insulin dose was decreased. Eventually he was changed to acetohexamide and finally to diet alone. After several months of this regimen, he was stabilized with diet alone. He had no clinical symptoms. There was no glycosuria and his blood glucose levels remained normal (86 mg% 2 hours p.c., November, 1972). He continued with this program.

It cannot be inferred that all diabetics can be treated in this fashion with the use of diet alone, nor is it certain how long these obviously adult-onset diabetics can remain in what appears to be a remission. However, with a greater effort on the part of the physician and with greater cooperation of the patient, it is amazing what might be accomplished even with the present imperfect tools of treatment. Certainly, in a highly motivated, cooperative group such as these pilots, the full impact of clinical diabetes as we know it today may be postponed and possibly in some cases permanently ameliorated.

Until we have more accurate information concerning the cause and ideal means of treatment of diabetes, it is important to make greater efforts to better treat our diabetics with the relatively crude tools of today.

The subject of remissions during diabetes has not been completely explored. Everyone accepts the remissive state in the juvenile and overlooks the fact that the adult remission may be more complete for a longer period. Pirart and Lauvaux (1971) have covered the subject in a most admirable fashion.

IMPROVED INSULIN DELIVERY SYSTEMS OF TOMORROW?

While the subject of improved systems for insulin delivery is discussed elsewhere, it is worthwhile to quickly review the possibilities.

While the transplant of the pancreas will probably be successful some day, at present it has been only a partial success because of rejection and other factors. The ultimate successful attempts will provide great research tools and give us important information. Transplants of the pancreas will probably never be a widespread factor in the treatment of diabetes because they will always involve formidable surgery. Furthermore, diabetics do not require a normal pancreas to live (and many have lived without active beta cells for most of their lifetime). Because of the vast number of diabetics in the world, it would be impractical to provide sufficient viable pancreases. The possibility of a true oral insulin is a hope for the future. There are many difficulties in the solution of this problem which may be dispelled if the practical synthesis of insulin becomes possible some day. This might permit the diabetic to orally ingest insulin according to his caloric intake. While not likely in the immediate future, it could be possible in these days of great scientific advances. An exotic possibility is the development of a glucose monitor as reported by Soeldner et al. (1973). This development received impetus from the reported new implantable sensor which could sense changes which could be correlated quite precisely with the glucose concentration in the body of the animal being monitored. In the laboratory this has taken place for long periods and the implanting of such a sensor with miniature computers and a small radiotransmitting station in a compact unit may be undertaken in human subjects within a year. Inevitably this will lead to the consideration of a complete artificial pancreas by these workers as well as Albisser et al. (1973) among others. This, however, may be a transitional stage en route to the ultimate goal. While complete pancreatic transplants have a high rejection rate and transplanting Islets of Langerhans likewise is difficult, apparently beta cell transplant can be accomplished more successfully. This has been done by a number of workers. Chick et al. (1973) as well as several others have been able to transplant beta cells into tissue culture and keep them growing for long periods of time. These tissue-culture living beta cells produce usable insulin in response to glucose and more recently have been successfully transplanted into rats closely related to the original donors of the beta cells. Apparently the intermediate stage of tissue culture is an important adjunct in this procedure. Summerlin et al. (1973) have found that cells of various types, when grown in tissue culture, lose much of their capacity to provoke rejection when transplanted into a different species. This evokes the exciting possibility that beta cells from experimental animals may some day be used in other animals and even in man. Then, for the first time, we shall be able to discuss intelligently the effects of 'good control'.

CONCLUSIONS

The world diabetes community is involved in much discussion about subjects concerning which we have few hard facts. The general feeling is that 'good control' is better for the patient than 'poor control'. Nearly everyone would like to offer better control to diabetic patients, but with unstable forms of diabetes this is difficult and sometimes nearly impossible to achieve with the present crude therapeutic tools. If one recalls that the non-diabetic *always* has a normal blood sugar, we then understand that there are no large numbers of really well-regulated diabetics. Certain groups of patients, however, who are well motivated and cooperative, have achieved good control of their diabetes. These special groups, such as airline pilots, have demonstrated the possibility of long periods of remission, sometimes with diet alone.

The Joslin Diabetes Foundation has for years awarded a medal to those patients who have had documented diabetes for 25 years without complications of any kind. More than 150 of these medals have been awarded. There is also a medal available for those who have had documented diabetes for 50 years or longer. More than 75 of these have been awarded, many to patients treated by other physicians. Some of these people had to live heroic lives in an attempt to live with their diabetes and indeed, if there is one common denominator among these persons, it is that most of them give a history of frequent hypoglycemic reactions. This does not indicate that hypoglycemic reactions are a goal, but with our imprecise therapeutic tools of today, the really 'well regulated' diabetic achieves normal blood chemistry with difficulty.

A great detriment to better care of diabetic patients now is the attitude of the physician who has become discouraged with the difficulties of diabetic treatment. In another field, for years it was widely taught that slightly elevated blood pressures were of no consequence and indeed somewhat elevated blood pressure levels were normal and acceptable in the aging. Now, with more knowledge of hypertension, the goals of treatment of high blood pressure have changed direction. Medical literature now emphasizes such titles as 'Is hypertension ever benign?'. The study of the Veterans Administration Cooperative Study (which won the Lasker Public Health Award in 1971), reported that the treatment of hypertension, even in its mildest forms, not only lowers blood pressure but significantly lessens the complications leading to death. These data were later published in a popular medical article: 'Even a little is too much'. Perhaps we are rapidly approaching the day in diabetes when the present 'laissez-faire' attitude of many physicians will be supplanted by the question: 'Is hyperglycemia ever benign?' and the thought that 'even a little is too much'.

REFERENCES

ALBISSER, A. M., LEIBEL, B. S., EWART, T., DAVIDOVAC, Z. and ZINGG, W. (1973): The artificial pancreas. *Diabetes, 22/Suppl. 1,* 294.

BLOODWORTH Jr., J. M. B., ENGERMAN, R. L., CAMERINI-DAVÁLOS, R. A. and POWERS, K. L. (1970): Variations in capillary basement membrane width produced by aging and diabetes mellitus. In: *Early Diabetes, Advances in Metabolic Disorders, Suppl. 1,* p. 279. Editors: R. A. Camerini-Dávalos and H. S. Cole. Academic Press, New York, N. Y.

BONDY, P. K. and FELIG, P. (1971): Relation of diabetic control to development of vascular complications. *Med. Clin. N. Amer., 55/4,* 889.

CAMERINI-DÁVALOS, R. A., BLOODWORTH Jr., J. M. B., LIMBURG, A., GORDON, A. L., COLE, H. S. and OPPERMANN, W. (1973): Deterioration of tolerance to glucose and progression of the microangiopathy: effect of treatment (preliminary report). In: *Early Diabetes, Advances in Metabolic Disorders, Suppl. 2,* p. 373. Editors: R. A. Camerini-Dávalos and H. S. Cole. Academic Press, New York, N. Y.

CHICK, W., LAURIS, V., FLEWELLING, J. H., ANDREWS, K. A. and WOODRUFF, J. M. (1973): Effects of glucose on beta cells in pancreatic monolayer cultures. *Endocrinology, 92/1,* 212.

CONSTAM, G. R. (1972): Contrôle du diabète et prevention des complications. *Journées Diabètologie, 13,* 313.

DANOWSKI, T. S., KHURANA, R. C., GONZALEZ, A. R. and FISHER, E. R. (1971): Capillary basement membrane thickness and pseudo-diabetes of myopathy. *Amer. J. Med., 51,* 757.

GABBAY, K. H. (1973): The sorbitol pathway and the complications of diabetes. *New Engl. J. Med., 288/16,* 831.

GABBAY, K. H. and O'SULLIVAN, J. B. (1968): The sorbitol pathway. Enzyme localization and content in normal and diabetic nerve and control. *Diabetes, 17/5,* 239.

KRALL, L. P. (1970a): Treatment of early diabetes. In: *Early Diabetes, Advances in Metabolic Disorders, Suppl. 1,* p. 395. Editors: R. A. Camerini-Dávalos and H. S. Cole. Academic Press, New York, N.Y.

KRALL, L. P. (1970b): Nutritional and genetic factors in the pathogenesis of diabetes mellitus. In: *Proceedings, VIII International Congress on Nutrition, Prague 1969,* pp. 376–378. Editors: J. Masek, K. Osancová and D. P. Buthbertson. International Congress Series No. 213, Excerpta Medica, Amsterdam.

KRALL, L. P. and PODOLSKY, S. (1971): Long-term clinical observations of diabetic retinopathy. In: *Proceedings, VII Congress of the International Diabetes Federation, Buenos Aires 1970,* pp. 268–275. Editors: R. R. Rodriguez and J. Vallance-Owen. International Congress Series No. 231, Excerpta Medica, Amsterdam.

LUNDBAEK, K. (1953): *Long-Term Diabetes. The Clinical Picture in Diabetes Mellitus of 15–25 Years' Duration with a Follow-Up of a Regional Series of Cases.* Munksgaard, Copenhagen.

MARBLE, A. (1967): Angiopathy in diabetes: an unsolved problem. *Diabetes, 16/12,* 825.

PIRART, J. and LAUVAUX, J. P. (1971): Remission in diabetes. In: *Diabetes Mellitus, Vol. II,* p. 443. Editor: E. Pfeiffer. Lehmanns Verlag, Munich.

SIPERSTEIN, M. D., UNGER, R. H. and MADISON, L. L. (1968): Studies of muscle capillary basement membranes in normal subjects, diabetic, and prediabetic patients. *J. clin. Invest., 47/9,* 1973.

SOELDNER, J. S., CHANG, K. W., HIEBERT, J. M. and AISENBERG, S. (1973): In-vitro and in-vivo experience with a miniature glucose sensor. *Diabetes, 22/Suppl. 1,* 294.

SOELDNER, J. S., GLEASON, R. E., KAHN, C. B., ROJAS, L. and MARBLE, A. (1967): Repetitive oral glucose tolerance testing in genetic prediabetics. In: *Abstracts, VI Congress of the International Diabetes Federation, Stockholm 1967,* p. 63. Editors: J. Östman, C. N. Hales, L. E. Miles and R. D. G. Milner. International Congress Series No. 140, Excerpta Medica, Amsterdam.

SPIRO, R. G. (1973): Biochemistry of the renal glomerular basement membrane and its alterations in diabetes mellitus.*New Engl. J. Med., 288/25,* 1337.

SUMMERLIN, W. T., MILLER, G. E. and GOOD, R. A. (1973): Successful tissue and organ allotransplantation without immunosuppression. Paper presented to: The American Society for Clinical Investigation, Atlantic City, N.J. 1973.

WHITE, P. (1956): The natural course and prognosis of juvenile diabetes. *Diabetes, 5/6,* 445.

WHITE, P. and GRAHAM, C. A. (1971): The child with diabetes. In: *Joslin's Diabetes Mellitus, 11th ed.,* Chapter 13, p. 339. Editors: A. Marble, P. White, R. F. Bradley and L. P. Krall. Lea and Febiger, Philadelphia, Pa.

WILKERSON, H. L. C. and KRALL, L. P. (1947): Diabetes in a New England town. *J. Amer. med. Ass., 135,* 209.

QUANTITATIVE STUDIES OF DIABETIC NEPHROPATHY AND THE GROWTH HORMONE HYPOTHESIS

K. LUNDBAEK

Aarhus Universitet, Kommunehospitalet, Aarhus, Denmark

Diabetic microangiopathy develops in all organs of the body but clinically it appears in only some organs. From the practical point of view, ocular and renal lesions are the most important (diabetic heart disease is probably a combination of diabetic microangiopathy, diabetic macroangiopathy and atherosclerosis) (Lundbaek, 1973).

Theoretically the renal lesions are of special interest because the capillary changes characterizing diabetic glomerulopathy can be studied morphologically with exact methods.

The following is a short summary of the results obtained in quantitative electron microscopic studies of normal and diabetic glomeruli by Ruth Østerby (1973a). This will be followed by a short presentation of the growth hormone hypothesis about diabetic vascular disease (Lundbaek et al., 1970, 1971). This hypothesis will finally have to be tested in a controlled clinical trial. Electron microscopic quantitation of the glomerular basement membrane will provide the best parameter in such a study.

QUANTITATIVE STUDIES OF VASCULAR CHANGES IN THE RENAL GLOMERULI

For a number of reasons the vascular wall of the renal glomeruli is the best choice for exact studies of diabetic angiopathy. However, after having decided to study renal capillaries, a number of other choices have to be made, which are both technical and clinical.

Technically it is clear that electron microscopy is mandatory and that a quantitative method has to be employed. This is, of course, not peculiar to diabetic vascular disease; it is recognized generally today that morphology has to be studied quantitatively. Moreover, it has been shown through Dr. Østerby's studies that quantification is possible, giving to morphology the same kind of precision that we are used to expect in physiology, clinical chemistry and physics.

Clinically the subproblem to be studied has to be selected. For many reasons some of the most obvious questions to be asked are: *When* does diabetic angiopathy appear, *how* does it develop, and how quickly?

Specifically for the glomerulus, and due to the confusion of earlier non-quantitative studies, it is necessary to ask: where in the glomerulus does it start? How does it develop in various parts? What comes first, peripheral changes or mesangial changes? Is there *cellular hypertrophy* that could explain basement membrane changes?

The decision to study the early time course of diabetic angiopathy in the kidney makes another choice necessary, namely the study of young diabetic patients. Only in classical juvenile diabetes can the clinical time of onset of the disease be determined with certainty.

In principle, Dr. Østerby's technique consists in measuring all relevant structures in a complete cross-section of a glomerulus, and in the construction of distribution curves from the values thus obtained for basement membrane thickness (Østerby, 1972a).

Figure 1 shows an electron micrograph from a renal glomerulus with 3 capillary walls. It is obvious that the basement membrane thickness varies very much, making quantitative studies mandatory.

Figure 2 shows a total cross-section of one glomerulus, photographed so as to give an impression of its size. It is a montage of about 60 individual electron micrographs. It is on such montages that measurements are carried out.

Figure 3 shows frequency distribution curves of glomerular basement membrane thickness in controls and in diabetic patients (cases after 1 month are the same as onset cases). Each curve is constructed on the basis of 500–2,000 measurements at regular intervals.

Figure 4 shows the same results as in Figure 3 after mathematical transformation of the values (Gundersen and Østerby, 1973). With the transformation used the basement membrane thickness is normally distributed, and the Gaussian scale cumulative frequency curves are therefore straight lines, well suited for statistical treatment. Inspection shows that there is no difference between controls and recent onset cases. Statistical analysis demonstrates a significant difference between recent onset cases and cases after 3.5–5 years of diabetes. Paired comparison also shows statistically significant differences between cases at onset and the cases after 1.5–2 years (Østerby, 1972a).

These results are quite clear-cut: At the moment when classical juvenile diabetes appears clinically the peripheral basement membrane of the renal glomerulus is normal. Thickening, demonstrable with this technique, is present after 1–2 years.

Some other interesting results of Dr. Østerby's work can be summarized as follows: (1) the basement membrane-like material of the mesangial areas is normal at the clinical start of juvenile diabetes. It increases *pari passu* with the thickening of the peripheral basement membrane (Østerby, 1973b). (2) The basement membrane changes develop uniformly all over the glomerulus, not particularly in the polar or the peripheral part, and not particularly in juxtamesangial areas or in areas far from the mesangial regions (Østerby, 1973c). (3) There is no hypercellularity in the early phase of diabetic glomerulopathy (Østerby, 1972b).

As for the pathogenic interpretation of these natural history data, the results obtained seem to indicate that the vascular changes are secondary to or the result of the metabolic disturbance characterizing diabetes mellitus. However, they do not allow any conclusions as to *what* element in the metabolic abnormality is responsible – high blood sugar itself or some resulting or co-related abnormal state of the cells or body fluids.

The studies that have been described here are from the kidney. However, there is no reason to doubt that they are also valid for blood vessels in the other organs of the body of diabetic patients.

THE GROWTH HORMONE HYPOTHESIS

The growth hormone hypothesis (Lundbaek et al., 1970, 1971) states that overpro-

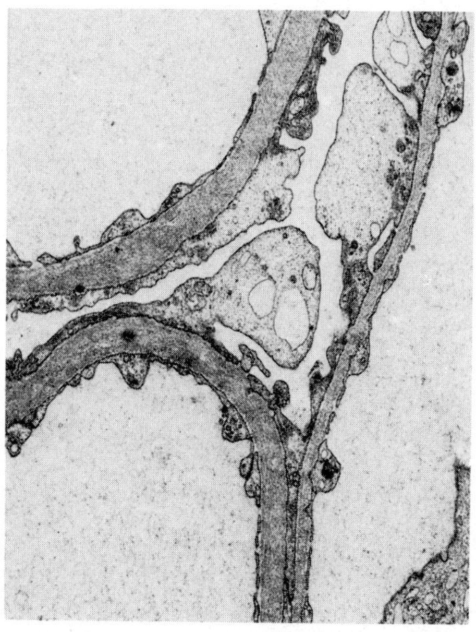

FIG. 1. A casual electron micrograph from a renal glomerulus.

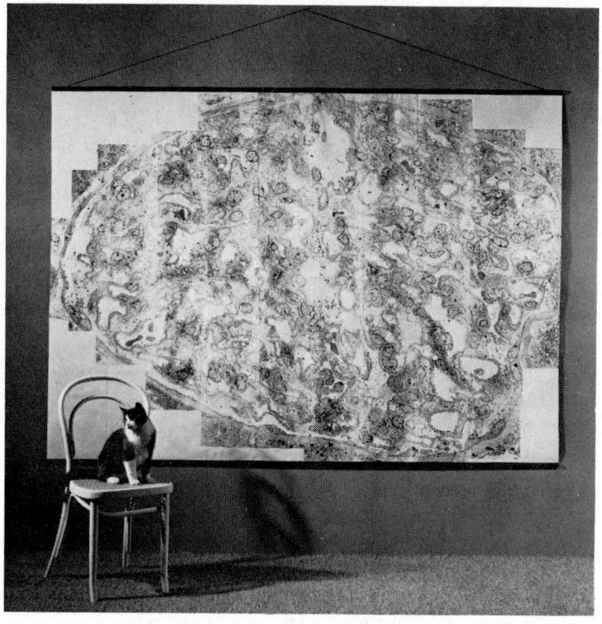

FIG. 2. Montage of electron micrographs forming a total cross-section of a renal glomerulus.

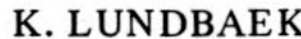

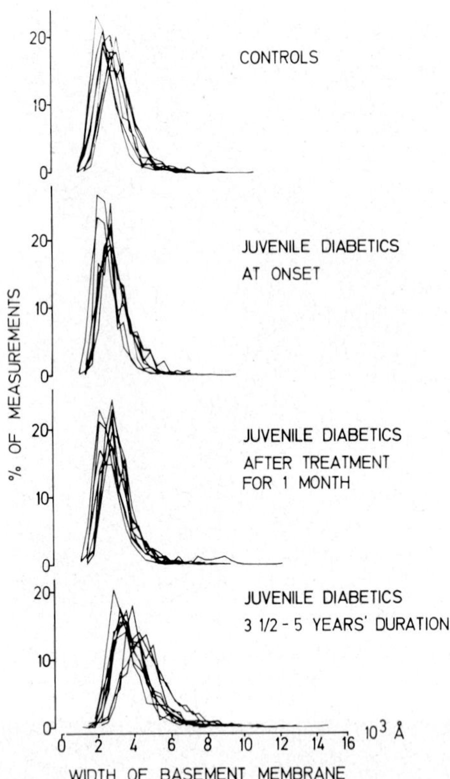

FIG. 3. Frequency distribution curves of glomerular basement membrane thickness.

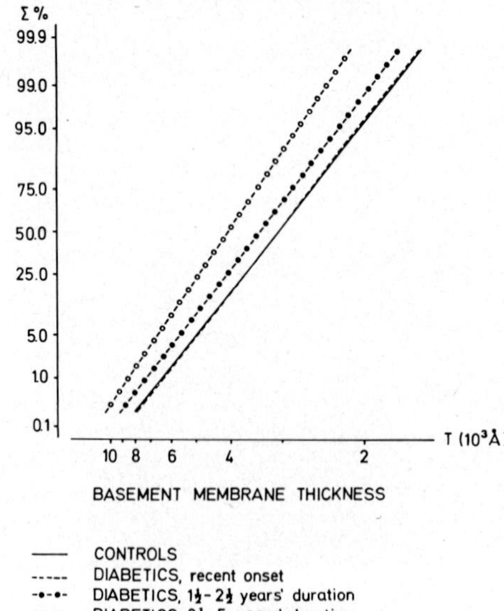

FIG. 4. Same results as Figure 3 after mathematical transformation (see text).

duction of growth hormone is a causal factor in the development of diabetic angiopathy. There are variants of this postulate, e.g. substituting 'a permissive factor' for 'a causal factor', or substituting 'high diurnal plasma growth hormone' for 'overproduction'.

The growth hormone hypothesis is a working hypothesis, not in any sense a theory. It is a tool for designing experiments and a pointer to further work.

This hypothesis is based on 2 facts: (1) the beneficial effect on angiopathy of growth hormone withdrawal, and (2) the high and fluctuating plasma growth hormone found in diabetic patients under ordinary daily life conditions.

The first point, the effect of growth hormone withdrawal, has been demonstrated in several careful studies of patients after complete or partial pituitary ablation. Our own controlled clinical trial was presented in great detail during the International Diabetes Congress in Stockholm 6 years ago (Lundbaek et al., 1967). Since that time half of the patients of our series have died. The groups are not suited for comparison any more, but the same tendency to better preservation of eye-sight and less development of rubeosis and glaucoma in the hypophysectomized patients is still to be seen – although less clearly than 5 years ago.

The beneficial result of pituitary ablation has also been shown in the careful study by Oakley et al. (1969) at the London Postgraduate School. Hypophysectomized patients are maintained on thyroid, steroid and gonadal hormones. Disregarding lactogenic hormone, the role of which is still obscure, these patients can be regarded as essentially growth hormone-ectomized patients.

The second point, oversecretion of growth hormone in diabetes, has been shown from the many experiments of Hansen (1972) in our laboratory. Early studies of young juvenile males demonstrated that the 24-hour plasma growth hormone level is 3–4 times higher and more fluctuant in diabetics than in comparable non-diabetics, and that the exercise-induced plasma growth hormone rise occurs earlier and is higher in diabetics (Hansen and Johansen, 1970; Hansen, 1970, 1971a). It was also shown that lowering of the blood sugar level reduces these abnormalities but only complete blood sugar normalization for several days is able to abolish it (Johansen and Hansen, 1971; Hansen, 1971b).

Lately the same phenomena have been found in young diabetic women and in elderly maturity-onset diabetics (see Figs 5 and 6) (Hansen, 1973a, b).

The growth hormone hypothesis puts together the hypophysectomy results and the plasma growth hormone studies (Lundbaek et al., 1970, 1971). If there is too much growth hormone circulating in diabetic patients during all the months and years while the slow development of angiopathy takes place, and if total removal of growth hormone – even late in the course of development – interferes to some extent with the further development of vascular damage, then growth hormone might be thought to be dangerous to diabetic blood vessels. This hypothesis found further support in the studies of Merimee et al. (1970), indicating that ateliotic growth hormone-deficient dwarfs, who have a mild type of diabetes, do not develop diabetic retinopathy.

It is not possible in practice to normalize blood sugar completely and constantly. Therefore the practical conclusion to be drawn from the growth hormone hypothesis is that growth hormone production should be suppressed.

Hypophysectomy is by no means ideal, and we are now trying to find a non-surgical way of suppressing growth hormone production.

We have tested orally about 50 psychotropic drugs of various types in the hope that one of these compounds, or a derivative, could influence the production of a growth hormone-stimulating factor from the hypothalamus. Only amitriptylene had an effect,

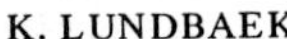

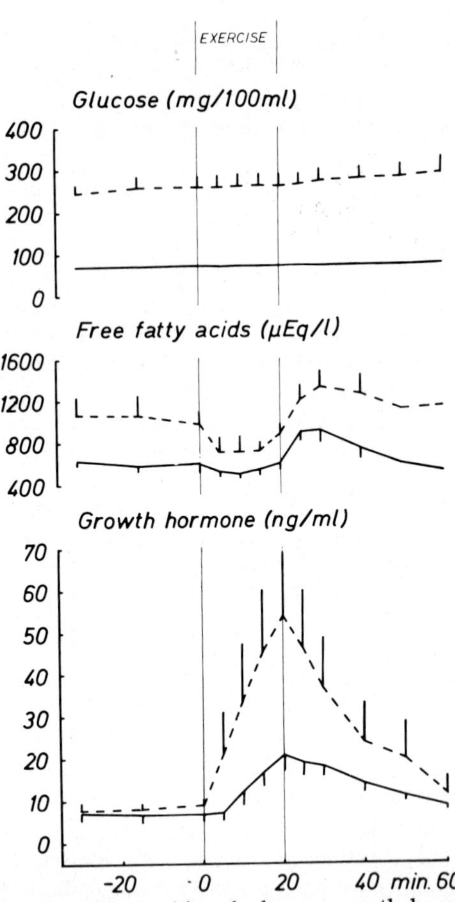

FIG. 5. Blood glucose, free fatty acid and plasma growth hormone, before, during and after a 20-minute exercise period (450 kg/min.) in 16 female juvenile diabetics (stippled) and in 20 comparable controls (fully drawn). Mean and S.E.M. are shown.

but it is much too weak even to justify trying molecular manipulations. The closely related drug imipramine, which has been shown to suppress sleep peaks (Takahashi et al., 1968), is inactive in the exercise test in diabetics. The same is true for chlorpromazine and medroxyprogesterone acetate, reported to suppress growth hormone in normals and acromegalics (Sherman et al., 1971; Kolodny et al., 1971). Pimozide, which has been reported to suppress growth hormone-releasing factor was inactive (Upton et al., 1973). Fenfluramine, administered intravenously, has been shown to suppress exercise-induced plasma growth hormone rise (Sulaiman and Johnson, 1973). It is inactive in the exercise test with diabetics when given orally.

Alpha blockade completely abolishes the abnormal rise of plasma growth hormone during exercise in diabetic patients, but only when given intravenously (Hansen, 1971c).

Preliminary data indicates that somatostatin, the naturally occurring hypothalamic growth hormone release-inhibiting factor (Brazeau et al., 1973) inhibits exercise-induced

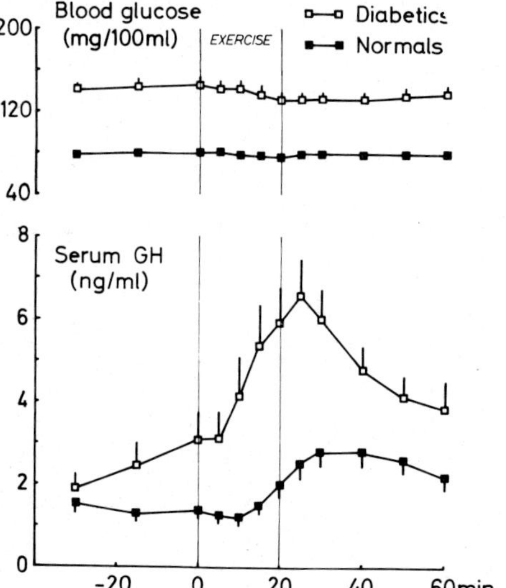

FIG. 6. Blood glucose and plasma growth hormone in 63 patients with maturity-onset diabetes (open squares) and in 31 comparable controls (closed squares). The exercise load was 350 kg/min. Mean and S.E.M. are shown.

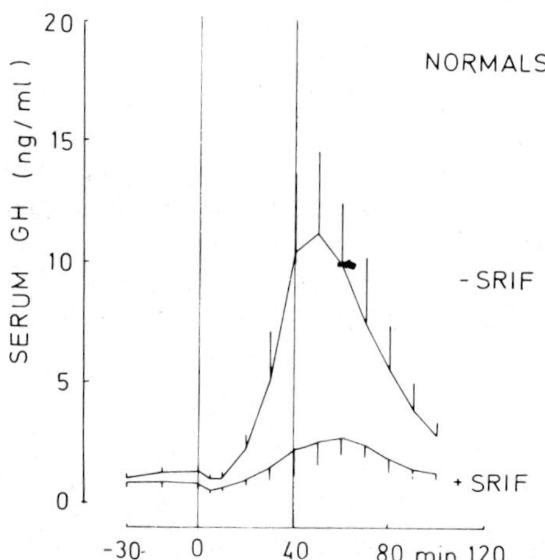

FIG. 7. Serum growth hormone in 7 normal, male subjects before, during and after exercise (450 kg/min.) with and without the infusion of somatostatin (SRIF). Mean and S.E.M. are shown.

plasma growth hormone rise when given intravenously to normal subjects and to diabetic patients (see Figs 7 and 8) (Hansen et al., 1973).

If a way can be found in which this compound, or one of its derivatives, can be administered in a clinically acceptable way, suppressing growth hormone production for

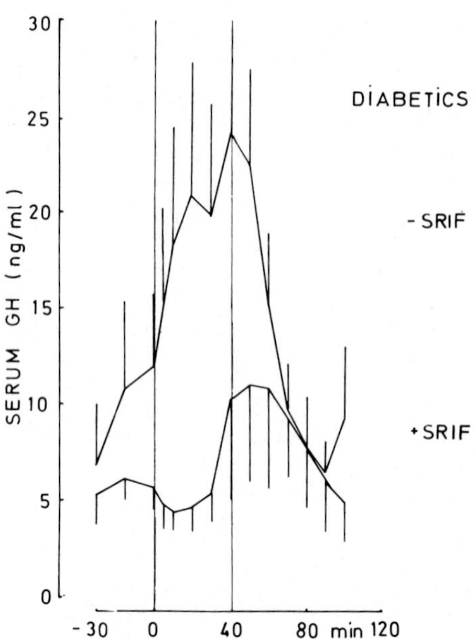

FIG. 8. Serum growth hormone in 9 male diabetics before, during and after exercise (450 kg/min.) with and without the infusion of somatostatin (SRIF). Mean and S.E.M. are shown.

reasonable periods of the day, its effect on the development of diabetic angiopathy will have to be tested in a controlled clinical trial. The vascular parameter of choice in such a study is the thickness of the peripheral basement membrane and the area of basement membrane-like material in the renal glomeruli, determined with the quantitative electron microscopic technique as described in the first part of this paper (Østerby, 1973).

REFERENCES

BRAZEAU, P., VALE, W., BURGUS, R., LING, N., BUTCHER, M., RIVIER, J. and GUILLEMIN, R. (1973): Hypothalamic polypeptide that inhibits the secretion of immunoreactive pituitary growth hormone. *Science, 179,* 77.

GUNDERSEN, H. J. G. and ØSTERBY, R. (1973): Statistical analysis of transformations leading to normal distribution of measurements of the peripheral glomerular basement membrane. *J. Microsc., 97,* 293.

HANSEN, A. P. (1970): Abnormal serum growth hormone response to exercise in juvenile diabetics. *J. clin. Invest., 49,* 1467.

HANSEN, A. P. (1971a): The effect of intravenous glucose infusion on the exercise-induced serum growth hormone rise in normals and juvenile diabetics. *Scand. J. clin. Lab. Invest., 28,* 195.

HANSEN, A. P. (1971b): Normalization of growth hormone hyperresponse to exercise in juvenile diabetics after 'normalization' of blood sugar. *J. clin. Invest., 50,* 1806.

HANSEN, A. P. (1971c): The effect of adrenergic receptor blockade on the exercise-induced serum growth hormone rise in normals and juvenile diabetics. *J. clin. Endocr., 33,* 807.

HANSEN, A. P. (1972): *Sereum Growth Hormone Patterns in Juvenile Diabetes. Dan med. Bull., 19,* Suppl. 1.

HANSEN, A. P. (1973a): Serum growth hormone patterns in female juvenile diabetics. *J. clin. Endocr., 36,* 638.

HANSEN, A. P. (1973b): Abnormal serum growth hormone response to exercise in maturity-onset diabetics. *Diabetes, 22,* 619.

HANSEN, A. P. and JOHANSEN, K. (1970): Diurnal patterns of blood glucose, serum free fatty acids, insulin, glucagon and growth hormone in normals and juvenile diabetics. *Diabetologia, 6,* 27.

HANSEN, A. P., ØRSKOV, H., SEYER-HANSEN, K. and LUNDBAEK, K. (1973): Some actions of growth hormone release inhibiting factor. *Brit. med. J., 3,* 523.

JOHANSEN, K. and HANSEN, A. P. (1971): Diurnal serum growth hormone levels in poorly and well-controlled juvenile diabetics. *Diabetes, 20,* 239.

KOLODNY, H. D., SHERMAN, L., SING, A., KIM, S. and BENJAMIN, F. (1971): Acromegaly treated with chlorpromazine. A case study. *New Engl. J. Med., 284,* 819.

LUNDBAEK, K. (1973): Diabetes and the heart. In: *Skandia International Symposium on Early Phases of Coronary Heart Disease,* pp. 215–222. Nordiska Bokhandeln, Stockholm.

LUNDBAEK, K., CHRISTENSEN, N. J., JENSEN, V. A., JOHANSEN, K., OLSEN, T. S., HANSEN, A. P., ØRSKOV, H. and ØSTERBY, R. (1970): Diabetes, diabetic angiopathy and growth hormone. *Lancet, 2,* 131.

LUNDBAEK, K., CHRISTENSEN, N. J., JENSEN, V. A., JOHANSEN, K., OLSEN, T. S., HANSEN, A. P., ØRSKOV, H. and ØSTERBY, R. (1971): The pathogenesis of diabetic angiopathy and growth hormone. *Dan. med. Bull., 18,* 1.

LUNDBAEK, K., MALMROS, R., ANDERSEN, H. C., RASMUSSEN, J. H., BRUNTSE, E., MADSEN, P. H. and JENSEN, V. A. (1967): Hypophysectomy for diabetic angiopathy. A controlled clinical trial. In: *Supplement, Proceedings of the Sixth Congress of the International Diabetes Federation, Stockholm, 1967,* p. 127. Editor: J. Östman. International Congress Series 172, Excerpta Medica, Amsterdam.

MERIMEE, T. J., FINEBERG, S. E., McKUSICK, V. A. and HALL, J. (1970): Diabetes mellitus and sexual ateliotic dwarfism: a comparative study. *J. clin. Invest., 49,* 1096.

OAKLEY, N. W., JOPLIN, G. F., KOHNER, E. M., BLACH, R., HARTOG, M. and FRASER, T. R. (1969): The treatment of diabetic retinopathy by pituitary implantation of radioactive yttrium. *U.S. PHS Publ., 1890,* 317.

ØSTERBY, R. (1972a): Morphometric studies of the peripheral glomerular basement membrane in early juvenile diabetes. I. Development of initial basement membrane thickening. *Diabetologia, 8,* 84.

ØSTERBY, R. (1972b): The number of glomerular cells and substructures in early juvenile diabetes. A quantitative electron microscopic study. *Acta path. microbiol. scand. A., 80,* 785.

ØSTERBY, R. (1973a): *Early Phases in the Development of Diabetic Glomerulopathy. A Quantitative Electron Microscopic Study.* Monograph, in preparation.

ØSTERBY, R. (1973b): A quantitative electron microscopic study of mesangial regions in glomeruli from patients with short-term juvenile diabetes mellitus. *Lab. Invest., 29,* 99.

ØSTERBY, R. (1973c): Morphometric studies of the peripheral glomerular basement membrane. II. Topography of the initial lesions. *Diabetologia, 9.* 108.

SHERMAN, L., KIM, S., BENJAMIN, F. and KOLODNY, H. D. (1971): Effect of chlorpromazine on serum growth hormone concentration in man. *New Engl. J. Med., 284,* 72.

SULAIMAN, W. R. and JOHNSEN, R. H. (1973): Effect of fenfluramine on human growth hormone release. *Brit. med. J., 2,* 329.
TAKAHASHI, Y., KIPNIS, D. M. and DAUGHADAY, W. H. (1968): Growth hormone secretion during sleep. *J. clin. Invest., 47,* 2079.
UPTON, G. V., CORBIN, A., MABRY, C. C. and HOLLINGSWORTH, D. R. (1973): The etiology of lipoatrophic diabetes. In: *Hypothalamic Hypophysiotropic Hormones. Proceedings of the Conference at Acapulco, Mexico, 1972,* p. 373. Editors: C. Gual and E. Rosemberg. International Congress Series No. 263, Excerpta Medica, Amsterdam.

HOW TO ACHIEVE BETTER DIABETIC CONTROL? STUDIES WITH INSULIN THREE TIMES A DAY

GEORGES TCHOBROUTSKY

Department of Diabetes, University of Paris, Hôtel-Dieu Hospital, Paris, France

Biochemical (Spiro and Spiro, 1971; Beisswenger and Spiro, 1973), morphological (Österby, 1971; Kilo et al., 1972), and clinical data (Lawrence, 1963; Colwell, 1966; Caird et al., 1969; Miki et al., 1969, 1972; Chazan et al., 1970; Dorf et al., 1971; Joplin et al., 1971; Constam, 1972; Pirart et al., 1972) strongly suggest that vascular changes in diabetes are related to the degree and the duration of hyperglycemia and/or insulin deficiency or their consequences. The development of diabetic angiopathy in secondary diabetes in man (Tutin et al., 1966) and of vascular changes in the retinae and glomerulae of laboratory animals with induced diabetes (Bloodworth et al., 1969; Cameron et al., 1971; Bloodworth and Engerman, 1973) also strongly suggests that microangiopathy in diabetes is not an independent inherited factor as claimed by some authors (Siperstein et al., 1968), but is related to the acquired disease and may be reduced or prevented by good control (Bloodworth and Engerman, 1973). Studies on the sorbitol pathway also indicated that functional and morphological changes in nerves and lenses (Gabbay, 1973) are directly related to elevated blood sugar levels.

Thus most diabetologists believe the best insurance against diabetic complications is optimum blood glucose control as recently emphasized by some authors (Rull et al., 1970; Marble, 1971; Constam, 1972; Fajans, 1972). The opinion that good control delays or prevents diabetic lesions is, however, not shared by all (Knowles, 1971; Ricketts, 1965), perhaps because clinical studies, even prospective ones, are very difficult to carry out (Kaplan and Feinstein, 1973).

HOW TO ACHIEVE IDEAL CONTROL?

Very early detection of the disease and strict normalization of blood sugar levels all day long would probably eradicate diabetes complications. These goals are still unrealistic, since (1) maturity-onset diabetes is discovered after years or decades of evolution with retinal changes frequently observed at the time of the diagnosis (Soler et al., 1969); (2) the treatment of obesity is disappointing (Control of Obesity, 1966); (3) oral hypoglycemic drugs do not control blood sugar levels in most long-term treated diabetic patients (Berchtold et al., 1971) and are perhaps not safe enough (University Group Diabetes Program, 1970); and (4) insulin-dependent diabetic patients cannot be perfectly treated with current methods because exogenous insulin is not given through the portal venous system and is not adapted to minute-to-minute changes of blood sugar levels.

Strict control of blood sugar has been obtained by pancreatic transplantations in man

(Lillehei et al., 1970) and will probably be achieved by artificial beta cell devices (Soeldner, 1972; Cahill et al., 1972; Bessman and Schultz, 1972; Soeldner et al., 1973; Albisser et al., 1973; Felts, 1973) or by isolated or cultured beta cell or islet implantations (Hegre et al., 1972; Summerlin et al., 1973; Reckard et al., 1973; Kumar et al., 1973; Leonard and Hegre, 1973).

Other attempts to prevent or delay vascular and nerve changes in diabetes have been made by suppressing growth hormone secretion either anatomically (Luft et al., 1955) or pharmacologically (Lundbaek, 1971), because of the permissive role of this hormone (Lundbaek, 1971), or by giving an aldose reductase inhibitor (Gabbay, 1973).

HOW TO APPROACH BETTER CONTROL IN INSULIN-TREATED PATIENTS WITH CURRENT METHODS

Until ideal treatments are available for all patients it is probably wise to strive for the best control and to seek more physiological insulin provision. Short-acting insulin is useful in improving the control of diabetic patients, even in unstable ones (Oakley et al., 1966; Metz et al., 1967; Service et al., 1970; Spathis, 1970; Vining and Strong, 1972; Kopf et al., 1973; Tchobroutsky et al., 1973). NPH plus regular insulin twice a day is widely used systematically or in unstable diabetic patients (Oakley et al., 1966, 1973; Forsham, 1967) and also during pregnancy (Pedersen, 1967; Oakley et al., 1973). Multiple daily injections of short-acting insulin before every meal have been advocated or suggested by several authors (Lawrence, 1963; Lukens, 1965; Deuil, 1967; Earl, 1968; Rull et al., 1970; Tchobroutsky et al., 1973).

We have studied the effects of divided doses of insulin given before the meals on blood sugar and plasma insulin levels (Kopf et al., 1973; Tchobroutsky et al., 1973). Because of French people's meal habits – a light breakfast and 2 main meals at lunch and dinner – we utilized short-acting insulin before breakfast and lunch and diphasic insulin or short-acting plus intermediate insulin before dinner.

The more daily injections the patient receives the lower the blood glucose levels and the greater the differences 2 hours after the beginning of lunch. The mean time of the maximal increase in blood glucose values was reached earlier when short-acting insulin was given just before the meal than with other kinds of insulin treatment, both in the general and in the randomized study where maximal efforts were made to achieve the best control in the ward (Figs 1 and 2). In both studies the daily urinary sugar excretions were significantly lower in patients treated with 3 daily injections of insulin, even when comparisons were made after daily insulin doses adjustment (Fig. 3). This indicates that probably a better control was achieved by multiple insulin injections not only after lunch but also during the 24-hour period.

In order to check the diurnal changes in blood sugar levels in diabetics treated with insulin 3 times a day we have taken blood samples every 15 minutes (or every hour between meals) in 7 subjects during 24 hours. These subjects were submitted the next day to i.v. insulin infusion for 1 to 4.5 days (Slama et al., 1973) (Fig. 4, Table 1). In these not particularly unstable patients a good mean control was achieved through the 24-hour period with insulin 3 times a day. With the pre-established program of insulin infusion no better results in terms of means were obtained. Generally speaking patients were more often hypoglycemic than hyperglycemic.

Plasma insulin levels were assayed after lunch in 38 lean normal and 30 insulin-

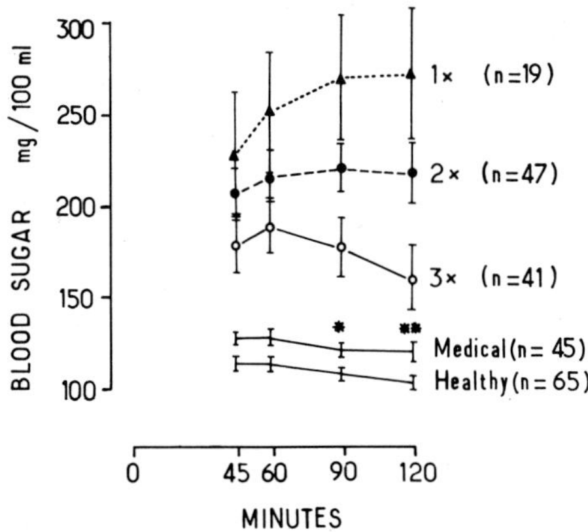

FIG. 1. Postprandial blood sugar values after the beginning of the meal in 107 insulin-treated diabetic patients and in 110 non-diabetic subjects (group A). 1X, 2X, 3X = number of daily injections of insulin. Values are means ± S.E.M. The more daily injections the patients receive the lower the blood sugar levels and the greater the differences 90 and 120 minutes after the beginning of lunch (* = $P < 0.05$; ** = $P < 0.01$). (From Kopf et al., 1973, by courtesy.)

dependent diabetic subjects taken from the first study on blood sugar levels. In insulin-treated subjects plasma insulin assays were performed only in patients treated for 4 weeks or less who had not developed detectable insulin antibodies (Fig. 5). Because all subjects were ketotic, young and thin at the beginning of the treatment, it may be assumed that mean endogenous insulin secretion was probably low. Insulin-treated diabetics have similar or slightly higher peripheral mean plasma insulin levels after lunch than non-diabetics. Patients receiving short-acting insulin just before lunch have the highest mean plasma insulin levels and the lowest blood sugar values. Thus it appears that higher than normal peripheral plasma insulin levels are necessary – at least 45–120 minutes after a meal – to lower blood sugar levels in insulin-treated patients.

Samples were not taken before the 45th minute after the beginning of the meal, but studies by Malherbe et al. (1969), Quabbe and Kliems (1969) and from our laboratory (Tchobroutsky, 1970; Hautecouverture et al., 1973) have shown that in young normal subjects the mean maximum plasma increase after a standardized lunch occurred 45 minutes after the beginning of the meal.

The fact that higher than normal peripheral plasma insulin levels are mandatory for blood glucose control in insulin-treated patients is also suggested by the results of a study we have done to compare healthy and perfectly controlled insulin-treated diabetic subjects submitted to moderate exercise in the afternoon 4 hours after lunch (Tchobroutsky et al., 1974). Diabetic patients received 3 daily insulin injections. Mean values of plasma glucose levels were not different between diabetics and non-diabetics but mean plasma insulin levels were about twice as high in diabetic than in non-diabetic subjects (Fig. 6).

It can be postulated that higher than normal peripheral plasma insulin levels in insulin-treated subjects indicate that normal portal insulin levels have probably been achieved by the treatment. In normal subjects portal insulin concentrations are higher than peripheral ones as shown for the first time by Blackard and Nelson (1970). Probably these high

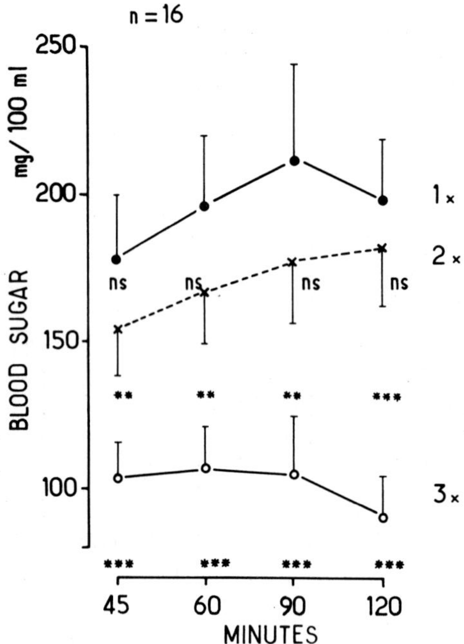

FIG. 2. Data obtained in 16 other diabetic patients already treated by insulin (group B). All patients were their own control during this study. The figure indicates the mean postprandial blood sugar values ± S.E.M. after the beginning of the midday meal according to the number of daily injections of insulin (1X, 2X or 3X). For each patient the order for administration of insulin was established at random. N.S. = non significant (1X versus 2X; ** = P <0.01 (2X versus 3X); *** = P <0.001 (general comparison). (From Kopf et al., 1973, by courtesy.)

concentrations of insulin are necessary for hepatic handling of glucose (Madison, 1969). The recent demonstration of endogenous insulin secretion during remissions or in mild forms of insulin-dependent diabetes (Foucar and Field, 1972; Block et al., 1973) also suggest that the portal delivery of insulin to the liver helps to achieve good diabetes control. In insulin-treated diabetics with very low or absent endogenous insulin secretion, it is quite certain that exogenous insulin injections lead to similar concentrations in portal and peripheral blood. If high concentrations of insulin in the portal blood are needed in insulin-treated subjects, large doses have to be administered at least before each meal. If insulin is not divided up throughout the day and if short-acting insulin is not used, hyperglycemia will occur during the meal periods.

LONG-TERM APPRECIATION OF THE MULTIPLE INSULIN INJECTION REGIMEN

A longer-term appreciation of blood sugar control in diabetic patients treated with insulin

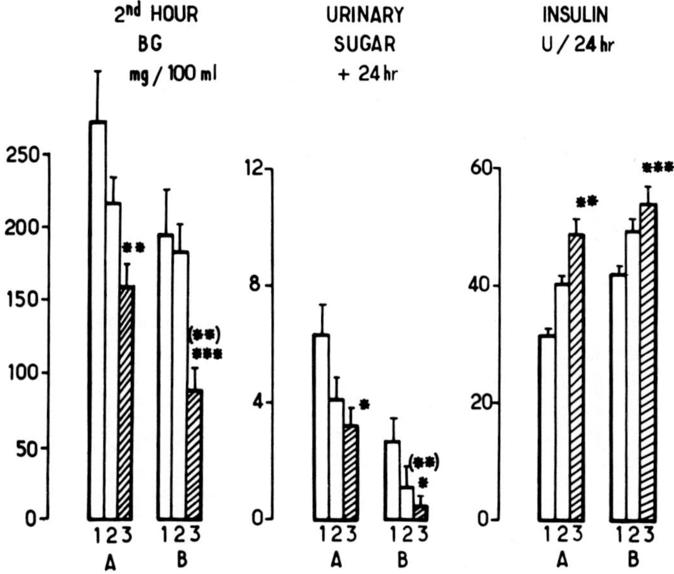

FIG. 3. Values for blood sugar levels 2 hours after the beginning of the lunch, for daily urinary sugar excretions and for daily administered insulin doses in the 107 insulin-treated patients (group A) and in the 16 additional diabetics (group B) according to the number of daily injections of insulin (1, 2, 3). Values are means ± S.E.M. The 24-hour glycosuria was calculated by adding the results of Clinitest estimation (0, +, ++, +++, ++++) made before the test-lunch, the dinner and the next morning * = P<0.05; ** = P <0.01; *** = P<0.001. Significance given in brackets refers to comparisons after daily insulin dose adjustment. (Based on data from Kopf et al., 1973.)

3 times a day was made in hospitalized pregnant women (Cassagne et al., 1973) and in outpatients (Goldgewicht et al., 1973).

A. Thirty-two pregnant women were investigated during the last 5 weeks before delivery. All were previously insulin-dependent diabetics and all received insulin 3 times a day, at least during the last 3 months; 238 blood sugar values were determined fasting and 196 after lunch (Fig. 7). The mean postprandial value was normal at 129 ± 4 mg/100 ml (for 40.2 ± 2.4 days per woman). The fasting (8 a.m.) overall mean value was higher than normal: 142 ± 4 mg/100 ml, probably in part because the evening injection was given too early in the ward. There was no perinatal death. Women had gained 9.6 ± 0.7 kg during pregnancy. Ten of them experienced hypoglycemia and in 2 episodes glucagon was necessary.

Of these 32 pregnant women 5 had previously been treated with insulin 3 times a day and 27 with a single injection. More experienced patients said that the good control obtained during pregnancy was due first of all to their own willingness to achieve the best control possible with scrupulous analysis of urinary sugar, an attentive follow-up of the diet and immediate and wise adaptations of insulin dosage. Secondly, all agreed that the multiple-injection technique was a very good way to achieve better control. Generally

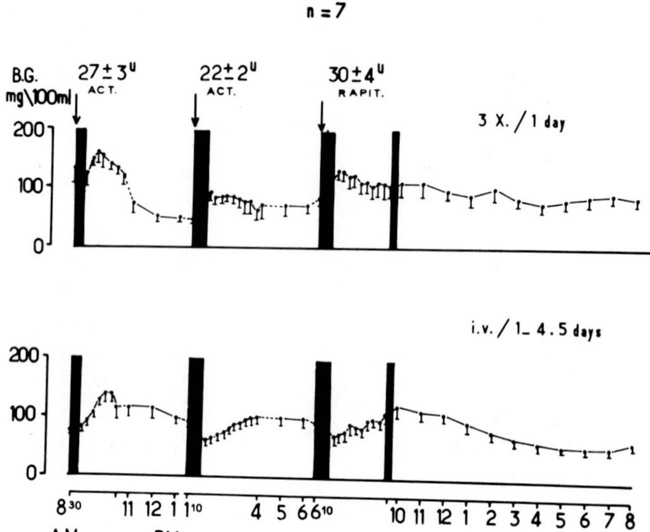

FIG. 4. Blood glucose levels in 7 insulin-dependent diabetic subjects treated with insulin 3 times a day (top) or continuous intravenous insulin infusion (bottom) at rate of 26 ± 4 mU per minute between meals and of 373 ± 58 mU per minute during the meal periods (black areas). Values are mean ± S.E.M. 'Act' = Actrapid novo (short-acting). 'Rapit' = Rapitard novo (mixture of short- and long-acting). (From Slama et al., 1973.)

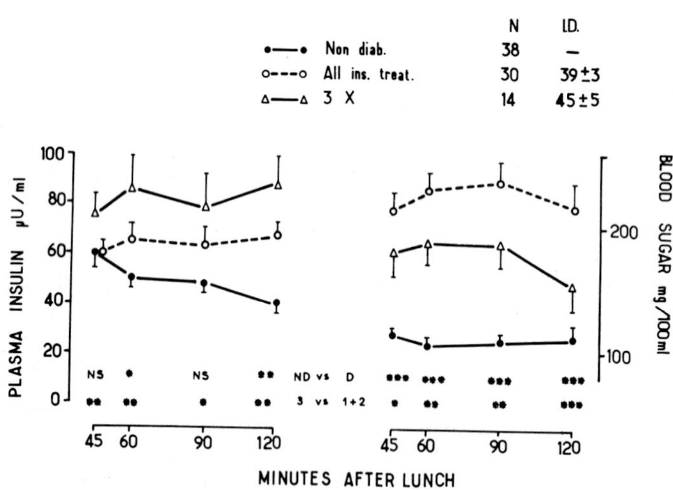

FIG. 5. Postprandial blood sugar (right) and plasma insulin (left) levels in 38 non-diabetic and 30 insulin-treated diabetic subjects (group A). Values are mean ± S.E.M. Values for the 14 patients treated by daily injections of insulin are given separately. I.D. = administered daily insulin doses; NS = non significant; * = $P<0.05$; ** = $P<0.01$; *** = $P<0.001$. (Based on data from Tchobroutsky et al., 1973.)

TABLE 1

Blood glucose values (mg/100 ml) in 7 diabetic patients submitted to insulin 3 times a day (3 injections) and to continuous intravenous insulin infusions (I.V.I.I.). Values are means ± S.E.M.

	Range		M.B.G.*		M.A.G.E.**		$M = \left| 10 \times \log \frac{BS}{80} \right|^3$***	
	3 injections	I.V.I.I.	3 injections	I.V.I.I.	3 injections	I.V.I.I.	3 injections	I.V.I.I.
A.C.	44 - 262	38 - 155	98 ± 7	87 ± 20	82 ± 3	43 ± 13[1]	12 ± 6	11 ± 3
P.M.	22 - 238	30 - 152	110 ± 9	86 ± 5[1]	116 ± 3	104 ± 2	31 ± 7	9 ± 3[2]
D.P.	29 - 235	23 - 228	80 ± 7	80 ± 16	94 ± 1	84 ± 18	21 ± 3	26 ± 6
H.S.	68 - 148	30 - 208	99 ± 4	99 ± 3	47 ± 1	69 ± 8	4 ± 2	8 ± 2
T.K.	32 - 185	32 - 139	94 ± 5	74 ± 4[3]	48 ± 5	45 ± 9	9 ± 3	7 ± 2
D.T.	25 - 142	18 - 137	83 ± 5	76 ± 16	51 ± 9	44 ± 9	20 ± 6	33 ± 13
B.A.	38 - 213	31 - 258	136 ± 6	127 ± 12	81 ± 5	76 ± 6	21 ± 4	34 ± 8
Mean ± S.E.M.			100 ± 7	89 ± 7	74 ± 10	66 ± 9	18 ± 5	17 ± 5

* M.B.G. = Diurnal (circadian) mean blood glucose level (Service et al., 1970).

** M.A.G.E. = Mean amplitude of glycemic excursions (Service et al., 1970).

*** M values expressed as the mean of 24 daily B.S. values according to Schlichtkrull et al. (1965) modified by Mirouze et al. (1963) and Service et al. (1970). Significance, P values: 1 = $P < 0.05$; 2 = $P < 0.01$; 3 = $P < 0.001$ (from Slama et al., 1973).

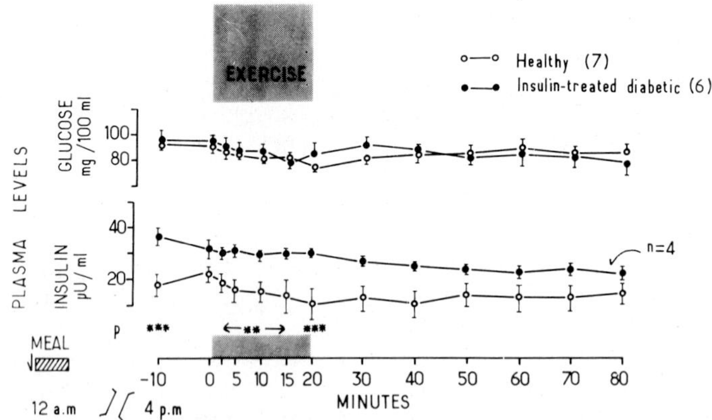

FIG. 6. Plasma levels of glucose and insulin in the afternoon before, during and after exercise in healthy subjects and insulin-treated diabetic men. Values are means ± S.E.M. Before and during exercise the mean plasma insulin values are significantly higher in diabetic than in healthy subjects. ** = P <0.01; *** = P <0.001. (From Tchobroutsky et al., 1974, by courtesy.)

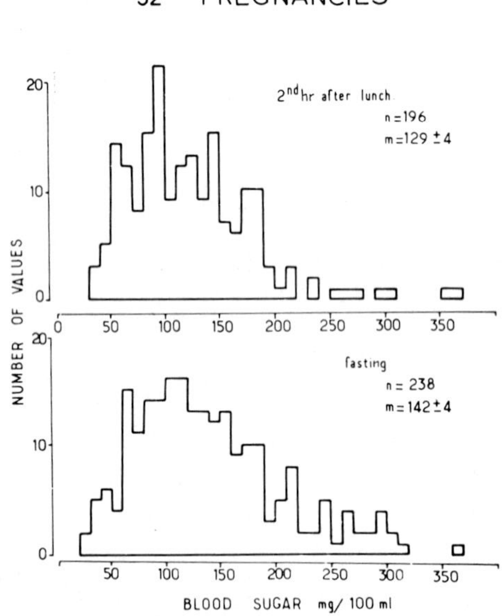

FIG. 7. Fasting and postprandial (2nd hour after lunch) blood sugar values in 32 hospitalized pregnant diabetic women the last 5 weeks before delivery. All women received 3 insulin injections per day (short-acting before breakfast and lunch, short-acting plus NPH or Rapitard (novo) before supper). (From Cassagne et al., 1973, by courtesy.)

speaking, when asked the question: 'is it easy to have 3 injections a day?' they replied: 'not easy but effective'.

Several months after delivery, of the 32 women studied, we lost track of 8, 3 asked for a single injection of insulin, 19 remained with a 3 injections regimen and 11 with 2 daily administrations of insulin for the sake of convenience or because of very small midday doses.

B. Since the end of 1969 all insulin-treated patients at the Hôtel-Dieu Hospital in Paris are systematically informed of this kind of treatment. Of 81 people who had accepted a 3 insulin injections regimen at least 2 years ago, we lost track of 33, mainly because they were living far from Paris. Thirty-eight out of the 48 who have been followed up are still treated with insulin 3 times a day.

Young and recently discovered diabetic subjects agree that such a regimen may be the closest to physiological patterns, but 2 years later there is no difference in attitude between patients under or over 40 years old nor between recent or long-term insulin-treated diabetics; 25 out of 51 and 17 out of 34 are still treated with insulin 3 times a day.

A long-term appreciation of blood sugar control in diabetic patients treated with insulin 3 times a day is obviously difficult. We observed that some long-term treated patients may be free of urinary sugar for most of the examinations. Slight hypoglycemia

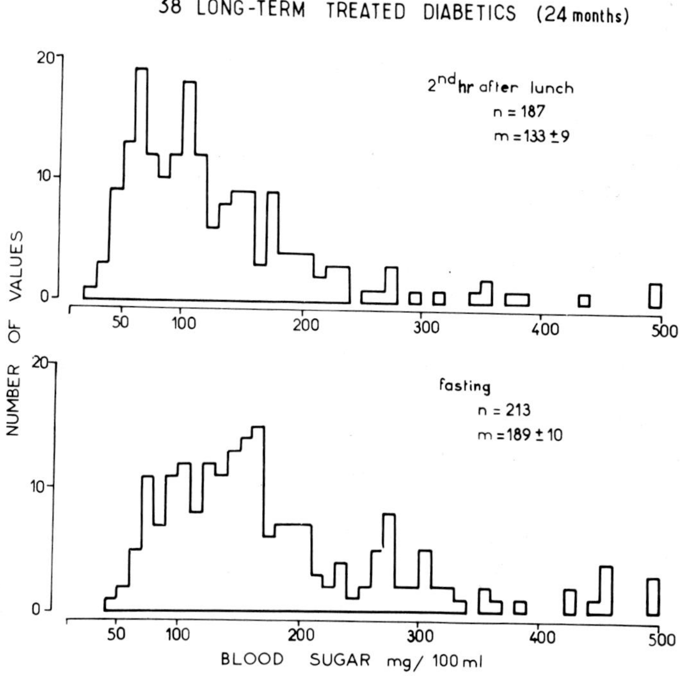

FIG. 8. Fasting and postprandial (2nd hour after lunch) blood sugar levels in 38 diabetic patients treated with insulin 3 times a day for 2 years. (From Goldgewicht et al., 1973, by courtesy.)

is not uncommon and obesity is to be carefully watched and prevented. For the 2-year period of follow-up the mean blood sugar levels were 189 ± 10 fasting, and 133 ± 9 2 hours after lunch (Fig. 8). Mean 24-hour glycosuria in these 38 patients was 25 ± 3 g.

CONCLUSION

Multiple injections of regular insulin before each meal (with intermediate insulin added for the night) was, in our experience, the most effective method for control of insulin-dependent diabetes during the postprandial and also the 24-hour periods.

Such a technique requires larger doses to be given and induces higher than normal plasma insulin levels, probably near the normal concentration of portal plasma insulin. About half of the patients who had accepted such an insulin regimen were still treated with insulin 3 times a day 2 years later.

REFERENCES

ALBISSER, A. M., LEIBEL, B. S., EWART, T., DAVIDOVAC, Z. and ZINGG, W. (1973): The artificial pancreas (abstract). *Diabetes, 22/Suppl. 1,* 294.

BEISSWENGER, P. J. and SPIRO, R. G. (1973): Studies on the human glomerular basement membrane. Composition, nature of the carbohydrate units and chemical changes in diabetes mellitus. *Diabetes, 22,* 180.

BERCHTOLD, P., BJÖRNTORP, P., GUSTAFSON, A., JONSSON, A. and FAGERBERG, S. E. (1971): Glucose tolerance, plasma insulin and lipids in diabetic subjects before and after treatment with a new sulfonylurea compound Ro. 6-4563. *Europ. J. clin. Pharmacol., 4,* 22.

BESSMAN, S. P. and SCHULTZ, R. D. (1972): Sugar electrode sensor for the 'artificial pancreas'. *Hormone Metabol. Res., 4,* 413.

BLACKARD, W. G. and NELSON, N. C. (1970): Portal and peripheral vein immunoreactive insulin concentrations before and after glucose infusion. *Diabetes, 19,* 302.

BLOCK, M. B., ROSENFIELD, R. L., MAKO, M. E., STEINER, D. F. and RUBENSTEIN, A. H. (1973): Sequential changes in beta-cell function in insulin-treated diabetic patients assessed by C-peptide immunoreactivity. *New Engl. J. Med., 288,* 1144.

BLOODWORTH Jr., J. M. B., ENGERMAN, R. L. and POWERS, K. L. (1969): Experimental diabetic microangiopathy. I. Basement membrane statistics in the dog. *Diabetes, 18,* 545.

BLOODWORTH Jr., J. M. B. and ENGERMAN, R. L. (1973): Diabetic microangiopathy in the experimentally-diabetic dog and its prevention by careful control with insulin (abstract). *Diabetes, 22/Suppl. 1,* 290.

CAHILL Jr., G. F., SOELDNER, J. S., HARRIS, G. W. and FOSTER, R. O. (1972): Practical developments in diabetes research. *Diabetes, 21/Suppl. 2,* 703.

CAIRD, F. I., PIRIE, A. and RAMSELL, T. G. (1969): *Diabetes and the Eye.* Blackwell Scientific Publications, Oxford.

CAMERON, D. P., LEUENBERGER, P., AMHERDT, M., PIRA, F., ORCI, L. and STAUFFACHER, W. (1971): Microvascular lesions including retinal aneurysms in chronic experimental diabetes (streptozotocin) (abstract). *Europ. J. clin. Invest., 1,* 365.

CASSAGNE, J., ASSAN, R. and TCHOBROUTSKY, G. (1973): The use of insulin three times a day in pregnant diabetic women. Submitted for publication.

CHAZAN, B. I., BALODIMOS, M. C., RYAN, J. R. and MARBLE, A. (1970): Twenty-five to forty-five years of diabetes with and without vascular complications. *Diabetologia, 6,* 565.

COLWELL, J. A. (1966): Effect of diabetic control on retinopathy. *Diabetes, 15,* 497.

CONSTAM, G. R. (1972): Contrôle du diabète et prévention des complications. In: *Journées de Diabétologie de l'Hôtel-Dieu,* pp. 314–320. Flammarion, Paris.

CONTROL OF OBESITY (1966): In: *Controversy in Internal Medicine, Vol. 1,* pp. 439–480. Editors: F. J. Ingelfinger, A. S. Relman and M. Finland. W. B. Saunders, Philadelphia.

DEUIL, R. (1967): La redécouverte de l'insuline ordinaire. *Presse Méd., 75,* 27.

DORF, A., BENNETT, P. H., BALLINTINE, E. J. and MILLER, M. (1971): Retinopathy in Pima indians: relationships to glucose level, duration of diabetes, and blood pressure in a population with a high prevalence of diabetes mellitus. *Diabetes, 20/Suppl. 1,* 352.

EARLL, J. M. (1968): Time for more physiologic management of diabetes. *Milit. Med., 133,* 39.

FAJANS, S. S. (1972): Current unsolved problems in diabetes management. *Diabetes, 21/Suppl. 2,* 678.

FELTS, P. W. (1973): Pancreas transplantation and the artificial pancreas: status of current experimental approaches. *South. med. J., 66,* 66.

FORSHAM, P. H. (1967): Insulin twice a day suggested for control. *J. Amer. med. Ass., 202,* 26.

FOUCAR, E. and FIELD, J. B. (1972): Effect of control of hyperglycemia on plasma insulin responses to various stimuli in newly diagnosed ketosis-prone diabetic patients. *J. clin. Endocr., 35,* 288.

GABBAY, K. H. (1973): The sorbitol pathway and the complications of diabetes. *New Engl. J. Med., 288,* 831.

GOLDGEWICHT, F., ASSAN, R. and TCHOBROUTSKY, G. (1973): A two years follow-up of diabetic patients treated with insulin three times a day. Submitted for publication.

HAUTECOUVERTURE, M., SLAMA, G., ASSAN, R. and TCHOBROUTSKY, G. (1973): Sex-related patterns in diurnal variations of plasma glucose and insulin levels. Submitted for publication.

HEGRE, O. D., WELLS, L. J. and LAZAROW, A. (1972): Insulin content of fetal rat pancreases grown in organ culture and subsequently transplanted into maternal hosts. *Diabetes, 21,* 193.

JOHNSSON, S. (1960): Retinopathy and nephropathy in diabetes mellitus. Comparison of the effects of two forms of treatment. *Diabetes, 9,* 1.

JOPLIN, G. F., BLACH, R. K., CHANG, H., ELKELES, R. S., FRASER, T. R., KOHNER, E. M. and OAKLEY, N. W. (1971): Treatability of diabetic retinopathy. In: *Diabetes, Proceedings of the Seventh Conference of the IDF,* pp. 276–280. Editors: R. R. Rodriguez and J. Vallance-Owen. International Congress Series No. 231, Excerpta Medica, Amsterdam.

KAPLAN, M. H. and FEINSTEIN, A. R. (1973): A critique of methods in reported studies of long-term vascular complications in patients with diabetes mellitus. *Diabetes, 22,* 160.

KILO, C., VOGLER, N. and WILLIAMSON, J. R. (1972): Muscle capillary basement membrane changes related to aging and diabetes mellitus. *Diabetes, 21,* 881.

KNOWLES Jr., H. C. (1971): Long-term juvenile diabetes mellitus and unmeasured diet. In: *Diabetes, Proceedings of the Seventh Conference of the IDF,* pp. 209–215. Editors: R. R. Rodriguez and J. Vallance-Owen. International Congress Series No. 231, Excerpta Medica, Amsterdam.

KOPF, A., TCHOBROUTSKY, G. and ESCHWEGE, E. (1973): Serial post prandial blood glucose levels in 309 subjects with and without diabetes. *Diabetes, 22,* 834.

KUMAR, D., PAYNE, J. E., OBERMAN, A. E., WARNER, N. E. and BERNE, T. V. (1973): Implantation of culture fetal dog pancreas into the anterior chamber of eye (abstract). *Diabetes, 22/Suppl. 1,* 322.

LAWRENCE, R. D. (1963): Treatment of 90 severe diabetics with soluble insulin for 20–40 years. Effect of diabetic control on complications. *Brit. med. J., 5373,* 1624.

LEONARD, R. J. and HEGRE, O. D. (1973): Reversal of diabetes in alloxanized rats following intraperitoneal implantation of dissociated neonatal pancreas (abstract). *Diabetes, 22/Suppl. 1,* 295.

LILLEHEI, R. C., SIMMONS, R. L., NAJARIAN, J. S., WEIL, R., UCHIDA, H., RUIZ, J. W., KJELLSTRAND, C. M. and GOETZ, F. C. (1970): Pancreatico-duodenal allotransplantation: Experimental and clinical experience. *Acta diabet. lat., 7,* 909.

LUFT, R., OLIVECRONA, H., IKKOS, D., KORNERUP, T. and LJUNGGREN, H. (1955): Hypophysectomy in man. Further experiences in severe diabetes mellitus. *Brit. med. J., 2,* 752.

LUKENS, F. D. W. (1965): The rediscovery of regular insulin. *New Engl. J. Med., 272,* 130.

LUNDBAEK, K. (1971): Growth hormone and diabetic angiopathy. In: *Blood vessel disease in diabetes mellitus,* V Capri Conference, pp. 344–370. Editors: K. Lundbaek and H. Keen. Il Ponte, Milan. Also in: *Acta diabet. lat., 8,* 1.

MADISON, L. L. (1969): Role of insulin in the hepatic handling of glucose. *Arch. intern. Med., 123,* 284.

MALHERBE, C., De GASPARO, M., De HERTOGH, R. and HOET, J. J. (1969): Circadian variations of blood sugar and plasma insulin levels in man. *Diabetologia, 5,* 397.

MARBLE, A. (1971): Long term diabetes and the effect of treatment. In: *Diabetes, Proceedings of the Seventh Conference of the IDF,* pp. 25–35. Editors: R. R. Rodriguez and J. Vallance-Owen. International Congress Series No. 231, Excerpta Medica, Amsterdam.

METZ, R., NICE, M. and LAPLACA, G. (1967): Evaluation of an eight-hour therapeutic regimen in uncontrolled diabetes. *Diabetes, 16,* 341.

MIKI, E., FUKUDA, M., KUZUYA, T., KOSAKA, K. and KAKAO, K. (1969): Relation of the course of retinopathy to control of diabetes, age, and therapeutic agents in diabetic japanese patients. *Diabetes, 18,* 773.

MIKI, E., KUZUYA, T., IDE, T. and NAKAO, K. (1972): Frequency, degree, and progression with time of proteinuria in diabetic patients. *Lancet, I,* 922.

MIROUZE, J., SATINGHER, A., SANY, C. and JAFFIOL, C. (1963): Coefficient d'efficacité insulinique. Coefficient M. de Schlichtkrull corrigé et simplifié par la technique de l'enregistrement glycémique continu. *Diabète, 6,* 267.

MOLNAR, G. D., TAYLOR, W. F. and LANGWORTHY, A. (1972): Plasma immunoreactive insulin (IRi) patterns in insulin-treated diabetics during continuous blood glucose (BG) monitoring. *Diabetes, 21/Suppl. 1,* 324.

OAKLEY, W., HILL, D. and OAKLEY, N. (1966): Combined use of regular and crystalline protamine (NPH) insulin in the treatment of severe diabetes. *Diabetes, 15,* 219.

OAKLEY, W. G., PYKE, D. A. and TAYLOR, K. W. (1973): *Diabetes and its Managements.* Blackwell Scientific Publications, Oxford.

ÖSTERBY, R. (1971): Course of diabetic glomerulopathy. In: *Blood Vessel Disease in Diabetes Mellitus,* pp. 179–191. Editors: K. Lundbaek and H. Keen. Il Ponte, Milan. Also in: *Acta diabet. lat., 8,* 1.

PEDERSEN, J. (1967): *The Pregnant Diabetic and Her Newborn. Problems and Management.* Munksgaard, Copenhagen.

PIRART, J., LAUVAUX, J. P. and VASSART, A. (1970): Evolution de la rétinopathie diabétique en fonction de la durée et du degré de contrôle du diabète. *Diabète, 20,* 209.

QUABBE, H. J. and KLIEMS, C. (1969): Glycémie et insuline plasmatiques sous l'in-

fluence du tolbutamide et du HB 419 chez des sujets normaux et diabétiques. In: *Journées de Diabétologie de l'Hôtel-Dieu,* pp. 301–309. Flammarion, Paris.
RECKARD, C. R., ZIEGLER, M. M. and BARKER, C. R. (1973): Islet transplantation in streptozotocin induced diabetes in rats (abstract). *Diabetes, 22/Suppl. 1,* 295.
RICKETTS, H. T. (1965): The influence of diabetic control on angiopathy. In: *On the nature and treatment of diabetes, Proceedings of the fifth Conference of the IDF,* pp. 588–600. Editors: B. S. Leibel and G. A. Wrenshall. International Congress Series No. 84, Excerpta Medica, Amsterdam.
RULL, J. A., CONN, J. W., FLOYD Jr., J. C. and FAJANS, S. S. (1970): Levels of plasma insulin during cortisone glucose tolerance tests in 'non diabetic' relatives of diabetic patients. *Diabetes, 19,* 1.
SERVICE, F. J., MOLNAR, G. D., ROSEVEAR, J. W., ACKERMAN, E., GATEWOOD, L. C. and TAYLOR, W. F. (1970): Mean amplitude of glycemic excursion, a measure of diabetic instability. *Diabetes, 19,* 644.
SCHLICHTKRULL, J., MUNCK, O. and JERSILD, M. (1965): The M-value, an index of blood sugar control in diabetics. *Acta med. scand., 177,* 95.
SIPERSTEIN, M. D., UNGER, R. H. and MADISON, L. L. (1968): Studies of muscle capillary basement membranes in normal subjects, diabetic, and prediabetic patients. *J. clin. Invest., 47,* 1973.
SLAMA, G., ASSAN, R. and TCHOBROUTSKY, G. (1973): Continuous intravenous insulin infusion for 1 to 5 days on 7 diabetic patients. Comparison with s.c. insulin three times a day. Submitted for publication.
SOELDNER, J. S. (1972): Summary of discussion. *Diabetes, 21/Suppl. 2,* 713.
SOELDNER, J. S., CHANG, K. W., HIEBERT, J. and AISENBERG, S. (1973): In vitro and in vivo experience with a miniature glucose sensor (abstract). *Diabetes, 22/Suppl. 1,* 294.
SOLER, N. G., FITZGERALD, M. G., MALINS, J. M. and SUMMERS, R. O. C. (1969): Retinopathy at diagnosis of diabetes, with special reference to patients under 40 years of age. *Brit. med. J., 3,* 567.
SPATHIS, G. S. (1970): Continuous monitoring of blood sugar in Brittle diabetics. *Diabetologia, 6,* 586.
SPIRO, R. G. and SPIRO, M. J. (1971): Effect of diabetes on the biosynthesis of the renal glomerular basement membrane. *Diabetes, 20,* 641.
SUMMERLIN, W. T., MILLER, G. E. and GOOD, R. A. (1973): Successful tissue and organ allotransplantation without immuno suppression (abstract). *J. clin. Invest., 52,* 83a.
TCHOBROUTSKY, G. (1970): Repas-test chez des sujets normaux et des diabétiques traités. *Presse Méd., 78,* 1359.
TCHOBROUTSKY, G., LENORMAND, M. E., MICHEL, G. and ASSAN, R. (1974): Lack of post-prandial exercise induced growth hormone secretion in normo-glycemic insulin-treated diabetic men. *Hormone metabol. Res.,* in press.
TCHOBROUTSKY, G., KOPF, A., ESCHWEGE, E. and ASSAN, R. (1973): Serial post prandial plasma insulin levels in 117 subjects with and without diabetes including insulin treated patients. *Diabetes, 22,* 825.
TUTIN, M., ROUSSELIE, F., RATHERY, M., BOUR, H. and DEROT, M. (1966): Angiopathies spécifiques dans les diabètes secondaires à des pancréatites et à des hémochromatoses (abstract). *Diabétologia, 2,* 223.
UNIVERSITY GROUP DIABETES PROGRAM (1970): A study of the effects of hypoglycemic agents on vascular complications in patients with adult-onset diabetes. *Diabetes, 19/Suppl. 2,* 830.
VINING Jr., K. K. and STRONG, L. E. (1972): The effectiveness of a highly structured diabetic control program on progress of proliferative diabetic retinopathy (abstract). *Diabetes, 21/Suppl. 1,* 382.

NEW DATA ON ISLET CELL TUMORS

MORPHOLOGICAL AND BIOCHEMICAL INVESTIGATIONS IN HUMAN INSULINOMAS AND GASTRINOMAS

W. CREUTZFELDT, R. ARNOLD, C. CREUTZFELDT, H. FRERICHS and N. S. TRACK

Department of Medicine, University of Göttingen, Göttingen, German Federal Republic

This report is based on the investigations of 32 pancreatic tumors found in patients with spontaneous hypoglycemia (insulinomas) and of 8 pancreatic tumors found in patients with the Zollinger-Ellison syndrome (gastrinomas). In all insulinomas insulin and in all gastrinomas gastrin has been extracted from the tumors. The content of insulin and proinsulin of the insulinomas has been correlated to the morphological findings. In addition subcellular fractionation and in vitro studies were performed in 7 insulinomas.

MORPHOLOGICAL INVESTIGATIONS

Insulinomas

The morphological diagnosis of an insulinoma has been made by
1. specific staining reaction
2. immunohistology
3. ultrastructural investigation.

Specific B-cell staining In the aldehyde-thionine stained sections only few tumors showed a very strong staining reaction similar to normal human islets of Langerhans. More frequently, only the capillary pole of the tumor cells reacted positively. In addition, many tumors showed a variable number of tumor cells which were not stained with aldehyde-thionine at all, suggesting that a number of tumor cells only store small amounts of insulin. In 9 of the 32 tumors less than 20% of the tumor cells reacted with aldehyde-thionine and 7 tumors showed no reaction. In the majority of the tumors the intensity of the staining reaction correlated with the concentration of insulin extracted from the tumors (Creutzfeldt et al., 1973b).

Immunohistology Using the peroxidase-labelled antibody method a positive reaction for insulin could be demonstrated in most insulinomas after fixation in Bouin's solution and embedding in paraffin (Arnold et al., 1972) (Fig. 1). It was noticed that the immunohistological reaction with insulin antibodies markedly decreased in the tumors one year after embedding in paraffin; however, not in the islets of the adjacent pancreas. This finding may explain why most authors (Federlin et al., 1969; Lacy and Williamson, 1960; Lacy, 1961; Misugi et al., 1970; Pfeiffer, 1967) could not demonstrate a positive im-

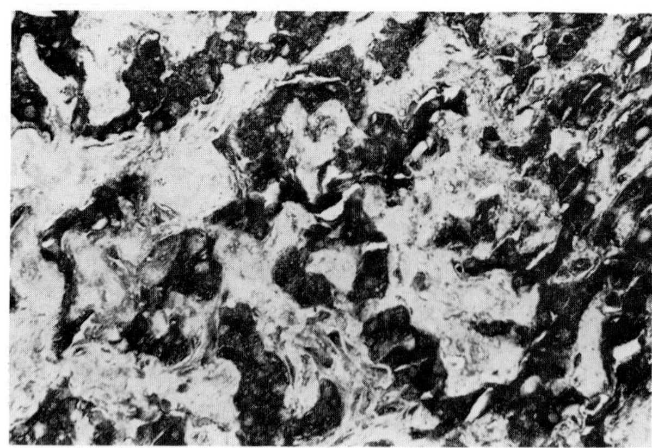

FIG. 1. Immunohistologic demonstration of insulin in a B-cell adenoma fixed in Bouin's fluid, embedded in paraffin. Incubation with 1/20 diluted anti-insulin serum; after washing incubation with 1/20 diluted peroxidase labelled anti-guinea pig γ-globulin from rabbit. The tumor shows numerous darkly stained insulin-containing cells. Magnification X 268.

munohistological reaction in insulinomas. Why the immunohistological reaction decreases only in B-cell tumors but not in normal pancreatic islets depending on the time elapsed between the paraffin embedding and the examination is not yet understood (Arnold et al., 1972). Some tumors which did not react with the aldehyde-thionine stain reacted positively with the peroxidase antibody method indicating the superiority of immunohistology in identifying insulin-producing tumor cells. Only in tumors with insulin concentration below 1.0 U/g was the immunohistological reaction negative. As with the aldehyde-thionine stain a variable number of tumor cells reacted positively with the peroxidase-labelled antibody indicating a different insulin content of the cells (Fig. 2). A

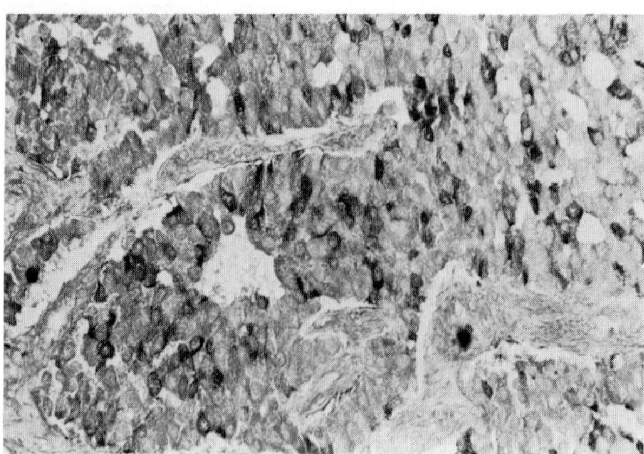

FIG. 2. Only few B-cells react in this tumor with an anti-insulin serum compared with Figure 1, whereas the majority of the cells remain unstained. Magnification X 268.

similar reaction could be achieved with porcine C-peptide antisera (Fig. 3) despite the fact that human and porcine C-peptide differ in 8 positions in the amino acid sequence (Ko et al., 1971). This finding is in agreement with the contention that insulin and C-peptide are retained in the B-cell in equimolar amounts (Rubenstein et al., 1969). None of the insulinomas reacted positively with glucagon antiserum.

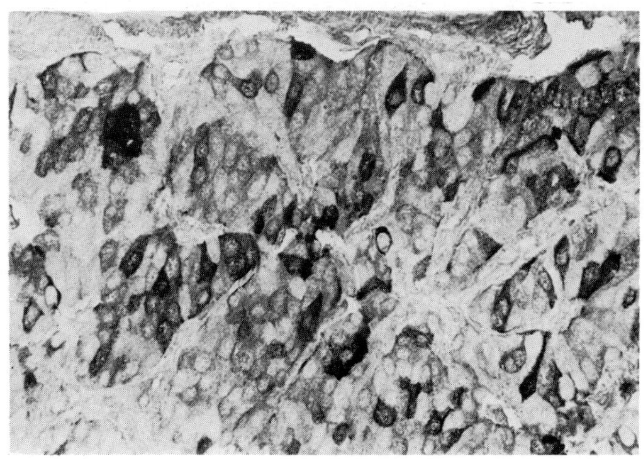

FIG. 3. Insulinoma after incubation with an anti C-peptide serum. Many cells react positively. Magnification X 268.

Ultrastructure Thirty of the 32 insulinomas were investigated ultrastructurally. The ultrastructural appearance of the tumors was not uniform. Even in individual cases the cells sometimes differed considerably in different areas of the tumor.

According to their ultrastructure, the 30 insulinomas can be categorized into the following 4 types (Creutzfeldt et al., 1973b):

1. Tumors with cells containing secretory granules typical for human islet beta cells (Fig. 4).
2. Tumors with cells containing typical and atypical secretory granules (Fig. 5).
3. Tumors with cells containing only atypical secretory granules (Fig. 6).
4. Tumors which only contain virtually agranular cells (Fig. 7).

In Types 3 and 4 the diagnosis of an insulinoma is not possible on ultrastructural grounds or with granule stains. Table 1 gives the frequency with which the different ultrastructural types were found. In addition, the IRI concentration is listed. From this it can be concluded that in the Type 1 tumors which are most frequent the IRI concentration is highest. The Type 4 tumors have the lowest insulin concentration. Types 2 and 3 are in between both these extremes. A correlation between ultrastructural findings and IRI concentration is more evident if the number of agranular cells is also accounted for: the more virtually agranular cells in a tumor, the lower the IRI concentration.

The frequent finding of atypical granules in insulinoma cells and the occurrence of virtually agranular tumors shows that ultrastructural analysis of a pancreatic endocrine tumor alone is insufficient for definite identification. Eight of the 30 tumors could not be identified as insulinomas by their ultrastructural appearance.

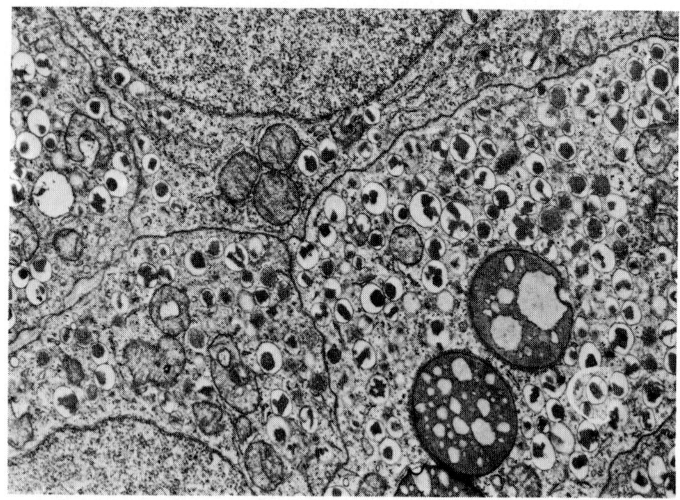

FIG. 4. Adjacent portions of 5 insulinoma cells showing typical beta-granules (Type 1 insulinoma). Crystalline, round and amorphous cores surrounded by an electron lucent space encompassed by a limiting membrane. One cell contains large lipid bodies. X 12,700.

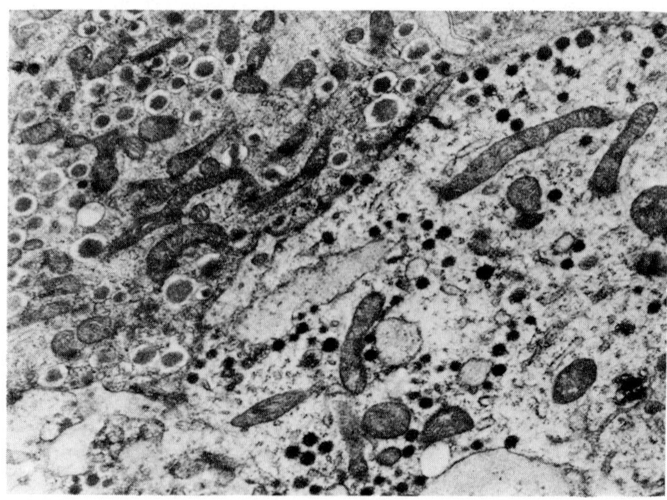

FIG. 5. Adjacent portions of 2 insulinoma cells, one showing typical beta-granules the other atypical granules (Type 2 insulinoma). X 12,700.

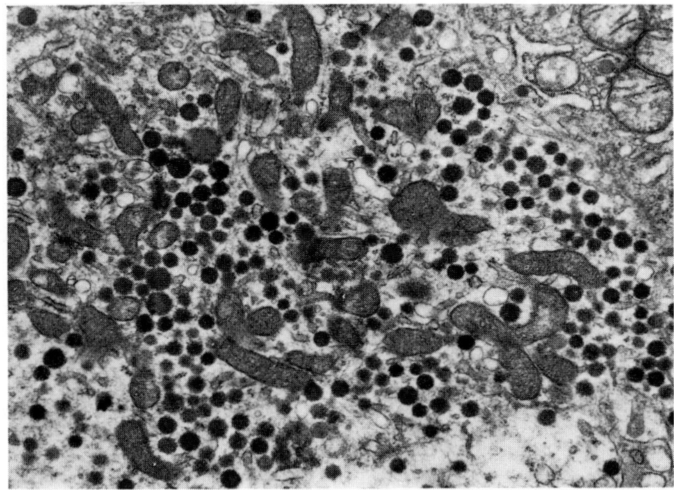

FIG. 6. Insulinoma cell with atypical granules, electron-dense spherical granules usually smaller than beta-granules with or without a tightly fitting membrane (Type 3 insulinoma). There is no similarity to the granules of normal islet A-cells (having an electrondense central core– or the granules of D-cells (which are larger and less electron dense). X 12,700.

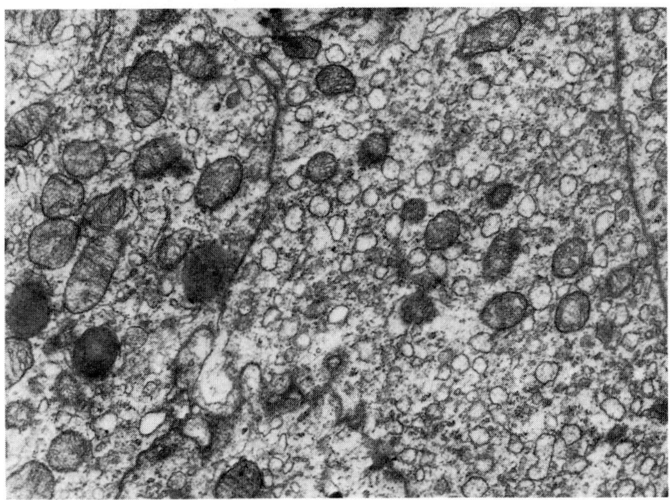

FIG. 7. Four adjacent portions of tumor cells of virtually agranular insulinoma-containing numerous small partially ribosome-coated vesicles containing some electron lucent amorphous material (Type 4 insulinoma). X 12,700.

TABLE 1
Categorization of 30 insulinomas according to the ultrastructural type of secretory granules

	Number of cases	Mean IRI concentration U/g (range)	Stainable with aldehyde-thionine	Immunohistological reaction for insulin
1. Tumors with typical β-granules	15	24.1 (3.6–88.9)	+	+
2. Tumors with typical and atypical β-granules	7	19.3 (4.8–43.2)	+	+
3. Tumors with atypical granules only	4	10.2 (1.7–16.3)	0	+
4. Virtually agranular tumors	4	0.5 (0.01–1.1)	0	0

Atypical secretory granules in human insulinomas have also been described by others (Bencosme et al., 1963; Greider and Elliott, 1964; Georgsson and Wessel, 1967) while most authors (Bencosme et al., 1963; Gusek and Kracht, 1961; Lacy and Williamson, 1960; Lacy, 1961; Lazarus and Volk, 1962) found normal B-cells. However, these reports are confined to single or few cases.

Other islet cells (A-cells and D-cells) were not identified in the tumors. However, in many tumors single cells were observed which resembled the enterochromaffin cells (EC-cells) found in the gastrointestinal mucosa and in carcinoid tumors. These EC-cells were most frequent in the 2 carcinomas.

Gastrinomas

Since contradictory findings have been reported on the morphology of gastrinomas some information shall be given about our observations in 8 gastrinomas, all investigated with silver impregnation, immunohistological and ultrastructural methods.

Silver impregnation The gastrin-producing cell of the human antrum can be stained by biochemical reactions which are not specific for the G-cells. The most reliable of these reactions is the silver impregnation according to Grimelius (1968). This silver impregnation gives positive results also in the islet A-cells, while the islet B- and D-cells are Grimelius-negative (Vassallo et al., 1972). Another widely used silver technique, the Davenport silver impregnation, is positive in the islet D-cells (Hellerström and Hellman, 1960) but not in the islet A-cells or the antral G-cells (Vassallo et al., 1972).

A positive Grimelius silver reaction in a gastrinoma is shown in Figure 8. All proven gastrinomas fixed in Bouin's solution contained Grimelius silver positive cells. However, the cells of the same tumors were Davenport silver negative. Thus, histochemically a close relationship between antral G-cells and gastrinomas is obvious while a relation between islet D-cells and these tumors could not be demonstrated.

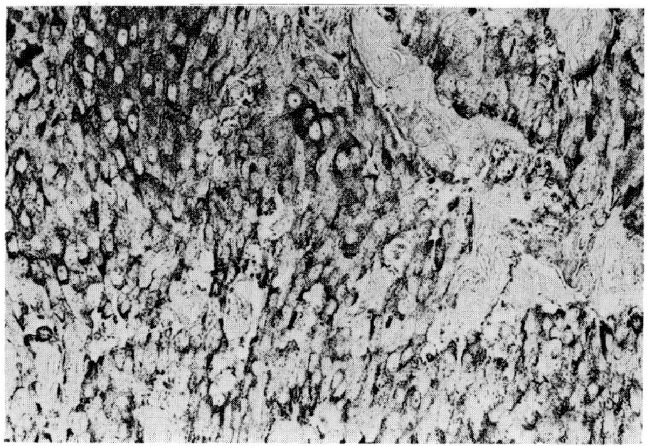

FIG. 8. Silver reactive cells in a pancreatic gastrinoma (Table 2, Case 1). Bouin's fixation, silver impregnation after Grimelius (1968). X 268.

Immunohistology Using the peroxidase-labelled antibody method a positive reaction for gastrin could be demonstrated in a proportion of cells in all 8 gastrinomas after fixation in Bouin's fluid (Fig. 9). With the same technique the human antral G-cells are easily demonstrated while no cells in the human pancreatic islets react positively (Creutzfeldt et al., 1971). Positive immunofluorescence of few pancreatic islet cells with labelled gastrin antiserum has been reported by Lomsky et al. (1970) in paraffin-embedded material and by Greider and McGuigan (1971) and Vassallo et al. (1972) only in fresh cryostat sections. These contradictions are not easily understood. Our findings suggest differences between the normal islet cells on one side and the G-cells of the antrum and the gastrinoma cells on the other, as also the Grimelius silver results have indicated.

In 5 of the 8 gastrinomas a proportion of the tumor cells reacted positively with anti-insulin serum (Fig. 10). In all 5 cases insulin could be extracted in significant amounts from the tumors. However, only in one case higher amounts were found (13.5 U/g). None of the tumors reacted with glucagon antiserum.

Ultrastructure Reports on the ultrastructural appearance of gastrinomas are contradictory (Vassallo et al., 1972). The identity of their secretory granules with A-cells (Greider and Elliott, 1964), D-cells (Thiery and Bader, 1966), antral G-cells (Creutzfeldt

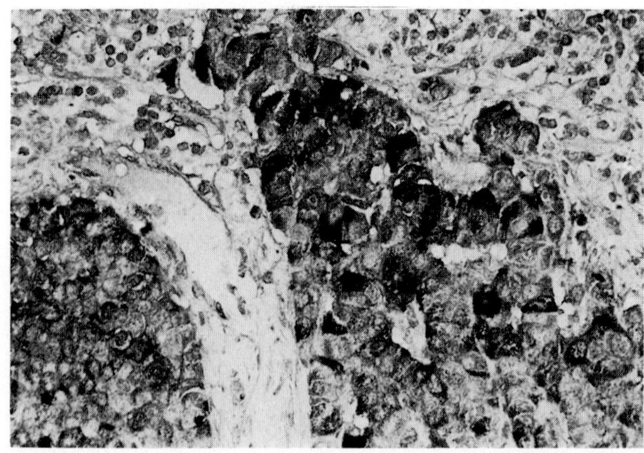

FIG. 9. Immunohistological demonstration of gastrin-producing cells in a pancreatic gastrinoma. Bouin's fixation, paraffin embedding (Table 2, Case 3). Incubation with 1/20 diluted anti-gastrin serum; after washing incubation with 1/20 diluted peroxidase labelled anti-guinea pig γ-globulin from sheep. $\times$ 268.

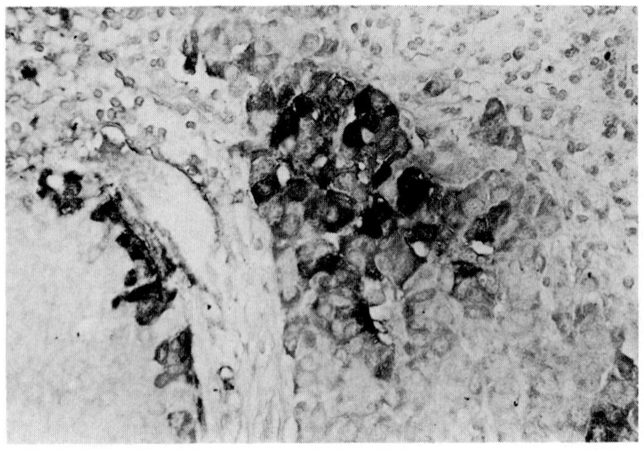

FIG. 10. Immunohistological demonstration of insulin-producing cells in the gastrinoma of Figure 9 (neighbouring serial section). Different cells react with insulin antiserum. Technique as Figure 1.

et al., 1971) and most recently abnormal islet D-cells (similar to gastrointestinal D_1-cells) (Vassallo et al., 1972) have been claimed. These different conclusions are based on the study of only a few cases. In our series of 8 gastrinomas 2 prominent types of cells have been found. In 3 cases typical G-cells of the antral G-cell type could be recognized (Fig. 11). Their granules were impregnated with silver grains when the Grimelius technique (Vassallo et al., 1971) was applied (Fig. 12) demonstrating their non-identity with islet D-cells.

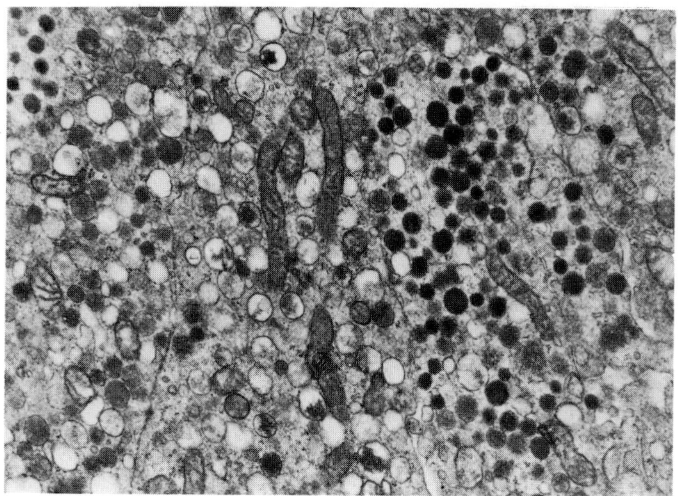

FIG. 11. Typical G-cell with granules of varying electron density in a pancreatic gastrinoma (Table 2, Case 4). X 12,700.

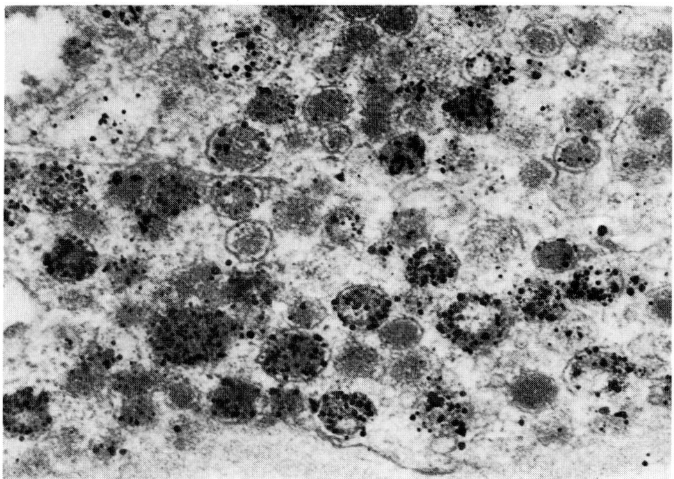

FIG. 12. Grimelius silver stain showing positively reacting tumor cells in a gastrinoma (Table 2, case 4). Karnovsky's fixative, silver impregnation according to Vassallo et al. (1971), post fixation with osmium. X 12,700.

In 4 cases the majority of the granulated tumor cells contained small round electron dense granules with tightly fitting or no discernible membranes (Fig. 13) similar to those described by Vassallo et al. (1972) as D_1-cells and possibly identical with the Type 4 islet cell of Deconinck et al. (1971). Also these granules were impregnated with Grimelius silver.

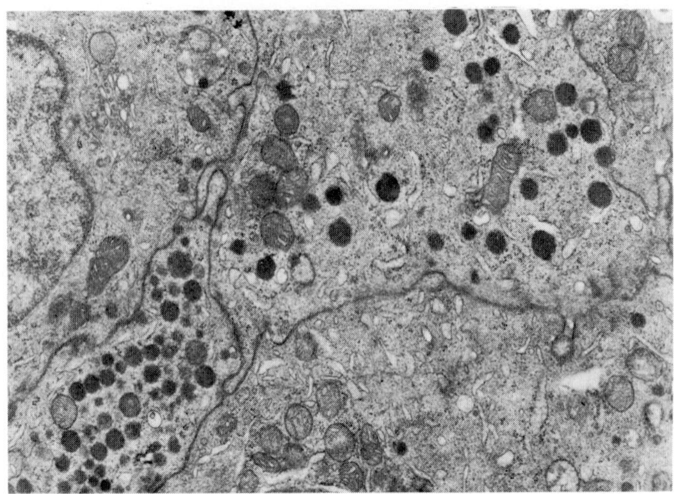

FIG. 13. Tumor cells containing small round electron-dense granules often with tightly encompassing limiting membranes in a pancreatic gastrinoma (Table 2, Case 3). Karnovsky's fixative, postfixation with osmium. × 12,700.

It may be discussed whether this type of peptide-secreting cell is a normal component of human pancreatic islets or a changed cell type or an undifferentiated precursor cell (Vassallo et al., 1972). On the other hand it has to be stressed that identical cells have been found in 11 out of 30 insulinomas (Creutzfeldt et al., 1973b). Therefore, the ultrastructural appearance of endocrine pancreatic tumors frequently does not allow their identification and does not justify any conclusions regarding their origin. It is possible that the endocrine tumors of the pancreas are derived from an undifferentiated stem cell of the ductular system and therefore can differentiate simultaneously into different cell types.

Table 2 compiles the morphological findings in the 8 gastrinomas. While the histochemical results are uniform the ultrastructural findings are not. The cells of one tumor even contained only beta granules.

BIOCHEMICAL INVESTIGATIONS

Insulin and proinsulin content in human insulinomas

Since the discovery of proinsulin different studies have demonstrated that patients with insulinomas have a higher percentage of proinsulin in their serum than normal persons (Goldsmith et al., 1969; Gorden and Roth, 1969; Gorden et al., 1971; Gutman et al., 1970; Melani et al., 1970; Creutzfeldt et al., 1973b). However, from only 3 single cases has the proinsulin content of insulinomas been reported (Gorden et al., 1971; Lindall et al., 1972; Melani et al., 1970). We have estimated the insulin concentration in 30 insulinomas and the percentage of proinsulin in 19 of these (Creutzfeldt et al., 1973b). Figure 14 demonstrates the wide range of the insulin concentration in the tumors in comparison

TABLE 2
Morphological findings in human gastrinomas

Case	Gastrin content (μg/g)	Grimelius silver	Davenport silver	Anti-gastrin serum	Ultrastructure (granule type)
1. Schm.	12.8	+	0	+	*G*
2. Ka.	0.5	+	0	+	D_1 (A, B, EC)
3. Bre.	25.6	+	0	+	D_1 (?G)
4. Stu.	8.0	+	0	+	*G* (?D,?D_1)
5. Dus.*	12.0	–	–	(+)	?D_1
6. Klau.	0.04	+	0	+	*G* (?D_1,?D)
7. Gei.	–	(+)	0	+	D_1 (EC)
8. Be.	0.3	0	0	(+)	B (!)

* = insufficient fixation
\+ = positive reaction
0 = negative reaction
– = not investigated

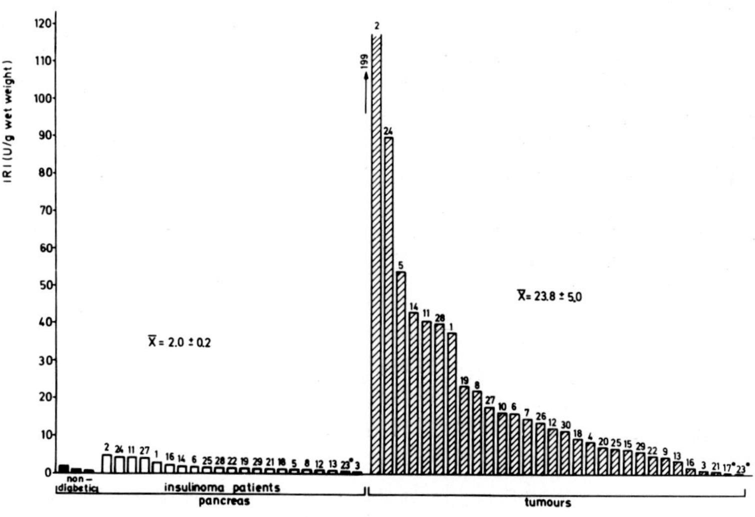

FIG. 14. Concentration of immunoreactive insulin (IRI) in the pancreas of 3 nondiabetics (black columns) and of 21 insulinoma patients (open columns) and in 30 insulinomas (hatched columns). Two cases with carcinoma are marked (•). The case numbers are written at the top of each column.

with the normal human pancreas. Only in one case was the insulin concentration of the tumor cells comparable with the concentration in the islet cells. The total insulin content of the tumors was, on average, lower than the insulin content of the pancreas (Fig. 15). Neither the insulin concentration nor the total content could be correlated with the severity of the hypoglycemic symptoms of the patient. The percentage of proinsulin was estimated by column chromatography of the extracts on Sephadex G-50. Figure 16 demonstrates that all tumors had a higher proinsulin percentage (5.3–22.0%) than the normal pancreas (1.7–4.8%). A near normal proinsulin percentage was found in the tumor with the highest insulin concentration. Generally the highest proinsulin percentages were in the tumors with the lowest insulin concentration. The serum levels of proinsulin were much higher than in the tumors of the same patients which may be explained by the longer half-life of proinsulin than insulin in the plasma (Rubenstein et al., 1972).

Correlation of these biochemical findings with the morphology of the tumors revealed the following: The more tumor cells reacting with aldehyde-thionine or with insulin antiserum the higher the insulin concentration. On the other hand, the fewer reactive cells present in an insulinoma the higher the proinsulin percentage in the extracts. The same correlation could be found in ultrastructural investigations regarding the number of secretory granules.

In the well granulated Type 1 insulinomas the insulin concentration was highest and the proinsulin percentage lowest while the virtually agranular Type 4 tumors had the lowest insulin concentration and the highest proinsulin percentages.

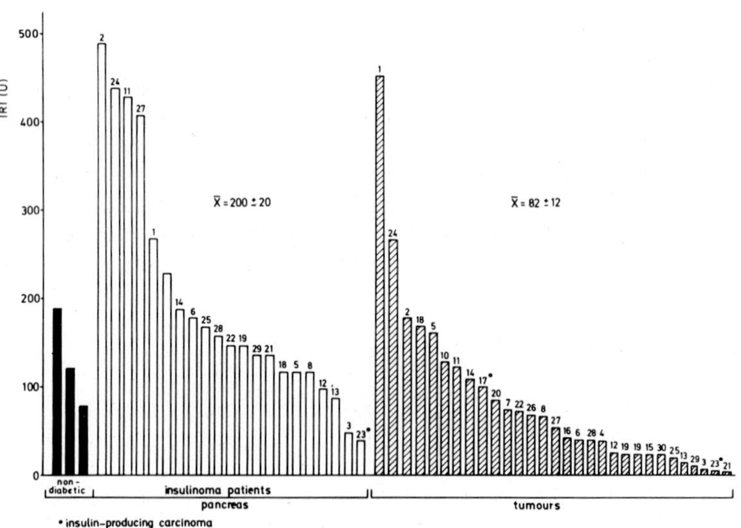

FIG. 15. Total IRI content of the pancreas of 3 non-diabetics and 21 insulinoma patients and of 30 insulinomas. For details see Figure 14.

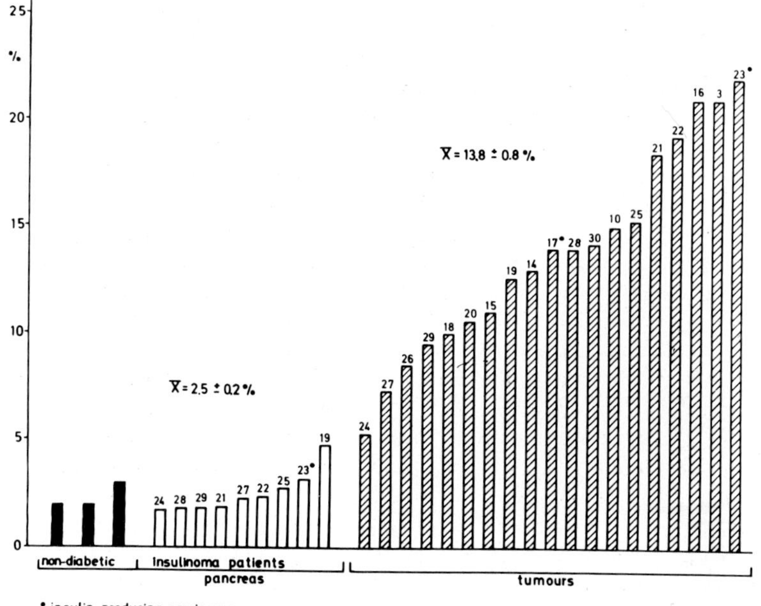

FIG. 16. Proinsulin-like components (PLC) as a percentage of the IRI concentration in the pancreas of 3 non-diabetics and 9 insulinoma patients and in 19 insulinomas. For details see Figure 14.

This finding suggested that the major defect in insulinomas was a decreased storage capacity resulting in uncontrolled insulin release in a proportion of the tumor cells. A defect storage mechanism would not only explain inappropriate insulin secretion with normal plasma glucose levels resulting in hypoglycemia but also the elevated proinsulin levels (Gorden et al., 1972; Rubenstein et al., 1972). Since the conversion of proinsulin to insulin takes place only in the Golgi apparatus and the secretory granules (Kemmler et al., 1972) a defect in storage capacity (i.e. granule formation) should lead to increased proinsulin levels.

Insulin and proinsulin turnover in human insulinomas

Subcellular fractionation and in vitro incorporation studies in 7 insulinomas are in agreement with this contention (Creutzfeldt et al., 1973a). Table 3 shows the percentage insulin distribution in tumor subcellular fractions from pulse and chase incubation samples. The S-100 contained approximately 40% of the immunoreactive insulin and a significantly higher proinsulin percentage than the secretory granule fraction. A similar situation can be produced experimentally by degranulating rat islets with tolbutamide pretreatment. Table 4 shows that also in degranulated rat islet tissue the percentage of IRI in the cytoplasm (i.e. in a non-granular form) increases significantly. These findings suggest that in degranulated B-cells an appreciable part of the insulin is present in a

TABLE 3

Percentage IRI distribution in tumor subcellular fractions from pulse and chase incubation samples. The percentage proinsulin is given in brackets in those fractions in which it was determined

Case	Incubation	Percentage of total IRI in				
		Cell debris	Mitochondria	Secretory granules	Microsomes	S-100
1. Ben.	Pulse	6	8	34	3	49
	Chase 1	7	11	29	2	51
	Chase 2	6	6	35	2	51
		6.3	8.3	32.6	2.3	50.3
2. Bök.	Pulse	5 (7)	16 (10)	40 (9)	2 (85)	37 (25)
	Chase 1	4	12	41 (12)	2	41 (30)
	Chase 2	3	18	43	2	34
		4.0	15.3	41.3	2.0	37.3
3. Kle.	Pulse	5	11	36	2	46 (52)
	Pulse	6 (18)	10 (16)	33 (18)	2 (81)	49 (57)
		5.5	10.5	34.5	2.0	47.5
4. Kön.	Pulse	3 (11)	18 (13)	40 (11)	4 (73)	35 (19)
5. Köt.	Pulse	4	21	43 (7)	1	31 (14)
6. Mur.	Pulse	7 (9)	14 (7)	36 (8)	2 (85)	41 (28)
	Chase 1	4	10	39 (10)	3	44 (32)
	Chase 2	6	9	38	4	43 (27)
		5.6	11.0	37.6	3.0	42.6
7. Schal.	Pulse	6 (13)	14 (13)	27 (15)	1 (92)	52 (63)
	Chase 1	4	13	28 (19)	2	53 (55)
	Chase 2	4	15	22	2	57
		4.6	14.0	25.6	1.6	54.0
Mean ±	4.7	13.8	36.3	2.2	42.5	
S.D.	1.1	4.4	6.0	0.9	8.5	

non-granular form, possibly in microvesicles. The release of IRI into the medium during 120 minutes incubation in 3.0 mg/ml glucose is much higher from insulinoma tissue (25–55% of the insulin content) compared to isolated human islets (5% of the insulin content) (Table 5).

TABLE 4
Percentage IRI distribution in rat pancreatic islet tissue subcellular fractions

Treatment	IRI U/g	Percentage of total IRI in				
		Cell debris	Mitochondria	Secretory granules	Microsomes	S-100
Control	2.1	9.2	13.4	68.5	3.2	5.7
	2.4	7.9	10.6	73.3	3.8	4.4
	2.3	8.4	9.3	74.5	2.9	4.9
m ± S.D.	2.2 ± 0.2	8.5 ± 0.7	11.1 ± 2.1	72.1 ± 3.1	3.3 ± 0.4	5.0 ± 0.7
Tolbutamide pretreatment	0.9	7.5	14.1	52.2	6.2	20.0
	1.2	9.5	16.2	46.9	4.8	22.6
	0.7	6.8	12.1	50.9	5.7	24.5
m ± S.D.	0.9 ± 0.3	7.9 ± 1.4	14.1 ± 2.1	50.0 ± 2.8	5.5 ± 0.7	22.3 ± 2.6
P value	< 0.005	n.s.	n.s.	< 0.001	< 0.01	< 0.001

The rate of proinsulin/insulin turnover was estimated by incubation of tissue from 7 insulinomas with 3.0 mg/ml glucose and ^{3}H-leucine (100 μC/ml) for a 15-minute pulse period. One third of the tissue was immediately homogenized in 0.3 M sucrose (pH 6.0), one third after 20 minutes chase (with leucine 375 μg/ml) and the remaining third after 80 minutes chase. Subcellular fractions were prepared by centrifugation and their identity was confirmed by ultrastructural examination. Figure 17 shows typical Sephadex G-50 radioactivity and IRI patterns of microsomal fractions from a pulse/chase experiment. The amount of newly synthesized proinsulin decreased over the chase period while the endogenous proinsulin remained relatively constant.

Figure 18 demonstrates typical Sephadex G-50 radioactivity and IRI pattern from the secretory granule sucrose gradient fraction 1.60 M from a pulse/chase experiment. No change in the percentage of endogenous proinsulin was apparent during the pulse and chase periods; however, a dramatic change in the radioactivity patterns was observed. The radioactivity decreased in the proinsulin peak and increased in the insulin peak during the chase period, indicating a conversion of newly synthesized proinsulin into insulin in the secretory granules.

Media samples of all 7 incubations were extracted and fractionated by G-50 column chromatography. In 5 of these labelled IRI was in the 15-minute pulse medium. The pulse and chase samples from a representative experiment are presented in Figure 19. In the 15-minute pulse medium only radioactive proinsulin was found along with endogenous proinsulin and insulin. This peak decreased over the chase period with a corresponding increase in the radioactive insulin peak.

TABLE 5
IRI release during incubations of insulinoma tissue and isolated human islets in 3.0 mg/ml glucose medium

A. Insulinoma tissue

Case	IRI content mU/mg	15 min. incubation (pulse period)		95 min. incubation (pulse and chase periods)	
		IRI release mU/mg	IRI release as % of IRI content	IRI release mU/mg	IRI release as % of IRI content
1. Ben.	13.6	1.81	13.3	5.91	43.4
2. Bök.	89.0	5.13	5.7	16.93	19.0
3. Kle.	11.5	1.42	12.3		
4. Kön.	6.0	0.48	8.0		
5. Köt.	81.1	7.12	8.7		
6. Mur.	17.9	1.09	6.1	3.69	20.6
7. Schal.	40.1	2.47	6.1	7.65	19.0

B. Isolated human islets

Case	IRI content mU	15 min. incubation (pulse period)		120 min. incubation (pulse and chase periods)	
		IRI release μU	IRI release as % of IRI content	IRI release μU	IRI release as % of IRI content
5. Köt.	17.4	91.2	0.5	847.5	4.8
6. Mur.	21.4	121.0	0.6	962.2	4.4

When isolated human pancreatic islets were pulsed for 60 minutes and chased for 60 minutes neither radioactive proinsulin nor insulin was released into the medium with the endogenous IRI. Also other available data concerning the turnover of IRI in various tissue preparations (Howell and Taylor, 1967; Howell et al., 1969; Sorenson et al., 1970; Kemmler and Steiner, 1970; Lazarus et al., 1970; Orci et al., 1971; Sando et al., 1972; Track et al., 1973) show that this turnover is much faster in human insulinomas.

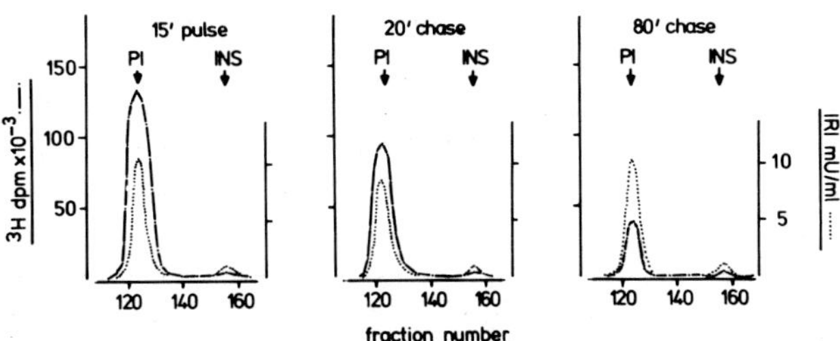

FIG. 17. Sephadex G-50 radioactivity (–•–•–) and IRI (•••••) patternss of microsomal fractions from a pulse/chase experiment. The elution positions of bovine proinsulin (PI) and human insulin (INS) are denoted above the G-50 patterns. The void volume of the column commenced at fraction 90. No significant radioactivity or IRI levels were detected before fraction 115.

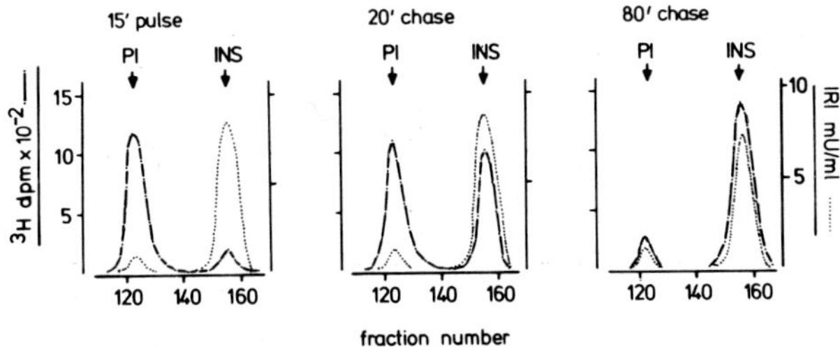

FIG. 18. Sephadex G-50 radioactivity (–•–•–) and IRI (•••••) patterns from the secretory granule sucrose gradient fraction 1.60 M from a pulse/chase experiment. Acid-ethanol extracts of the 1.60 M sucrose fractions were chromatographed upon Sephadex LH-20 and then upon Sephadex G-50 to separate proinsulin from insulin. The elution positions of bovine proinsulin (PI) and human insulin (INS) are denoted above the G-50 patterns. The void volume of the column commenced at fraction 90. No significant radioactivity or IRI levels were detected before fraction 115.

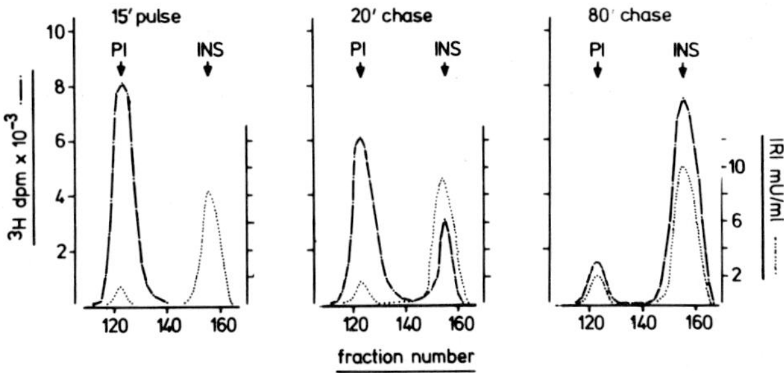

FIG. 19. Sephadex G-50 radioactivity (–•–•–) and IRI (•••••) patterns of media samples from a pulse/chase experiment. Only one-third of the pulse sample was chromatographed to compensate for the three-fold excess of incubated tissue compared to the 2 chase periods. The elution positions of bovine proinsulin (PI) and human insulin (INS) are denoted above the G-50 patterns. The void volume of the column commenced at fraction 90. No significant radioactivity or IRI levels were detected before fraction 115.

CONCLUSION

1. The morphological diagnosis of the type of an endocrine pancreatic tumor has to be based on hormone extraction and immunohistological investigations. Specific staining methods for B-cells give negative results in 20% of the insulinomas. No specific staining methods are available yet for G-cells. The ultrastructural appearance of the secretory granules allows the correct diagnosis only in 70% of insulinomas and in the minority of gastrinomas. Different peptide-producing cells can be identified immunohistologically and ultrastructurally in the same tumor, especially in the case of gastrinomas. It is suggested that endocrine pancreatic tumors originate from immature stem cells in the ductular system rather than from the pancreatic islets.
2. Human insulinomas have the capacity for an increased turnover of proinsulin and insulin compared to normal pancreatic islets. This increased turnover does not necessarily mean an increased rate of biosynthesis. The simplest explanation for this phenomenon would be uncontrolled hormone release from and/or decreased storage capacity in the tumor cells. This means a shortened granule phase during which less proinsulin can be converted into insulin. This could explain the high percentage of proinsulin found in insulinoma tissue and in the plasma of insulinoma patients.

The concept that the major defect of insulinoma cells is a disturbed storage and release mechanism and not pathological biosynthesis of the hormone, can explain all the so far known clinical, morphological and biochemical observations.

REFERENCES

ARNOLD, R., DEUTICKE U., FRERICHS, H. and CREUTZFELDT, W. (1972): Immunohistologic investigations of human insulinomas. *Diabetologia, 8,* 250.

BENCOSME, S. A., ALLEN, R. A. and LATTA, H. (1963): Functioning pancreatic islet cell tumours studied electron microscopically. *Amer. J. Path., 42,* 1.

CREUTZFELDT, W., ARNOLD, R., CREUTZFELDT, C., FEURLE, G. and KETTERER, H. (1971): Gastrin and G-cells in the antral mucosa of patients with pernicious anemia, acromegaly and hyperparathyroidism and in a Zollinger-Ellison tumour of the pancreas. *Europ. J. clin. Invest., 1,* 461.

CREUTZFELDT, C., TRACK, N. S. and CREUTZFELDT, W. (1973a): In vitro studies of the rate of proinsulin and insulin turnover in seven human insulinomas. *Europ. J. clin. Invest., 3,* 371.

CREUTZFELDT, W., ARNOLD, R., CREUTZFELDT, C., DEUTICKE, U., FRERICHS, H. and TRACK, N. S. (1973b): Biochemical and morphological investigations of 30 human insulinomas. *Diabetologia, 9,* 217.

DECONINCK, J. F., POTVLIEGE, P. R. and GEPTS, W. (1971): The ultrastructure of the human pancreatic islets. I. The islets of adults. *Diabetologia, 7,* 266.

FEDERLIN, K., RAPTIS, S., BEYER, J. and PFEIFFER, E. F. (1969): Immunhistologische Untersuchungen und der Nachweis von Serum- und Tumor-Insulin beim Insulinom. In: *15. Symposium der Deutschen Gesellschaft für Endokrinologie,* pp. 415–417. Editor: J. Kracht. Springer Verlag, Berlin – Heidelberg – New York.

GEORGSSON, G. and WESSEL, W. (1967): Vergleichende elektronenmikroskopische Untersuchungen normaler menschlicher Pankreasinseln und eines hormonell aktiven Inselzellcarcinoms mit Hyperinsulinismus. *Z. Krebsforsch., 69,* 70.

GOLDSMITH, S., YALOW, R. and BERSON, S. A. (1969): Significance of human plasma insulin sephadex fractions. *Diabetes, 18,* 834.

GORDEN, P. and ROTH, J. (1969): Circulating insulins. *Arch. intern. Med., 123,* 237.

GORDEN, P., SHERMAN, B. and ROTH, J. (1971): Proinsulin-like component of circulating insulin in the basal state and in patients and hamsters with islet cell tumours. *J. clin. Invest., 50,* 2113.

GORDEN, P., ROTH, J., FREYCHET, P. and KAHN, R. (1972): The circulating proinsulin-like components. *Diabetes, 21/Suppl. 2,* 673.

GREIDER, M. H. and ELLIOTT, D. W. (1964): Electron microscopy of human pancreatic tumours of islet cell origin. *Amer. J. Path., 44,* 663.

GREIDER, M. H. and McGUIGAN, J. E. (1971): Cellular localization of gastrin in the human pancreas. *Diabetes, 20,* 389.

GRIMELIUS, L. (1968): A silver nitrate stain for a_2-cells in human pancreatic islets. *Acta Soc. Med. upsalien., 73,* 243.

GUSEK, W. and KRACHT, J. (1961): Elektronenmikroskopische Befunde am Inselorgan. In: *7. Symposium der Deutschen Gesellschaft für Endokrinologie,* p. 109. Editor: K. Oberdisse. Springer Verlag, Berlin – Heidelberg – New York.

GUTMAN, R., LAZARUS, N. R., PENHOS, J., RECANT, L. and FAJANS, S. S. (1970): Circulating proinsulin-like material in patients with functioning insulinomas. *New Engl. J. Med., 284,* 1003.

HELLERSTRÖM, C. and HELLMAN, B. (1960): Some aspects of silver impregnation of the islets of Langerhans in the rat. *Acta endocr. (Kbh.), 35,* 518.

HOWELL, S. L. and TAYLOR, K. W. (1967): The secretion of newly synthesized insulin in vitro. *Biochem. J., 102,* 922.

HOWELL, S. L., KOSTIANOVSKY, M. and LACY, P. E. (1969): Beta granule formation in isolated islets of Langerhans. A study by electron microscopic radioautography. *J. Cell Biol., 42,* 695.

KEMMLER, W. and STEINER, D. F. (1970): Conversion of proinsulin to insulin in a subcellular fraction form rat islets. *Biochem. biophys. Res. Commun., 41,* 1223.

KEMMLER, W., PETERSON, J. D., RUBENSTEIN, A. H. and STEINER, D. F. (1972): On the biosynthesis, intracellular transport and mechanism of conversion of proinsulin to insulin and C-peptide. *Diabetes, 21/Suppl. 2,* 572.

KO, A. S. C., SMYTH, D. G., MARKUSSEN, J. and SUNDBY, F. (1971): The amino acid sequence of the C-peptide of human proinsulin. *Europ. J. Biochem., 20,* 190.

LACY, P. E. (1961): Electron microscopy of beta cells of pancreas. *Amer. J. Med., 31,* 851.

LACY, P. E. and WILLIAMSON, J. R. (1960): Electron microscopic and fluorescent antibody studies of islet cell adenomas. *Anat. Rec., 136,* 227.

LAZARUS, S. S. and VOLK, B. W. (1962): Histochemical and electron microscopic studies of a functioning insulinoma. *Lab. Invest., 11,* 1279.

LAZARUS, N. R., TANESE, T., GUTMAN, R. and RECANT, L. (1970): Synthesis and release of proinsulin and insulin by human insulinoma tissue. *J. clin. Endocr., 30,* 273.

LINDALL, A. W., WONG, E. T., SORENSON, R. L. and STEFFES, M. W. (1972): Proinsulin and insulin content of subcellular fractions from an islet adenoma. *J. clin. Endocr., 34,* 718.

LOMSKY, R., LANGR, F. and VORTEL, V. (1970): Immunohistological demonstration of gastrin in mammalian islets of Langerhans. *Nature (Lond.), 223,* 618.

MELANI, F., RYAN, W. G., RUBENSTEIN, A. H. and STEINER, D. F. (1970): Proinsulin secretion by a pancreatic beta cell adenoma: proinsulin and C-peptide secretion. *New Engl. J. Med., 283,* 713.

MISUGI, K., HOWELL, S. L., GREIDER, M. H., LACY, P. E. and SORENSON, G. D. (1970): The pancreatic beta cell. *Arch. Path., 89,* 97.

ORCI, L., LAMBERT, A. E., KANAZAWA, Y., AMHERDT, M., ROULLIER, C. and RENOLD, A. E. (1971): Morphological and biochemical studies of B-cells of fetal rat endocrine pancreas in organ culture. Evidence for (pro)insulin biosynthesis. *J. Cell Biol., 50,* 565.

PFEIFFER, E. F. (1967): Die Immunologie des Insulins. *Verh. Dtsch. Ges. inn. Med., 72,* 811.

RUBENSTEIN, A. H., CLARK, J. L., MELANI, F. and STEINER, D. F. (1969): Secretion of proinsulin C-peptide by pancreatic beta cells and its circulation in blood. *Nature (Lond.), 224,* 697.

RUBENSTEIN, A. H., BLOCK, M. B., STARR, J., MELANI, F. and STEINER, D. F. (1972): Proinsulin and C-peptide in blood. *Diabetes, 21/Suppl. 2,* 661.

SANDO, H., BORG, J. and STEINER, D. F. (1972): Studies on the secretion of newly synthesized proinsulin and insulin from isolated rats islets of Langerhans. *J. clin. Invest., 51,* 1476.

SHERMAN, B. M., PEK, S., FAJANS, S. S., FLOYD, J. C. and CONN, J. W. (1972): Plasma proinsulin in patients with functioning pancreatic islet cell tumours. *J. clin. Endocr., 35,* 271.

SORENSON, R. L., STEFFES, M. W. and LINDALL, A. W. (1970): Subcellular localization of proinsulin to insulin conversion in isolated rat islets. *Endocrinology, 86,* 88.

THIERY, J. P. and BADER, J. P. (1966): Ultrastructure des îlots de Langerhans du pancréas humain normal et pathologique. *Ann. endocr. (Paris), 27,* 625.

TRACK, N. S., FRERICHS, H. and CREUTZFELDT, W. (1973): Release of newly synthesized proinsulin and insulin from granulated and degranulated isolated rat islets (abstract). *Diabetologia, 9,* 93.

VASSALLO, G., CAPELLA, C. and SOLCIA, E. (1971): Grimelius' silver stain for endocrine cell granules as shown by electron microscopy. *Stain Technol., 46,* 7.

VASSALLO, G., SOLCIA, E., BUSSOLATI, G., POLAK, J. M. and PEARSE, A. G. E. (1972): Non-G-cell gastrin-producing tumours of the pancreas. *Virchows Arch. Abt. B Zellpath., 11,* 66.

NEW DATA ON NON-B CELL TUMORS OF THE PANCREAS

S. BONFILS

Unité de Recherches de Gastroentérologie, INSERM, Hôpital Bichat, Paris, France

In the past 15 years, at least 4 new syndromes have been associated with non-B cell tumors: Zollinger-Ellison syndrome or gastrinoma; watery diarrhea hypokalemic syndrome (WDHA or Verner Morrison syndrome); glucagonoma with diabetes; mixed endocrinopathies with polyhormonal secretion from a solitary islet tumor. This paper will only deal with the first 3 syndromes mentioned above.

There is a strong tendency to classify tumors of the pancreatic islets by linking the clinical syndrome with the hormone secreted by each type of tumor. Unfortunately the WDHA syndrome represents a failure in this logical attitude: neither the hormone nor the type of cell capable of secreting this unknown substance have been so far definitely characterized. Furthermore some islet tumors are not hormone-secreting, their clinical course being exclusively related to tumor growth and metastases, usually in the liver.

It still remains that radioimmunoassay represents, at the present time, a great improvement in diagnostic certainty, specially for gastrinoma; and for the future, with the expected technical improvements and increase in specificity, the best chance for an accurate and better understanding of the pathophysiological mechanisms.

ZOLLINGER-ELLISON SYNDROME (ZES)

Clinical basis of the diagnosis

It is now known that the clinical presentations of the ZES are extremely varied. These included relapsing ulcer, some forms of duodenal ulcer, multiple ulcers, abnormally situated ulcers, multiple endocrine adenomas, or severe diarrhea. Thus, originally a quite different diagnosis may be made.

Sex and age All the authors (Bonfils and Bader, 1970; Ellison and Wilson, 1964) agree that these 2 factors have no bearing upon diagnosis. The male sex predominates slightly (60% of cases). The age of onset of symptoms is in most cases between 20 and 50 years. The extreme age limits in published cases are 9 and 90 years.

Length of history and presenting symptoms The sudden onset of symptoms is not often observed, contrary to what was originally believed (Zollinger and Ellison, 1955), and 80% of patients had symptoms for more than one year before the diagnosis was made. In our series of 53 cases this percentage was only 62%, suggesting that more frequent use of laboratory tests would speed up diagnosis.

Abdominal pain believed to be due to an ulcer was noted in 75% of cases. The ulcer was fairly often accompanied by vomiting (25% of cases), hemorrhage (melena 22%, hematemesis 19%) and acute perforation (18%)

Diarrhea This symptom is of diagnostic and physiopathological interest. According to Ellison and Wilson (1964), 36% of patients had diarrhea at some stage of the disease: in 12% of these the ulcer preceded diarrhea, in 18% diarrhea preceded the ulcer, and in 7% there was diarrhea without ulcer.

We believe that diarrhea in the ZES is even more frequent than would appear from the published series. Careful questioning in our personal series led to its finding in 81% of cases, of which 16% had no ulcer. In one half of these cases, diarrhea was the first symptom (Bonfils and Bader, 1970).

The following clinical presentations may be distinguished: (1) simple diarrhea sometimes evolving by acute bouts with fairly long periods of remission; (2) steatorrhea with and without ulcer, resembling sprue and improved by anticholinergic drugs; (3) massive diarrhea with low serum potassium.

The mechanism of the diarrhea is predominantly due to the increased secretion of hydrochloric acid as shown by suppression of the diarrhea by aspiration of the gastric secretions and by evidence of a very low fecal pH (sometimes around 2.0). This acid hypersecretion (a) irritates the intestine locally, (b) creates mucosal changes in the small intestine, (c) disturbs enzymatic processes within the intestinal lumen, causing malabsorption, and (d) has a diluting effect upon intestinal content owing to voluminous gastric secretions.

Clinical criteria for diagnosis The clinical features leading to the diagnosis of ZES are as follows:

1. Peptic ulcer having a very malignant course and leading to one or more fruitless surgical operations, which were followed early by an anastomotic ulcer, often resulting in perforation. The localization of the ulcer is usually marginal, jejunal or duodenal, more rarely gastric or esophageal. Multiple ulcers have been observed in 42% of cases. This clinical picture, which is all the more suggestive when there are several operative failures, was present in about half the cases collected by Ellison and Wilson and in one fourth of our own cases.

2. Common duodenal ulcer of long duration with high basal secretion lately resistant to medical treatment.

3. Peptic ulcer, presenting one or more of the following features: (a) site outside of the stomach or duodenal bulb; (b) multiplicity of ulcers; (c) diarrhea as associated symptom; (d) endocrine syndrome; (e) malignant metastases in the liver or lungs.

4. Lack of peptic ulcer, the ZES being exclusively manifested by either various types of diarrhea or by multiple endocrine syndromes, often familial in nature.

Statistical repartition (Dubrasquet et al., 1973) appears in Figure 1, involving 74 cases with clinical suspicion of ZES: 44 with tumors (macroscopic tumor and/or microadenoma), 9 with islet cell hyperplasia, 21 with no macroscopic or microscopic pancreatic abnormalities.

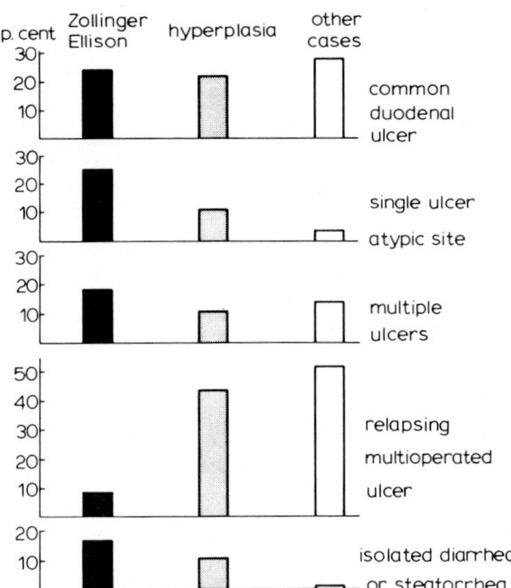

FIG. 1. Clinical course in 74 patients suspected of ZES: distribution in 3 groups according to the final operative and histological diagnosis.

Zollinger-Ellison syndrome in multiple endocrine adenomatosis

The ZES is often considered as part of multiple endocrine adenomatosis (MEA I) usually known as Wermer's syndrome. Hyperparathyroidism is the most common associated endocrine abnormality; pituitary, adrenal, thyroid and ovarian tumors are less common. Insulinoma, as a separate pancreatic anatomical lesion, is a member of the syndrome.

Following Wermer's original descriptions, the familial incidence of MEA I has been repeatedly emphasized, suggesting inheritance as an autosomal dominant with high but variable expressivity (Wermer, 1963). Another familial disease, MEA II, is characterized by the potential association of pheochromocytoma, medullary carcinoma of the thyroid and hyperparathyroidism but does not include pancreatic tumors.

One out of 4 to 5 ZES was characterized as a part of MEA (Table 1). The distribution of organ involvement and most common clinical features were recently compiled by Croisier et al. (1971). Their findings differ slightly from our personal series owing to the gastrointestinal symptoms, on which our patients were selected.

The presenting symptoms in various individuals differ markedly, depending on the glands involved and on the functional activity of the adenoma. In cases collected by Ballard et al. (1964), the history was dominated by peptic ulcer in 21 cases; in 16 patients the presenting symptom was hypoglycemia and parathyroid syndrome attracted attention in 8 cases.

Tumor of one organ may also modify the clinical manifestations caused by tumors of other endocrine organs: for example, resection of one or more parathyroid adenomas improved symptoms of peptic ulcer and decreased gastric acid secretion when ZES was also present; this beneficial effect appears to be due to reduction of hypercalcemia.

Discrepancies between the clinical signs and symptoms and the pathological findings

TABLE 1
Statistical data on multiple endocrine adenomatosis (MEA I or Wermer's syndrome)

Wermer's syndrome		
	169 Cases from the literature (Croisier et al., 1971)	Personal cases (N)
Pancreas	84%	14
Parathyroids	87.5%	6
Peptic ulcer and/or diarrhea	61.5%	14
Pituitary	51%	4
Adrenal cortex	41.5%	4
Thyroid	26.5%	2
Hypoglycemia	26%	3
Number of endocrine glads (other than non-B pancreatic cells) involved in cases of ZES		
1 Endocrine gland	54%	9
2 Endocrine glands	27%	4
3 Endocrine glands	19%	1

led Ballard et al. (1964) to conclude that in ZES the frequency of MEA is greater than generally supposed.

A broader spectrum of pathophysiological interferences could result from antral gastrin cell participation in inter-endocrine relationships: this new field was opened by recent reports of G-cell hyperplasia in several clinical states: duodenal ulcer with acid hypersecretion, gastric ulcer with pyloric obstruction, primary hyperparathyroidism without acid hypersecretion or ulcer disease, and acromegaly with or without enhanced gastric secretory activity (Creutzfeldt et al., 1971).

Some cases of clinically suspected ZES with elevated blood gastrin were found to be accompanied by hyperplasia of the antral G-cells. The usual lack of complete pancreatic examination and the only assessment of cellular density in antral mucosal biopsies makes pathophysiological interpretation very difficult.

Gastric hypersecretion

The diagnostic importance of studies of gastric secretion in ZES is considerable: permanence of tumoral hormone liberation results in a near maximal secretory stimulation and in an increase in the cell masses, both phenomena being more marked for acid than for pepsin (Neuburger et al., 1972).

Various criteria have been proposed for discriminating ZES cases among large ulcer population: basal acid output >15 mEq/hr, acid concentration >100 mEq/l and low pepsin/acid correlation (K 25 < 40). Comparison of 20 cases of ZES with 495 duodenal ulcers leads us to conclude that neither an acid concentration > 100 mEq/l nor an acid output ⩾ 15 mEq/hr is sufficiently discriminatory when taken alone because they were respectively found in 8.2% and 6% duodenal ulcers (Bernades et al., 1973).

However, their association in the same secretory study strongly increases the suspicion of this diagnosis because it was found in 60% of ZES cases and in only 2.8% of duodenal ulcers. The most valuable modification of those criteria taken alone is the presence of a basal acid output > 18 mEq/hr which was found in 60% of ZES cases and in 2.4% of duodenal ulcer cases. In any case a low pepsin/acid correlation (K 25) improves the suspicion of the diagnosis. The most characteristic secretory status of the ZES consists of an association of a basal acid output > 18 mEq/hr, a basal acid concentration > 100 mEq/l and K 25 < 35 which is found in 55% of ZES cases and only in 0.6% of duodenal ulcers without stenosis.

Blood gastrin measurement

The ulcerogenic tumor in the ZES produces gastrin, and the demonstration of elevated levels of circulating gastrin can point directly to the diagnosis. More precisely, the development of sensitive radioimmunoassay technics for gastrin has allowed a definitive diagnosis to be made much earlier, and thus patients may be operated on sooner.

As more patients with ulcer disease are studied, it is likely that many patients with less overt clinical manifestations of the ZES will be recognized. Already several gastrinoma patients have been found with only moderate basal acid hypersecretion and only moderately elevated serum gastrin values. Such patients will provide a diagnostic challenge since their basal gastrin concentrations may overlap basal and certainly postprandial values obtained in some patients with duodenal ulcer disease, especially those with vagotomy.

Likewise, provocative tests have been of great help in following up problem cases and cases with atypical manifestations of the syndrome.

Fasting blood-gastrin concentrations other than in ZES Normal gastrin concentrations vary among various laboratories (Table 2) using different assay methods and different standards (Accary and Bonfils, 1973; Ganguli and Hunter, 1972; Hansky and Cain, 1969; McGuigan and Trudeau, 1972; Stadil et al., 1971). Among the several assays now being reported, normal mean values for basal gastrin concentration have been 15 to 120 pg/ml with a few apparently normal subjects having values in the range of 200–300 pg/ml.

In the various series reported to date, there have been no large differences in fasting gastrin concentrations between normal subjects and those with duodenal ulcer, with mean values between groups usually varying by less than 20 pg/ml, either higher or lower.

Gastrin values usually are elevated in patients with hypochlorhydria; in cases of achlorhydria with or without pernicious anemia, they tend to average between 500 and 1000 pg/ml and thus overlap the values found in the ZES.

TABLE 2
Serum gastrin concentrations in fasting subjects

Authors	Normal subjects		Duodenal ulcer		Pernicious anemia	
	Mean ± S.E.M.	No	Mean ± S.E.M.	No	Mean ± S.E.M.	No
Hansky	32 ± 4.3	93	16 ± 1.5	72	1036 ± 215	21
McGuigan	85 ± 9.8	35	78 ± 6.7	55	997 ± 182	29
Ganguli	105 ± 7	113	91 ± 6	27	1167 ± 147	51
Stadil	52 ± 4.6	120	50 ± 2.4	103	912 ± 163	36
Accary and Bonfils	15 ± 2.2	38	23 ± 1.9	85	385 ± 152	14

Fasting blood gastrin in ZES Patients with well-documented ZES usually have serum gastrin concentrations more than 10 times higher than the normal range, often greater than 1,000 pg/ml. However, several series have included patients with values between 2 and 4 times the normal level. Many of these patients have had intact stomachs. Even lower values have been found in some patients who have had total gastrectomy, excision of a parathyroid adenoma, or partial excision of the gastrin-secreting tumor. Some of these values have fallen in the normal range. However, most patients with ZES continue to have markedly increased serum gastrin concentrations after total gastrectomy, subtotal pancreatectomy, or removal of parathyroid adenomas.

The prognosis of patients with residual tumor after total gastric secretion seems relatively good and there are many reports of long survival in patients with known metastatic disease. Friesen et al. (1970) have suggested that removal of the stomach may result in regression of metastasis because of loss of gastric factor affecting pancreatic islet cells.

Passaro et al. (1972) studied 4 patients with the ZES, 2 of whom had low serum gastrin levels (67 and 3 pg/ml) after substantiated total gastrectomy, while in the other 2, with high serum gastrin levels (3,250 and 2,000 pg/ml), there was evidence of incomplete gastrectomy, i.e., no squamous epithelium histologically at the upper margin of the resected stomach and the presence of acid-secreting (pH 1) mucosa by placement of pH electrode at the distal esophagus. They interpreted this finding as evidence in support of a gastric factor in the genesis of the ZES.

Other patients have been reported by Wilson et al. (1971) to have high levels of serum gastrin many years after total gastrectomy; a concentration of serum gastrin greater than 5,000 pg/ml was observed in a patient 13 years after total gastrectomy. It would seem unlikely, therefore, that measurement of serum gastrin concentrations in general will afford any direct prognostic information, as has been suggested, although an abrupt and persistent fall in serum gastrin levels after operation would certainly appear to be a good prognostic sign.

Our own series of 7 cases shows that the normal blood gastrin level after surgery could be found in cases without metastasis following tumor excision whatever the gastric surgical procedure. After total gastrectomy alone, no significant change in blood gastrin was observed within a follow-up period of 4 months (case 1) and one year (case 6) (Table 3).

TABLE 3
Comparison of pre-operative and post-operative fasting blood gastrin level in 7 cases of Zollinger-Ellison syndrome

	Age	Sex	Liver metastasis	Blood gastrin (pg/ml)	Surgical procedure: Gastrectomy	Surgical procedure: Tumor excision	Post-operative blood gastrin (pg/ml)
Case 1	75	F	0	15,000	Partial	0	189
Case 2	42	M	0	520	Partial	+	64
Case 3	38	M	0	450	Total	+	5
Case 4	35	F	0	375	Total	+	23
Case 5	50	F	+	350	Total	0	165
Case 6	42	F	+	300	Total	0	180
Case 7	31	M	+	140	Total	0	200

Provocative tests using gastrin radioimmunoassay for ZES diagnosis and postoperative follow-up As indicated above, several ZES patients have been found with only a moderate increase in fasting blood gastrin. Likewise, after operation some cases demonstrated a noticeable decrease without definite normalization. In both circumstances a need for sensitization of hormonal dosage is obvious, using dynamic studies.

Two agents, calcium and secretin, may selectively increase serum gastrin concentrations in patients with gastrinoma. In normal subjects and in patients with duodenal ulcer, calcium is a moderate stimulant of acid secretion, while in patients with the Zollinger-Ellison syndrome the stimulation by calcium may be pronounced (Trudeau and McGuigan, 1969). Calcium infusion may increase serum gastrin values in normal and ulcer subjects, but the increases are only approximately 2 times basal levels after a 3-hr infusion of 4 mg/kg/hr. In response to an infusion of 5 mg/kg/hr (15 mg/kg i.v., 3 hours infusion) patients with gastrinoma have shown marked increases in serum gastrin, usually to stimulated values greater than 1,000 pg/ml (Passaro et al., 1972).

Current observations pointed out that (1) routine fasting gastrin levels during the postgastrectomy follow-up period may be inaccurate for identifying patients with retained functioning tumor, and (2) the calcium-stimulated gastrin survey may provide a more effective means for such detection and be a helpful tool in evaluating the concept of tumor regression after 'target organ' removal. The main interest of the provocative test using secretin is the opposite reactions of gastrinoma to any other physiological or pathological condition, where it was repeatedly shown that exogenous secretin decreases basal acid output, gastric secretory response to endogenous or exogenous gastrin, fasting and postprandial serum gastrin levels (Hansky et al., 1971).

Contrary to these observations, ZES patients exhibit, in response to exogenous secretin, an unexpected increase in both serum gastrin levels and basal acid secretion. Secretin has been variably administered as a continuous infusion of graded dosage and as a single injection (from 1 to 3 units/kg). The percentage of false negative response has not, so far, been determined (Bradley and Galambos, 1972).

Some kind of gastrin release has been assumed as explanation in spite of the fact that this phenomenon is dose-related (Schrumpf et al., 1973).

Bioassays using blood or urine are by comparison to gastrin measurement of little interest. However, large statistical studies as well as long-term postoperative follow-up suggest that bioassays could still be helpful in some clinical problems as possibly reflecting hormonal changes other than gastrin hypersecretion (Dubrasquet et al., 1973).

WDHA SYNDROME

Verner and Morrison, in 1958, described 2 cases of non-B islet cell tumors of the pancreas in which the patients had died from the effects of severe watery diarrhea and hypokalemia without any evidence of peptic ulcer. Absence of free acid in gastric secretion was demonstrated later, but represents the best clinical test for distinguishing this group from cases of diarrhea associated with the Zollinger-Ellison syndrome. The diarrhea is generally so severe that Matsumoto et al. (1966) called it 'pancreatic cholera'. 'WDHA' syndrome is another term denoting the main features of watery diarrhea, hypokalemia and achlorhydria. This group represents approximately 5% of all those with hormone-producing non-B islet cell tumors of the pancreas (Verner, 1968). Approximately 2/5 of these tumors were malignant by the time of surgery or autopsy. Neither specific staining nor ultrastructure studies allowed characterization of a specific cell type (Martin et al., 1974).

There has been considerable speculation regarding the probable humoral mechanisms underlying the clinical features. Zollinger's group have suggested that secretin may be responsible. Barbezat and Grossman, on the other hand, speculated that combined production of gastrin and glucagon might be involved. No gastrin has been found by bioassay of tumor extracts but gastrin-like material (PSU) has been found in urine samples from one case (Gjone et al., 1970).

More recently Elias et al. (1972) described a case of pancreatic cholera with a non-B islet cell tumor of the pancreas producing the enterogastrone, gastric inhibitory polypeptide; evidence was obtained by immunofluorescence technique.

Regarding clinical manifestations, the tremendous volume of stool combined with massive potassium loss can be illustrated by the average daily amount of 5.8 litres in a group of 20 patients (Kraft et al., 1970). Likewise potassium losses averaged 350 mEq/24 hr during acute diarrheal episodes and could be responsible for alterations in glucose metabolism (fasting hyperglycemia, diabetic type results on glucose tolerance test). Of the patients 80% have elevated levels of serum calcium and one half of these values were greater than 12 mg%. Alterations in magnesium balance might explain hypercalcemia, the magnesium-deficient state constantly occurring in diseases with prolonged diarrhea.

Corticosteroid therapy was claimed to improve water and electrolyte losses in WDHA syndrome: actually, in 7 reported patients, one had a definite improvement, 2 others experienced only temporary remission and 4 were not improved. Only surgical removal of the tumor led to definite cure.

GLUCAGONOMA

Glucagon-secreting tumors are extremely rare and in the few reported glucagonomas there have been no consistent clinical features. McGavran et al. (1966) reported the first proven case. The patient was a 42-year-old female with mild diabetes mellitus and bulbous eczematoid dermatitis. Pancreatic alpha cell carcinoma with metastasis in the right lobe of the liver was present; tumor extract showed a large amount of immunoreactive glucagon (14 μg per gram of tissue). Fasting plasma glucagon content ranged from 36 to 55 ng/ml (normal $<$ 2 ng).

Yoshinaga et al. (1966) described a similar case with insulin-requiring diabetes, a palpable mass in the left upper abdomen and elevated glucagon-like activity in the serum. They referred to 2 other examples of alpha cell tumor associated with diabetes mellitus and another case with elevated glucagon-like activity in the tumor extract but in which diabetes was not found.

Several unexplained aspects have been described in glucagonomas including abnormalities of liver functions, amenorrhea, skin rash, hemolytic anemia, and edema.

Hyperglucagonemia was recently mentioned in MEA, the significance of which would depend on whether an alpha cell tumor of the pancreas is found or not. The well-documented case of Croughs et al. (1972) is characterized by the occurrence of a benign glucagonoma and 'primary' hyperthyroidism in a patient presenting with Cushing's syndrome due to an adrenal adenoma and galactorrhea. Serum levels of glucagon-like immunoreactivity were slightly elevated before pancreatic surgery and within normal limits thereafter; biological and immunological investigations of the tumor extract demonstrated the presence of enormous amounts of pancreatic glucagon.

The presence of a large amount of glucagon-like immunoreactivity in a hormone-secreting renal tumor (Gleeson et al., 1971), although exceptional, raises the question of radioimmunoassay specificity for clinical diagnosis. Evidence has been given that enteroglucagon alone was responsible from the lack of effect on plasma glucose and insulin levels in the rat and its failure to combine with an antiserum which only reacts with pancreatic glucagon.

To summarize some of the current problems raised by non-B cell pancreatic tumors, the different kinds of information relating to hormone hypersecretion have been listed comparably (Table 4). The most frequent syndrome, i.e. ZES, is obviously the best

TABLE 4
Evidence of hormone hypersecretion in non-B islet cell tumors

	Gastrinoma	Glucagonoma	WDHA
Target organ hyperfunction	+	0	0
Bioassay	+	0	0
Blood radioimmunoassay	+	+ (–)	0
Tissue and cell structures	0	+	0
Selective staining	0	+	0 (+)
Tumor extract (bioassay or radioimmunoassay)	+	+	0 (+)
Recovery after tumor excision	+	+	+

known and is almost ideal for logical pathophysiology. However, even here, obscurities as well as contradictory data make further biochemical and radioimmunological studies indispensable for improved diagnosis and understanding in individual cases.

REFERENCES

ACCARY, J. P. and BONFILS, S. (1973): Apport du dosage radioimmunologique de la gastrine en pathologie digestive. *Nouv. Presse méd., 2,* 41.

BALLARD, H. S., FRAME, B. and HARTSOCK, R. J. (1964): Familial multiple endocrine adenoma-peptic ulcer complex. *Medicine, 43,* 481.

BERNADES, P., MIGNON, M., BENSALEM, R., DUBRASQUET, M., BADER, J. P. and BONFILS, S. (1973): Basal acid secretion and pepsin acid ratio in the diagnosis of Zollinger-Ellison syndrome. *Digestion, 9,* 1.

BONFILS, S. and BADER, J. P. (1970): The diagnosis of Zollinger-Ellison syndrome with special reference to the multiple endocrine adenomas. In: *Progress in Gastroenterology, Vol. II,* pp. 332–355. Editor: G. B. Jerzy Glass. Grune and Stratton, New York, N.Y.

BRADLEY, E. L. and GALAMBOS, J. T. (1972): Failure of a secretin feed-back loop in the Zollinger-Ellison syndrome. The 'gastric factor' revisited. *Amer. J. Digest. Dis., 17,* 939.

CREUTZFELDT, W., ARNOLD, R. and CREUTZFELDT, C. (1971): Gastrin and G-cells in the antral mucosa of patients with pernicious anemia, acromegaly and hyperthyroidism and in a Zollinger-Ellison tumor of the pancreas. *Europ. J. clin. Invest., 1,* 461.

CROISIER, J. C., AZERAD, E. and LUBTZKI, J. (1971): L'adénomatose polyendocrinienne (Syndrome de Wermer). *Sem. Hôp., 47,* 494.

CROUGHS, R. J. M., HULSMANS, H. A. M., ISREEL, D. E., HACKENG, W. H. L. and SCHOPMAN, W. (1972): Glucagonoma as part of the polyglandular adenoma syndrome. *Amer. J. Med., 52,* 690.

DUBRASQUET, M., BONFILS, S., BADER, J. P., MARTIN, E. and SERGENT, D. (1973): Essai biologique des urines (test PSU) pour le diagnostic et la surveillance post-opératoire du syndrome de Zollinger-Ellison. *Acta gastroentérol. Belg., 36,* 438.

ELIAS, E., BLOOM, S. R., WELBOURN, R. B., KUZIO, M., POLAK, J. M., PEARSE, A. G. E., BOOTH, C. C. and BROWN, J. C. (1972): Pancreatic cholera due to production of gastric inhibitory polypeptide. *Lancet, 2,* 791.

ELLISON, E. H. and WILSON, D. D. (1964): Reappraisal and evaluation of 260 registered cases. *Ann. Surg., 160,* 512.

FRIESEN, S. R., BOLINGER, R. E. and PEARSE, A. G. E. (1970): Serum gastrin levels in malignant Zollinger-Ellison syndrome after total gastrectomy and hypophysectomy. *Ann. Surg., 172,* 504.

GANGULI, P. C. and HUNTER, W. M. (1972): Radio-immunoassay of gastrin in human plasma. *J. Physiol., 220,* 499.

GJONE, E., FRETHEIM, B., NORDÖY, A., JACOBSEN, C. D. and ELGJO, K. (1970): Intractable watery diarrhoea, hypokalaemia and achlorhydria associated with pancreatic tumour containing gastric secretory inhibitor. *Scand. J. Gastroenterol., 5,* 401.

GLEESON, M. H., BLOOM, S. R., POLAK, J. M., HENRY, K. and DOWLING, R. H. (1971): Endocrine tumour in kidney affecting small bowel structure, motility and absorptive function. *Gut, 12,* 773.

HANSKY, J. and CAIN, M. D. (1969): Radioimmunoassay of gastrin in human serum. *Lancet, 2,* 1388.

HANSKY, J., SOVENY, C. and KORMAN, M. G. (1971): Effect of secretin on serum gastrin as measured by immunoassay. *Gastroenterology, 61,* 62.

KRAFT, A. R., TOMPKINS, R. K. and ZOLLINGER, R. M. (1970): Recognition and management of the diarrheal syndrome caused by non-beta islet cell tumors of the pancreas. *Amer. J. Surg., 119,* 163.

MARTIN, E., DUBOIS, J. C., LACOURBE, R., DUCHESNE, G. and BONFILS, S. (1974): Tumeur endocrine du pancréas avec choléra pancréatique (WDHA): données histologiques et ultrastructurales. *Arch. Franç. Mal. Appar. Dig.,* in press.

McGAVRAN, M. H., UNGER, R. H., RECANT, L., POLK, H. C., KILO, C. and LEVIN, M. E. (1966): A glucagon-secreting alpha-cell carcinoma of the pancreas. *New Engl. J. Med., 274,* 1408.

McGUIGAN, J. E. and TRUDEAU, W. L. (1972): Serum gastrin levels before and after vagotomy and pyloroplasty or vagotomy and antrectomy. *New Engl. J. Med., 286,* 184.

MATSUMOTO, K. K., PETER, J. B. and SCHULTZE, R. G. (1966): Watery diarrhea and hypokalemia associated with pancreatic islet cell adenoma. *Gastroenterology, 50,* 231.

NEUBURGER, P., LEWIN, M. and BONFILS, S. (1972): Parietal and chief cell populations in 4 cases of the Zollinger-Ellison syndrome. *Gastroenterology, 63,* 937.

PASSARO Jr., E., BASSO, N. and WALSH, J. H. (1972): Calcium challenge in the Zollinger-Ellison syndrome. *Surgery, 72,* 60.

SCHRUMPF, E., PETERSEN, H., BERSTAD, A., MYREN, J. and ROSENLUND, B. (1973): The effect of secretin on plasma gastrin in the Zollinger-Ellison syndrome. *Scand. J. Gastroenterol., 8,* 145.

STADIL, F., REHFELD, J. F. and THAYSEN, E. H. (1971): Variations in the concentrations of serum gastrin in the Zollinger-Ellison syndrome. In: *Gastrointestinal Hormones,* pp. 125–129. Editor: E. H. Thaysen. Munksgaard, Copenhagen.

TRUDEAU, W. L. and McGUIGAN, J. E. (1969): Effects of calcium on serum gastrin levels in the Zollinger-Ellison syndrome. *New Engl. J. Med., 281,* 862.

VERNER, J. V. (1968): Clinical syndromes associated with non-insulin producing tumors of the pancreatic islets. In: *Non Insulin Producing Tumors of the Pancreas,* pp. 165–183. Editors: L. Demling and R. Ottenjann. Thieme, Stuttgart.

WERMER, P. (1963): Endocrine adenomatosis and peptic ulcer in a large kindred. *Amer. J. Med., 35,* 205.

WILSON, S. D., SCHULTE, W. J. and MEADE, R. C. (1971): Longevity studies following total gastrectomy in children with the Zollinger-Ellison syndrome. *Arch. Surg., 103,* 108.

YOSHINAGA, T., OKUNO, G., YOSHITAKE, D., TSUJII, T. and NISHIKAWA, M. (1966): Pancreatic A-cell tumor associated with severe diabetes mellitus. *Diabetes, 15,* 709.

ZOLLINGER, R. M. and ELLISON, E. M. (1955): Primary peptic ulceration of the jejunum associated with islet cell tumors of the pancreas. *Ann. Surg., 142,* 709.

CHEMOTHERAPY OF MALIGNANT INSULINOMAS WITH STREPTOZOTOCIN

LAWRENCE E. BRODER and STEPHEN K. CARTER

NCI-VA Oncology Branch and Cancer Therapy Evaluation Branch,
Division of Cancer Treatment, National Cancer Institute,
Washington, D.C. and Bethesda, Md., U.S.A.

Pancreatic islet cell tumors, both benign and malignant, are quite rare tumors. Indeed, through 1960, less than 1000 cases had been reported in the world literature (Levin, 1968). In one large series encompassing 398 cases (Howard et al., 1950) 10% were found to be malignant, 12% were thought to be questionably malignant, while 78% were benign. That islet cell carcinoma is particularly rare is indicated by data from a large Cancer Registry in the United States (Moldow and Connelly, 1968) where the incidence was less than 1 per 100,000 population. Nevertheless, the highly malignant potential of pancreatic islet cell carcinoma is well recognized. Previous reports (Laurent et al., 1971) have indicated that about 70% are accompanied by metastases. When metastases are present at diagnosis, the disease has characteristically been rapidly fatal (Bell, 1957; Duff, 1942; McIntosh et al., 1960). Furthermore, a review of the literature of islet cell carcinoma with metastases through 1950 (Howard et al., 1950) indicated a median survival of less than 10 months from symptoms to death. From these data, the need for effective chemotherapy is quite clear.

Prior to the advent of streptozotocin (NSC-85998), the medical treatment of inoperable islet cell carcinoma has been less than adequate. Alloxan, an islet cell toxin, has been utilized, but the results have generally been poor (Brunschweig et al., 1944; Zimmer, 1964). The use of classical antitumor cytotoxic compounds such as tubercidin, mechlorethamine, or 5-fluorouracil has yielded only uncertain responses (Longmire, 1968). In a recent review of the use of streptozotocin in islet cell carcinoma (Broder and Carter, 1973), 5-fluorouracil was used as prior therapy in 12 cases, of which 3 patients responded. Other drugs have been used to effectively control the hypoglycemic symptoms resulting from the hypersecretion of insulin. These include glucocorticoids and adrenocorticotropin (Brown et al., 1952; Baumgartner and Reynolds, 1955) and glucagon (Landau et al., 1958; Roth et al., 1958). Both these agents have temporarily ameliorated the symptoms of hypoglycemia but have not shown any lasting effect in terms of tumor responses. Diazoxide, a benzothiadiazine compound, has been effectively utilized in the control of hypoglycemic symptoms (Ernest et al., 1965; Graber et al., 1966; Hunt, 1966) perhaps by decreasing the secretion of insulin by the tumors (Bleicher et al., 1964) but has not produced lasting tumor regression.

That streptozotocin not only effectively controlled hypoglycemic symptoms but also caused a measurable decrease in tumor size was first demonstrated by Murray-Lyon et al. (1968). Streptozotocin is a broad-spectrum antibiotic belonging to the nitrosourea group of compounds. It was originally isolated and purified from a *Streptomyces acromogenes* fermentation broth (Vavra et al., 1960) but since its initial discovery from biological material, the drug's structure has been elucidated and confirmed by chemical synthesis (Herr et al., 1967). Structurally it is composed of a nitrosourea moiety with a methyl group attached on one end and a glucosamine on the other as shown in comparison with 2 other clinically useful nitrosourea compounds – 1-3-bis(2-chloroethyl)-1-nitrosourea (BCNU) and 1-(2-chloroethyl)-3-cyclohexyl-1-nitrosourea (CCNU) (Fig. 1).

Following the demonstration of the drug's activity in preclinical animal tumor systems, the drug was further developed by the Division of Cancer Treatment, National Cancer Institute, National Institutes of Health in preparation for clinical trials. This development included the elucidation of drug action, animal toxicology data, and pharmacology. There have been several recent reports on the effects of streptozotocin on mammalian as well as bacterial cells. In bacterial cells, it has been observed (Reusser, 1971) that the drug induces rapid degradation of deoxyribonucleic acid (DNA) in actively dividing or resting *Bacillus subtilis* cells apparently through a specific interaction with cytosine containing mononucleotides. Similar experiments were carried out in *E. coli* (Rosenkranz and Carr, 1970) which demonstrated a 50% inhibition of DNA synthesis at a concentration of 10^{-3} M. In mammalian cells, utilizing the National Cancer Institute's primary tumor screen murine leukemia 1210, studies done in tissue culture confirmed the effects on DNA synthesis (Bhuyan, 1970). Furthermore, an exponential cell kill pattern was obtained in vitro, suggesting that streptozotocin, like other nitrosoureas, is not phase-specific and probably affects cells in all stages of the cell cycle. The cell cycle non-specificity of the agent can best be explained by the observation in these studies that the drug affects the synthesis of other subcellular constituents such as ribonucleic acid (RNA) and protein synthesis. As a result of these biochemical actions of the drug, in vivo activity of streptozotocin in the murine leukemia 1210 system produces a maximum increase in life span of affected animals of about 60% (Carter et al., 1971), at a dose of 80 mg/kg body weight. Other experimental tumor systems in which streptozotocin is effective include sarcoma 180, Ehrlich carcinoma, leukemia L5178y, and Walker carcinosarcoma 256 (Carter et al., 1971).

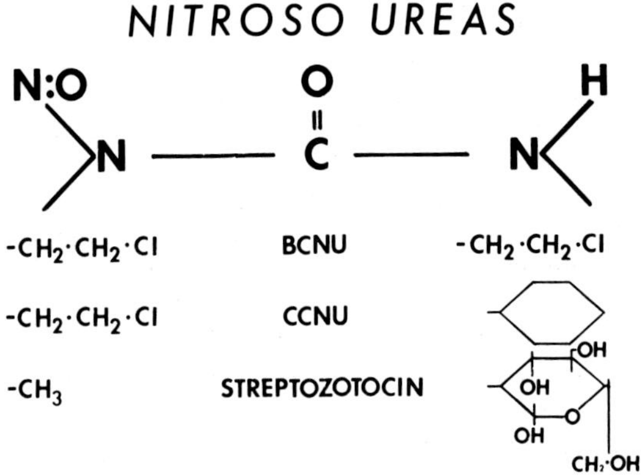

FIG. 1. The structure of streptozotocin compared with 2 other clinically useful nitrosourea compounds, BCNU and CCNU.

Prior to the initiation of clinical trials with any new anticancer drug, the toxicity of the compound must be studied in 2 large animal species. The Division of Cancer Treatment regularly utilizes the beagle hound and the rhesus monkey. In both species the drug was found to be diabetogenic (Carter et al., 1971). At a dose of 50 mg/kg body weight of streptozotocin, i.v. chemical and histologic evidence of hepatotoxicity was noted and a diabetic syndrome developed. At this dosage level in monkeys, permanent diabetes was produced and one animal died in irreversible diabetic ketoacidosis. Multiple repeated doses of drug consistently confirmed sparing of the bone marrow and gastrointestinal mucosa. A focal interstitial nephritis was found in several animals but was unaccompanied by elevation of blood urea nitrogen (BUN) or creatinine levels. Interestingly, in both the rat and mouse, pretreatment with nicotinamide prior to streptozotocin protects against the diabetogenicity of the compound (Schein and Loftus, 1968). Nicotinamide is also effective in preventing streptozotocin-induced diabetes in the dog and monkey but does not alleviate the hepatotoxic action of the drug in either species (Broder and Carter, 1971). As will be pointed out later in this paper, the diabetogenic action of streptozotocin has not been a major problem in clinical usage and no patient receiving the drug has developed irreversible diabetes.

Pharmacological data was developed in both small and large animal studies. In mice, the serum half-life of streptozotocin after an i.v. injection of 200 mg/kg was approximately 5 minutes, with no drug measurable by 2 hours. From i.v. infusion studies in dogs, the degradation rate has been estimated to be 5 mg/min. (White, 1963). The drug is not absorbed at all from the gastrointestinal tract of the dog regardless of dosage. Subcutaneous absorption has only been studied in mice and was found to be very efficient. Tissue distribution has been studied in the mouse, rat, cat, monkey, and dog and in all species the drug was found to be markedly concentrated in the liver and kidney (Broder and Carter, 1971).

The unique diabetogenic properties observed in the preclinical toxicology studies pointed the way toward trials in metastatic insulinoma. Such an approach, utilizing specific organ toxicity in large animal studies to predict possible activity in unusual human tumors, had also been successful in the case of Lysodren (mitotane, ortho-para′-DDD). In that case, adrenal atrophy first seen in dogs led to positive clinical trials in adrenal cortical carcinoma (Hutter and Kayhoe, 1966). In 1968, Murray-Lyon et al. first utilized streptozotocin in the successful treatment of a patient with metastatic insulinoma and demonstrated the drug's effectiveness both in relieving hypoglycemic symptoms and in producing measurable tumor regression. Since then there have been 13 additional case reports describing the efficacy of streptozotocin in the treatment of this disease (Sadoff, 1969; Arnould et al., 1969; Blackard et al., 1970; Liaw et al., 1970; Stanley et al., 1970; Taylor et al., 1970; Vogel et al., 1970; Cunningham et al., 1971; Schreibman et al., 1971; Smith et al., 1971; Vogel, 1971; Bruns et al., 1971; Dahl and Mengshoel, 1973). The Cancer Therapy Evaluation Branch of the Division of Cancer Treatment, National Cancer Institute, has collected an additional 38 cases for a total of 52 evaluable patients which forms the basis of this report. Much of this data has been recently reported (Broder and Carter, 1973) and an attempt will be made here to summarize the important features of the data.

Because streptozotocin remains an investigational drug unavailable from a commercial source, the Cancer Therapy Evaluation Branch is solely responsible for its distribution and clinical evaluation. All patients in the series were treated by experienced investigators in the field, most of them being associated with large treatment centers. Since streptozotocin is only available for the treatment of malignant disease, all patients in the series had inoperable or metastatic islet cell carcinoma, biopsy-proven. Three patients were inevaluable due to lack of data confirming tissue diagnosis and were excluded. The data was evaluated separately for functional tumors (those which were biochemically active) and for non-functional tumors (those without biochemical documentation of function). Evidence of biochemical function included hypoglycemia or symptoms thereof, hyperinsulin levels (usually determined by radioimmunoassay techniques), or elevations of other hormones.

The general clinical characteristics of the patients are given in Table 1. The median age for all patients was 52 years with similar medians for either functional or non-functional tumors. In an earlier review (Howard et al., 1950) the median age for the functional tumor patients was about 10 years younger. The disease primarily was found in white people (90% of cases), however, selection factors may have played a role. There were about equal numbers of males and females with equal distribution around the median. Earlier series (Howard et al., 1950) had indicated a predominance of males, but no reasonable explanation has been found to explain this minor difference. The predominant location of the primary tumor in the tail of the pancreas concurs with previous reports in which the body and tail are most frequently involved (Laurent et al., 1971). The disease behaves typically like a carcinoma spreading locally or via lymphatics, but due to the pancreatic venous blood flow via the portal vein, liver metastases were noted in more than 90% of cases.

The hormonal characteristics of the functional cases as well as the symptoms of the entire group of patients are given in Table 2. About three-quarters of the patients evaluable demonstrated elevated insulin levels and in 4 of the patients the insulin was characterized as proinsulin. Understandably, the majority of symptoms were related to hyperinsulinism and manifested as hypoglycemia. The presence of proinsulin-secreting tumors has been attributed to a deficiency of the enzyme or enzymes necessary for converting proinsulin to insulin in tumor tissue (Taylor et al., 1970). One patient presented with diabetes and probably corresponds to the ordinary 'diabetic risk' (Laurent et al., 1971). Elevation of other hormones in association with elevated insulin levels were seen in 4 additional patients. In one case a multiple hormone-producing tumor was reported. Two patients had elevated adrenocorticotropin or cortisol but Cushing's syndrome was not reported. Hormonal syndromes such as Cushing's, carcinoid, and polyglandular syndrome have been previously reported (Levin, 1968; Ballard et al., 1964). The elevated glucagon levels could not be correlated with a specific syndrome and data to support the diagnosis of a malignant glucagonoma such as alpha cell tumor histology was lacking. Islet cell tumors have been known to produce more than one hormone simultaneously and multiple endocrine syndromes have been reported. One wonders if these tumors are pluripotential and should be termed peptide-secreting carcinoma as has been suggested (Murray-Lyon et al., 1968). Only one patient in the series could be classified as a Zollinger-Ellison syndrome as defined as the association of peptic ulceration and islet cell tumors (Zollinger and Ellison, 1956). The observed association of islet cell tumors of the pancreas with diarrhea and hypokalemia (Priest and Alexander, 1957; Verner and Morrison, 1958) could not be documented, perhaps due to inadequate data on serum potassium levels, although diarrhea was a prominent symptom.

The streptozotocin used in this review is available from the Cancer Therapy Evaluation Branch, Division of Cancer Treatment, National Cancer Institute, Bethesda, Maryland. It is supplied in lyophilized form and is reconstituted with sodium chloride injection USP.

TABLE 1
Patient population of metastatic islet cell carcinoma treated with streptozotocin[a]

Data	No. of patients[b]	Percent
Total entered	55	100
Total evaluable	52/55	94
Functional tumors	41/52	79
Non-functional tumors	11/52	21
Sex		
Male	27/52	52
Female	25/52	48
Race		
White	41/45	90
Negro	1/45	2
Oriental	3/45	8
Age (years)		
Median	54 yr	
Site of tumor		
Head	6/45	13
Body	8/45	18
Tail	19/45	42
More than 2 areas or undetermined	12/45	27
Metastases		
Abdomen	8/52	15
Liver	48/52	92
Lymph nodes	10/52	19
Gastrointestinal	4/52	8
Other	2/52	4

a. Summarized from Broder and Carter (1973).
b. The denominator contains only evaluable patients for the characteristic described.

The drug is stable in solution for at least 48 hours and has generally been given as a rapid i.v. injection or in an infusion. Table 3 describes the dose and route of administration. The majority of the patients received the drug i.v., while 8 patients received the drug primarily intra-arterially (i.a.). Of the patients 90% received the drug on a weekly dosage schedule, and slightly better than half of the cases received maintenance therapy (therapy maintained for more than 6 weeks or additional course of therapy within one year).

TABLE 2
Hormonal characteristics and presenting symptoms in islet cell carcinoma patients treated with streptozotocin[a]

Data	No. of patients[b]	Percent
Hormone		
Insulin elevated	26/35	74
Insulin normal	1/35	3
Gastrin only	1/35	3
ACTH[c] or cortisol	2/35	6
Insulin + gastrin	2/35	6
Insulin + glucagon	2/35	6
Insulin + glucagon + gastrin	1/35	3
Presenting symptoms		
Hypoglycemia	37/41	90
GI[d] ulceration	7/48	15
Diarrhea	5/48	10
Diabetes	1/48	2
Abdominal pain	4/48	8
Abdominal mass	1/48	2
Melena	1/48	2
Fever	1/48	2

a. Summarized from Broder and Carter (1973).
b. The denominator contains only evaluable patients for the characteristic described.
c. Adrenocorticotropin.
d. Gastrointestinal.

Prior therapy consisting of surgery, radiotherapy or chemotherapy was given to about half of the cases; 37% had a palliative or resective procedure. Prior chemotherapy was given to about 40% of the cases with the majority receiving antimetabolites. Radiotherapy was given to only one patient. Concomitant diazoxide therapy was used in about 40% of cases but any change in dosage of the drug during the evaluation period made the case unevaluable for response.

The patients with functional tumors were evaluated for both biochemical as well as objective tumor response while non-functional tumors were evaluable only for tumor regression. In either case (biochemical or objective measurable response) a complete response (CR) was a complete return to normal of biochemical abnormality or complete regression of tumor. A biochemical response was usually associated with a measurable response and vice versa. A partial response was defined as a more than 25% return of the abnormality (either biochemical or measurable tumor) toward normal. Table 4 describes the response rates in the various categories. A subjective response (amelioration of

TABLE 3
Dose and route of administration of streptozotocin in islet cell carcinoma patients[a]

Dose	Median range of dose (g/m^2)	No. of patients[b]	Percent
		Intravenous (44 patients)	
Initial	0.6–1.0	22/37	59
Maximum	1.1–2.0	16/37	43
Total	8.1–10.0	20/37	54
		Intra-arterial (8 patients)	
Initial	0.6–1.0	3/4	
Maximum	6.1–8.0	3/4	
Total	10.1–40.0	4/4	

a. Summarized from Broder and Carter (1973).
b. The denominator contains only evaluable patients for the characteristic described.

symptoms without biochemical documentation) was not considered in the overall response rate. Responses lasting less than one month were considered no response. As can be seen, in the functional tumor patients a biochemical response was observed in 64% while a measurable response was seen in 50%. Of the non-functional tumor patients 5 of 8 (63%) had a measurable response; 3 of 4 patients with proinsulin-secreting tumors responded biochemically. The patient with Zollinger-Ellison syndrome did not respond. Isolated responses were seen in the multihormonal producing tumor patients. All patients with biochemical responses had amelioration of hypoglycemic symptoms. The duration of response could only be adequately evaluated in the functional tumor patients. The biochemical responders remained in remission for about 10 months while the measurable disease responders remained in remission for about 13 months. In 18 patients treated on a weekly intravenous schedule, serial fasting insulin levels were available. The median time to onset of insulin response was about 17 days while that to maximum response was about 35 days. The onset of response occurred at about a total dose of 2 g/m^2 while the maximum response occurred at about a total dose of 4 g/m^2.

Survival data indicated that, at least with streptozotocin therapy, the disease was not as rapidly fatal as had previously been reported (Bell, 1957; Duff, 1942; McIntosh et al., 1960). The survival rate was determined by the Life Table Method (Cutler and Ederer, 1968) and median survival data was determined at the 50% survival rate. The median duration of survival of about 30 months (Table 5) from symptoms to last follow-up compares favorably with that reported by Howard et al. (1950), where a median survival from symptoms to death of 10 months was observed in a similar group of patients. Undoubtedly, more recent advances in diagnosis, surgery, and supportive care may ac-

TABLE 4
Response of metastatic islet cell carcinoma patients treated with streptozotocin functional tumors[a]

Category of response	No. of patients[b]	Percent	Median response duration (months)
Biochemical response			
Complete	10/39	26	
Partial (> 50%)	11/39	28	
Partial (25–50%)	4/39	10	
Subjective	1/39	2	
No response	13/39	33	
Total responses	25/39	64	10+[c]
Measurable disease			
Response			
Complete	5/30	17	
Partial (> 50%)	6/30	20	
Partial (25–50%)	4/30	13	
No response	15/30	50	
Total responses	15/30	50	13+[d]

a. Summarized from Broder and Carter (1973).
b. The denominator contains only evaluable patients for the characteristic described.
c. Median derived from 21 evaluable patients.
d. Median derived from 10 evaluable patients.

count for some of the difference observed. There were no significant differences in survival between male and female patients or between functional and non-functional tumor patients. That streptozotocin has a profound impact on survival can be obtained by analyzing the differences in survival rate and duration between the responders and the non-responders. From diagnosis to last follow-up, a significant increase in survival rate at one year (95% confidence level) was observed for the responders as compared to the non-responders. These differences were reflected in the median survival of responders of about 42 months versus that for non-responders of about 17 months. These data held for both biochemical or measurable disease responders. Complete as well as partial responders did about equally well in survival rate. However, the median duration of survival was appreciably better for the complete responders. Patients with long-lasting duration of symptoms had appreciably better survival time from diagnosis to last follow-up as did patients on continuous therapy. By definition, however, these patients were selected, since their characteristics would contribute to longer survivals. In neither of the latter categories was there an appreciable difference in survival rate.

TABLE 5
Survival rate and median survival duration in islet cell carcinoma patients treated with streptozotocin[a]

Category	No. of patients	Survival rate at one year (%)	Median survival time (months)
Responders	33	94[b]	42
vs.			
non-responders	16	57	17
Biochemical resp.	26	92[b]	42
vs.			
biochemical non-resp.	13	48	5
Meas. dis. resp.	19	100[b]	42
vs.			
meas. dis. non-resp.	18	70	22
Complete responders	14	100	88+
vs.			
partial responders	19	89	40
vs.			
non-responders	16	57	17

a. Summarized from Broder and Carter (1973).
b. Significantly different at the 95% confidence level.

The acute and chronic toxicity of streptozotocin is outlined in Table 6. Acutely, nausea and vomiting were the predominant symptoms, occurring in 94% of evaluable patients. Other gastrointestinal toxicity included diarrhea in 10% of evaluable patients.

Chronic toxicity involved the renal, hepatic and hematologic systems. Proteinuria was predominant, occurring in the second to third week of drug therapy on a weekly drug administration schedule. This was usually reversible upon discontinuance of the agent. Changes in glomerular filtration rate reflected in decrease in creatinine clearance or elevation of BUN occurred in about 25% of cases. The animal toxicology studies had predicted a reversible nephritis which may have accounted for the tubular defects, both renal tubular acidosis and the Fanconi syndrome, that were seen clinically in about 15% of cases. At somewhat higher dosages, others (Sadoff, 1970) observed a higher incidence of renal abnormalities such as azotemia. Anuria in both Sadoff's as well as this series was observed in about 10% of cases and is generally irreversible. Five patients had fatal renal failure which seemed to be related to both high single dosages of drug as well as i.a. administration.

Hepatic toxicity was reflected usually in transient and mild abnormalities of liver function studies, the most consistent of which were elevations in transaminases. Elevations in alkaline phosphatase were observed in 12%. Liver function abnormalities were reversible upon discontinuance of drug therapy. Sadoff observed a 50% abnormality of liver function, an incidence which is somewhat less than in this series. It is conceivable

TABLE 6
Toxicity of streptozotocin in islet cell carcinoma patients[a]

Toxicity	No. of patients[b]	Percent
No toxicity	1/52	2
Gastrointestinal	45/48	94
Nausea and vomiting	45/48	94
Diarrhea	5/48	10
Renal	30/46	65
Proteinuria	18/35	51
Decreased creatinine clearance	6/23	26
Fatal renal toxicity	5/46	11
Hepatic	33/49	67
Elevated SGOT	13/49	27
Elevated alkaline phosphatase	6/49	12
Hematologic	10/50	20
Anemia	7/49	14
Leukopenia	3/49	6
Thrombocytopenia	1/50	4
Fatal hematological toxicity	1/50	2
Other		
Insulin shock	11/52	22
Reversible glucose intolerance	3/52	6

a. Summarized from Broder and Carter (1973).
b. Denominator contains only evaluable patients for the characteristic described.

that the high incidence of liver metastases in the present series of cases may have contributed to a higher degree of hepatotoxicity.

Hematologic toxicity was seen in about 20% of cases and was primarily manifested as a falling hematocrit. Anemia, however, is not an uncommon complication of malignancy in general and probably played a role in the analysis of the results. Only one patient had fatal hematological toxicity consisting of pancytopenia after an unusually large single dose of drug.

In a more recent study (Sadoff, 1972) the effect of streptozotocin on glucose tolerance has been evaluated. That study revealed a reversible mild to moderate abnormality in 9 of 15 patients studied. Insulin was required in no patients. Only 3 patients in our series demonstrated glucose intolerance for an incidence of 6%. No case of irreversible diabetes mellitus has been reported to date.

SUMMARY

Pancreatic islet cell carcinoma, although a rare tumor, metastasizes readily and causes significant morbidity due to the hypoglycemia caused by hyperinsulinism. Previously, medical therapy has relied on classical anticancer agents which are less than effective and hyperglycemic agents such as adrenal steroids, glucagon, and diazoxide, which produce no lasting tumor regressions. Streptozotocin, which was shown to be cytotoxic to the beta cell in large animal studies, was successfully used in the treatment of a patient with islet cell carcinoma in 1968, and is now considered the treatment of choice for inoperable or metastatic disease. The drug is a nitrosourea antibiotic which appears to act by inhibition of DNA synthesis.

We have confirmed the previous literature reports on the effectiveness of streptozotocin in islet cell carcinoma by demonstrating an overall response rate of about 60% with a concomitant significant increase in survival rate in the responders. In patients with functional tumors, elevated insulin levels respond to therapy in about 2–3 weeks when the drug is given on a weekly schedule with the maximum response in about 5 weeks. The onset and maximum responses occur at total doses of 2 g/m^2 and 4 g/m^2 respectively. The median duration of response is about one year. Partial as well as complete responses contribute measurably to survival rate and duration.

Toxicity may be acute as manifested by gastrointestinal symptoms or chronic, affecting the renal, hepatic, and hematological systems. The most disturbing toxic effect is renal, which may be unpredictable but appears to be primarily related to high single doses of drug as well as intra-arterial administration. Currently, the Cancer Therapy Evaluation Branch is recommending a dose of 1 g/m^2/week i.v. The drug should be discontinued if progressive renal function abnormalities develop. Hepatic toxicity was mild and reversible. No appreciable hematological toxicity developed at recommended dosages.

In view of the responses seen in the non-functional tumors, the activity of the drug in animal tumors systems, the similarity of the agent to the nitrosourea compounds, and the relative lack of hematological toxicity, current investigations are underway in other malignancies. Preliminary activity has been noted in pancreatic adenocarcinoma as well as malignant carcinoid tumors but little or no activity has been seen in bronchogenic carcinoma or other gastrointestinal malignancies (Broder and Carter, 1971).

Currently, the drug is limited to investigational usage only in patients with malignant disease. Studies are planned for combinations of streptozotocin with other anticancer drugs in view of the relative lack of hematological toxicity.

ACKNOWLEDGEMENT

We are indebted to the following physicians for the patient reports and follow-up without which this analysis would not have been possible: P. W. Adams, Y. Arnould, M. Austoni, E. O. Balasse, A. D. Bird, W. G. Blackard, C. L. Brown, V. W. Bruns, J. H. Burrows, J. A. Bruner, G. P. Canellos, N. T. Caputo, G. R. Cunningham, A. Dahl, E. T. Davidson, G. Duchesne, J. W. Ensinck, O. Enstreom, S. S. Fajans, W. S. Fletcher, G. Fonken, N. R. Freeman, P. Gorden, Y. Goto, J. G. Hazen, F. Hermann, B. Hoogstraten, S. Hsu, G. D. Kerr, D. Klaassen, I. Krakoff, H. Lebowitz, H. E. Lessner, K. Lundbaek, A. S. Mason, D. S. J. Maw, C. G. Moertel, D. A. D. Montgomery, I. M. Murray-Lyon, J. O'Donnell, A. Ohnedam, A. Piard, L. Sadoff, P. Schreibman, O. Sejer-Hansen, N. N. Stanley, S. G. Taylor, I. Toien, T. S. Tolloczko, M. Tzagournis, T. T. Vogel, F. Welland, R. H. Williams, F. E. Zimmer and R. M. Zollinger.

REFERENCES

ARNOULD, Y., OOMS, H. and BASTENIE, P. A. (1969): Treatment of insulinoma with streptozotocin. Letter to the editor. *Lancet, 1,* 1210.

BALLARD, H. S., FRAME, B. and HARTSTOCK, R. J. (1964): Familial multiple endocrine adenoma-peptic ulcer complex. *Medicine, 43,* 481.

BAUMGARTNER, C. J. and REYNOLDS, J. L. (1955): Functioning metastases from islet cell tumor of pancreas; control with corticotropin (ACTH). *Arch. Surg., 70,* 793.

BRODER, L. E. and CARTER, S. K. (1971): Streptozotocin, Clinical Brochure. National Cancer Institute, Bethesda.

BRODER, L. E. and CARTER, S. K. (1973): Pancreatic islet cell carcinoma: results of therapy with streptozotocin in 52 patients. *Ann. intern. Med., 79,* 101.

BRODER, L. E. and CARTER, S. K. (1973): Pancreatic islet cell carcinoma. I. Clinical features of 52 patients. *Ann. intern. Med., 79,* 108.

BELL, E. T. (1957): Carcinoma of the pancreas. *Amer. J. Path., 33,* 499.

BHUYAN, B. K. (1970): The action of streptozotocin on mammalian cells. *Cancer Res., 30,* 2017.

BLACKARD, W. G., GARCIA, A. R. and BROWN Jr., C. L. (1970): Effect of streptozotocin in qualitative aspects of plasma insulin in a patient with a malignant islet cell tumor. *J. clin. Endocr., 31,* 215.

BLEICHER, S. I., CHOWDHURY, F. and GOLDNER, M. G. (1964): Thiazide therapy in hypoglycemia of metastatic insulinoma (abstract). *Clin. Res., 12,* 456.

BROWN, H., HARGREAVES, H. P. and TYLER, F. H. (1952): Islet-cell adenoma of pancreas; metabolic studies on patients treated with corticotropin and cortisone. *Arch. intern. Med., 89,* 951.

BRUNS, V. W., MEHNERT, E., BIBERGEIL, H. and HEGEWALD, G. (1971): Metastatic islet cell carcinoma. Experience of treatment with streptozotocin. *Endokrinologie, 58,* 193.

BRUNSCHWEIG, A., ALLEN, J. G., OWENS Jr., F. M. and THORTON, T. F. (1944): Alloxan in treatment of insulin producing islet cell carcinoma of pancreas. *J. Amer. med. Ass., 124,* 212.

CARTER, S. K., BRODER, L. E. and FRIEDMAN, M. (1971): Streptozotocin and metastatic insulinoma. *Ann. intern. Med., 74,* 445.

CUNNINGHAM, G. R., QUICKEL Jr., K. E. and LEBOVITZ, H. E. (1971): The use of insulin dynamics in the evaluation of streptozotocin therapy of malignant insulinomas. *J. clin. Endocr., 33,* 530.

CUTLER, S. J. and EDERER, F. (1968): Maximum utilization of the life table method in analyzing survival. *J. chron. Dis., 8,* 699.

DAHL, A. A. and MENGSHOEL, S. (1973): Hyperinsulinism due to metastasizing insulinoma treated with diazoxide and streptozotocin. *T. norske Laegeforen.,* in press.

DUFF, G. L. (1942): The pathology of islet cell tumors of the pancreas. *Amer. J. Med. Sci., 203,* 437.

ERNEST, M., MITCHELL, M. L., RABEN, M. S. and GILBOA, Y. (1965): Control of hypoglycemia with diazoxide and human growth hormone. *Lancet, 1,* 628.

GRABER, A. L., PORTE, D. and WILLIAMS, R. H. (1966): Clinical use of diazoxide and mechanism for its hyperglycemic effects. *Diabetes, 15,* 143.

HERR, R. R., JAHNKE, H. K. and ARGOUDELIS, A. (1967): The structure of streptozotocin. *J. Amer. chem. Soc., 89,* 4808.

HOWARD, J. M., MOSS, N. H. and RHOADS, J. E. (1950): Collective review: Hyperinsulinism and islet cell tumors of the pancreas with 398 recorded tumors. *Int. Abstr. Surg., 90,* 417.

HUNT, P. S. (1966): Adult hypoglycemia associated with neoplasia. A report of three cases with a note on the use of diazoxide. *Aust. New Zeal. J. Surg., 35,* 295.

HUTTER Jr., A. M. and KAYHOE, D. E. (1966a): Adrenal cortical carcinoma, clinical features of 138 patients. *Amer. J. Med., 41,* 572.
HUTTER Jr., A. M. and KAYHOE, D. E. (1966b): Adrenal cortical carcinoma; results of treatment with op'DDD in 138 patients. *Amer. J. Med., 41,* 581.
LANDAU, B. R., LEVINE, H. J. and HERTZ, R. (1958): Prolonged glucagon administration in a case of hyperinsulinism due to disseminated islet-cell carcinoma. *New Engl. J. Med., 259,* 286.
LONGMIRE, W. P. (1968): Islet cell tumors of the pancreas. *Ann. intern. Med., 68,* 203.
LAURENT, J., DEBRY, G. and FLOQUET, J. (1971): *Hypoglycaemic Tumours.* Excerpta Medica, Amsterdam.
LEVIN, M. E. (1968): Endocrine syndromes associated with pancreatic islet cell tumors. *Med. Clin. N. Amer., 52,* 295.
LIAW, K. Y., WEI, T. C. and HSU, S. C. (1970): Treatment of malignant insulinoma with streptozotocin. *J. Surg. Soc. (China), 3,* 62.
McINTOSH, H. W., ROBERTSON, H. R., WALTERS, W. and RANDALL, R. V. (1960): Functioning islet cell carcinoma of the pancreas with metastases and prolonged survival. *Arch. Surg., 80,* 1021.
MOERTEL, C. G., REITEMEIER, R. J., SCHUTT, A. J. and HAHN, R. G. (1971): Phase II study of streptozotocin (NSC-85998) in the treatment of advanced gastrointestinal cancer. *Cancer Chemo Rep., 55,* 303.
MOLDOW, R. E. and CONNELLY, R. R. (1968): Epidemiology of pancreatic cancer in Connecticut. *Gastroenterology, 55,* 677.
MURRAY-LYON, I. M., EDDLESTON, A. L. W. F., WILLIAMS, R., BROWN, M., HOGBIN, B. M., BENNETT, A., EDWARDS, J. C. and TAYLOR, K. W. (1968): Treatment of multiple-hormone-producing malignant islet-cell tumor with streptozotocin. *Lancet, 2,* 895.
REUSSER, F. (1971): Mode of action of streptozotocin. *J. Bact., 105,* 580.
ROSENKRANZ, H. S. and CARR, H. S. (1970): Differences in the action of notrosomethylurea and streptozotocin. *Cancer Res., 30,* 112.
ROTH, H., THIER, S. and SEGAL, S. (1958): Zinc glucagon in the management of refractory hypoglycemia due to insulin-producing tumors. *New Engl. J. Med., 274,* 493.
SADOFF, L. (1969): Effects of streptozotocin in a patient with islet cell carcinoma. *Diabetes, 18,* 675.
SADOFF, L. (1970): Nephrotoxicity of streptozotocin (NSC-85998). *Cancer Chemother. Rep., 54,* 457.
SADOFF, L. (1972): Patterns of intravenous glucose tolerance and insulin response before and after treatment with streptozotocin (NSC-85998). *Cancer Chemother. Rep., 56,* 61.
SCHEIN, P. S. and LOFTUS, S. (1968): Streptozotocin: Depression of mouse liver pyridine nucleotides. *Cancer Res., 28,* 1501.
SCHREIBMAN, P. H., DE KOLIREN, L. G. and ARKY, R. A. (1971): Metastatic insulinoma treated with streptozotocin. *Ann. intern. Med., 74,* 399.
SMITH, C. K., STOLL, R. W., VANCE, J., RICKETTS, H. and WILLIAMS, R. H. (1971): Treatment of malignant insulinoma with streptozotocin. *Diabetologia, 7,* 118.
STANLEY, N. N., MARKS, V., KREEL, L. and McINTYRE, N. (1970): Streptozotocin treatment of malignant islet cell tumor. *Brit. med. J., 3,* 562.
TAYLOR, S. G., SCHWARTZ, T. B., ZANNINI, J. Z. and RYAN, W. G. (1970): Streptozotocin therapy for metastatic insulinoma. *Arch. intern. Med., 126,* 654.
VAVRA, J. J., DeBOER, C., DIETZ, A., HANKA, L. J. and SOKOLSKI, W. T. (1960): Streptozotocin, a new antibacterial antibiotic. *Antibiot. Ann., 7,* 230.
VERNER, J. V. and MORRISON, A. R. (1958): Islet cell tumor and a syndrome of refractory watery diarrhea and hypokalemia. *Amer. J. Med., 25,* 374.

VOGEL, T. T., MOTT, V., MINTON, J. P. and ZOLLINGER, R. M. (1970): The effect of streptozotocin on glucose and insulin levels in advanced insulinoma. *Int. Cancer Congr. Abstr., 10,* 533.

VOGEL, T. T. (1971): Notes on streptozotocin in metastatic insulinoma. *J. Surg. Oncol., 3,* 481.

WHITE, F. R. (1963): Streptozotocin. *Cancer Chemother. Rep., 30,* 49.

ZIMMER, F. E. (1964): Islet cell carcinoma treated with alloxan. *Ann. intern. Med., 61,* 543.

ZOLLINGER, R. M. and ELLISON, E. H. (1955): Primary peptic ulcerations of the jejunum associated with islet cell tumors of the pancreas. *Ann. Surg., 142,* 709.

ORIGIN AND MORPHOLOGY OF ISLET CELL TUMORS WITH SINGLE OR MULTIPLE HORMONE PRODUCTION

CHR. HEDINGER

Department of Pathology, University of Zurich, Switzerland

Islet cell tumors of the pancreas can be very varied with regard to their structure, their growth tendency, especially their inclination to metastasize, and their function. The diagnosis of such tumors is made more difficult because it often involves tumors with multiple endocrine activities. The tumors can be formed from one cell type producing different hormones, or, which is probably most often the case, from various cell types with different endocrine activities. Finally, multiple, different hormone-producing tumors appear in the pancreas.

I first want to speak about pure tumors, then about tumors with combined endocrine activities, and finally about multiple tumors of the pancreas.

What do we actually know about *pure tumor forms*? Table 1 shows you the most important types. Probably at this time the *B cell tumors* are the best characterized. They are derived from the B cells of the islets of the pancreas. Their increased insulin activity leads to a relatively clear, definitive clinical picture. In approximately 85% of the cases you find adenomas compared to 10% carcinomas. Microadenomatoses, that is, tumor-like growths in all or almost all islets, make up approximately 5% (Laroche et al., 1968).

TABLE 1

Pancreatic lesions with single endocrine activity

Cell type	Hormone	Hyperplasia	Adenomatosis	Adenoma	Carcinoma
B	Insulin	?	5%	85%	10%
A (A_2)	Glucagon	(+)		++	+
G, D (A_1)	Gastrin	10%		30%	60%
? 'Verner-Morrison' 'WDHA'	Secretin? GIP? VIP?	~10%		30%	60%
Argentaffin cell	5-HT	(+)			~100%

These microadenomatoses have to be distinguished from the so-called hyperplasias with a relative increase of B cells in the islets of the pancreas with a normal or augmented number of islets. Despite good characterization of B cell tumors, there are still many unsolved problems. Is a definite hyperinsulinism always due to a tumor or can it be due to a hyperplasia of the B cell system? Such cases have been published. However, a hidden adenoma which may be outside the pancreas must often be considered (see Filipi and Higgins, 1973). Is there a transition from normal B cells into B cell hyperplasias, microadenomatoses, adenomas, and carcinomas, and where should the line be drawn? We find this problem not only in islet cell tumors but also in most tumors of the endocrine organs.

In all other tumors of the islet system with predominantly single hormonal activity, the difficulties of morphological classification are even greater. Therefore, the term *non-B cell tumor* is frequently used. Besides the morphological assessment of their endocrine activity, the diagnosis of malignancy may also be difficult.

Glucagon-producing tumors are relatively rare. They are derived from the A cells, or more precisely, from the A-2 cells because the expression A-1 cell is also used for the G or D cell. Such tumors cause clinical signs of diabetes mellitus. In the relatively few diagnosed cases, glucagon-producing tumors appear to be more often malignant than insulinomas, but they are less often malignant than the gastrin-producing tumors (Bretholz and Steiner, 1973). Morphologically, they can hardly be distinguished from the B cell tumors aside from their special granulation. Exceptionally, microadenomatoses with excessive glucagon activity can also occur (Lomsky et al., 1969).

More important are the *gastrin-producing tumors,* the so-called G cell tumors. They are also called A-1 cell tumors by certain authors. They do not seem to occur as often as B cell tumors but appear essentially more often than the so-called glucagonomas. The granules of these tumor cells are less characteristic than the B and A-2 granules. They are mainly round and of different size and density. The tumor cells are related to the so-called D cells and A-1 cells of the pancreas, but their identities are still disputed (Vassallo et al., 1972). In approximately 60% of Zollinger-Ellison cases with lesions of the pancreas, malignant tumors are found, adenomas in 30%, and microadenomatoses or hyperplasias in 10%. However, even malignant tumors may be accompanied by microadenomatoses (Ellison and Wilson, 1964). Not every case of Zollinger-Ellison syndrome is based on a tumor or hyperplasia of the G cells in the pancreas. G cell hyperplasias or tumors of the stomach may also be found (Polak et al., 1972). Stephens (1973) has therefore just proposed the classification, shown in Table 2, of the different forms of Zollinger-Ellison syndrome.

TABLE 2

Classification of the different forms of Zollinger-Ellison syndrome (Stephens, 1973)

Pancreatic:	Zollinger-Ellison syndrome
	Type I: D cell hyperplasia
	Type II: Tumor
Gastric:	Pseudo-Zollinger-Ellison syndrome
	Type I: G cell hyperplasia
	Type II: G cell tumor

The basic lesions in the *Verner-Morrison syndrome, the so-called WDHA syndrome* (*w*atery *d*iarrhea, *h*yperkalemia, *a*chlorhydria) (Marks et al., 1967) is still obscure. Up to now relatively few cases have been published and in several cases no adequate pancreas lesions could be found. Definite statements concerning the type of tumors, therefore, cannot be made at present. According to Marks et al. (1967) and Schoenemann (1972), 50% of the corresponding tumors are malignant. Kraft et al. (1970) found the same distribution as in the Zollinger-Ellison syndrome. The origin of these cells is not yet clearly determined. This syndrome is also pathogenetically obscure. At one time an overproduction of secretin or even glucagon was thought to be responsible (see Zollinger et al., 1968), but today the assumption of abnormal GIP production (*g*astric *i*nhibitory *p*olypeptide) or VIP production (*v*asoactive *i*ntestinal *p*eptide) seems to be more probable (Elias et al., 1972; Bloom et al., 1973).

Finally, in this group of endocrine-active pancreatic tumors, we should discuss the *carcinoids.* The occurrence of carcinoids in the pancreas has been known for a long time (Feyrter, 1943; Dollinger et al., 1967; Gordon et al., 1971). Recently, particular attention has been paid to a special form of such tumors, the so-called carcinoid-islet cell tumors, because of their combined endocrine activity. They are always considered potentially malignant tumors except for the carcinoids of the appendix and similar tumors of the bronchial system. Actually, in the pancreas transitions are known from the highly differentiated carcinoids to the small cell anaplastic carcinomas of the oat cell type (see Patchefsky et al., 1972).

More important than pancreatic tumors which only produce one hormone are *tumors with multiple endocrine activities.* Figure 1 gives the most important combinations known at this time. Tumors with combined insulin and gastrin secretion, glucagon- and gastrin-producing tumors, and finally tumors which show B cell, G cell, and A cell

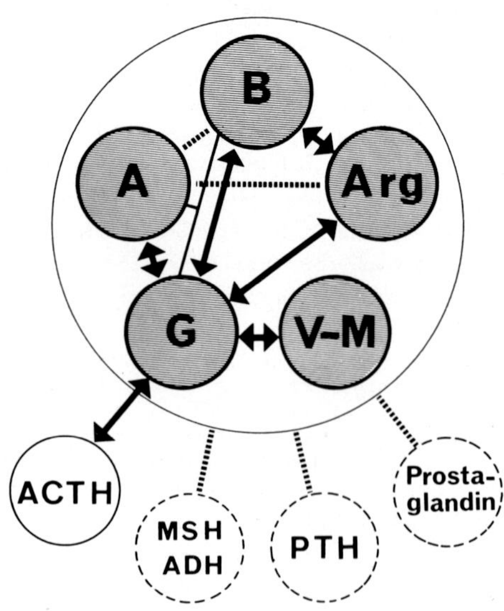

FIG. 1. Pancreatic tumors with multiple endocrine activity. Most important combinations. (B: B cell, A: A cell, G: G cell, V-M: Verner-Morrison, Arg: argentaffin cells, PTH: parathyroid hormone.)

activities have definitely been demonstrated. Combinations of Zollinger-Ellison syndrome with the Verner-Morrison syndrome seem to exist. However, different combinations are not yet fully proven. Within the past few years special attention has been paid to the occurrence of argentaffin cells in islet cell tumors, that is, the so-called carcinoid-islet cell tumors. The emphasis on these types of tumors seems especially reasonable to mention in Brussels, as Gepts et al. (1960) have already published a paper about a similar tumor. Of the new combinations of pancreatic tumors which have been seen within the past few years, one of the most typical seems to be the gastrin-producing tumor with ACTH activity and Cushing's syndrome (see Modlinger et al., 1972; Rawlinson, 1973).

Finally, there are *multiple adenomas with different endocrine activities* in the pancreas. With such combinations one must always think about the possibility of a general adenomatosis of the endocrine system, for example, the Wermer syndrome. Pancreatic tumors are found in 87% of the cases with this disease (see Steiner and Heitz, 1973).

Despite the variety of the hormonal activity in the above tumors, the *light microscopic picture* is relatively similar. The tumors are mostly trabecular but may have glandular structures. With proper fixation it is generally possible to identify them as B or non-B cell tumors. With special methods, particularly silver stainings, the non-B cell tumors can be further differentiated. In tumors with carcinoid-like structures the possibility of combined endocrine activity with serotonin production must be taken into consideration. If there are band-like formations, the so-called ribbon patterns, a polyadenomatosis of type Steiner I must be suspected. However, the histological structure itself does not permit a definite conclusion of endocrine activity. Very endocrine-active tumors are often not or are only slightly granulated so that a diagnosis cannot be made by special granular stainings. The advantages of electron microscopic and immunohistological techniques in making a diagnosis have been discussed by Creutzfeldt (this Volume, pp. 681–700).

The histological diagnosis of malignancy is very difficult. Obviously, cell anaplasia gives rise to the possibility of malignancy. However, in benign tumors, as a result of abnormal functional activity, cellular and nuclear irregularities may be seen. This type of degenerative anaplasia is very common in tumors of many other endocrine glands. Invasive growth of tumors in the surrounding pancreatic tissue may also be seen in adenomas. Therefore, metastases are the only reliable sign of malignancy.

Adenomas and carcinomas can be considerably vascularized, which is important for the angiographic diagnosis. The stroma is often very hyalinized. Sometimes large amyloid deposits can be found. It seems to be a special amyloid (Pearse et al., 1972) and not the ordinary substance of the primary or secondary amyloidosis. Such amyloid-producing tumors have a tendency to calcify which is again important for the radiological diagnosis. Amyloid production can occur in tumors with various types of endocrine activity. All these tumors are histologically comparable to the medullary carcinomas of the thyroid with amyloid deposits.

How can the appearance of such similarly structured tumors with different, often combined, endocrine activity be explained? Many years ago, Feyrter (1953) set up the theory that the argentaffin cells, which have to be considered as the stem cells of the carcinoids, are only a part of a more extensive system of peripheral endocrine cells. Not all of these cells are silver positive. However, in ordinary stainings the cytoplasm of these cells is particularly bright. Therefore, Feyrter called the system of these peripheral endocrine cells 'Helle Zellen' system. Pearse (1968) created the term APUD cells. The initial letters APUD are derived from *a*mine *p*recursor *u*ptake and *d*ecarboxylation. The newly created amines are stored in specific cytoplasmic granules and can be identified by special stainings, mainly by fluorescence techniques. With the fluorescence method, Pearse and Polak (1971) and Pearse et al. (1973) were able to demonstrate on mice embryos that such cells emigrate early from the neural crest to the ventral region. Around the 9th day they are seen in the developing foregut and its derivatives, particularly in the pancreas; and in later stages, up to the 12th day, in the lower gastrointestinal tract. That these embryonal APUD cells are precursors of almost all endocrine active polypeptide-producing cells has not yet been fully proven. However, the APUD theory explains the interrelationship of these endocrine cells. Table 3 shows the elements attributed to the APUD cell system by Pearse et al. (1972). If all these cells can be the starting points of combined tumors, then the possibilities are those shown in Figure 2. In the upper half we have the cells with proven polypeptide hormone formation; in the lower half (broken lines) the cells with speculative polypeptide hormone formation. As this figure shows, many different endocrine tumors with varied hormonal activity can result, especially in the region of the pancreas, stomach, and duodenum.

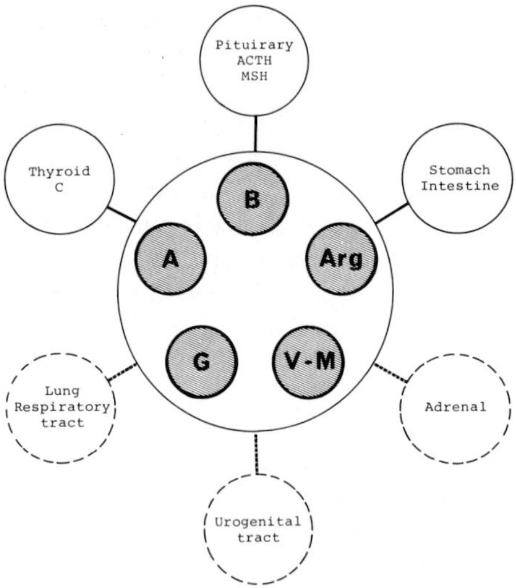

FIG. 2. Possibilities of tumors with combined endocrine activity (for further information see text).

SUMMARY

The pancreas may be the site of primary lesions with single or multiple hormone production. Special emphasis is given to the basic lesions and their relative frequency in the different pancreatic endocrine syndromes. The stem cells of endocrine-active pancreatic tumors belong to the group of the so-called APUD cells. Therefore, it is not surprising that we find tumors with combined hormonal activity. Taking into account that there are many other APUD cells, there may still be other unknown endocrine syndromes.

TABLE 3
Cells and hormones attributed to the APUD cell system (Pearse et al., 1972)

Cell	Hormone
Pituitary c, m (corticotroph/melanotroph)	ACTH/MSH
Pancreatic islet B (β)	Insulin
Pancreatic islet A (α_2)	Glucagon
Pancreatic islet D (δ, α_1)	Gastrin
Thyroid and ultimobranchial C	Calcitonin
Stomach G	Gastrin
Stomach A	Enteroglucagon
Intestine L (EG)	Enteroglucagon
Intestine S	Secretin
Stomach D	(Enterogastrone)
Stomach EC	(Incretin)
Stomach EC-like	(Fundin)
Intestinal EC	(Motilin)
Intestinal X	(CCK-PZ)
Carotid body type 1	(Glomin)
Melanoblast/melanocyte	(Nigrin)
Adrenal A	(Medullarin)
Adrenal NA	(Neuraleistin)
Lung, trachea, bronchi, P	(Pneumokinin)
Urogenital tract, U	(Urogastrone)

In brackets: known hormones doubtfully attributed or hypothetical hormones not yet identified.

REFERENCES

BLOOM, S. R., POLAK, J. M. and PEARSE, A. G. E. (1973): Vasoactive intestinal peptide and watery diarrhoea syndrome. *Lancet, II,* 14.

BRETHOLZ, A. and STEINER, H. (1973): Les insulomes. Intérêt d'un diagnostic morphologique précis. *Virchows Arch. Path. Anat. Abt. A, 359,* 49.

DOLLINGER, M. R., RATNER, L. H., SHAMOIAN, C. A. and BLACKBOURNE, B. D. (1967): Carcinoid syndrome associated with pancreatic tumors. *Arch. intern. Med., 120,* 575.

ELIAS, E., BLOOM, S. R., WELBOURN, R. B., KUZIO, M., POLAK, J. M., PEARSE, A. G. E., BOOTH, C. C. and BROWN, J. C. (1972): Pancreatic cholera due to production of gastric inhibitory polypeptide. *Lancet, II,* 791.

ELLISON, E. H. and WILSON, S. D. (1964): The Zollinger-Ellison Syndrome. Reappraisal and evaluation of 260 registered cases. *Ann. Surg., 160,* 512.

FEYRTER, F. (1943): Über das Inselorgan des Menschen. *Ergebn. allg. Path. path. Anat., 36,* 3.

FEYRTER, F. (1953): *Über die Peripheren Endokrinen (Parakrinen) Drüsen des Menschen.* Wilhelm Maudrich, Wien, Düsseldorf.

FILIPI, C. J. and HIGGINS, G. A. (1973): Diagnosis and management of insulinoma. *Amer. J. Surg., 125,* 231.

GEPTS, W., DESNEUX, J. J. and HENROTIN, E. (1960): Tumeur insulaire à cellules argento-réductrices (carcinoïdes). *Acta gastroenterol. belg., 23,* 162.

GORDON, D. L., CHANG LO, M. and SCHWARTZ, M. A. (1971): Carcinoid of the pancreas. *Amer. J. Med., 51,* 412.

HEITZ, P., STEINER, H., HALTER, F., EGLI, F. and KAPP, J. P. (1971): Multihormonal, amyloid-producing tumour of the islets of Langerhans in a twelve year old boy. Clinical, morphological and biochemical data and review of the literature. *Virchows Arch. Path. Anat. Abt. A, 353,* 321.

LAROCHE, G. P., FERRIS, D. O., PRIESTLEY, J. T., SCHOLZ, D. A. and DOCKERTY, M. B. (1968): Hyperinsulinism. Surgical results and management of occult functioning islet cell tumor: review of 154 cases. *Arch. Surg., 96,* 763.

LOMSKY, R., LANGR, F. and VORTEL, V. (1969): Demonstration of glucagon in islet cell adenomas of the pancreas by immunofluorescent technics. *Amer. J. clin. Pathol., 51,* 245.

KRAFT, A. R., TOMPKINS, R. K. and ZOLLINGER, R. M. (1970): Recognition and management of the diarrheal syndrome caused by nonbeta islet cell tumors of the pancreas. *Amer. J. Surg., 119,* 163.

MARKS, I. N., BANK, S. and LOUW, J. H. (1967): Islet cell tumor of the pancreas with reversible watery diarrhea and achlorhydria. *Gastroenterology, 52,* 695.

MODLINGER, R. S., NICOLIS, G. L., PERTSEMLIDIS, D. and GABRILOVE, J. L. (1972): Cushing syndrome and avascular necrosis of bone associated with carcinoid-islet cell tumor of the pancreas. *Cancer, 30,* 782.

PATCHEFSKY, A. S., SOLIT, R., PHILLIPS, L. D., CRADDOCK, M., HARRER, W. V., COHN, H. E. and KOWLESSAR, O. D. (1972): Hydroxyindole-producing tumors of the pancreas. *Ann. intern. Med., 77,* 53.

PEARSE, A. G. E. (1968): Common cytochemical and ultrastructural characteristics of cells producing polypeptide hormones (the APUD series) and their relevance to thyroid and ultimobranchial C cells and calcitonin. *Proc. Roy. Soc. Med. Ser. B, 170,* 171.

PEARSE, A. G. E. (1969): The cytochemistry and ultrastructure of polypeptide hormone-producing cells of the APUD series, and the embryologic, physiologic and pathologic implications of the concept. *J. Histochem. Cytochem., 17,* 303.

PEARSE, A. G. E. and POLAK, J. M. (1971): Neural crest origin of the endocrine polypeptide (APUD) cells of the gastrointestinal tract and pancreas. *Gut, 12,* 783.

PEARSE, A. G. E., EWEN, S. W. B. and POLAK, J. M. (1972): The genesis of apud-amyloid in endocrine polypeptide tumours: histochemical distinction from immunamyloid. *Virchows Arch. Zellpath. Abt. B, 10,* 93.

PEARSE, A. G. E., POLAK, J. M. and HEATH, C. M. (1973): Development, differentiation and derivation of the endocrine polypeptide cells of the mouse pancreas. Immunofluorescence, cytochemical and ultrastructural studies. *Diabetologia, 9,* 120.

POLAK, J. M., STAGG, B. and PEARSE, A. G. E. (1972): Two types of Zollinger-Ellison syndrome: immunofluorescent, cytochemical and ultrastructural studies of the antral and pancreatic gastrin cells in different clinical states. *Gut, 13,* 501.

RAWLINSON, D. G. (1973): Electron microscopy of an ACTH-secreting islet cell carcinoma. *Cancer, 31,* 1015.

SCHOENEMANN, J. (1972): Das Verner-Morrison-Syndrom (pankreatische Cholera). Übersicht über 53 Fälle der Literatur und 3 eigene Beobachtungen. *Dtsch. Gesundh.-Wes., 27,* 1782.

STEINER, H. and HEITZ, P. (1973): Die pluriglandulären endokrinen Regulationsstörungen. In: *Endokrine Organe. Spezielle Pathologische Anatomie.* Editors: W. Doerr, G. Seifert. and E. Uehlinger. Springer, Berlin, Heidelberg, New York. In press.

STEPHENS, E. (1973): Zollinger-Ellison Syndrome reclassified. *Brit. med. J., 2,* 180.

VASSALLO, G., SOLCIA, E., BUSSOLATI, G., POLAK, J. M. and PEARSE, A. G. E. (1972): Non-G cell gastrin-producing tumours of the pancreas. *Virchows Arch. Zellpath. Abt. B, 11,* 66.

ZOLLINGER, R. M., TOMPKINS, R. K., AMERSON, J. R., ENDAHL, G. L., KRAFT, A. R. and MOORE, F. T. (1968): Identification of the diarrheogenic hormone associated with non-beta islet cell tumors of the pancreas. *Ann. Surg., 168,* 502.

CIRCULATING PROINSULIN IN PATIENTS WITH ISLET CELL TUMORS*

ARTHUR H. RUBENSTEIN, MARY E. MAKO, JEROME I. STARR, DOOJUNG J. JUHN and DAVID L. HORWITZ

Department of Medicine, The University of Chicago, Chicago, Ill., U.S.A.

The diagnosis of insulin-secreting beta cell tumors of the pancreas continues to be a formidable challenge, despite the introduction of new methods which facilitate their identification (Marks and Rose, 1965; Laurent et al., 1971; Koutras and White, 1972). The clinical symptoms and signs of this condition have been reviewed on numerous occasions and the frequency of psychiatric and neurologic presentations has been stressed. The importance of having a high incidence of suspicion has been repeatedly documented, for many examples of delayed or erroneous diagnoses are recorded in the literature.

The preoperative diagnosis of insulinomas was originally based upon the patient's blood sugar response to various procedures designed to stress the gluco-regulatory system. These include the demonstration of symptomatic hypoglycemia during fasting or following provocative tests (Fajans and Conn, 1959), such as the administration of tolbutamide, l-leucine and glucagon. The introduction of methods for the measurement of serum insulin in 1960 (Yalow and Berson, 1960) complemented the value of blood glucose determinations and proved invaluable in differentiating the hypoglycemia of hyperinsulinism from other etiological causes. Elevated serum insulin concentrations after a short (overnight) or more prolonged (72-hour) fast, particularly in relation to the simultaneously measured blood sugar level, is frequently present in these subjects, especially if multiple samples are obtained. In addition, an excessive insulin rise following the administration of tolbutamide, leucine or glucagon may occur (Floyd et al., 1964).

Although a definitive diagnosis of an insulinoma can usually be made using these methods, there are a number of patients in whom the blood sugar and insulin values are of borderline significance and the diagnosis remains uncertain. It is under these circumstances that the estimation of serum proinsulin may be of help in determining the presence of an islet cell tumor. In this paper we will review the published information regarding circulating proinsulin levels in subjects with insulinomas and compare our experience with 19 such patients. In addition, we have studied the metabolism of endogenous proinsulin in some of these patients before and after the surgical removal of their tumors.

* Supported by grants from the National Institutes of Health (AM-13941) and the Pfizer Company, New York, N.Y.

MEASUREMENT OF INSULIN AND PROINSULIN-LIKE COMPONENTS (PLC) IN SERUM

Although it would be advantageous to measure human proinsulin and its intermediate fractions by direct immunoassay in unextracted serum, this has not been possible. The reasons lie in the cross-reactivity of proinsulin with insulin, on the one hand, and the C-peptide on the other. As all 3 of these peptides have been identified in the circulation, a preliminary step is required to separate them from each other. The most commonly used approach has involved gel filtration of serum followed by measurement of the column fractions in the insulin immunoassay. In our initial studies we extracted serum insulin and proinsulin into acid ethanol and separated the 2 peptides by gel filtration on a Bio-Gel P-30 column equilibrated in 3 M acetic acid (Melani et al., 1970a). The initial reason for choosing this technique was the reluctance to gel filter serum in neutral or alkaline buffers in which polymerization or aggregation of insulin might occur. In fact, this does not appear to be a problem. Another advantage is the ability to extract large volumes of serum and yet separate the hormones on relatively small columns. Furthermore, it is easier to characterize the separated proinsulin and insulin under these conditions when most of the other serum proteins have been removed. The most obvious disadvantage of the method is the length of time required for the procedure and the limitation on the number of samples that can be analyzed by one laboratory.

Roth et al. (1968) have separated proinsulin and insulin on 1 X 50 cm columns of Sephadex G-50, fine, equilibrated in a veronal buffer containing human serum albumin, rabbit fraction II and toluene. One or two ml of serum is applied directly to the column, fraction sizes of 1.0 to 1.5 ml collected and 0.4 to 0.8 ml aliquots taken for immunoassay. We have modified this method to use a column of Bio-Gel P-30, equilibrated in the borate buffer which we use in the immunoassay. Fractions can be collected directly into the immunoassay tubes, thus obviating the need for further pipetting at this stage. The void volume is determined by the elution position of ^{125}I-albumin or blue dextran 2000, while the salt peak is marked by Na ^{125}I. The column is calibrated with tracers of ^{125}I-proinsulin and ^{125}I-insulin. Because certain preparations of these labelled hormones may not elute identically with the native proteins, it may be preferable to determine the characteristics of the column by assaying the elution position of unlabelled insulin (2 ng) and proinsulin (2 ng).

When serum is directly applied to the columns, essentially complete recoveries have been obtained. In order to calculate the absolute level of proinsulin and insulin, fractions of the earlier eluting peak are read from a human proinsulin standard (Fig. 1), while those comprising the second peak are measured against a human insulin standard (Fig. 1). As the supply of human proinsulin is limited at present, many investigators have expressed the values of proinsulin in terms of the insulin standard (Fig. 2).

REVIEW OF THE LITERATURE

Serum PLC has been measured in a number of patients with islet cell tumors, but it is difficult to compare the results reported by different investigators. One reason lies in the varying time intervals after eating at which the blood samples were drawn, for it is well established that both the serum proinsulin concentration and proinsulin:insulin ratio differ in the fasted and fed state (Melani et al., 1970a). Secondly, although it has proven

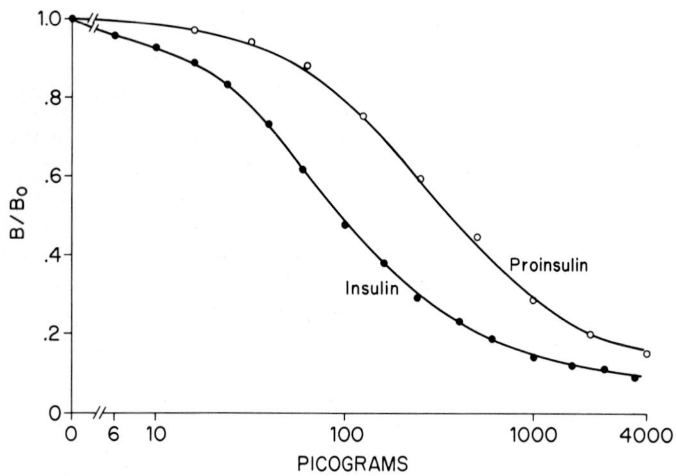

FIG. 1. Standard curves of human insulin and human proinsulin. The assay system utilizes guinea pig insulin antiserum (1:550,000) and a tracer of porcine ^{125}I-insulin.

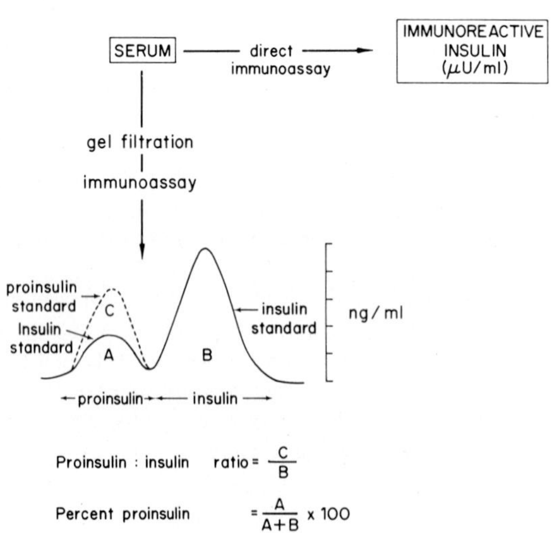

FIG. 2. Schematic method for measuring proinsulin-like components and insulin in serum. The direct immunoassay provides the total serum immunoreactive insulin concentration (IRI). After gel filtration, the early eluting component can be measured against the human insulin standard (A) or human proinsulin standard (C). Most authors have expressed the proinsulin as a percent of the total IRI i.e. $\left(\frac{A}{A+B} \times 100\right)$.

useful to express proinsulin and insulin as a percentage of the total insulin-like immunoreactivity in plasma, certain problems are inherent in this approach. Because of the limited availability of human proinsulin most investigators have measured the individual fractions of both the proinsulin and insulin peaks after gel filtration of plasma against a standard of human insulin. The potential errors in this method lie in the variable underestimation of the PLC concentration and have been discussed in detail previously (Rubenstein et al., 1972a). Finally, the use of different techniques for the separation and measurement of serum PLC has resulted in a wide range of values for these polypeptides in healthy subjects (Kitabchi et al., 1971), and thus the significance of similarly abnormal levels in pathological states may vary from one laboratory to another. In order to standardize the results as far as possible, we have quoted the PLC concentration and its percentage of the total immunoreactive insulin from values measured from human insulin standards.

Gorden and Roth (1970) studied 2 patients with histologically proven islet cell carcinomas and liver metastases. Their percentage PLC 200 minutes after a small meal was 18 and 37%. After tolbutamide administration, the percentage PLC in the latter patient fell to 3% of the total immunoreactive insulin (IRI), while that of the former subject was, 35% 2 hours after oral glucose. These findings highlight the importance of standardizing the sampling conditions for interpreting the PLC results. In healthy subjects the percentage PLC was less than 5% at 15–30 minutes after glucose and then rose 2–8-fold to reach 5 to 29% of the plasma insulin at 90–120 minutes. Goldsmith et al. (1969) observed values of PLC between 24 and 55% of IRI in a patient with a beta cell tumor after tolbutamide or glucagon stimulation, whereas a single sample from another such patient showed only 5%. The plasma PLC values from a variety of other patients taken under similar conditions was consistently below 20%.

The effect of streptozotocin on the relative concentrations of PLC and insulin were studied by Blackard et al. (1970) in a 68-year-old woman with an islet cell carcinoma. Prior to treatment, PLC represented 36, 32 and 53% of total IRI at 1, 2 and 3 hours after glucose. Following treatment with streptozotocin, the percentage PLC fell to 21, 22, and 27% at the same time intervals. Values of normal subjects studied in this laboratory did not contribute more than 30% of the total IRI, but the sampling times were not stated. Although the authors comment on the possible relationship of the lower PLC percentages to the absence of hypoglycemia after streptozotocin therapy, it is difficult to interpret its significance in the light of the different patterns of insulin secretion in the 2 tests. In this regard, Pearson et al. (1972) have also studied the response of PLC to streptozotocin in a 56-year-old man with an inoperable islet cell carcinoma. Administration of the drug over a short- (1.5 g in minutes) or long-term (9 g within 8 weeks) period did not affect either plasma total IRI or percentage PLC. It is of interest that the levels of both increased in parallel with clinical progression of the tumor, the percentage PLC rising from 14 to 80%. A very high concentration of PLC in a patient with an islet cell carcinoma who responded dramatically to streptozotocin therapy has been reported by Taylor et al. (1970).

Relative PLC concentrations of greater than 40% have been reported by Lazarus et al. (1970) and Melani et al. (1970b) in fasting sera from 2 patients with islet cell adenomas. In the latter patient the levels of both PLC and insulin rose after tolbutamide, but the increase in PLC at 15–30 minutes was proportionately less than that in insulin. At this time the concentration of proinsulin represented only 36% of the total IRI. At 1, 2 and 3 hours the proportion of PLC rose above the fasting value to 62%, 59% and 67% respectively. Six months postoperatively, the PLC was less than 10% of the IRI 20 minutes after tolbutamide. The proinsulin extracted from the adenoma was markedly elevated (27%) compared to that of the normal pancreas (2–9%) (Rastogi et al., 1970; Sando et al., 1972; Sando and Grodsky, 1973). Gorden et al. (1971b) found basal PLC ranging from 26 to 79% in 5 patients with beta cell tumors (normal values were below 30%). Four of these patients had islet cell carcinomas and showed high basal PLC percentages (38, 46, 53 and 78%). After release of insulin with tolbutamide or streptozotocin, PLC changed in a similar direction to that observed in non-tumor subjects whose insulin secretion was stimulated by tolbutamide or other agents. Percent PLC was high when total insulin concentrations were low, but fell to low levels when insulin was acutely released, the rise in total IRI being almost entirely due to the release of insulin. Ten days of treatment with diazoxide in one of these patients did not change the total IRI level or the percentage proinsulin.

A large group of patients with insulinomas was studied by Gutman et al. (1971). Ten had adenomas and one a carcinoma with liver metastases. The PLC percentage varied between 3 and 71% at 10–20 minutes after tolbutamide in 8 patients (normal subjects had less than 20%), and basal values of 28, 29 and 89% were noted in the remaining 3. Two of the 11 patients showed no significant elevation of PLC concentration or percentage in the post-tolbutamide samples. One of the patients with 71% PLC was examined 10 months after partial pancreatectomy and circulating PLC was undetectable in a sample obtained 15 minutes after tolbutamide. Similar results were described in a further 21 patients (19 adenomas, 2 carcinomas) by Sherman et al. (1972). The percentage PLC in fasting samples of patients with adenomas comprised 8 to 78% (mean 37%) of their total IRI and in 20 of the 21 the absolute level of PLC (1 to 110 μU/ml) exceeded the highest value found in healthy subjects (2.2 μU/ml). These authors confirmed the previously reported findings that tolbutamide, leucine and arginine caused an increase in total IRI which was mainly due to the insulin component. As a result of the greater rise in insulin compared to PLC, the percentage PLC decreased from 37% in the fasting state to 16% at the time of maximal insulin response. This figure contrasts with a mean PLC percentage of 4% in control subjects following tolbutamide. The 2 patients with malignant tumors had 62 and 76% PLC, and in one no increase in plasma IRI occurred in response to provocative stimuli.

The serum PLC values in a patient with an islet cell adenoma have also been measured using an enzyme, insulin-specific protease, which degrades the circulating insulin component but leaves the PLC intact. Although PLC comprised almost 50% of total IRI, the significance of this observation is uncertain, considering that fasting values of 26 to 75% were found in control subjects (Kitabchi et al., 1971).

Elevated PLC has also been measured in the plasma of Syrian hamsters bearing islet cell tumors (Gorden et al., 1971b). When tumor slices were incubated in vitro, both insulin and proinsulin were secreted into the medium. Although raising the glucose concentration from 1 to 3 mg/ml resulted in an increased secretion of both components, glucagon and tolbutamide led to the release mainly of insulin and a decrease in percentage PLC. It thus appears that this tumor will prove to be a useful model to compare with islet cell tumors of man.

PLC IN NINETEEN PATIENTS WITH ISLET CELL TUMORS

The basal total immunoreactive insulin, proinsulin and percentage proinsulin in 17 patients with beta cell adenomas and in 2 with carcinomas are shown in Figure 3. The blood was drawn after an overnight fast (8–10 hours) in the majority of the patients, but in 4 a shorter period without food was necessary because of the occurrence of hypoglycemic symptoms. Eleven patients had IRI values which fell within the range of our 46 control subjects (4.5 to 22.4 μU/ml, and 7 were within 2 S.D. of the mean (19.2 μU/ml). This finding highlights again the frequency with which slightly elevated IRI levels are observed in this condition and points to the importance of obtaining repeated samples in each patient and the need to correlate the IRI with the simultaneous blood glucose concentration.

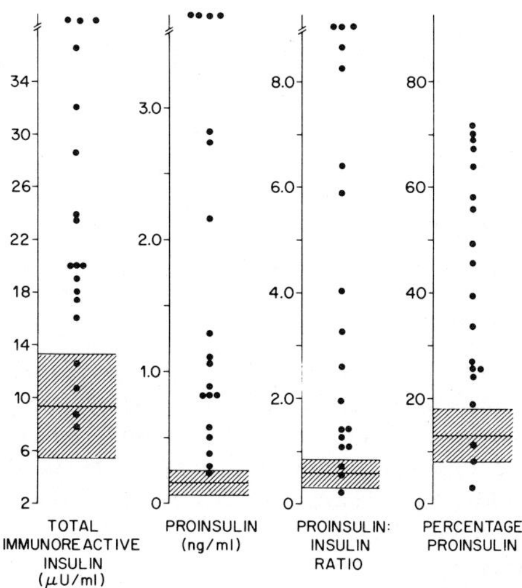

FIG. 3. Basal total immunoreactive insulin (IRI), proinsulin-like components, proinsulin:insulin ratio and percentage proinsulin in 19 patients with islet cell tumors. The mean ± 1 S.D. of 46 control subjects is shown in the hatched area.

The absolute basal proinsulin concentrations varied between 0.23 and 17.48 ng/ml. Only 3 patients overlapped the normal range (0.038–0.45 ng/ml), having values of 0.23, 0.27 and 0.4 ng/ml. The percentage proinsulin ranged from 2.9 to 71 (normal values being 4.6–22.8 with a mean of 13.2%). Four of the insulinoma group fell within this normal range. When the results of the 3 subjects with normal proinsulin concentrations were analyzed, one showed an elevated percentage proinsulin, one had an abnormally high IRI value, while the third had levels of both IRI and PLC at the upper limit of normal. These findings indicate that measurement of PLC in those patients with marginally elevated, or normal, IRI values may be of considerable diagnostic help, and that analysis of basal PLC levels in addition to those of the blood glucose and IRI may provide an important lead to the presence of an insulinoma. The great variability in the patterns of circulating components which react in the insulin immunoassay in these patients is shown in Figure 4.

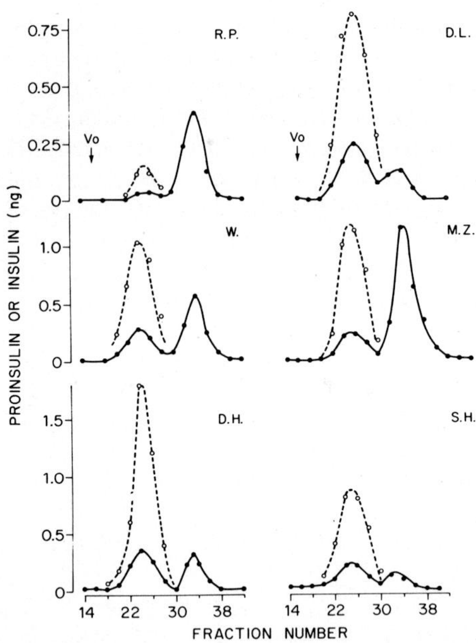

FIG. 4. Gel filtration patterns of proinsulin-like components and insulin in a control subject (top left) and 5 patients with islet cell tumors. The sera were gel-filtered on Bio-Gel P-30 columns equilibrated in a borate-albumin buffer and measured in the insulin immunoassay. The dotted line represents the PLC values read from the human proinsulin standard. Note the different scales on the ordinate.

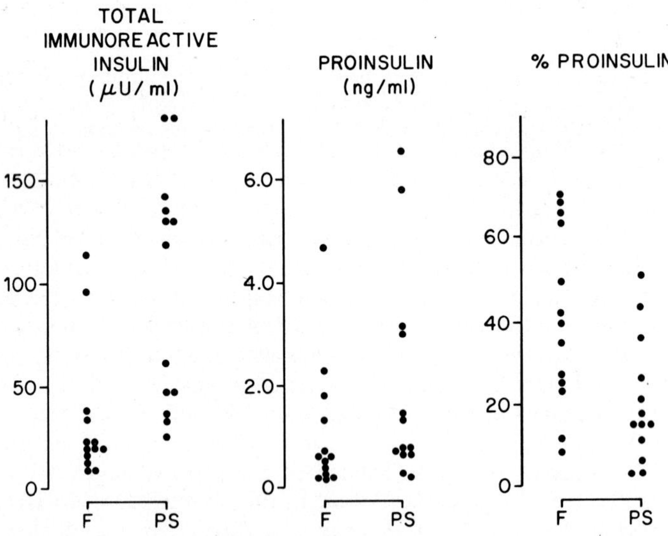

FIG. 5. Basal and poststimulated (PS) total immunoreactive insulin, proinsulin and percentage proinsulin values in 13 patients with insulinomas.

A comparison of the results of basal and stimulated values in 13 of the patients is shown in Figure 5. The stimulated measurements were carried out on samples with peak IRI concentrations during provocative tests. The stimuli varied in different patients and included oral and intravenous glucose, tolbutamide, leucine and glucagon. During an oral glucose tolerance test, the percentage proinsulin of all control subjects decreased to below 8%, and 4 of the 13 insulinoma patients had values within this range.

These results are very similar to those of Sherman et al. (1972) who described 3 of 21 islet cell tumor patients with basal IRI concentrations within their normal range, but only one with a normal proinsulin concentration. Four subjects had percentage PLC which overlapped their controls. As in our data, a number of additional patients had values in these 3 categories which were only marginally abnormal. However, 5 of 7 patients with fasting IRI of 20 μU/ml or less had an elevated percentage proinsulin (3 were only marginally increased), and 6 had raised PLC concentrations (one with a very small increase). The authors believed that in 2 of these 7 patients, the finding of a high PLC would have been of additional diagnostic aid. The measurement of PLC following the administration of tolbutamide did not provide further information of diagnostic significance.

We have also measured basal PLC in 9 of our patients after surgical removal of their tumors. The total IRI was within the normal range in all subjects, but the PLC concentration remained abnormal in one and the percentage PLC fell, but did not reach normal values in another. These latter 2 samples were obtained within a short time of the operation and further studies on these patients are planned.

DIFFERENTIATION OF ADENOMA FROM CARCINOMA

We have considered the possibility that serum PLC estimations may be useful in differentiating benign beta cell tumors from carcinomas. The basal PLC percentage was 58 and 70 in the 2 patients with malignant tumors in our series, but values in this range (above 50%) were also noted in 5 subjects with adenomas. Similar results were found by Sherman et al. (1972) (2 patients with malignant tumors had percentage PLC of 62 and 76, while 5 adenoma cases also had values higher than 50%). The patient with a malignant tumor had the highest percentage PLC (89%) in the study of Gutman et al. (1971), while Gorden et al. (1971) reported values of 38, 46, 53 and 78% in 4 such patients. Although Blackard et al. (1970) did not measure basal PLC, the percentage 2 hours after oral glucose was 53%. The finding of Pearson et al. (1972) is also of interest in this regard, because the percentage PLC in their patient with an islet cell carcinoma rose to 80% over an 8-week period. The authors concluded that the percentage PLC may rise as loss of tumor differentiation occurs. Nevertheless, as many drugs and continuous glucose infusions were administered during this time, the results should be interpreted with caution. Very high PLC values in a further 2 patients with carcinomas have also been reported by Taylor et al. (1970) and Lazarus et al. (1970).

These results suggest that most patients with malignant islet cell tumors do have a markedly elevated percentage PLC. However, a significant number of subjects with adenomas also fall into this high range. On the other hand it seems that the finding of a low percentage PLC in a patient with an islet cell tumor does favor the diagnosis of a benign lesion.

CHARACTERIZATION OF CIRCULATING PROINSULIN-LIKE COMPONENTS

In most studies PLC has been measured after gel filtration of sera on Sephadex or Bio-Gel columns equilibrated in acetic acid, borate or veronal buffers. Because of its higher molecular weight, PLC elutes before insulin and may be identified in either the insulin or human C-peptide immunoassays. However, these methods do not differentiate the 2 chain proinsulin intermediates (Steiner et al., 1968) from the single chain precursor and additional techniques are required to demonstrate their presence in the circulation.

Lazarus et al. (1972) have described the presence of a proinsulin intermediate, in addition to proinsulin, in the serum of a patient with a surgically-documented carcinoma of the pancreatic islets. The fasting total IRI concentration was approximately 1000 μU/ml and the percentage PLC was 85%. An acid alcohol extract of serum was electrophoresed on polyacrylamide gel and 3 peaks were identified. Two of these had mobilities corresponding to insulin and proinsulin, while the third peak ran in an intermediate position. The authors suggested that the migration behavior of this peak was compatible with desdipeptide proinsulin. Although the biological activity of the PLC was almost 50% that of insulin, it is difficult to be certain of this result because of problems in standardizing the proinsulin components.

In addition to this intermediate form, other components which react in the insulin assay have been identified in sera of patients with islet cell tumors. Thus Gorden et al. (1971) have described a proinsulin-like component which eluted ahead of the proinsulin marker on a 1.5 X 90 cm column of Sephadex G-50 in a subject with an islet cell carcinoma. The PLC isolated from this patient's serum did not cross-react identically with a porcine insulin standard, whereas dilutions of plasma PLC from healthy subjects and other patients with tumors were indistinguishable from the porcine standard in this assay system. Its biological activity was 3 times greater than porcine proinsulin and it was converted to insulin by exposure to trypsin. It is of interest that the serum insulin component also did not exhibit immunological identity with a porcine insulin standard. Because of the small amounts of material available, further characterization was not achieved.

Yet another form of immunoreactive insulin, which has been named 'big, big insulin' has recently been described in the plasma of an insulinoma suspect by Yalow and Berson (1973). This component has a molecular weight of approximately 100,000, is immunochemically identical to human insulin, is more basic than porcine or human insulin and is rapidly transformed by trypsin to an insulin-like component. In several samples from this particular patient, virtually all the insulin immunoreactivity was present in the form of this high molecular weight protein. In other sera significant amounts of insulin, but not proinsulin, were detected. Gel filtration of acid-alcohol extracts of 2 islet cell adenomas and a normal pancreas revealed a small quantity (0.7–1.0%) of a similar component.

The presence of a similar, but probably not identical, component in an acid-ethanol extract of an insulinoma was described by Melani et al. (1970b). This material which eluted in the void volume of the Bio-Gel P-30 column, comprised 10% of the total immunoreactive insulin-like material. It reacted in the C-peptide assay but was not converted to insulin or proinsulin by trypsin.

In our studies on insulinoma patients, we have noted variable amounts of material eluting in the void volume of Bio-Gel P-30 columns which reacts with insulin antibodies (Fig. 6). The origin and significance of this component is still uncertain and further work is necessary in order to characterize it fully.

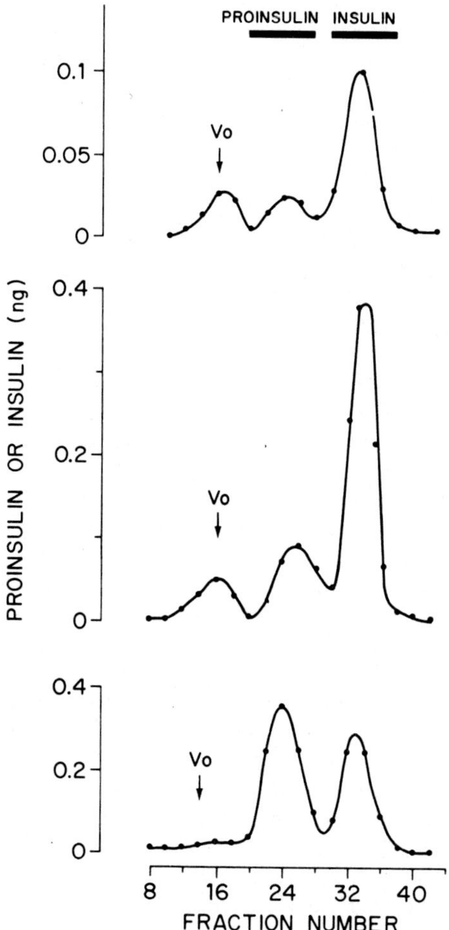

FIG. 6. Gel filtration patterns of sera from 3 patients with islet cell tumors. The samples in the upper and middle panel show 3 peaks which react in the insulin assay system. The second peak represents proinsulin-like components, and the third insulin. The nature of the large molecular weight, early eluting peak is uncertain. The lower panel, shown for contrast, demonstrates the absence of this material in another patient.

DIFFERENTIAL DIAGNOSIS

Obese patients with hyperinsulinemia had higher fasting concentrations of proinsulin and a greater absolute increase after glucose than did control subjects (Melani et al., 1970a). Since the high levels of PLC coexisted with raised insulin concentrations, the relative proportions of the 2 fractions were generally in the same range observed in normal subjects and would not be difficult to distinguish from insulinoma patients. Gorden and Roth (1969) have shown that the proportion of PLC is higher than normal in some obese subjects and acromegalics at 15–30 minutes after oral glucose. However, only a relatively minor part of the observed hyperinsulinism in these patients can be explained by the elevation of PLC and the fasting percent PLC was well within the normal range (Gorden et al., 1971b).

These are 2 situations in which a significant elevation of basal PLC has been recorded. Gorden et al. (1972) showed that in 6 patients with severe hypokalemia of diverse etiologies, the PLC formed a greater proportion of the total IRI in the basal and post-stimulated state. These subjects were glucose intolerant, exhibited delayed and low insulin responses, and the high PLC percentage was at least partly a result of their insulinopenic state. Correction of the hypokalemia reversed this abnormality. Secondly, Mako et al. (1973) have pointed out that the absolute concentration and percentage PLC in the basal state in patients with chronic renal failure are markedly elevated and that the values may overlap those found in subjects with islet cell tumors. The reason for this finding lies in the critical role of the kidney as the major organ involved in proinsulin degradation (Katz and Rubenstein, 1973). These 2 conditions should thus be excluded when abnormalities of PLC are being used to aid in the diagnosis of insulinomas.

Goldsmith et al. (1969) found that the serum PLC comprised less than 20% of the total IRI in patients with a variety of disorders characterized by glucose intolerance and insulin insensitivity (myotonic dystrophy, hypertriglyceridemia, uremia and myxedema). However, it should be noted that in this study plasma samples with high insulin levels obtained after glucose, tolbutamide, arginine or glucagon stimulation were specifically chosen and fasting levels have not been measured.

Great interest has been expressed in the possibility that an altered proinsulin:insulin ratio might occur in patients with diabetes mellitus. Initial results in a limited number of both normal weight and obese patients with mild diabetes characterized only by glucose intolerance, demonstrated basal and postglucose responses indistinguishable from control subjects (Melani et al., 1970a; Gorden and Roth, 1970; Gorden et al., 1971b). More recently Duckworth et al. (1972), using the insulin-specific protease to measure proinsulin, reported that both obesity and carbohydrate intolerance were associated with slightly increased PLC levels, but that the coexistence of the 2 conditions, especially in older diabetics, was marked by significantly elevated PLC concentrations and a rise in the PLC:IRI ratio. Notwithstanding these findings, it is unlikely that the values in most diabetics will overlap those of insulinoma patients, especially when other methods for measuring PLC are used.

The PLC levels in reactive hypoglycemia have been measured by Gutman et al. (1971) and Duckworth and Kitabchi (1972). The 3 patients in the former study had normal levels, but 2 patients in the latter investigation showed high PLC values during the oral glucose tolerance test in which hypoglycemia occurred. However, the basal levels appeared normal, thus providing a ready means of differentiating them from insulinoma patients. Moreover, the finding was not reproduced in repeat testing.

METABOLISM OF PLC AND INSULIN IN PATIENTS WITH ISLET CELL TUMORS

We have previously reported (Katz and Rubenstein, 1973) that the metabolic clearance rate of bovine insulin in rats is 16.4 ± 0.4 ml/min., while that of bovine proinsulin is much slower (6.7 ± 0.3 ml/min.). However, this study as well as other studies (Stoll et al.,

1971; Izzo et al., 1971; Tompkins et al., 1971) which demonstrated prolongation of the half disappearance time of proinsulin compared to insulin have used heterologous insulin preparations. Because inter-species differences in the structure of proinsulin are considerably greater than that of insulin (Tager and Steiner, 1972) we felt that it was important to confirm these results using the homologous species of proinsulin in man. Because sufficient human proinsulin is not yet available for infusion studies, we investigated the metabolism of endogenous proinsulin and insulin in 3 patients following surgical removal of islet cell tumors. Sequential serum specimens from a peripheral vein were obtained during and at short time intervals following the surgical removal of their tumors.

A representative result in a patient with markedly elevated concentrations of insulin and proinsulin prior to the removal of the islet cell tumor is shown in Figure 7. Insulin reached low levels by 20 minutes, but proinsulin fell to a considerably lesser degree and continued to decline in the later samples.

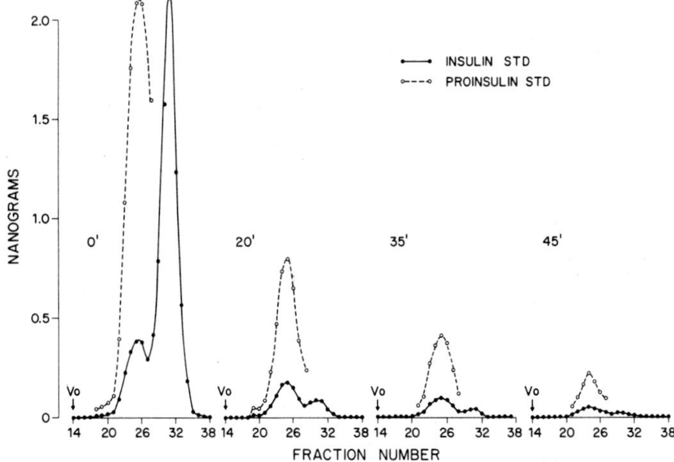

FIG. 7. Gel filtration patterns of sera from a patient following removal (at 20, 35 and 45 minutes) of an islet cell tumor. The closed circles represent the concentrations measured against the human insulin standard, while the open circles are the concentration of the fractions in the proinsulin peak read from the human proinsulin standard.

The disappearance of insulin and proinsulin, expressed as a percent of their initial values, is shown in Figure 8. The disappearance of insulin was more rapid than proinsulin in each patient. The half disappearance times for proinsulin and insulin are shown in Figure 9. The mean value of proinsulin was 17.2 minutes, which was more than 3 times as long as the mean for insulin (4.8 minutes).

We have also measured PLC and insulin in simultaneously drawn portal and systemic samples in 2 patients prior to removal of their insulinomas. The difference in insulin levels between these 2 sites was much greater than proinsulin (Fig. 10). Thus, the portal systemic ratio of insulin ranged between 5 and 22, while that of proinsulin was approximately 2 (Fig. 11). We have previously demonstrated that bovine insulin is metabolized more rapidly than proinsulin by the isolated rat liver (Rubenstein et al., 1972b) and the relative portal-systemic concentrations of the 2 polypeptides undoubtedly reflects this

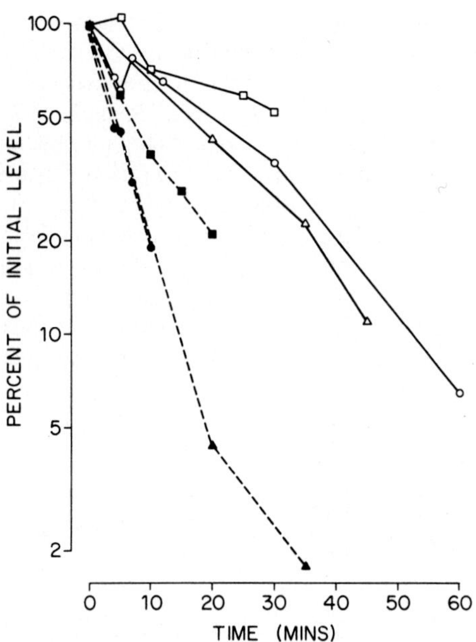

FIG. 8. The disappearance of insulin and proinsulin in 3 patients following surgical removal of their islet cell tumors. The concentration of these polypeptides immediately before removal of the tumors is shown as 100% and the subsequent samples are expressed as a percentage of this value. The insulin values are shown in closed and the proinsulin in open symbols.

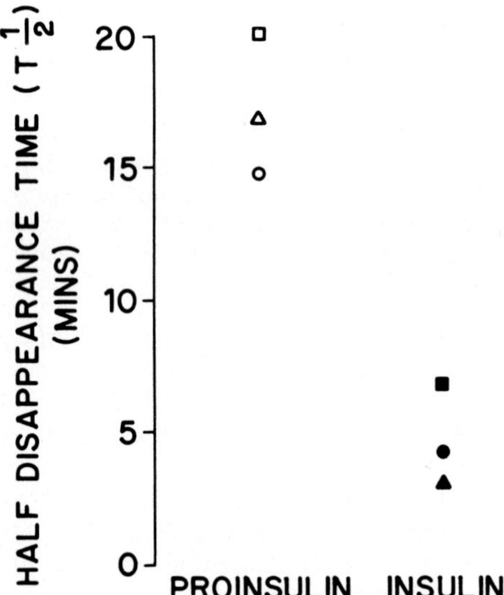

FIG. 9. The half-disappearance times of proinsulin and insulin following removal of islet cell tumors in 3 patients. The mean value for proinsulin was 17.2 minutes, and for insulin 4.8 minutes.

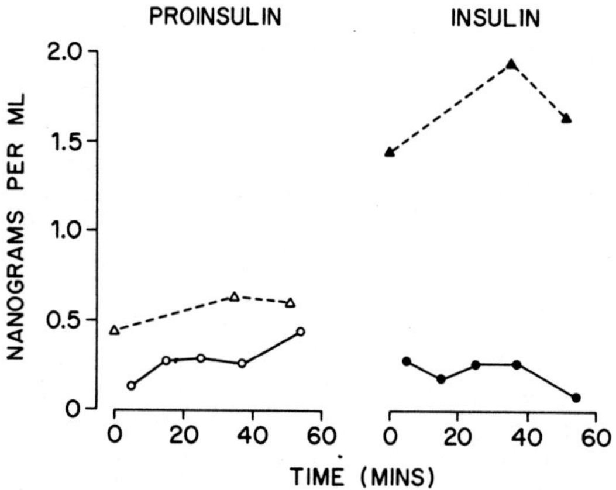

FIG. 10. Concentrations of proinsulin (left panel) and insulin (right panel) in portal (triangles) and peripheral (circles) blood. The samples were obtained during an operation for removal of an islet cell tumor.

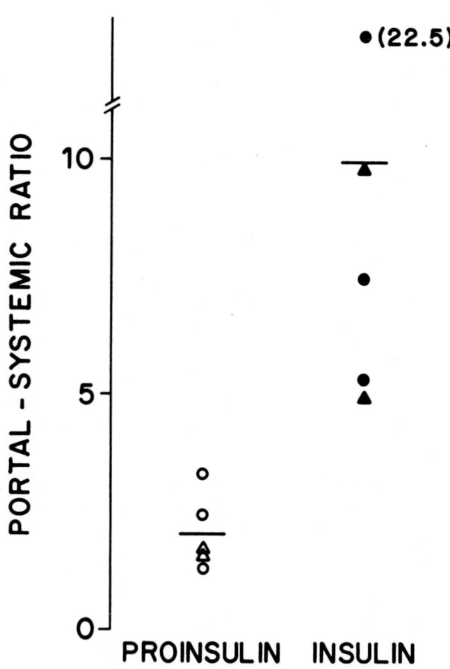

FIG. 11. Portal-systemic ratio of proinsulin (left) and insulin (right) in 2 patients with islet cell tumors. The samples were obtained during operations to remove the tumors. The 3 samples from one patient are shown in triangles and the 2 samples from the other patient are in circles.

differential extraction. Essentially similar results have been reported by Sherman et al. (1972) in 2 insulinoma patients. The percentage IRI in the portal vein was 8 and 9%, while that in the splenic artery was 34 and 24% respectively.

These differences in hepatic uptake and peripheral metabolism of proinsulin and insulin are sufficient to account for their steady state serum levels and explain the marked difference in their pancreatic and serum ratios. Furthermore, these results indicate that caution must be shown before attributing changes in the peripheral proinsulin:insulin ratio to varying secretion by the pancreatic beta cells.

SUMMARY

1. The serum PLC concentration and percentage of total immunoreactive insulin are frequently elevated in patients with insulinomas. This abnormality may aid in establishing the diagnosis, especially in subjects in whom the total IRI is only marginally raised.
2. Patients with hypokalemia and chronic renal failure may also show abnormally high serum PLC levels.
3. The peripheral metabolism of proinsulin is slower than insulin, thus contributing to the higher proinsulin:insulin ratio in the posthepatic circulation compared to the beta cell.

ACKNOWLEDGEMENTS

We wish to thank the many physicians who sent us blood samples from their patients.

REFERENCES

BLACKARD, W. G., GARCIA, A. R. and BROWN, C. L. (1970): Effect of streptozotocin on qualitative aspects of plasma insulin in a patient with a malignant islet cell tumor. *J. clin. Endocr., 31,* 215.

DUCKWORTH, W. C. and KITABCHI, A. E. (1972): Hyperproinsulinemia in hypoglycemic subjects. *Hormone Metabol. Res., 4,* 133.

DUCKWORTH, W. C., KITABCHI, A. E. and HEINEMANN, M. (1972): Direct measurement of plasma proinsulin in normal and diabetic subjects. *Amer. J. Med., 53,* 418.

FAJANS, S. S. and CONN, J. W. (1959): An intravenous tolbutamide test as an adjunct in the diagnosis of functioning pancreatic islet cell adenomas. *J. Lab. clin. Med., 54,* 811.

FLOYD, J. C., FAJANS, S. S., KNOPF, R. F. and CONN, J. W. (1964): Plasma insulin in organic hyperinsulinism: comparative effects of tolbutamide, leucine and glucose. *J. clin. Endocr., 24,* 747.

GOLDSMITH, S. J., YALOW, R. S. and BERSON, S. A. (1969): Significance of human plasma insulin Sephadex fractions. *Diabetes, 18,* 340.

GORDEN, P., FREYCHET, P. and NANKEN, H. (1971a): A unique form of circulating insulin in human islet cell carcinoma. *J. clin. Endocr., 33,* 983.

GORDEN, P. and ROTH, J. (1970): Plasma insulin: fluctuations in the 'Big' insulin component in man after glucose and other stimuli. *J. clin. Invest., 48,* 2225.

GORDEN, P., SHERMAN, B. and ROTH, J. (1971b): Proinsulin-like component of circulating insulin in the basal state and in patients and hamsters with islet cell tumors. *J. clin. Invest., 50,* 2113.

GORDEN, P., SHERMAN, B. M. and SIMOPOULOS, A. P. (1972): Glucose intolerance with hypokalemia: an increased proportion of circulating proinsulin-like component. *J. clin. Endocr., 34,* 235.

GUTMAN, R. A., LAZARUS, N. R., PENHOS, J. C., FAJANS, S. S. and RECANT, L. (1971): Circulating proinsulin-like material in functioning insulinomas. *New Engl. J. Med., 284,* 1003.

IZZO, J. L., RONCONE, A. and IZZO, M. J. (1971): Disposition of I^{131}-proinsulin. *Diabetes, 20/Suppl. 1,* 333.

KATZ, A. I. and RUBENSTEIN, A. H. (1973): Metabolism of proinsulin, insulin and C-peptide in the rat. *J. clin. Invest., 52,* 1113.

KITABCHI, A. E., DUCKWORTH, W. C., BRUSH, J. S. and HEINEMANN, M. (1971): Direct measurement of proinsulin in human plasma by the use of an insulin-degrading enzyme. *J. clin. Invest., 50,* 1792.

KOUTRAS, P. and WHITE, R. R. (1972): Insulin-secreting tumors of the pancreas. *Surg. Clin. N. Amer., 52,* 299.

LAURENT, M., DEBRY, G. and FLOQUET, M. (1971): *Hypoglycaemic Tumours.* Excerpta Medica, Amsterdam.

LAZARUS, N. R., GUTMAN, R. A., PENHOS, J. C. and RECANT, L. (1972): Biologically active circulating proinsulin-like materials from an islet cell carcinoma patient. *Diabetologia, 8,* 131.

LAZARUS, N. R., TANESE, T., GUTMAN, R. and RECANT, L. (1970): Synthesis and release of proinsulin and insulin by human insulinoma tissue. *J. Clin. Endocr., 30,* 273.

MAKO, M. E., BLOCK, M., STARR, J., NIELSEN, E., FRIEDMAN, E. and RUBENSTEIN, A. (1973): Proinsulin in chronic renal and hepatic failure: a reflection of the relative contribution of the liver and kidney to its metabolism. *Clin. Res., 21,* 631.

MARKS, V. and ROSE, F. C. (1965): *Hypoglycemia.* Blackwell Scientific Publications, Oxford.

MELANI, F., RUBENSTEIN, A. H. and STEINER, D. F. (1970a): Human serum proinsulin. *J. clin. Invest., 49,* 497.

MELANI, F., RYAN, W. G., RUBENSTEIN, A. H. and STEINER, D. F. (1970b): Proinsulin secretion by a pancreatic beta cell adenoma: proinsulin and C-peptide secretion. *New Engl. J. Med., 283,* 713.

PEARSON, M. J., LARKINS, R. G. and MARGIN, F. I. R. (1972): 'Big' insulin and the treatment of an islet cell carcinoma with streptozotocin. *Metabolism, 21,* 551.

RASTOGI, G. K., LETARTE, J. and FRASER, T. R. (1970): Proinsulin content of pancreas in human fetuses of healthy mothers. *Lancet, 1,* 7.

ROTH, J., GORDEN, P. and PASTAN, I. (1968): 'Big insulin'; new component of plasma insulin detected by immunoassay. *Proc. nat. Acad. Sci. U.S.A., 61,* 138.

RUBENSTEIN, A. H., BLOCK, M. B., STARR, J. I., MELANI, F. and STEINER, D. F. (1972a): Proinsulin and C-peptide in blood. *Diabetes, 21/Suppl. 2,* 661.

RUBENSTEIN, A. H., POTTENGER, L., MAKO, M., GETZ, G. and STEINER, D. F. (1972b): Metabolism of proinsulin and insulin by the liver. *J. clin. Invest., 51,* 912.

SANDO, H., BORG, J. and STEINER, D. F. (1972): Studies on the secretion of newly synthesized proinsulin and insulin from isolated rat islets of Langerhans. *J. clin. Invest., 51,* 1476.

SANDO, H. and GRODSKY, G. M. (1973): Dynamic synthesis and release of insulin and proinsulin from perifused islets. *Diabetes, 22,* 354.

SHERMAN, B. M., PEK, S., FAJANS, S. S., FLOYD, J. C. and CONN, J. W. (1972): Plasma proinsulin in patients with functioning pancreatic islet cell tumors. *J. clin. Endocr., 35,* 271.

STEINER, D. F., HALLUND, O., RUBENSTEIN, A. H., CHO, S. and BAYLISS, C. (1968): Isolation and properties of proinsulin, intermediate forms, and other minor components from crystalline bovine insulin. *Diabetes, 17,* 725.

STOLL, R. W., TOUBER, J. L., WINTERSCHEID, L. C., ENSINCK, J. W. and WILLIAMS, R. H. (1971): Hypoglycemic activity and immunological half-life of porcine insulin and proinsulin in baboons and swine. *Endocrinology, 88,* 714.

TAGER, H. S. and STEINER, D. F. (1972): Primary structures of the proinsulin connecting peptides of the rat and the horse. *J. biol. Chem., 247,* 7936.

TAYLOR, S. G., SCHWARTZ, T. B., ZANNINI, J. J. and RYAN, W. W. (1970): Streptozotocin therapy for metastatic insulinoma. *Arch. intern. Med., 126,* 654.

TOMPKINS, C. V., SRIVASTAVA, M. C., SONKSEN, P. H. and WABARRO, J. D. N. (1971): A comparative study of the distribution and metabolism of monocomponent human insulin and porcine proinsulin in man. *Biochem. J., 125,* 64.

YALOW, R. S. and BERSON, S. A. (1960): Immunoassay of endogenous plasma insulin in man. *J. clin. Invest., 39,* 1157.

YALOW, R. S. and BERSON, S. A. (1973): 'Big, big insulin'. *Metabolism, 22,* 703.

INDEX OF AUTHORS

SUBJECT INDEX

Prepared by W. van Westering, M.D., Amsterdam